D1476516

Insulin Resistance and Polycystic Ovarian Syndrome

CONTEMPORARY ENDOCRINOLOGY

P. Michael Conn, SERIES EDITOR

INSULIN RESISTANCE AND POLYCYSTIC OVARIAN SYNDROME

PATHOGENESIS, EVALUATION, AND TREATMENT

Edited by

EVANTHIA DIAMANTI-KANDARAKIS, MD, PhD

Endocrine Section of First Department of Internal Medicine, Athens University School of Medicine, Athens, Greece

JOHN E. NESTLER, MD

Division of Endocrinology and Metabolism, Department of Internal Medicine, Medical College of Virginia, Virginia Commonwealth University, Richmond, VA

DIMITRIOS PANIDIS, MD, PhD

Division of Endocrinology and Human Reproduction, Second Department of Obstetrics and Gynaecology, Aristotle University of Thessaloniki, Thessaloniki, Greece

RENATO PASQUALI, MD

Endocrinology Unit, Department of Internal Medicine and Gastroenterology and C.R.B.A., S.Orsola-Malpighi Hospital, Alma Mater Studiorum University of Bologna, Bologna, Italy

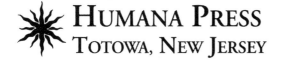

HUMANA PRESS
TOTOWA, NEW JERSEY

This publication is printed on acid-free paper. ⬚∞

ANSI Z39.48-1984 (American National Standards Institute) Permanence of Paper for Printed Library Materials.

Cover design by Karen Schulz

Production Editor: Jennifer Hackworth

For additional copies, pricing for bulk purchases, and/or information about other Humana titles,contact Humana at the above address or at any of the following numbers: Tel: 973-256-1699; Fax: 973-256-8341; E-mail: orders@ humanapr.com or visit our website at http://humanapress.com

Photocopy Authorization Policy:

10 9 8 7 6 5 4 3 2
eISBN 13: 978-1-59745-310-3

Library of Congress Cataloging-in-Publication Data
Insulin resistance and polycystic ovarian syndrome / edited by Evanthia Diamanti-Kandarakis, MD, PhD, John E. Nestler, MD, Dimitrios Panidis, MD, PhD, and Renato Pasquali, MD
        p. ; cm. -- (Contemporary endocrinology)
        Includes bibliographical references and index.
        ISBN 978-1-58829-763-1 (alk. paper)
1. Hypertension--Endocrine aspects. 2. Hypertension--Pathophysiology. 3. Hormones--Therapeutic use. I. Carey, Robert M. II. Series: Contemporary endocrinology (Totowa, N.J.: Unnumbered)
[DNLM: 1. Hypertension--physiopathology. 2. Hypertension--therapy. 3. Autacoids--therapeutic use. 4. Hormones--therapeutic use. WG 340 H998 2007]
RC685.H8H7692 2007
616.1'32--dc22
2007005797

Preface

"The natural flights of the human mind are not from pleasure to pleasure but from hope to hope"

Samuel Johnson, The Rambler no 2.

In this text, our hope is to highlight the recent transition of the polycystic ovary syndrome (PCOS) from an infertility disorder whose diagnosis was based on ovarian tissue histology to a more complex clinical entity—namely, a metabolic disorder in which insulin resistance plays a central role.

Research into PCOS has advanced at a dizzyingly fast pace over the past two decades, but not without substantial controversy. Despite great advances, even the definition of the syndrome remains in dispute, illustrating that many basic aspects of the syndrome remain unresolved.

However new dilemmas have been posed despite the fact that the intensified world wide research has elucidated new aspects of the syndrome contributing to the expansion of scientific knowledge. Because of the central role of insulin resistance in the syndrome, it is increasingly clear that PCOS is not simply a reproductive disorder, but a metabolic disorder that places women with the syndrome at markedly high risk for the development of glucose intolerance and, arguably, cardiovascular disease.

The editors have made every effort to provide an up-to-date and balanced overview of PCOS, paying special attention to the central role of insulin resistance in the syndrome's pathogenesis and in the management of its reproductive and metabolic abnormalities.

It is important to note that we are still searching a way out of the labyrinth in the aetiology of this enigmatic syndrome, despite significant advances in the field of molecular medicine, genetics, and pharmacogenomics.

The editors, in this joined effort, hope that the reader will discover a valuable thought-provoking and stimulating text, as we all felt during the preparation of the book.

E. Diamanti-Kandarakis MD, PhD
J. E. Nestler MD
D. Panidis MD, PhD
R. Pasquali MD

Acknowledgments

We owe a debt of thanks to everyone who has contributed to the preparation of this book.

We are extremely fortunate to have the outstanding contributions from distinguished co-authors and research leaders. Without their enthusiasm and hard work this project would not have been possible.

We are privileged to have reviewed their chapters, seeing their preliminary data and learning from their exciting areas of research.

We are particularly grateful to the editorial staff at Humana Press, especially to Richard Lansing.

Additional thanks to Miss Theodouli Piscopou for her outstanding, tireless, impecable secretarial work. Finally, we cannot thank enough our families and friends for their invaluable support and tolerance during the long hours of work in order to materialize this task.

Contents

Contributors

LAUREN ANTLER, BA • *Morgan Stanley's Children's Hospital of New York-Presbyterian, New York, NY*

YVES ARDAENS, MD • *Department of Radiology, Hopital Jeanne de Flandre, Centre Hospitalier et Universitaire de Lille, France*

RICARDO AZZIZ, MD, MPH, MBA • *Department of Ob/Gyn, Cedars-Sinai Medical Center, and Departments of Ob/Gyn and Medicine, The David Geffen School of Medicine at UCLA, Los Angeles, CA*

ANDREW A. BREMER, MD, PhD • *Department of Pediatrics, University of California, San Francisco, CA*

FRANK J. BROEKMANS, MD, PhD • *Department of Reproductive Medicine and Gynecology, University Medical Center, Utrecht, The Netherlands*

GOLDY CARBUNARU, MD • *University of Illinois Hospital, Department of Pediatrics, Chicago, IL*

ENRICO CARMINA, MD • *Department of Clinical Medicine, University of Palermo, Palermo, Italy*

R. JEFFERY CHANG, MD • *Department of Reproduction Medicine, School of Medicine, University of California, San Diego, CA*

GEORGE CHROUSOS, MD, FACP • *First Department of Pediatrics, Athens University Medical School, Athens, Greece*

GEORGE CREATSAS, MD • *Endocrine Unit, Second Department of Obstetrics and Gynecology, Aretaieion Hospital, Medical School of Capodistriakon Athens University, Athens, Greece*

MAREK DEMISSIE, MD, PhD • *Division of Endocrinology and Molecular Medicine, The Feinberg School of Medicine, Northwestern University, Chicago, IL*

DIDIER DEWAILLY, MD • *Department of Endocrine Gynaecology and Reproductive Medecine, Hopital Jeanne de Flandre, Centre Hospitalier et Universitaire de Lille, France*

EMMANUEL DIAKOMANOLIS, MD • *Alexandra Hospital, Athens, Greece*

EVANTHIA DIAMANTI-KANDARAKIS, MD, PhD • *Endocrine Section of First Department of Internal Medicine, Athens University School of Medicine, Athens, Greece*

ANTONI J. DULEBA, MD • *Department of Obstetrics/Gynecology, Yale University School of Medicine, New Haven, CT*

ANDREA DUNAIF, MD • *The Division of Endocrinology and Molecular Medicine, The Feinberg School of Medicine, Northwestern University, Chicago, IL*

DAVID A. EHRMANN, MD • *Department of Medicine, University of Chicago, Chicago, IL*

HÉCTOR F. ESCOBAR-MORREALE, MD, PhD • *Department of Endocrinology, Hospital Ramón y Cajal, Department of Medicine, Universidad de Alcalá, Madrid, Spain*

STEPHEN FRANKS, MD • *Institute of Reproductive and Developmental Biology, Wolfson and Weston Research Centre for Family Health, Imperial College London, Hammersmith Hospital, London, UK*

BART C. J. M. FAUSER, MD, PhD • *Department of Reproductive Medicine and Gynecology, University Medical Center, Utrecht, The Netherlands*

WALTER FUTTERWEIT, MD, FACP • *Division of Endocrinology, Mount Sinai School of Medicine, New York, NY*

ALESSANDRA GAMBINERI, MD • *Endocrinology Unit, Department of Internal Medicine and Gastroenterology and C.R.B.A., S.Orsola-Malpighi Hospital, Alma Mater Studiorum University of Bologna, Bologna, Italy*

NEOKLIS A. GEORGOPOULOS, MD • *Department of Obstetrics and Gynecology, Division of Reproductive Endocrinology, Patras Medical School, Patras, Greece*

SUSANNE HAHN, MD • *Endokrinologikum Ruhr, Center for Metabolic and Endocrine Diseases, Bochum, Germany*

MARY HORLICK, MD • *Morgan Stanley's Children's Hospital of New York-Presbyterian, New York, NY*

DANIELA JAKUBOWICZ, MD • *Division of Reproductive Endocrinology, Department of Medicine Hospital de Clinicas Caracas, Venezuela*

ONNO E. JANSSEN, MD • *Division of Endocrinology, Metabolism and Molecular Medicine, Department of Medicine, The Feinberg School of Medicine, Northwestern University, Chicago, IL*

SOPHIE JONDARD, MD • *Department of Endocrine Gynecology and Reproductive Medicine, Hospital Jeanne de Flandre, Centre Hospitalier et Universitaire de Lille, France*

GREGORY KALTSAS, MD, FRCP • *Department of Pathophysiology, Athens University Medical School, Athens, Greece*

FAHRETTIN KELEŞTIMUR, MD • *Department of Endocrinology, Erciyes University Medical School, Kayseri, Turkey*

PINAR H. KODAMAN, MD, PhD • *Department of Obstetrics/Gynecology, Yale University School of Medicine, New Haven, CT*

CAROLINA KOLIOPOULOS, MD • *Endocrine Unit, Second Department of Obstetrics and Gynecology, Aretaieion Hospital, Medical School of Capodistriakon Athens University, Athens, Greece*

JOOP S. E. LAVEN, MD, PhD • *Center of Reproductive Medicine, Erasmus Medical Center, Rotterdam, The Netherlands*

RICHARD S. LEGRO, MD • *Department of Obstetrics and Gynecology, Pennsylvania State University College of Medicine, Hershey, PA*

NATASHA LEIBEL, MD • *Morgan Stanley's Children's Hospital of New York-Presbyterian, New York, NY*

LENORE S. LEVINE, MD • *Morgan Stanley's Children's Hospital of New York-Presbyterian, New York, NY*

XIMENA LOPEZ, MD • *Department of Pediatrics, University of Illinois Hospital, Chicago, IL*

DJURO MACUT, MD, PhD • *Institute of Endocrinology, Diabetes and Diseases of Metabolism, Belgrade, Serbia*

NICK S. MACKLON, MD, PhD • *Department of Reproductive Medicine and Gynecology, University Medical Center, Utrecht, The Netherlands*

GEORGE MASTORAKOS, MD • *Endocrine Unit, Second Department of Obstetrics and Gynecology, Aretaieion Hospital, Medical School of Capodistriakon Athens University, Athens, Greece*

WALTER L. MILLER, MD • *Department of Pediatrics, University of California, San Francisco, CA*

L. J. MORAN, BSc, MBCHB, MD, FRACOG, FRACP • *CSIRO Human Nutrition, South Australia, Australia*

SHAHLA NADER, MD • *Departments of Obstetrics, Gynecology, and Reproductive Sciences and Internal Medicine, The University of Texas Medical School, Houston, TX*

JOHN E. NESTLER, MD • *Division of Endocrinology and Metabolism, Department of Internal Medicine, Medical College of Virginia, Virginia Commonwealth University, Richmond, VA*

R. J. NORMAN, BSc, BND • *Research Centre for Reproductive Health and Repromed, The Queen Elizabeth Hospital, University of Adelaide, South Australia, Australia*

SHARON E. OBERFIELD, MD • *Morgan Stanley's Children's Hospital of New York-Presbyterian, New York, NY*

FRANCESCO ORIO, JR., MD, PhD • *Department of Molecular and Clinical Endocrinology & Oncology, University "Federico II", Naples, Italy*

UBERTO PAGOTTO, MD, PhD • *Endocrinology Unit, Department of Internal Medicine and Gastroenterology and C.R.B.A., S.Orsola-Malpighi Hospital, Alma Mater Studiorum University of Bologna, Bologna, Italy*

STEFANO PALOMBA, MD • *Department of Obstetrics and Gynecology, University "Magna Graecia", Catanzaro, Italy*

SONGYA PANG, MD • *University of Illinois Hospital, Department of Pediatrics, Chicago, IL*

DIMITRIOS PANIDIS, MD, PhD • *Division of Endocrinology and Human Reproduction, Second Department of Obstetrics and Gynaecology, Aristotle University of Thessaloniki, Thessaloniki, Greece*

RENATO PASQUALI, MD • *Endocrinology Unit, Department of Internal Medicine and Gastroenterology and C.R.B.A., S.Orsola-Malpighi Hospital, Alma Mater Studiorum University of Bologna, Bologna, Italy*

YANN ROBERT, MD • *Department of Radiology, Hopital Jeanne de Flandre, Centre Hospitalier et Universitaire de Lille, France*

CYNTHIA S. RYAN, MD • *Clinical Fellow, Division of Endocrinology and Metabolism, Medical College of Virginia, Virginia Commonwealth University, Richmond, VA*

SUSMEETA T. SHARMA, MBBS • *Division of Endocrinology and Metabolism, Virginia Commonwealth University, Richmond, VA*

MIRIAM SILFEN, MD • *Morgan Stanley's Children's Hospital of New York-Presbyterian, New York, NY*

SUSANNE TAN, MD • *Division of Endocrinology, Department of Medicine, University Hospital of Essen Medical School, Essen, Germany*

BASIL TARLATZIS, MD, PhD • *Unit for Human Reproduction, First Department of Obstetrics and Gynecology, Aristotle University of Thessaliniki, Greece*

ANN E. TAYLOR, MD • *Pfizer Global Research and Development, Groton, CT*

VINCENZO TOSCANO, MD • *Dipartimento di Fisiopatologia Medica, University of Rome La Sapienza, Rome, Italy*

KÜRŞAD ÜNLÜHIZARCI, MD • *Department of Endocrinology, Erciyes University Medical School, Kayseri, Turkey*

VALENTINA VICENNATI, MD • *Endocrinology Unit, Department of Internal Medicine and Gastroenterology and C.R.B.A., S.Orsola-Malpighi Hospital, Alma Mater Studiorum University of Bologna, Bologna, Italy*

DEBORAH S. WACHS, MD • *Department of Reproduction Medicine, School of Medicine, University of California, San Diego, CA*

BULENT O. YILDIZ, MD • *Department of Internal Medicine, Endocrinology and Metabolism Unit, Hacettepe University Faculty of Medicine, Ankara, Turkey*

FULVIO ZULLO, MD • *Department of Obstetrics and Gynecology, University "Magna Graecia", Catanzaro, Italy*

I PATHOPHYSIOLOGY – GENETICS OF INSULIN RESISTANCE IN PCOS

1

Polycystic Ovary Syndrome
Definitions and Epidemiology

Bart C. J. M. Fauser, MD, PhD,
Frank J. Broekmans, MD, PhD,
Joop S. E. Laven, MD, PhD,
Nick S. Macklon, MD, PhD,
and Basil Tarlatzis, MD, PhD

CONTENTS

Summary

It is of interest to realize that polycystic ovary syndrome (PCOS) has moved from a histology diagnosis of ovarian tissue to a heterogeneous clinical syndrome (characterized by abnormal menstrual cyclicity, infertility, hirsutism, and obesity), to a reproductive endocrine abnormality with elevated serum luteinizing hormone and androgen levels and, finally, to a metabolic disease characterized by hyperinsulinemia and dyslipidemia. This altered emphasis may have major implications for patient diagnosis and management, with a shift of focus from ovarian abnormalities and ovulation induction for infertility toward the prevention of long-term health consequences. This change is also represented by the involvement of other medical specialists in addition to gynecologists such as general practitioners, pediatricians, dermatologists, medical endocrinologists, and even cardiologists.

A consensus workshop organized in 2003 in Rotterdam, The Netherlands, agreed to broaden the previous National Institutes of Health criteria for diagnosing PCOS by including the ultrasound diagnosis of polycystic ovaries. This wider definition will encompass a broader spectrum of this heterogeneous condition, facilitating future metabolic and genetic studies.

From: *Contemporary Endocrinology: Insulin Resistance and Polycystic Ovarian Syndrome:*
Pathogenesis, Evaluation, and Treatment
Edited by: E. Diamanti-Kandarakis, J. E. Nestler, D. Panidis, and R. Pasquali © Humana Press Inc., Totowa, NJ

Key Words: PCOS; diagnosis; epidemiology; polycystic ovary syndrome.

INTRODUCTION

Polycystic ovary syndrome (PCOS) is a heterogeneous condition that is associated with the following clinical features: oligo/amenorrhea (caused by chronic oligo/anovulation), acne or hirsutism (resulting from hyperandrogenemia), infertility, and finally, obesity. This condition is considered the major enigma in reproductive medicine, affecting up to 7% of the female population. The clustering of PCOS in families suggests a genetic basis. Although multiple gene polymorphisms or mutations may subserve a similar clinical condition, it is generally believed that hyperandrogenism and insulin resistance represent the central endocrine and metabolic abnormalities in PCOS. The occurrence of obesity may elicit a clinical phenotype in women predisposed to develop PCOS or aggravate the clinical picture in women with a mild form of the syndrome. Recent observations establish PCOS as a polygenic condition, where multiple genes and gene–environment interactions are central in the development of a clinical phenotype. Because of the increased prevalence of obesity in the Western world, it is to be expected that the incidence of PCOS will rise even further.

The association between bilateral polycystic ovaries and amenorrhea, hirsutism, and infertility was first described by Stein and Leventhal (1). The treatment of choice was initially ovarian wedge resection, which provided material for morphological confirmation of the diagnosis. A collection of clinical data from more than 1000 patients with morphologically proven Stein-Leventhal disease firmly established the frequent occurrence of oligo/amenorrhea, infertility, hirsutism, and obesity in these women (2). After the conversion from a morphological diagnosis to a clinical syndrome, the introduction of hormone assays in clinical practice allowed an assessment of the frequency of reproductive endocrine abnormalities in these women, such as elevated serum luteinizing hormone (LH) and androgen concentrations (3,4). Subsequently, the first reports of insulin resistance in PCOS appeared (5), as well as the noninvasive assessment of ovarian morphology by ultrasound (6). In recent years, the occurrence of hypertension and an abnormal lipid profile has also been established in these women.

During different stages of life, women with PCOS may seek medical care for different reasons (Fig. 1). For childhood obesity or abnormal menstrual bleeding during puberty or adolescence, patients may visit a general practitioner or a pediatrician. For complaints of hirsutism, a dermatologist may be approached. During reproductive life, a gynecologist may be visited for menstrual cycle abnormalities, infertility, or complications during pregnancy. Finally, the internist may be consulted for obesity or signs of type 2 diabetes (*see also* Table 1). A recent survey suggests that the cost related to diabetes care in PCOS exceeds by far the expenses in relation to infertility treatment (7).

All these complaints are evidence of the extremely heterogeneous spectrum of the same condition, i.e., PCOS. For obvious reasons, various diagnostic procedures are chosen by the medical specialist depending on the primary complaint of the patients. The focus on metabolic conditions seems a reasonable approach in women presenting with diabetes complaints, whereas a transvaginal ultrasound scan represents the key diagnostic procedure in a woman in need of medical intervention for anovulatory infertility.

PCOS throughout life

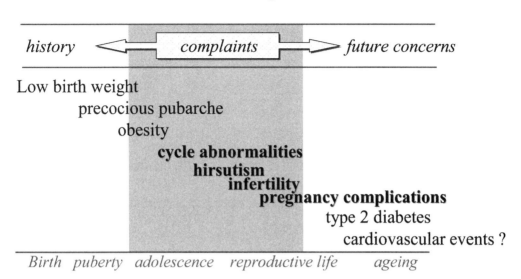

Fig. 1. Medical concerns associated with polycystic ovary syndrome throughout life.

Table 1
Various Complaints for Which PCOS Women Might Seek Medical Intervention
by Different Specialists

Complaint	Medical doctor
Cycle abnormalities during adolescence	GP, Pediatrician
Cycle abnormalities during reproductive life	GP, Gynecologist
Hirsutism	Dermatologist
Infertility	Gynecologist
Pregnancy complications	Obstetrician
Obesity	Internist
Late-onset diabetes	Internist
Cardiovascular disease	Cardiologist

EPIDEMIOLOGY

All studies performed to date on the prevalence of PCOS in the general population applied the 1990 National Institutes of Health (NIH) criteria for diagnosis, which included both oligo/amenorrhea and either biochemical or clinical evidence of hyperandrogenemia. Although populations studied varied (Caucasian, European, black, and white Americans), as did inclusion criteria for the studies (blood donors, preemployment check-up), the reported prevalences are remarkably similar and are between 6.5 and 6.8% (Table 2) *(8–11)*. A substantially increased prevalence of PCOS has been reported for women who presented with gestational diabetes and type 2 diabetes. As discussed later, the incidence of PCOS will rise even further when more recent, wider inclusion criteria for diagnosis are applied.

Table 2
Prevalence of PCOS (Diagnosed According to NIH Criteria) in Different Populations

Population/ethnicity	Sample size	Prevalence	Reference
Lesbos, Greek Island Free medical examination Age 17–45 years	192	6.8%	Diamanti-Karamanlis, 1999 (10)
Caucasian, Spain Blood donors Age 18–45 years	154	6.5%	Asuncion, 2000 (11)
Preemployment physical, United States	400	6.6%	Azziz, 2004 (8)
56% black, 42% white, 2% other 18–45 years			Knochenhauer, 1998 (9)

HOW TO DIAGNOSE PCOS?

At the end of a workshop organized by the NIH in 1990, it was decided that PCOS should be diagnosed on the basis of both hyperandrogenemia (clinical or biochemical) and chronic oligo- or anovulation (12). In addition, it was noted that known etiologies for hyperandrogenemia or ovulatry dysfunction needed to be excluded, rendering PCOS a diagnosis of exclusion. As stated by the participants, this conclusion was based on an anonymous questionnaire among the predominantly US participants, and, therefore, does not qualify for the term "consensus." Over the years, it had become increasingly evident that the NIH "consensus" criteria for PCOS were not universally accepted, despite the fact that "chronic hyperandrogenic anovulation" as the central clinical entity of PCOS has been advocated strongly by several investigators (see also Table 3).

Some US investigators continued to use elevated LH as the hallmark for diagnosis, whereas others primarily focused on establishing metabolic abnormalities, such as insulin resistance. In contrast, many European investigators focused on the ultrasound diagnosis of polycystic ovaries (PCO), and some UK investigators advocated that the anatomic presence of PCO alone would suffice for PCOS diagnosis.

ROTTERDAM CONSENSUS ON DIAGNOSTIC CRITERIA FOR PCOS

Some years ago, Professor Tarlatzis and myself concluded that the literature was becoming increasingly diverse, with many conflicting results. Results from one study in patients with PCOS often could not be confirmed by others. This was no real surprise because all groups used different criteria for defining PCOS. We therefore approached both US (ASRM) and European (ESHRE) societies to sponsor a closed consensus workshop. The majority of principal investigators of groups that had contributed significantly to this area of research were invited and agreed to participate (for names of all participants, see the conference report). An unconditional grant provided by NV Organon, along with sponsorship from the previously mentioned societies, enabled us to organize an one and a half-day workshop in Hotel New York, Rotterdam, The Netherlands, in May 2003. For each separate topic under discussion, four investigators were invited

Table 3
Powerful Statements From Comments/Editorials on PCOS Diagnosis and Significance

"Physicians traditionally approach PCOS with tunnel vision, seeing only those aspects of the disorder that are relevant to their specialty." *(18)*

"Gratifying to see a shift away from disease to syndrome, which confirms the notion of PCOS as a collection of signs, symptoms and endocrine disturbances." *(19)*

"It has become painfully apparent that it is not only the Atlantic Ocean that divides North America from Europe, but also the definition and diagnosis of PCOS." *(20)*

"PCOS is a diagnosis of exclusion in which other causes of oligo-ovulation or hyperandrogenemia are ruled out." *(21)*

"Diagnostic criteria in PCOS are at a cross road between consensus-based and evidence-based guidelines." *(22)*

"The 1990 NIH meeting was not designed to be a consensus meeting and there was no overall consensus about how the disorder should be diagnosed." *(23)*

"The misleading and simplified term PCOS, pre-programs bias in future studies." *(24)*

"It remains to be demonstrated whether the additional phenotypes created by the Rotterdam criteria actually represent patients with PCOS." *(25)*

"New diagnostic guidelines represent important progress because they are more flexible and permit us to make the diagnosis in patients who where previously excluded from the syndrome." *(26)*

"The 2003 Rotterdam consensus criteria define a population of patients inclusive of those previously diagnosed as having PCOS according to the 1990 NIH criteria." *(27)*

"There is a marked difference between endocrinologists and gynaecologists in diagnosis and management of PCOS." *(28)*

"There are three clinical phenotypes of PCOS which do not represent forms of the same metabolic disorder." *(29)*

"Findings indicate a trend among pediatric endocrinologists toward earlier work-up of menstrual irregularities in teenagers." *(30)*

beforehand to screen the literature, introduce the topic during the meeting, and structure the subsequent discussion with the other participants. Discussions were subsequently summarized, specifically indicating where consensus was reached among all participants. Controversial issues were again discussed. At the end of the meeting, the scientific committee generated conclusions based on these statements, and prepared a manuscript that was subsequently amended and agreed on by all participants.

Overall, the approach was chosen to acknowledge the fact that PCOS involves a heterogeneous condition, and that not all criteria needed to be fulfilled for the diagnosis. The NIH criteria of hyperandrogenemia and oligo/anovulation remained, but the ultrasound picture of PCO was added to the diagnostic criteria. It was suggested that PCOS could be diagnosed in cases where at least two of these three criteria are present. Hence, NIH criteria for PCOS are widened rather than replaced by the new consensus criteria (Fig. 2, Table 4). The approach of considering various features that are not all required for the diagnosis is new in reproductive medicine. However, such an approach is applied in other areas of medicine, such as the diagnosis of the metabolic syndrome where at least three out of five criteria (hypertension, increased abdominal circumference, low high-density lipoprotein cholesterol, high triglycerides, or impaired fasting glucose) would suffice for establishing the diagnosis.

PCOS diagnosis

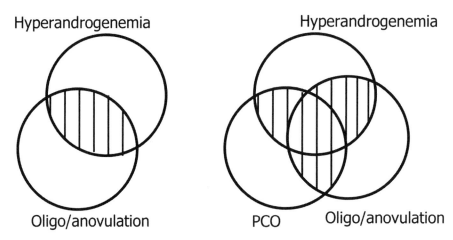

Fig. 2. Polycystic ovary syndrome diagnostic criteria according to the 1990 NIH criteria and the 2003 Rotterdam consensus criteria.

Table 4
Possible Combinations of Features for PCOS Diagnosis
According to 2003 Rotterdam Consensus

Oligo/amenorrhea	Hyperandrogenemia	PCO	Comments
+	+		Classical NIH criteria for PCOS diagnosis
+		+	PCOS, without hyperandrogenemia
	+	+	PCOS, with normo-ovulatory cycles
+	+	+	Inclusive, all

Oligo/Anovulation

It had already been described by Stein and Leventhal that corpora lutea can be observed in classical PCO. Hence, ovulation may sometimes occur in these women, and some oligomenorrheic women may occasionally ovulate and conceive spontaneously. In addition, under the new Rotterdam guidelines, PCOS can also be diagnosed in regularly cycling women (Table 4). Bleeding in oligomenorrheic women can either represent a withdrawal bleed (after ovulation) or a breakthrough bleed resulting from continued unopposed estrogen exposure. It remains unknown to what extent ovulations occur in women presenting with oligomenorrhea.

Anovulation represents one of the most frequent causes of infertility. The diagnostic work-up includes serum assays for follicle-stimulating hormone (FSH) and estradiol (E_2). In approx 85% of anovulatory women, FSH and E_2 levels are within the normal range (World Health Organization group 2 [WHO 2]) (Fig. 3). PCOS represents the most frequent diagnosis in these women *(13)*. In fact, approx 70% of WHO 2 women

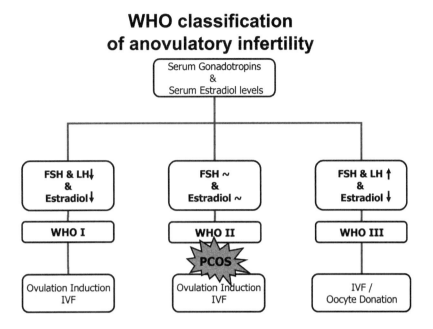

Fig. 3. Polycystic ovary syndrome is part of the heterogeneous World Health Organization group 2 of anovulatory infertility.

present with PCO and 61% with elevated androgen levels *(14)*. For obvious reasons, additional endocrine investigations should be performed in these women to exclude other endocrine abnormalities, such as late-onset 21-hydroxylase deficiency, androgen-producing tumors, or hyperprolactinemia.

HYPERANDROGENEMIA

The clinical manifestations of androgen excess are hirsutism and/or acne. However, distinct ethnic differences are reported for hirsutism, and the objective scoring of the severity of hirsutism is not easy. The direct assessment of free testosterone (T) (after ammonium sulfate precipitation or equilibrium dialysis) or the calculation of free T from determinations of sex-hormone binding globulin and total T were considered the more sensitive methods of assessing hyperandrogenemia. In addition, the role of other androgens, such as androstenedione or dehydroepiandrosterone-sulfate, remains unclear. Reference data in well-characterized control populations are mostly lacking.

Polycystic Ovaries

Consensus was reached in Rotterdam regarding the ultrasound criteria in order to diagnose PCO with sufficient specificity and sensitivity. As published in a separate paper, the most powerful ultrasound criteria included the presence of 12 or more follicles measuring 2–9 mm in diameter in at least one ovary or an ovarian volume of greater than 10 cm^3 *(see also* Table 5) *(15)*.

Although PCOS frequently coincides with both elevated serum LH levels and insulin resistance, these abnormalities do not represent useful diagnostic tools for PCOS. Discussion continues regarding the relevance of elevated LH for infertility treatment

Table 5
Consensus Regarding Ultrasound Assessment of Polycystic Ovaries

At least one of the following criteria should be present (in at least one ovary):
- ≥12 follicles (assessed in longitudinal, transverse, and antero-posterior cross sections), 2–9 mm diameter (mean of 3 sections)
- Ovarian volume greater than 10 cm^3 (0.5 × length × width × thickness)

What should be omitted:
- Follicle distribution
- Stroma volume or echogenicity

The transvaginal approach should be preferred wherever possible
These PCO criteria do not apply to women using oral contraceptives
Scanning in regularly menstruating women should be performed during the early follicular phase
Ultrasound may be helpful in the prediction of infertility therapy outcome

Adapted from ref. *15.*

and the possible relationship of elevated LH to risk of miscarriage. In addition, the pulsatile nature and brief half-life of LH render it difficult to obtain a reliable estimate based on a single blood sample. Finally, incidental ovulation and rise in progesterone may induce lower LH levels because of steroid-negative feedback. Insulin resistance occurs in up to 60% of women with PCOS (approximately threefold more compared with the general population), and is suggested to be a key feature in ovulatory dysfunction in these women. Indeed, the improvement of insulin sensitivity by means of lifestyle, weight reduction, or insulin-sensitizing drugs can ameliorate these abnormalities. It remains uncertain what should be considered the preferred test to diagnose insulin resistance in clinical practice.

CONCLUSIONS/FUTURE AVENUES

The consensus manuscript was published simultaneously in the January 2004 issue of both *Human Reproduction (16)* and *Fertility & Sterility (17)* in an attempt to secure maximum exposure to the scientific community and to show that this consensus is indeed supported by both societies. This was a unique event in the history of both journals.

With the Rotterdam consensus, new clinical conditions can be diagnosed as PCOS, i.e., regularly cycling women with PCO and hyperandrogenemia or anovulatory women with PCO but normal androgens (*see also* Table 4). This will undoubtedly give rise to PCOS being diagnosed more frequently and to PCOS encompassing an even more heterogeneous patient group (*see also* Fig. 2). Some clinical investigators continue to have conceptual difficulty with the heterogeneous nature of the syndrome, and prefer to consider PCOS as a single gene disease. They prefer to focus on hyperandrogenemia as the central hallmark of all PCOS. It should be realized that in the face of the absence of a gold standard for diagnosis it is not going to be possible to evaluate characteristics of diagnostic tests such as false-positive (the diagnosis suggesting the presence of the condition, in the absence of the disease) or false-negative (the test being negative despite the fact that the disease is present). By definition, a syndrome suggests a hetero-geneous clinical condition and it should be accepted that different complaints during different stages in life require different diagnostic approaches. For obvious reasons, cycle abnormalities in an adolescent girl require different diagnostic procedures compared with a woman attending a physician for type 2 diabetes later in life. Again, both clinical conditions are very likely to be associated with PCOS.

The overall prevalence of PCOS in the general population will be substantially higher using the new Rotterdam diagnostic criteria, and may be as high as 10%. This will require additional studies because ultrasound was not performed in most of the epidemiology studies performed to date.

Several editorials and original papers have specifically addressed the Rotterdam consensus criteria, and most—but certainly not all—acknowledged the fact that progress was made (*see also* Table 3). A Google Scholar search performed on October 13, 2005 established 472 citations of both consensus papers, which causes us to believe that acceptance of the Rotterdam diagnostic criteria in the scientific community is good. We can only hope that fertility journals and referees will continue to insist on the Rotterdam criteria for PCOS diagnosis to be mentioned specifically in the materials and methods section of the manuscripts. This will certainly help the homogeneity of future studies related to PCOS in terms of etiology, outcomes of infertility treatments, long-term health consequences, and genetic background.

KEY POINTS

- PCOS is a notoriously heterogeneous condition (i.e., a syndrome).
- PCOS can be diagnosed in women presenting with a wide spectrum of complaints in different phases in life, from precocious puberty at the beginning of reproductive life to type 2 diabetes at the end of reproductive life.
- Diagnostic procedures should be adjusted according the patient's complaints.
- Diagnostic test characteristics cannot be assessed in terms of false-positive or false-negative in the phase of a lack of a gold standard for the condition.
- For these reasons, the Rotterdam consensus criteria seems a reasonable approach for diagnosing PCOS.
- The Rotterdam consensus should be regarded as work in progress.
- We need new data concerning phenotype and prognosis of PCOS based on the Rotterdam consensus before a possible revision of the Rotterdam consensus can be discussed in a meaningful way.

REFERENCES

1. Stein IF, Leventhal ML. Amenorrhea associated with bilateral polycystic ovaries. Am J Obstet Gynecol 1935;29:181–191.
2. Goldzieher JW, Axelrod LR. Clinical and biochemical features of polycystic ovarian disease. Fertil Steril 1963;14:631–653.
3. Yen SS, Vela P, Rankin J. Inappropriate secretion of follicle-stimulating hormone and luteinizing hormone in polycystic ovarian disease. J Clin Endocrinol Metab 1970;30:435–442.
4. Lobo RA, Goebelsmann U. Effect of androgen excess on inappropriate gonadotropin secretion as found in the polycystic ovary syndrome. Am J Obstet Gynecol 1982;142:394–401.
5. Dunaif A. Insulin resistance and the polycystic ovary syndrome: mechanism and implications for pathogenesis. Endocr Rev 1997;18:774–800.
6. Adams J, Polson DW, Franks S. Prevalence of polycystic ovaries in women with anovulation and idiopathic hirsutism. Br Med J (Clin Res Ed) 1986;293:355–359.
7. Azziz R, Marin C, Hoq L, Badamgarav E, Song P. Health care-related economic burden of the polycystic ovary syndrome during the reproductive life span. J Clin Endocrinol Metab 2005;90:4650–4658.

8. Azziz R, Woods KS, Reyna R, Key TJ, Knochenhauer ES, Yildiz BO. The prevalence and features of the polycystic ovary syndrome in an unselected population. J Clin Endocrinol Metab 2004;89:2745–2749.

9. Knochenhauer ES, Key TJ, Kahsar-Miller M, Waggoner W, Boots LR, Azziz R. Prevalence of the polycystic ovary syndrome in unselected black and white women of the southeastern United States: a prospective study. J Clin Endocrinol Metab 1998;83:3078–3082.

10. Diamanti-Kandarakis E, Kouli CR, Bergiele AT, et al. A survey of the polycystic ovary syndrome in the Greek island of Lesbos: hormonal and metabolic profile. J Clin Endocrinol Metab 1999;84:4006–4011.

11. Asuncion M, Calvo RM, San Millan JL, Sancho J, Avila S, Escobar-Morreale HF. A prospective study of the prevalence of the polycystic ovary syndrome in unselected Caucasian women from Spain. J Clin Endocrinol Metab 2000;85:2434–2438.

12. Dunaif A, Givens JR, Haseltine F, Merriam G. The Polycystic Ovary Syndrome. Boston: Blackwell Scientific; 1992.

13. The ESHRE Capri Workshop Group. Anovulatory infertility. Hum Reprod 1995;10:1549–1553.

14. Laven JS, Imani B, Eijkemans MJ, Fauser BC. New approach to polycystic ovary syndrome and other forms of anovulatory infertility. Obstet Gynecol Surv 2002;57:755–767.

15. Balen AH, Laven JS, Tan SL, Dewailly D. Ultrasound assessment of the polycystic ovary: international consensus definitions. Hum Reprod Update 2003;9:505–514.

16. The Rotterdam ESHRE/ASRM-Sponsored PCOS Consensus Workshop Group. Revised 2003 consensus on diagnostic criteria and long-term health risks related to polycystic ovary syndrome (PCOS). Hum Reprod 2004;19:41–47.

17. Rotterdam ESHRE/ASRM-Sponsored PCOS Consensus Workshop Group. Revised 2003 consensus on diagnostic criteria and long-term health risks related to polycystic ovary syndrome. Fertil Steril 2004;81:19–25.

18. Nestler JE. Polycystic ovary syndrome: a disorder for the generalist. Fertil Steril 1998;70:811–812.

19. Balen A, Michelmore K. What is polycystic ovary syndrome? Are national views important? Hum Reprod 2002;17:2219–2227.

20. Homburg R. What is polycystic ovary syndrome? Hum Reprod 2002;17:2495–2499.

21. Azziz R. Androgen excess is the key element in polycystic ovary syndrome. Fertil Steril 2003;80: 252–254.

22. Legro RS. Diagnostic criteria in polycystic ovary syndrome. Semin Reprod Med 2003;21:267–275.

23. Lobo RA. What are the key features of importance in polycystic ovary syndrome? Fertil Steril 2003; 80:259–261.

24. Geisthovel F. A comment on the European Society of Human Reproduction and Embryology/American Society of Reproductive Medicine consensus of the polycystic bovarian syndrome. Reprod Biomed Online 2003;7:602–605.

25. Azziz R. PCOS: a diagnostic challenge. Reprod Biomed Online 2004;8:644–648.

26. Carmina E. Diagnosis of polycystic ovary syndrome: from NIH criteria to ESHRE-ASRM guidelines. Minerva Ginecol 2004;56:1–6.

27. Azziz R. Diagnostic criteria for polycystic ovary syndrome: a reappraisal. Fertil Steril 2005;83: 1343–1346.

28. Cussons AJ, Stuckey BG, Walsh JP, Burke V, Norman RJ. Polycystic ovarian syndrome: marked differences between endocrinologists and gynaecologists in diagnosis and management. Clin Endocrinol (Oxf) 2005;62:289–295.

29. Chang WY, Knochenhauer ES, Bartolucci AA, Azziz R. Phenotypic spectrum of polycystic ovary syndrome: clinical and biochemical characterization of the three major clinical subgroups. Fertil Steril 2005;83:1717–1723.

30. Guttmann-Bauman I. Approach to adolescent polycystic ovary syndrome in the pediatric endocrine community in the USA. J Pediatr Endocrinol Metab 2005;18:499–506.

2 Insulin Resistance

Definition and Epidemiology in Normal Women and Polycystic Ovary Syndrome Women

Renato Pasquali, MD
and Alessandra Gambineri, MD

CONTENTS

Summary

Insulin resistance and hyperinsulinemia are key features of women with polycystic ovary syndrome (PCOS), particularly in the presence of obesity. This has important effects in the pathophysiology of this disorder and contributes largely to its changing aspects throughout the lifespan. Insulin excess does in fact have a direct responsibility in favoring androgen excess and oligo-anovulation in PCOS. On the other hand, insulin resistance represents the main pathophysiological event leading to the development of the metabolic syndrome, which affects almost 50% of women with PCOS.

Insulin resistance and the metabolic syndrome probably represent different entities and, therefore, should not be used as a synonym. Although there are no epidemiological data, it appears that the incidence of insulin resistance in PCOS exceeds the prevalance expected in the general population. On the other hand, although prevalence largely depends on the method used, insulin resistance in PCOS appears to be even higher in the presence of obesity, particularly the abdominal phenotype. Insulin resistance may be found, however, even in some normal-weight women with PCOS. Notably,

From: *Contemporary Endocrinology: Insulin Resistance and Polycystic Ovarian Syndrome:*
Pathogenesis, Evaluation, and Treatment
Edited by: E. Diamanti-Kandarakis, J. E. Nestler, D. Panidis, and R. Pasquali © Humana Press Inc., Totowa, NJ

the larger the number of criteria used to define the metabolic syndrome, the higher the probability that affected women are insulin resistant.

Recognition of these abnormalities in PCOS women may be of relevance for both treatment and preventive strategies. It is in fact well defined that PCOS itself, and even more so in the presence of obesity and a positive family history, may increase individual susceptibility to an early development of T2DM.

Key Words: PCOS; insulin resistance; glucose intolerance; type 2 DM; metabolic syndrome.

INTRODUCTION

The polycystic ovary syndrome (PCOS), one of the most common causes of ovulatory infertility, affects 4–7% of women (1). Over the years this syndrome has been defined in different ways. In 1990, the National Institutes of Health established the new diagnostic criteria for this disorder, which were based on the presence of hyper-androgenism and chronic oligo-anovulation, with the exclusion of other causes of hyperandrogenism such as adult-onset congenital adrenal hyperplasia, hyperprolactinemia, and androgen-secreting neoplasms. More recently, a consensus conference held in Rotterdam, in 2003, reexamined the 1990 criteria and admitted the opportunity of including ultrasound morphology of the ovaries among the diagnostic criteria of the syndrome. Moreover, it established that at least two of the diagnostic criteria proposed, i.e., oligo-anovulation, clinical and/or biochemical signs of hyperandrogenism, and polycystic ovaries at ultrasound, were sufficient to make the diagnosis (2).

However, debate is still continuing in relation to which criteria should be used to define PCOS. In fact, it is quite broadly accepted that PCOS may have a genetic component, although specific genes defining individual or ethnic susceptibility to develop the syndrome have not been discovered yet, despite the great research effort in this area (3). In addition, there is consistent clinical evidence that clinical features of PCOS may change throughout lifespan, starting from adolescence to post-menopausal age (1). However, no effort has been made to define differences in the phenotype and clinical presentation according to age. One major concern in the definition of PCOS is related to the fact that insulin resistance and hyperinsulinemia are present in the majority of women with PCOS (4,5), as obesity is, particularly the abdominal phenotype (6). Metabolic derangements (hyperinsulinemia, insulin resistance, and obesity) have in fact important effects in the pathophysiology of PCOS and largely contribute to the changing aspects of this disorder throughout lifespan. Insulin excess has in fact a direct responsibility in determining ovarian androgen production and increasing their availability in the target tissues through different mechanisms, i.e., a synergistic stimulatory effect with luteinizing hormone on ovarian steroidogenetic enzyme activity, and an inhibition of sex hormone-binding globulin (SHBG) synthesis and secretion from the liver (5). Insulin resistance per se may be responsible for the development of compensatory hyperinsulinemia. It also represents the main pathophysiological event leading to the development of the metabolic syndrome, which is largely prevalent in PCOS women (7), thereby increasing the risk for development of type 2 diabetes mellitus (T2DM) and, possibly, cardiovascular disease (CVD) in these patients. The presence of obesity could also have a pathophysiological responsibility in the development not only of the insulin resistant state and the associated metabolic abnormalities, but also of hyperandrogenism and associated clinical consequences, such as menstrual disturbances and infertility *(6)*.

Although these metabolic alterations are not included in the definition of PCOS, nonetheless there is clear clinical evidence that the growing epidemic of obesity and associated comorbidities may play a relevant role in increasing the prevalence of PCOS worldwide. In addition, the important impact of the so-called "metabolic way" of treating PCOS (by lifestyle modifications and short-term and long-term use of insulin sensitizers) has improved major signs of the syndrome, such as menstrual disturbances, oligo-anovulation, and infertility, as well as major metabolic disorders, therefore, suggesting strongly the important role of these factors in the pathophysiology of PCOS, related to both its diagnosis and its clinical management.

HOW TO DEFINE INSULIN RESISTANCE: FROM RESEARCH TO A CLINICAL SETTING

Insulin resistance can be defined as a reduced biological effect of insulin for any given concentration of insulin. The definition and accurate quantification of insulin resistance are important and a number of methods are available for its evaluation *(8)*. Because there are basic mathematical principles common to various methods and each of them has well known advantages and limitations, their use should depend on the major aim of each particular study. From a general point of view, they can be divided into two principal classes, those used for research purposes and those available for epidemiological and clinical evaluations.

Three major factors control the overall glucose tolerance of an individual: the amount of circulating insulin; the biological effect of insulin (insulin sensitivity, S_i); and the impact of glucose itself on its own disposal, regardless of insulin action and glucose sensitivity (S_g, or glucose effectiveness). The measurement of S_g is particularly applicable in conditions of severe insulin resistance with associated relative insulin deficiency, such as in type 2 diabetes. Because a close relationship exists between insulin sensitivity and insulin secretion, particularly at the early phase of insulin release, in quantification of the contribution of absolute insulin secretion on glucose tolerance measurement of both S_i and insulin secretion must be known. S_i represents, however, a quantitative measurement of the biological effect of insulin measurement of insulin resistance is the reciprocation of S_i, therefore, this factor needs to be considered when comparing different methodologies *(9)*. Finally, because insulin action takes place in numerous tissue sites (the liver, skeletal muscle, and adipose tissue), whole body measurements of S_i represent a composite. Differentiation of the insulin effect at each tissue level therefore requires extra-experimental procedures *(8)*.

Insulin sensitivity can be evaluated in vivo by using either complex techniques or mathematical models based on simple tests. For in vivo assessment of S_i, the hyperinsulinemic euglycemic clamp technique represents the gold standard procedure *(10)*. With this technique, insulin concentrations are maintained elevated by using a constant insulin infusion, and plasma glucose is maintained constant by a variable intravenous glucose infusion. The glucose infusion rate necessary to maintain euglycemia during the clamp represents the net effect of insulin on glucose metabolism. The average glucose infusion rate during the last hour of the clamp is often termed the *m*-value. An insulin resistant state is defined when the glucose disposal rate is reduced.

Another method used to analyze insulin sensitivity is the minimal model. This is based on a complex computer modeling analysis of the glucose and insulin profiles obtained following the frequently sampled iv glucose tolerance test (FSIVGTT), which has undergone several modifications over the years *(10,11)*. This test provides information on S_i, S_g, and early phase insulin secretion, as well as glucose tolerance (K_g).

Because of the complexity of these approaches, which are usually reserved for clinical research, a great effort has been made in the search for simpler tests. Many tests have in fact been produced in the last decade as nondynamic measurements of S_i, and because of their simplicity they have been widely used in both epidemiological and clinical studies. Most of these tests, which include fasting insulin alone, the homeostasis assessment method ([HOMA]: [fasting glucose, mmol/L × fasting insulin, mIU/mL]/25) *(12)* and the quantitative insulin-sensitivity check index (QUICKI: 1/[log insulin fasting + log glucose fasting]) have been extensively reviewed *(13,14)*. These tests are simple to perform, and are based on fasting insulin concentrations and glucose levels alone. However, even these simple procedures need to be carried out in carefully standardized conditions if reliable measurements of insulin resistance are to be obtained. Many factors must be controlled, such as the accuracy of the insulin assay performed, and processing of samples before assay *(8)*. It should also be emphasized that once a significant defect of insulin secretion exists, the value of these measurement is poor and can be misleading.

THE PCOS AS A STATE OF INSULIN RESISTANCE: FROM COMPLEX TO SIMPLE TESTS

The majority of clinical studies performed so far have shown that most women with PCOS are characterized by a condition of insulin resistance, with a wide interindividual variability *(1,4,5)*. Several factors influence this variability, chiefly including body weight, family history for T2DM, and ethnicity *(4,5)*. In fact, obese women with PCOS, particularly those with the abdominal obesity phenotype, are usually more insulin resistant and more hyperinsulinemic than their normal-weight counterpart *(6)*. Both fasting and glucose-stimulated insulin concentrations are significantly higher in obese than in non-obese PCOS subgroups *(4–6)*. Accordingly, studies examining insulin sensitivity by means of different methods, such as the euglycemic hyperinsulinemic clamp technique, the FSIVGTT, and the insulin tolerance test (ITT), have further demonstrated that almost all obese PCOS women had significantly lower insulin sensitivity than their non-obese PCOS counterparts and, therefore, a more severe insulin resistant state *(4–6)*.

Simpler indices derived from the measurement of fasting glucose and insulin concentrations have been proposed as a surrogate of more complex tests such as the clamp technique. Both the HOMA and QUICKI indices have been shown to significantly correlate with S_i (measured by the clamp technique or the FSIVGTT) in non-obese, obese, and T2DM patients *(15)*. However, when each group was analyzed separately, the correlation coefficient was low, particularly in non-obese individuals, although in some studies it reached significant values *(15)*.

In many studies performed in PCOS women, HOMA and QUICKI were used as markers of insulin resistance. They commonly confirmed that, compared to appropriate age- and weight-matched controls, PCOS women are more insulin resistant, regardless of the method used to measure insulin sensitivity *(16)*. In a group of normal-weight and obese PCOS women, Carmina and Lobo *(17)* found that insulin resistance, as measured by the kinetic disappearance rate (k_{itt}) during an ITT or HOMA or QUICKI, was detectable in approx 80% of women and in 95% of those who were obese, and that there was a significant correlation between HOMA ($r = -0.48$; $p < 0.01$), or QUICKI ($r = 0.65$; $p < 0.01$) with k_{itt}. These results have not, however, been supported by recent studies, which did not show a significant correlation between *m*-value and HOMA or QUICKI values in a group of normal-weight, overweight, and obese PCOS women *(18)*. Although these unexpected results could be explained by the low insulin rate (40 mU/m^2/minute), as the same authors observed, it should be noted that even the high correlation previously found in non-PCOS insulin resistant patients by Katz et al. *(13)* may be owed to the very high rates of insulin infusion (120 mU/m^2/minute) used. By contrast, Ciampelli et al. *(19)* found that in PCOS patients a highly significant correlation existed between *m*-values and an index derived from basal glucose and insulin ([$0.137 \times$ Sib] + Si 120]/2), where "Sib" is the sensitivity index measured in the basal state, and "Si120" is calculated on the basis of values obtained at 120 minutes during an oral glucose tolerance test (OGTT, using C-peptide values rather than insulin values) proposed by Avignon et al. *(20)*.

These data therefore imply that these mathematical indices should be applied with caution in different insulin resistant populations, particularly in PCOS patients, and should not be considered *a priori* equivalent to the euglycemic clamp technique. According to recent data, which, however, need to be confirmed, it appears that the evaluation of insulin secretion during an OGTT may provide a reliable and simple way to evaluate insulin sensitivity in vivo *(21)*. Notably, however, even if this approach appears to be adequate for clinical investigation, it can be used much less sufficient in epidemiological studies, where mathematical indices such as HOMA or QUICKI could be used.

PREVALENCE OF THE METABOLIC SYNDROME IN THE GENERAL POPULATION

Sensitivity to insulin-mediated glucose disposal varies widely in the general population. Several studies have in fact demonstrated that, at least in apparently healthy nondiabetic individuals, insulin-mediated glucose disposal varies by approximately six- to eightfold and that, despite this great variability, insulin is secreted in sufficient amounts to prevent decompensation of glucose homeostasis *(22,23)*. Increased β-cell insulin secretion represents an effort by the body to face the peripheral defect of insulin action, to preserve normal glucose tolerance. When insulin-resistant individuals cannot maintain the necessary degree of compensatory hyperinsulinemia to overcome the insulin resistant state, impaired glucose tolerance, or T2DM develop.

In 1988, Reaven proposed that individuals who displayed this cluster of abnormalities associated with insulin resistance and compensatory hyperinsulinemia were at significant risk for CVD *(23)*. Interestingly, a clear description of the constellation of metabolic abnormalities representing a risk for CVD was first described more than 20 years ago by an Italian group of researcher from Padua, although they did not describe the central pathophysiological role of insulin resistance *(24)*. Insulin resistance is not a disease in itself, but rather a pathophysiological abnormality that increases the likelihood that other abnormalities could cluster together. These include glucose intolerance, dyslipidemia, endothelial dysfunction, procoagulant factors, hemodynamic changes, low-grade inflammation, abnormal serum uric acid *(25)*, and several hormonal derangements, such as low or high testosterone in men and women, respectively *(26)*, and some degree of hypothalamic–pituitary–adrenal axis abnormal functions *(27)*. This implies that epidemiological data on the prevalence of insulin resistance in different populations or ethnicities is difficult to define, particularly if the aforementioned difficulties in the definition of insulin resistance by simple methods are taken into account.

Over the last 15 years, the concept underlying the common aggregation of major abnormalities associated with an insulin resistant state has emerged as a unique entity, the so-called metabolic syndrome. Although the concept that insulin resistance is ontologically different from the metabolic syndrome, nonetheless for many years these two conditions have been often used more or less as synonymous. This issue is, however, a matter of great controversy at the present time. One of the reasons is certainly represented by the difficulty of measuring the insulin resistance state and the need for more reliable parameters defining the risk for CVD diseases. Another practical implication is related to the easier possibility of defining the metabolic syndrome in epidemiological studies, provided that geographical and cultural differences, ethnicity and lifestyle habits are taken into consideration, because these factors are important determinants of the heterogeneity in the prevalence of both insulin resistance and the metabolic syndrome among different populations worldwide. Researchers have used various terms to describe the cluster of abnormalities that make up the metabolic syndrome. Consequently, the lack of a standard definition has also greatly impeded the efforts to determine the prevalence of this syndrome and, furthermore, the establishment of a surveillance system. Overall, these definitions propose the collection of very simple parameters, mostly based on a clinical approach. The major differences between these definitions are represented by the appropriate levels of each parameter included in the definition, modifiable if necessary according to ethnic variability, and the potential inclusion of a simple marker of insulin resistance in the definition. After the first definition (the so-called syndrome X) proposed by Reaven *(23)*, which described the metabolic syndrome as the co-occurrence of resistance to insulin-mediated glucose uptake, hyperinsulinemia, increased very low-density lipoproteins, decreased high-density lipoproteins (HDL)-cholesterol and hypertension, many other definitions are now available (Table 1).

Particular attention has been paid to the National Cholesterol Education Program expert Panel on Detection, Evaluation and Treatment of High Blood Cholesterol in Adults (NCEP/ATP III) report *(28)*, which includes a practical definition based on clinical simple parameters. Several reports had estimated the prevalence of the metabolic syndrome indirectly, on that of the insulin resistance syndrome. They included studies performed in both adults and children or adolescents, which have been recently reviewed by Ford *(29)*. Based on these studies, the estimate of the prevalence of the metabolic syndrome has been reported to range from 4.6 to 29.4%,

Table 1
Definition of the Metabolic Syndrome According to Different Criteria
(WHO, EGIR, ATPIII, and IDF)

WHO 1999 *(33)*

Diabetes or impaired fasting glycemia or impaired glucose tolerance or insulin resistance (under hyperinsulinemic and euglycemic conditions, glucose uptake in lowest 25%) plus two or more of the following:

- Obesity: body mass index >30 kg/m² or waist:hip ratio (WHR) >0.9 (male) or >0.85 (female)
- Dyslipidemia: tryglicerides ≥1.7 mmol/L or HDL cholesterol <0.9 (male) or <1.0 (female) mmol/L
- Hypertension: blood pressure ≥140/90 mmHg
- Microalbuminuria: albumin excretion ≥20 µg/minute

EGIR 1999 *(37)*

Insulin resistance (defined as hyperinsulinemia, top 25% of fasting insulin values among the nondiabetic population) plus two or more of the following:

- Central obesity: waist circumference ≥94 cm (male) or ≥80 cm (female)
- Dyslipidemia: tryglicerides >2.0 mmol/L or HDL cholesterol <1.0 mmol/L
- Hypertension: blood pressure ≥140/90 mmHg and or medication
- Fasting plasma glucose ≥6.1 mmol/L

NCEP/ATPIII *(28)*

Three or more of the following:

- Central obesity: waist circumference >102 cm (male) or >88 cm (female)
- Hypertrygliceridemia: tryglicerides >1.7 mmol/L
- Low HDL cholesterol: <1.0 mmol/L (male) or <1.3 mmol/L (female)
- Hypertension: blood pressure ≥135/85 mmHg or medication
- Fasting plasma glucose ≥6.1 mmol/L

IDF 2005 *(25)*[b]

Central obesity: waist circumference[a]—ethnicity specific (*see* Table 1 Appendix) plus two or more of the following:

- Raised tryglicerides: >1.7 mmol/L or specific treatment for this lipid abnormality
- Reduced HDL cholesterol: <1.03 mmol/L (male) <1.29 mmol/L (female) or specific treatment for this lipid abnormality
- Raised blood pressure: systolic ≥130 mmHg or diastolic ≥85 mmHg or treatment of previously diagnosed hypertension
- Raised fasting plasma glucose: fasting plasma glucose ≥5.6 mmol/L or previously diagnosed type 2 diabetes. If above 5.6 mmol/L oral glucose test is strongly recommended, but is not necessary to define presence of syndrome

[a]If body mass index is over 30 kg/m², central obesity can be assumed and waist circumference does not need to be measured.
[b]Please *see* Table 1 Appendix.

Table 1 Appendix
Ethnic-Specific Values for Waist Circumference

	Euripides Sub-Saharan Africans Eastern Mediterranean and Middle East (Arab) population	*South Asian Ethnic South Central Americans*	*Chinese*	*Japanese*
Male	94 cm	90 cm	90 cm	85 cm
Female	80 cm	80 cm	80 cm	90 cm

but comparison is difficult because of the different definition criteria, demographic variability, and geographical heterogeneity. Moreover, many of these studies were performed before the appearance of the NCEP/ATP III report. Notably, the introduction of the NCEP/ATP III criteria have introduced a great advantage, because they allow investigators to determine the prevalence of the metabolic syndrome using the same criteria, therefore improving cross-study comparisons and prevalence estimates. Results from the National Health and Nutrition Survey III have documented a prevalence rate of the metabolic syndrome of 23% in the adult US population, with peak values of more than 40% in subjects aged 60 years or more, with significant ethnic differences *(30)*. In other studies, the prevalence rate was found to range from 13 to 55% *(28)*. The main reasons for these large differences were again ethnicity and sex.

More recently, the American College of Endocrinology (ACE) released a position statement on what it refers to as the "insulin resistance syndrome" *(31)*. This document reported a list of four factors described as "identifying abnormalities" of the syndrome, including increased triglycerides, reduced HDL-cholesterol, elevated blood pressure, increased fasted, and postlast 2-hour glucose levels. Other factors, such as obesity, gestational diabetes, family history of diabetes, hypertension, or CVDs, age greater than 40 years and a sedentary lifestyle were also listed, although they were not considered as factors classifying the syndrome. The list of the four principal factors was described as a simple method of identifying individuals who are likely to be insulin-resistant. The most important difference with other criteria in the ACE definition *(31)* was the absence of obesity as a factor. In addition, the ACE statement did not include fasting insulin levels because of the lack of standardized measurement method making interlaboratory comparison difficult and the lack of evidence that increased insulin levels per se, in the absence of other factors, can predict the development of CVDs.

Several studies performed in US populations have compared the prevalence of the metabolic syndrome estimated by the criteria proposed by both the NCEP/ATP III and the World Health Organization (WHO) *(32,33)*. Results of the NHANES III showed that the prevalence rate using these two criteria was more or less similar *(34)*. In another study performed using data from the Framingham Offspring Study and the San Antonio Heart Study *(35)*, it was found that the NCEP/ATP III criteria produced somewhat higher estimates, with minor differences according to ethnicity, and no difference in men.

There are also many studies that were performed to estimate the prevalence of the metabolic syndrome in worldwide populations (including the US population), which have been reviewed recently *(36)*. They were carried out by means of different criteria, particularly the NCEP/ATP III and the WHO criteria. Several studies also used the criteria proposed by the European Group for the Study of Insulin Resistance (EGIR), which are based on data collected in European individuals *(37)* and many studies used combinations of these criteria. Among other intuitive reasons previously reported, these different approaches are responsible for the great heterogeneity of prevalence data among these studies. Using the NCEP/ATP III criteria, and considering only individuals aged more than 20 years, prevalence rates have been estimated to range from 8 to 24% in men and from 7 to 46% in women *(36)*. A more recent study, performed in a nationally representative sample of 15,540 Chinese adults, aged 35–74 years, Gu et al. *(38)* found that the age-standardized prevalence of the metabolic syndrome was (as defined by the NCEP/ATP III criteria), 9.8 and 17.8% in men and women, respectively, whereas the age-standardized prevalence of overweight or obesity was 26.9 and 31.1%, respectively. These data further indicate that excess body weight represents an important although not exclusive factor, with all the metabolic and CVD risk factors included in the definition of the metabolic syndrome. An important note on the data coming from all the reports on the prevalence of the metabolic syndrome by the EGIR group is that they are all taken from comparative studies in European populations and undertaken by the EGIR itself *(37)*. From a general point of view, prevalence rates using these criteria are lower in comparison with the NCEP/ATP III criteria, with a significantly higher prevalence in men, with some exceptions *(36)*. Overall, prevalence rates reported by the EGIR range from 10 to 20% for men and 10 to 15% for women.

HOW THE DEFINITION OF THE METABOLIC SYNDROME OVERLAPS THAT OF INSULIN RESISTANCE

As previously reported, the NCEP/ATP III report designated a cluster of related CVD risk factors as a definition of the metabolic syndrome, and stated that "this syndrome is closely linked to insulin resistance" *(28)*. Insulin resistance and/or compensatory hyperinsulinemia are undoubted CVD risk factors *(23)*. On the other hand, although insulin resistance is believed to be the basic pathophysiological alteration leading to the metabolic syndrome, neither assessment of insulin resistance nor hyperinsulinemia were among the criteria proposed by the NCEP/ATP III report. This omission was justified by the lack of adequate sensitivity and specificity of the different insulin assays used in clinical practice and other potential limitations. This is of importance, because there are patients with the metabolic syndrome who are unlikely to have insulin resistance and vice versa *(37)*.

There are several other considerations emphasizing why different definitions of the metabolic syndrome and of insulin resistance may in some way represent different entities and they should not therefore be used as synonyms *(39)*. In fact, many studies indicate that relatively new indices related to both insulin resistance and the CVD may also be useful predictive tools or useful additions to the definition of the metabolic syndrome *(39)*. These indices include markers of low-grade inflammation, which is currently suggested to play a major role in atherogenesis development. In fact, recent studies have shown that a relationship exists between inflammatory markers and indices of insulin resistance, both in subjects with the metabolic syndrome and in those with T2DM and obesity *(39)*, as well as in those with PCOS *(40)*. It is now well established that there is a strong and consistent inverse association between adiponectin and both insulin resistance and inflammatory markers *(39)*. In addition, adiponectin is also inversely related with other CVD risk factors, clustering all definitions of the metabolic syndrome *(39)*. Several other molecules and factors (such as fibrinogen, plasminogen activator inhibitor [PAI]-1, and so on) have also been found to be closely associated to insulin resistance, metabolic syndrome risk factors and risk of CVD *(39)*. The reasons supporting the possibility that the phrase "insulin resistance" may not adequately describe the hallmark of the metabolic syndrome or vice versa, even though insulin resistance may represent a component or a main pathophysiological factor of the metabolic syndrome itself, have been recently and extensively discussed by Kahn et al. in a provocative report which the readers should refer to for further details to understand the fundamental issues of the debate (39). Therefore, the attempt to define the metabolic syndrome as a result of a simple unifying pathophysiological process is problematic. This can be simply documented by the fact that there are very few studies that have described the relationship between reliable measurements of insulin resistance and all of the components of each cluster used to define the metabolic syndrome. One example of these studies is the report by Cheal et al. (41). The authors investigated a large group of healthy volunteers with different anthropometric and metabolic characteristics, and insulin resistance was defined as being in the top tertile of the steady-state plasma glucose during the combined octreotide-insulin-glucose test (42). They found that, although insulin resistance and the presence of the metabolic syndrome were significantly associated ($p < 0.001$) with the sensitivity and positive predictive values equal to 46 and 76%, respectively. It should be noticed that the presence of overweightness with high triglycerides, low HDL-cholesterol, or elevated blood pressure were the most common factors included in the diagnosis of the metabolic syndrome itself.

Despite these limitations, it is quite clear that the presence of the metabolic syndrome includes a high proportion of subjects with an insulin resistance state. Therefore, with some caution, it could be argued that measurement of the metabolic syndrome may be a justified method of detecting insulin resistant individuals, although some of them may be lost in the analysis. This is particularly important not only in the general population and in diabetic subjects, but also in women suffering from PCOS.

INSULIN RESISTANCE AND THE METABOLIC SYNDROME IN PCOS

Insulin Resistance

Insulin resistance in women with PCOS is more common than in the general population (1). It should, however, be emphasized that the majority of the studies have simply demonstrated that, in comparison to adequate control groups, insulin resistance, as measured by different techniques or methods, was more common in PCOS. There are no studies focusing on the prevalence of insulin resistance in PCOS. One study by Azziz et al. (43) examined the clinical features of more than 1000 consecutive women with androgen excess, and found that 716 of them had PCOS and were characterized, as a group, by hyperinsulinemia and insulin resistance. Interestingly, 60% of them were obese, which raises the possibility that obesity per se may be an amplifier of this metabolic derangement. Many other studies have in fact reported that insulin resistance is very common in the presence of obesity, particularly the abdominal phenotype (4–6). On the other hand, insulin resistance may be present even in PCOS with normal weight (4–6). The common thought is that obesity and PCOS have an additive deleterious effect on insulin sensitivity, by mechanisms that have still not been adequately defined and could be partly different (4,5,44). Reports on the prevalence of insulin resistance in women with PCOS are not homogeneous, depending on the sensitivity and specificity of the test employed. Because of the lack of epidemiological studies, available data refer to clinical studies performed in different centers worldwide and including only PCOS patients attending each institution for medical problems or personal complaints, particularly hirsutism, menstrual abnormalities, infertility, or obesity.

Both fasting and glucose-stimulated insulin concentrations are usually significantly higher in PCOS than in non-PCOS controls *(4–6)*. Accordingly, studies examining insulin sensitivity by using different methods, such as the euglycemic hyperinsulinemic clamp technique, the FSIVGTT or the ITT have demonstrated that PCOS women had significantly lower insulin sensitivity compared to age- and weight-matched controls. In addition, they demonstrated that almost all obese PCOS women have some degree of insulin resistance, whereas this abnormality is present in more than half their non-obese PCOS counterparts (*see* extensive revision in refs. *4–6*).

Interestingly, however, some studies found some degree of deficiency in the first phase of insulin secretion in selected groups of PCOS women with obesity investigated in the United States *(14,45)*, which were not confirmed by other studies performed in Europe *(46,47)*. A more recent study using the FSIVGTT technique has produced additional data in European PCOS women, showing that in those with normal weight, insulin sensitivity and β-cell function is preserved, whereas glucose effectiveness (which is the insulin-independent glucose uptake) may be decreased *(48)*.

At variance, other relevant papers did not confirm decreased insulin sensitivity in PCOS, particularly in the normal weight subjects. In addition, these papers raised several questions regarding the opportunity of evaluating potential confounding factors, which, if not considered, can lead to false-positive results. Holte et al. *(49)* reported that some differences in the insulin sensitivity index (ISI), defined as the ratio of the glucose disposal rate (S_i) to the insulin concentrations at the end of a euglycemic hyperinsulinemic clamp, was present only in subjects with high body mass index values. Interestingly, while examining insulin sensitivity (measured by the FSIVGTT) in relation to the presence of a heredity risk for T2DM, Ehrmann et al. *(45)* were not able to find any difference in ISI between obese PCOS and controls in affected women with a negative family history, whereas it was present in those with a positive one. Morin-Papunen et al. *(50)* found that, compared to adequate control groups, only obese PCOS women were more insulin resistant, without any difference between normal weight PCOS and controls. More recently, these findings have been confirmed by another study *(51)*. Among potential factors explaining these different findings, dietary factors *(52)*, heredity, or pattern of fat distribution (in both obese and non-obese women) should therefore be considered in all studies performed in this field.

As reported in the previous paragraph, there are several concerns related to the identity of the definition of the metabolic syndrome and that of insulin resistance. As emphasized by the EGIR group, these conditions should be considered separately. On the other hand, it has been shown that the greater the number of factors defining the metabolic syndrome, the higher the probability that affected subjects are insulin resistant *(41)*. This indicates the need to carefully collect the data for each parameter and if necessary to include some other parameters in the definition of the metabolic syndrome. Considering the lack of studies on this particularly important field in PCOS, we investigated the prevalence of insulin resistance measured by simple mathematical tests and insulin concentrations in a cohort of 289 women with PCOS and we compared the data with those observed in a sample of normal weight healthy controls. We also investigated how many PCOS women with the metabolic syndrome according to the NCEP/ATP III criteria were insulin resistant (as defined by the same parameters previously reported), in comparison to PCOS women without the metabolic syndrome

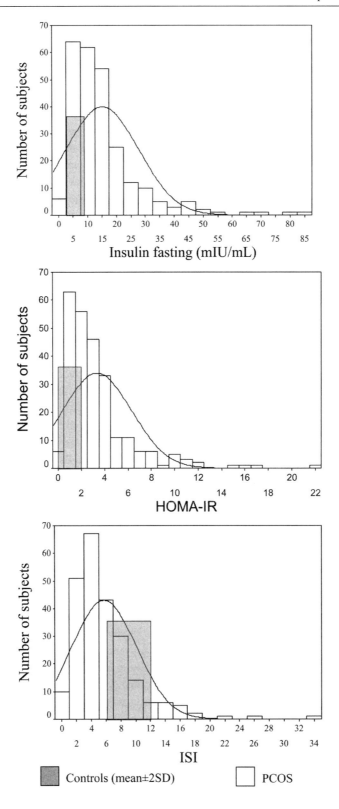

(therefore with only two or fewer criteria). Figure 1 shows the distribution of fasting insulin levels, HOMA and ISI applied to the OGTT (ISI_{OGTT}) *(53)*. Collectively, 55% of PCOS women had fasting insulin values higher than 2SD those observed in the control group, 37% had higher HOMA values, and 49.5% had higher IS_I, which indicates that approx 40–50% of PCOS subjects were insulin resistant, based on these measurements. These findings are in agreement with the prevalence of the metabolic syndrome, according to previously reported data *(54)*. When PCOS subjects were classified as having or not having the metabolic syndrome, according to the NCEP/ATP III criteria, we found that in the former, higher (than 2SD those found in the controls) fasting insulin was present in 87.3%, higher HOMA in 74.6% and higher ISI in 79.4%, compared to 54.7% ($p < 0.001$), 32.8% ($p < 0.001$), and 56.7% ($p < 0.001$), respectively, of those without the metabolic syndrome (Table 2). Notably, there was no difference in age values between the two groups, whereas body mass index was significantly higher in the former (37.2 ± 5.4 vs 27.5 ± 5.2 kg/m^2; $p < 0.001$). From these data it, therefore, appears that insulin resistance is present at least in 70–85% of women with PCOS.

GLUCOSE INTOLERANCE, THE METABOLIC SYNDROME, AND T2DM

Undoubtedly, aggravation of insulin resistance in the long term may represent an important factor in the development of glucose intolerance states in PCOS *(55,56)*. Clinical studies have in fact shown that glucose intolerance is present at the first clinical examination, in as many as 30–40% of obese PCOS women in the United States *(4)* and, probably, to a lesser extent in those living in Europe *(47)*, whereas it is uncommon in their normal-weight counterparts *(4,47)*. In any case, the prevalence rate for impaired glucose tolerance in the population of obese PCOS subjects appears to be higher than that reported in population-based studies on the incidence of glucose intolerance in women of similar ages *(57)*, although cross-sectional or longitudinal epidemiological studies are lacking. These findings indicate that obesity may contribute to determine the insulin resistant state and may impair glucose tolerance in PCOS. Although insulin resistance seems to play a determining role in the development of diabetes, the presence of insulin resistance does not immediately imply a concomitant alteration of glucose tolerance. In fact, most obese insulin-resistant PCOS women still have a normal glucose tolerance state. On the other hand, it has recently been found that PCOS women with impaired glucose tolerance or type 2 diabetes are significantly more insulin-resistant and hyperinsulinemic than those with normal glucose tolerance, regardless of the presence of obesity *(47)*. It has also been reported that the development of states of glucose intolerance can be predicted to a certain extent, because there are early markers such as low birth-weight in PCOS subjects *(47)*, as well as in the general population *(58,59)*.

Fig. 1. Prevalence of insulin resistance as measured by simple tests (fasting insulin levels, HOMA, ISI_{OGTT}) among PCOS women. Data are represented as tentiles of distribution. The gray area refers to data (mean ± 2SD) obtained in normal weight healthy women.
Age (years): controls: 28.8 ± 5.8, PCOS: 24.9 ± 6.5 ($p =$ NS)
Body mass index (kg/m^2): controls: 20.8 ± 2.1, PCOS: 30.1 ± 7.5 ($p < 0.001$)
Fasting glucose (mg/dL): controls: 81.1 ± 7.9, PCOS: 87.3 ± 10.1 ($p = 0.001$)
Fasting insulin (mIU/mL): controls 6.9 ± 1.5, PCOS: 15.1 ± 612.6 ($p < 0.001$)
HOMA: controls: 1.40 ± 0.76, PCOS: 3.33 ± 1.48 ($p < 0.001$)
ISI: controls: 9.00 ± 1.66, PCOS: 5.73 ± 4.39 ($p < 0.001$)

Table 2
Association Between Insulin Resistance (as Defined by Simple Tests
[Fasting Insulin Levels, HOMA, ISI]) in PCOS Women
With or Without the Metabolic Syndrome[a]

	General data and metabolic parameters in the two groups		
	Without MS (n = 137)	*With MS* (n = 63)	p-*value*
Age (years)	23.9 ± 5.8	25.9 ± 7.9	0.074
Body mass index (kg/m^2)	27.5 ± 5.2	37.2 ± 5.4	<0.001
Glucose, fasting (mg/mL)	85.6 ± 10.5	95.7 ± 18.2	<0.001
Insulin, fasting (mIU/mL)	10.9 ± 7.7	24.2 ± 18.2	<0.001
HOMA	2.36 ± 1.93	5.87 ± 5.18	<0.001
ISI	7.74 ± 4.49	3.10 ± 3.29	<0.001
	Number of subjects (%) with hyperinsulinemia and insulin resistance		
	Without MS (n = 137)	*With MS* (n = 63)	*Chi-square test*
High (>2 SD) fasting insulin	75/137 (54.7%)	55/63 (87.3%)	<0.001
High (>2 SD) HOMA	45/137 (32.8%)	47/63 (74.6%)	<0.001
Low (<2SD) ISI$_{OGTT}$	64/137 (46.7%)	50/63 (79.4%)	<0.001

[a]Defined according to the NCEP ATP III criteria (*see* Table 1 for details). Each parameter was defined as abnormal when values exceeded 2SD those observed in a normal-weight healthy control group (*see* legend to Fig. 1).

Prospective studies in PCOS women also found that insulin resistance tends to worsen over time together with an increment of insulin and C-peptide response to an oral glucose challenge, and that, in several cases, glucose intolerance is diagnosed *(55,56)*. Taken together, these findings strongly support the role of insulin resistance in the development of altered glucose tolerance states in PCOS women.

Particularly if they are obese, PCOS women may also present with a more athero-genic lipoprotein pattern profile, which is characteristic of the metabolic syndrome and is strongly associated with the presence of insulin resistance. A greater reduction of HDL-cholesterol, together with a higher increase of both triglycerides and total- and LDL-cholesterol levels were in fact observed in obese respectively to normal-weight PCOS women, particularly when the abdominal obesity phenotype was present *(6)*.

Some recent studies used the NECP/ATPIII criteria to assess the prevalence of the metabolic syndrome in PCOS women. Glueck et al. *(60)* studied 138 PCOS patients and found a prevalence rate of 46%, whereas, more recently, Apridonidze et al. *(7)* found a prevalence of 43% by retrospectively reviewing the medical charts of 106 PCOS women attending the Endocrine Clinic of Richmond, VA. Both these studies, described a prevalence of the metabolic syndrome in PCOS nearly twofold higher than that reported in the general population investigated in the cited NHANES III report *(61)*, matched for age and body weight. Apridonidze et al. *(7)* also described higher free testosterone and lower SHBG levels in those women with the metabolic syndrome with respect to those without it, as well as a higher prevalence of acanthosis nigricans and with family history for PCOS. These results were in accordance with a cross-sectional population-based study conducted by Korhonen et al. *(62)* who reported a different concentration of some sex hormones between premenopausal women with and without the NCEP/ATPIII defined metabolic syndrome.

Studies in American *(63,64)*, Asian *(65)*, and Italian *(47)* subjects have also shown that women with PCOS have an increased risk for the selective development of impaired glucose tolerance and T2DM, with a tendency to early development of glucose intolerance states, when compared to the general population. We recently analyzed 200 selected PCOS women from the Mediterranean area and we found that 18% were characterized by the absence of any criteria of the metabolic syndrome, 51% had at least two criteria, and 31% met the three criteria according to the NCEP/ATPIII recommendations. Therefore, collectively, 82% of PCOS women had at least one feature of the metabolic syndrome, a finding consistent with a very large presence of single or grouped metabolic abnormalities in this disorder. Compared to those without any criteria, the other two groups were progressively more obese and had a higher prevalence of the abdominal pattern of fat distribution. In addition, women presenting with the metabolic syndrome were characterized by higher systolic and diastolic blood pressure, higher pulse rate, greater frequency of liver enzyme abnormalities, worsened insulin resistance, higher glycosylated hemoglobin, and a more severe hyperandrogenemia (higher free androgen index and lower SHBG concentrations) with respect to those without the metabolic syndrome (unpublished data). Taken together, these findings demonstrate that the prevalence of the metabolic syndrome and T2DM in women with PCOS is higher than that of the general population, regardless of ethnicity and geographical area. They also indicate a strong association between the metabolic syndrome and the hyperandrogenic state. Moreover, the apparent difference in the prevalence of T2DM among studies performed in the US and European populations suggests that environmental factors may play a dominant role in determining individual susceptibility to metabolic disorders, which is probably more important than genetic background, as supported by recent long-term epidemiological studies demonstrating that the appearance of type 2 diabetes can be prevented by adequate lifestyle interventions, focusing on dietary habits and increased physical activity *(66,67)*.

FUTURE AVENUES OF INVESTIGATION

From the theoretical point of view, it is hypothesized that the worldwide epidemia of obesity and the metabolic syndrome may explain the suggested increasing prevalence of PCOS, although this should be investigated in large multicenter cross-sectional epidemiological studies.

In addition, there is the need to further clarify the prevalence of both insulin resistance and the metabolic syndrome in women with PCOS of different ethnicities and living in different countries of the world.

Molecular mechanisms responsible for insulin resistance in PCOS and the potential impact of obesity and multiple environmental and genetic factors require more intensive investigation.

In addition, the need for carefully conducted clinical studies, aimed at identifying the most reliable and relatively simple methods to define insulin resistance in a clinical setting, are warranted.

Finally, PCOS subjects being exposed to a high risk of developing T2DM and, possibly, CVDs, the role of insulin resistance, hyperinsulinemia, and the metabolic syndrome require more attention in both epidemiological and clinical longitudinal studies. This may be achieved by defining preventive strategies targeted in women suffering from PCOS.

KEY POINTS

- Insulin resistance and the metabolic syndrome are commonly present in PCOS women, particularly those with obesity and the abdominal phenotype.
- Obesity amplifies the expression of both insulin resistance and the metabolic syndrome.
- Although insulin resistance and the metabolic syndrome represent different entities, the higher the number of criteria used to define the metabolic syndrome, the larger the presence of insulin resistance in affected women.
- Because of these metabolic abnormalities, women with PCOS have an increased risk of developing type 2 diabetes.

REFERENCES

1. Ehrmann DA. Polycystic ovary syndrome. N Engl J Med 2005;352:1223–1236.
2. The Rotterdam ESHRE/ASRM-Sponsored PCOS Consensus Workshop Group. Revised 2003 consensus on diagnostic criteria and long-term health risks related to polycystic ovary syndrome (PCOS). Hum Reprod 2004;19:41–47.
3. Legro RS. The genetics of obesity: lessons for polycystic ovary syndrome. Ann NY Acad Sci 2000; 900:193–202.
4. Dunaif A. Insulin resistance and the polycystic ovary syndrome: mechanisms and implications for pathogenesis. Endocr Rev 1997;18:774–800.
5. Poretsky L, Cataldo NA, Rosenwaks Z, Giudice LC. The insulin-related ovarian regulatory system in health and disease. Endocr Rev 1999;20:535–582.
6. Gambineri A, Pelusi C, Vicennati, Pagotto U, Pasquali R. Obesity and the polycystic ovary syndrome. Int J Obes Relat Metab Dis 2002;26:883–896.
7. Apridonidze T, Essah P, Iourno MJ, Nestler JE. Prevalence and characteristics of the metabolic syndrome in women with PCOS. J Clin Endocrinol Metab 2005;90:1929–1935.
8. Beck-Nielsen H, Alford F, Hother-Nielsen O. Insulin resistance in glucose disposal and production in man with specific reference to metabolic syndrome and type 2 diabetes. In: Kumar S, O'Railly S, eds. Inb Insulin Resistance. New York: John Wiley and Sons Ltd., 2000, pp.155–178.
9. Radziuk J. Insulin sensitivity and its measurement: structural commonalities among the methods. J Clin Endocrinol Metab 2000;85:4426–4433.
10. Bergman RN, Finegood DT, Ader M. Assessment of insulin sensitivity in vivo. Endocr Rev 1985;6:45–86.
11. Weber KM, Martin IK, Best JD, Alford FP, Boston RC. Alternative methods for minimal model analysis of intravenous glucose tolerance data. Am J Physiol 1989;256:E524–E535.
12. Mattews Dr, Hosker JP, Rudenski AS, Naylor BA, Treacher DF, Turner RC. Homeostasis model assessment: insulin resistance and B-cell function from fasting plasma glucose and insulin concentrations in man. Diabetologia 1985;28:412–419.
13. Katz A, Nambi SS, Mater K, et al. Quantitative insulin sensitivity check index: a simple, accurate method for assessing insulin sensitivity in humans. J Clin Endocrinol Metab 2000;85:2402–2410.
14. Dunaif A, Finegood DT. β-cell dysfunction independent of obesity and glucose intolerance in the polycystic ovary syndrome. J Clin Endocrinol Metab 1996;81:942–947.
15. Hrebicek J, Janout V, Malincikova J, Horakova D, Cizek L. Detection of insulin resistance by simple quantitative insulin sensitivity check index QUICKI for epidemiological assessment and prevention. J Clin Endocrinol Metab 2002;87:144–147.
16. Reaven GM. The metabolic syndrome or the insulin resistance syndrome? Different names, different concepts, and different goals. Endocrinol Metab Clin N Am 2004;33:283–303.

17. Carmina E, Lobo R. Use of fasting blood to assess the prevalence of insulin resistance in women with polycystic ovary syndrome. Fertil Steril 2004;82:661–665.
18. Diamanti-Kandarakis E, Kouli C, Alexandraki K, Spina G. Failure of mathematical indices to accurately assess insulin resistance in lean, overweight, or obese women with polycystic ovary syndrome. J Clin Endocrinol Metab 2004;89:1273–1276.
19. Ciampelli M, Leoni F, Cucinelli F, et al. Assessment of insulin sensitivity from measurements in the fasting state and during an oral glucose tolerance test in polycystic ovary syndrome and menopausal patients. J Clin Endocrinol Metab 2005;90:1398–1406.
20. Avignon A, Boegner C, Mariano-Goular D, Colette C, Monnier L. Assesment of insulin sensitivity from plasma insulin and glucose in the fasting or post oral glucose-load state. In J Obes Rel Metab Dis 1999;23:512–517.
21. Mari A, Pacini G, Brazzale AR, Ahren B. Comparative evaluation of simple insulin sensitivity methods based on the oral glucose tolerance test. Diabetologia 2005;48:748–751.
22. Yeni-Konshian H, Carantoni M, Abbasi F, Reaven GM. Relationship between several surrogate estimates of insulin resistance and quantification of insulin-mediated glucose disposal in 4090 healthy, nondiabetic volunteers. Diabetes Care 2000;23:171–175.
23. Reaven GM. Insulin resistance in human disease. Diabetes 1988;37:1595–1607.
24. Avogaro P, Crepaldi G, Enzi G, Tiengo A. Associazione di iperlipidemia, diabete mellito e obesità di medio grado. Acta Diabetol Lat 1967;4:36–41.
25. International Diabetes Federation: the IDF worldwide definition of the metabolic syndrome. Available from http://www.cdc.gov/nchs/about/major/nhanes/nhanes/99-02.htm. Accessed 18 May 2005.
26. Wu FC, von Eckardstein A. Androgens and coronary artery disease. Endocr Rev 2003;24:183–217.
27. Bjorntorp P, Rosmond R. The metabolic syndrome-a neuroendocrine disorder. Br J Nutr 2000;83: S49–S57.
28. Executive Summary of the Third Report of The National Cholesterol Education Program (NCEP) Expert Panel on Detection, Evaluation, and Treatment of High Blood Cholesterol in Adults (Adult Treatment Panel III). JAMA 2001;285:2486–2497.
29. Ford ES. Prevalence of the metabolic syndrome in US population. Endocrinol Metab Clin N Am 2004;33:333–350.
30. Resnick HE. Strong Heart Study Investigators: metabolic syndrome in American Indians. Diabetes Care 2002;25:1246–1247.
31. American College of Endocrinology Task Force on the Insulin Resistance Syndrome. American College of Endocrinology Position Statement on the Insulin Resistance Syndrome. Endocr Pract 2002;9:236–252.
32. Alberti K, Zimmet P. Definition, diagnosis and classification of diabetes mellitus and its complications. Part 1: diagnosis and classification of diabetes mellitus. Report of a WHO consultation. Diab Med 1998;15:539–553.
33. World Heath Organization. Definition, diagnosis and classification of diabetes mellitus and its complications. Part 1: diagnosis and classification of diabetes mellitus. Geneva (Switzerland): Department of Noncommunicable Disease Surveillance; 1999.
34. Ford ES, Giles WH. A comparison of the prevalence of the metabolic syndrome using two proposed definitions. Diabetes Care 2003;26:575–581.
35. Meigs JB, Wilson PW, Nathan DM, D'Agostino RB Sr. Williams K, Haffner SM. Prevalence and characteristics of the metabolic syndrome in the San Antonio Heart and Framingham Offspring Studies. Diabetes 2003;52:2160–2167.
36. Cameron AJ, Shaw JE, Zimmet PZ. The metabolic syndrome: prevalence in worldwide populations. Endocrinol Metab Clin N Am 2004;33:351–375.
37. Balkau B, Charles MA. Comment on the provisional report from the WHO consultation. European Group for the Study of Insulin Resistance (EGIR). Diab Med 1999;16:442–443.
38. Gu D, Reynolds K, Wu X, Chem J, et al. InterASIA Collaborative Group. Prevalence of the metabolic syndrome and overweight among adults in China. Lancet 2005;365:1398–1405.
39. Kahn R, Ferrranini E, Buse J, Stern M. The metabolic syndrome: time for a critical rappraisal. Joint statement from the American Diabetes Association and the European Association for the study of Diabetes. Diabetes Care 2005;28:2289–2304.
40. Orio F Jr. Palomba S, Cascella T, et al. The increase of leukocytes as a new putative marker of low-grade chronic inflammation and early cardiovascular risk in polycystic ovary sindrome. J Clin Endocrinol Metab 2005;90:2–5.

41. Cheal KL, Abbasi F, Lamendola C, McLaughlin T, Reaven GM, Ford ES. Relationship to insulin resistance of the adult treatment panel III diagnostic criteria for identification of the metabolic syndrome. Diabetes 2004;53:1195–1200.

42. Greenfield MS, Doberne L, Kraemer F, Tobey T, Reaven GM. Assessment of insulin resistance with insulin suppression test and the euglycemic clam. Diabetes 1981;30:387–392.

43. Azziz JR, Sanchez LA, Knochenhauer ES, et al. Androgen excess in women: experience with over 1000 consecutive patients. J Clin Endocrinol Metab 2004;89:453–462.

44. Cibula D. Is insulin resistance an essential component of PCOS? Hum Reprod 2004;19:757–759.

45. Ehrmann DA, Sturis J, Byrne MM, Karrison T, Rosenfield RL, Polonsky KS. Insulin secretory defects in polycystic ovary syndrome. Relationship to insulin sensitivity and family history of non-insulin-dependent diabetes mellitus. J Clin Invest 1995;96:520–527.

46. Holte J, Bergh T, Berne C, et al. Restored insulin sensitivity but persistently increased early insulin secretion after weight loss in obese women with polycystic ovary syndrome. J Clin Endocrinol Metab 1995;80:2586–2593.

47. Gambineri A, Pelusi C, Manicardi E, et al. Glucose intolerance in a large cohort of mediterranean women with polycystic ovary syndrome: phenotype and associated factors. Diabetes 2004;53: 2353–2358.

48. Gennarelli G, Roveri R, Novi F, et al. Preserved insulin sensitivity and β-cell activity, but decreased glucose effectiveness in normal weight women with polycystic ovary syndrome. J Clin Endocrinol Metab 2005;90:3381–3386.

49. Holte J, Bergh Ch, Berglund L, Litthell H. Enhanced early phase insulin response to glucose in relation to insulin resistance in women with polycystic ovary syndrome. J Clin Endocrinol Metab 1994;78: 1052–1058.

50. Morin Papunen LC, Vahkonen I, Koivunen RM, Ruokonen A, Tapanainen JS. Insulin sensitivity, insulin secretion and metabolic and hormonal parameters in healthy women and women with polycystic ovary syndrome. Hum Reprod 2004;15:1266–1274.

51. Vrbikova J, Cibula D, Dvorakova K, et al. Insulin sensitivity in women with polycystic ovary syndrome. J Clin Endocrinol Metab 2004;89:2942–2945.

52. Wijeyartne CN, Balen AH, Barth JH, Belchetz PE. Clinical manifestation and insulin resistance (IR) in polycystic ovary syndrome (PCOS) among South Asians and Caucasians: is there a difference? Clin Endocrinol (Oxf) 2002;57:343–350.

53. Matusda M, De Fronzo RA. Insulin sensitivity indices obtained from oral glucose tolerance testing. Diabetes Care 1999;22:1462–1470.

54. Pasquali R, Patton L, Pagotto U, Gambineri A. Metabolic alterations and cardiovascular risk factors in the polycystic ovary syndrome. Min Ginecol 2005;57:79–85.

55. Pasquali R, Patton L, Pagotto U, Gambineri A. Metabolic alterations and cardiovascular risk factors in the polycystic ovary syndrome. Min Ginecol 2005;57:79–85.

56. Pasquali R, Gambineri A, Anconetani B, et al. The natural history of the metabolic syndrome in young women with the polycystic ovary syndrome and the long-term effect of oestrogen-progestagen treatment. Clin Endocrinol (Oxf) 1999;50:517–527.

57. Legro RS, Gnatuk CL, Kunselman AR, Dunaif A. Changes in glucose tolerance over time in women with polycystic ovary syndrome: a controlled study. J Clin Endocrinol Metab 2005;90:3236–3242.

58. Harris MI, Hadden WC, Knowler WC. Prevalence of diabetes and impaired glucose tolerance and plasma glucose levels in the US population aged 20-74. Diabetes 1987;36:523–534.

59. Hofman PL, Cutfiled WS, Robinson EM, et al. Insulin resistance in short children with intrauterine growth retardation. J Clin Endocrinol Metab 1997;82:402–406.

60. Phillips DI. Insulin resistance as a programmed response to fetal undernutrition. Diabetologia 1996;39:1119–1122.

61. Glueck CJ, Papanna R, Wang P, Goldemberg N, Sieve-Smith L. Incidence and treatment of metabolic syndrome in newly referred women with confirmed polycystic ovarian syndrome. Metabolism 2003; 52:908–915.

62. US Department of Health and Human Services (DHHS). National Center for Health Statistics. Third National Health and Nutrition Examination Survey, 1988-1994, NHANES III. 1996. Hyattsville, MD, Center for Disease Control and Prevention. Ref type: Data File.

63. Kohronen S, Hippelainen M, Vanhala M, Heinonen S, Niskanen L. The androgenic sex hormone profile is an essential feature of metabolic syndrome in premenopausal women: a controlled community-based study. Fertil Steril 2003;79:1327–1334.

64. Legro RS, Kunselman AR, Dodson WC, Dunaif A. Prevalence and predictions of the risk of type 2 diabetes mellitus and impaired glucose tolerance in polycystic ovary syndrome: a prospective, controlled study in 254 affected women. J Clin Endocrinol Metab 1999;84:165 169.
65. Ehrmann DA, Barnes RB, Rosenfield RL, Cavaghan MK, Imperial J. Prevalence of impaired glucose tolerance and diabetes in women with polycystic ovary syndrome. Diabetes Care 1999;22:141–146.
66. Weerakiet S, Srisombut C, Bunnag P, Sangtong S, Chuangsoongnoen N, Rojanasakul A. Prevalence of type 2 diabetes mellitus and impaired glucose tolerance in Asian women with polycystic ovary syndrome. Int J Gynaecol Obstet 2001;75:177–184.
67. Norris SL, Zhang X, Avenell A, et al. Long-term effectiveness of lifestyle and behavioral weight loss interventions in adults with type 2 diabetes: a meta-analysis. Am J Med 2004;117:762–774.
68. Kanaya AM, Narayan KM. Prevention of type 2 diabetes: data from recent trials. Prim Care 2003;30: 511–526.

3 The Insulin Resistance of Polycystic Ovary Syndrome

Marek Demissie, MD, PhD, Richard S. Legro, MD, and Andrea Dunaif, MD

CONTENTS

Summary

Insulin resistance is a common feature of polycystic ovary syndrome (PCOS). Affected women are at high risk of impaired glucose tolerance and type 2 diabetes mellitus. The insulin resistance in PCOS is due to a postbinding defect in insulin signaling associated with constitutive serine phosphorylation of the insulin receptor and downstream signaling proteins secondary to a yet unidentified serine kinase. The insulin resistance is selective, affecting the metabolic due, but not mitogenic actions of insulin in some tissues. Such a defect might lead to increased susceptibility to factors inducing insulin resistance present in vivo, such as free fatty acids and cytokines.

Key Words: PCOS; insulin resistance; insulin receptor; hyperandrogenism; obesity; beta-cell function; adipocyte; skeletal muscle.

HYPERANDROGENISM AND INSULIN RESISTANCE

The association between glucose intolerance and hyperandrogenism was first described in 1921 by Achard and Thiers as "the diabetes of bearded women." It is now well established that is a common feature of polycystic ovary syndrome (PCOS). The metabolic aspects of this syndrome include insulin resistance, obesity, lipid abnormalities, and an increased risk for impaired glucose tolerance and type 2 diabetes mellitus (*1–5*).

Burghen et al. (*6*) showed that women with PCOS had higher basal and postglucose insulin levels in comparison to weight- and age-matched control women. Euglycaemic clamp studies have demonstrated that women with PCOS are substantially more insulin resistant than unaffected women of comparable BMI and body composition (*7–9*).

From: *Contemporary Endocrinology: Insulin Resistance and Polycystic Ovarian Syndrome:
Pathogenesis, Evaluation, and Treatment*
Edited by: E. Diamanti-Kandarakis, J. E. Nestler, D. Panidis, and R. Pasquali © Humana Press Inc., Totowa, NJ

Insulin resistance was independent of obesity and glucose intolerance *(10,11)*. In addition to decreased insulin sensitivity, an intrinsic pancreatic β-cell secretory dysfunction leading to an excessive compensatory insulin secretion has been suggested in PCOS *(12)*.

MOLECULAR PATHWAYS IN INSULIN ACTION

The insulin receptor is a protein tyrosine kinase receptor that exists as a dimer in the absence of ligand. Binding of insulin can initiate two distinct postreceptor signaling pathways that propagate the insulin signal downstream. Tyrosine autophosphorylation increases the insulin receptor tyrosine kinase activity, whereas serine phosphorylation inhibits it. One pathway, involving phosphorylation of a 130-kDa polypeptide, called insulin receptor substrate (IRS)-1 and activation of phosphatidylinositol (PI)-3-kinase is necessary for mediating metabolic effects of insulin. Phosphorylated IRS-1 binds PI-3-kinase causing a 10-fold stimulation in its kinase activity and consequently the rapid rise in phosphoinositides in insulin-stimulated cells. The increase in phosphoinositides leads to recruitment of protein kinase B (PKB or AKT) to the membrane. The N-terminal region of this kinase contains a PH domain, which binds to plasma membrane phosphoinositides. Once localized to the membrane, PKB is phosphorylated and released into the cytosol where it mediates many effects of insulin, including stimulation of glucose uptake and stimulation of glycogen synthesis (Fig. 1) *(13,14)*.

The second signaling pathway involves the phosphorylation of Shc and activation of Ras, Raf, MEK, and mitogen-activated protein (MAP) kinases (Erk 1 and 2) and contributes to the nuclear and mitogenic effects of insulin (Fig. 1) *(13)*.

Molecular Defects in Insulin Action in PCOS

There were no mutations of insulin receptor or defects in insulin-binding suggesting the existence of a postreceptor defect in insulin action in PCOS *(15–17)*. The inhibition of insulin signaling was related to constitutively excessive serine phosphorylation of the insulin receptor β-subunit by a factor extrinsic to the insulin receptor (actually a serine/threonine kinase yet to be identified). This defect is selective, affecting metabolic but not mitogenic actions of insulin *(10)*.

A critical point in understanding the role of insulin resistance in PCOS was to determine whether the insulin receptor abnormalities are present in the key insulin target tissues-adipocytes and skeletal muscles.

Studies in adipocytes have shown no aberrations in insulin receptor number or affinity compared to weight-matched control women *(7)*. However, the presence of postbinding defect in insulin signaling in adipocytes of women with PCOS was suggested by decreased insulin-mediated glucose transport and reduction in the abundance of GLUT4 glucose transporters *(18)*. Additionally, an enhanced lipolytic effect of catecholamines in visceral fat cells of PCOS women (subcutaneous abdominal adipocytes are resistant to catecholamine-induced lipolysis) can contribute to insulin resistance by increasing free fatty acids (FFA) release directly into the portal circulation *(19)*.

Because skeletal muscle glucose transport normally accounts for approx 85% of whole body insulin-stimulated glucose uptake a defective step in this pathway is central for characterization of PCOS-related insulin resistance. In contrast to skin fibroblasts, many of the defects in glucose metabolism vanish in skeletal muscle cells from women with PCOS in long-term culture suggesting existence of extrinsic

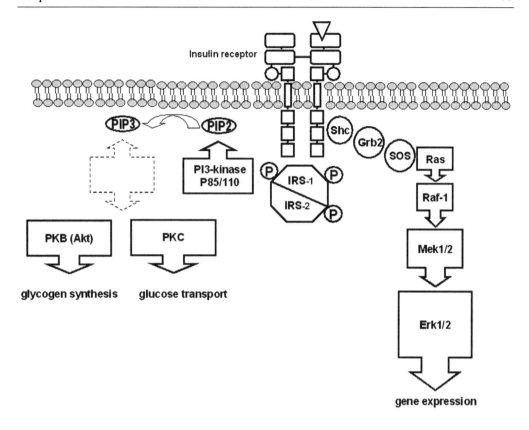

Fig. 1. Insulin signaling pathways in skeletal muscle. Explanations in the text.

circulating factors presumably produced in adipose tissue (FFA, TNF-α, or other adipocytokines). FFA have been shown to produce insulin resistance in muscles and liver in healthy individuals *(20)*.

Studies in vivo have demonstrated a postreceptor defect in IRS-1 mediated activation of PI3-kinase activity in skeletal muscle in parallel with decreased insulin-stimulated glucose uptake in PCOS *(21)*. Some defects in insulin signaling persist in cultured skeletal muscle cells. An increase in basal and insulin-stimulated glucose transport and GLUT-1 abundance in cultured myotubes from women with PCOS has been shown. As the IRS-1 abundance was significantly increased in PCOS it resulted in significantly decreased PI3-kinase activity when normalized for IRS-1. Increased phosphorylation of Ser-312 (an inhibitory site on IRS-1) in PCOS may contribute to the previously mentioned abnormality. Cultured skeletal muscle cells from women with PCOS also exhibit decreased insulin signaling via IRS-2 *(22)*. Furthermore, we have recently found that mitogenic pathways are constitutively activated in PCOS skeletal muscle (both in vivo and in culture) and that MAP kinase may be contributing to increased Ser-312 phosphorylation of IRS-1 in PCOS. MAP kinase modulation of the Ser-312 phosphorylation in myotubes from control women suggests that this pathway may play a role in normal feedback of insulin signaling and contribute to resistance to insulin's metabolic actions in PCOS *(23)*.

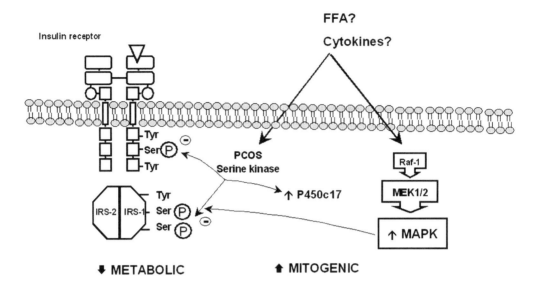

Fig. 2. Insulin resistance in some polycystic ovary syndrome (PCOS) tissues (e.g., skin fibroblasts) results from the constitutive serine phosphorylation of the insulin receptor secondary to an as yet unidentified serine kinase. The insulin resistance is selective, affecting the metabolic but not mitogenic actions of insulin. Serine phosphorylation of P450c17 (CYP 17), the rate-limiting enzyme for androgen biosynthes increases its activity. It is possible that the same serine kinase phosphorylates the insulin receptor, producing insulin resistance, and P450c17, producing hyperandrogenemia. Cytokines and free fatty acids (FFA) can activate intracellular serine kinases and might play a role in the pathogenesis of PCOS. It is possible that the serine kinase phosphorylates downstream signaling molecules, such as insulin receptor substrates (IRS)-1 or -2, further compromising insulin signaling. Constitutive activation of MAP kinase in PCOS skeletal muscle may be contributing to increased Ser-312 phosphorylation of IRS-1. MAP kinase modulation of the Ser-312 phosphorylation in myotubes from control women suggests that this pathway may play a role in normal feedback of insulin signaling and contribute to resistance to insulin's metabolic actions in PCOS. Minus symbols (–) denote serine phosphorylation, which inhibits signal transduction. Reproduced with permission from Andrea Dunaif.

FUTURE AVENUES

Only in recent decades has the association between insulin resistance and PCOS become well known. As a result of this discovery, our knowledge regarding the pathogenesis and clinical consequences of PCOS has increased greatly. Insulin resistance in PCOS is a complex phenomenon and it is likely that the combination of several molecular defects lead to its development. Future studies should examine the crosstalk between classic insulin targets (adipose tissue, liver, and skeletal muscles) and other systems such as the autonomic nervous system and the immune system. A more comprehensive understanding of insulin receptor function, postreceptor pathways, and their relationships to other metabolic pathways and the inflammatory cascade could lead to the development of new treatment strategies for PCOS.

KEY POINTS

- Insulin resistance in PCOS is due to a postbinding defect in signaling that persists in cultured skin fibroblasts and is associated with constitutive serine phosphorylation of the insulin receptor.

- The insulin resistance in PCOS is selective, affecting the metabolic but not mitogenic actions of insulin.
- Cytokines and FFA can activate intracellular serine kinases and might play a role in the pathogenesis of PCOS.
- Constitutive activation of MAP kinase in PCOS skeletal muscle may be contributing to increased Ser-312 phosphorylation of IRS-1 and may play a role in normal feedback of insulin signaling and contribute to resistance to insulin's metabolic actions in PCOS.

REFERENCES

1. The Rotterdam ESHRE/ASRM-Sponsored PCOS consensus workshop group. Revised 2003 consensus on diagnostic criteria and long-term health risks related to polycystic ovary syndrome (PCOS). Hum Reprod 2004;19:41–57.
2. Sam S, Dunaif A. Polycystic ovary syndrome: syndrome XX? Trends Endocrinol Metab 2003;14: 365–370.
3. Legro RS, Kunselman AR, Dodson WC, Dunaif A. Prevalence and predictors of risk for type 2 diabetes mellitus and impaired glucose tolerance in polycystic ovary syndrome: a prospective, controlled study in 254 affected women. J Clin Endocrinol Metab 1999;84:165–169.
4. Polson DW, Adams J, Wadsworth J, Franks S. Polycystic ovaries: a common finding in normal women. Lancet 1988;1:870–872.
5. Legro RS, Kunselman AR, Dodson WC, Dunaif A. Prevalence and predictors of risk for type 2 diabetes mellitus and impairedglucose tolerance in polycystic ovary syndrome: a prospective, controlled study in 254 affected women. J Clin Endocrinol Metab 1999;84:165–169.
6. Burghen GA, Givens JR, Kitabchi AE. Correlation of hyperandrogenism with hyperinsulinism in polycystic ovarian disease. J Clin Endocrinol Metab 1980;50:113–116.
7. Dunaif A, Segal KR, Shelley DR, Green G, Dobrjansky A, Licholai T. Evidence for distinctive and intrinsic defects in insulin action in polycystic ovary syndrome. Diabetes 1992;41:1257–1266.
8. Chang RJ, Nakamura RM, Judd HL, Kaplan SA. Insulin resistance in nonobese patients with polycystic ovarian disease. J Clin Endocrinol Metab 1983;57:356–359.
9. Dunaif A, Segal KR, Futterweit W, Dobrjansky A. Profound peripheral insulin resistance, independent of obesity, in polycystic ovary syndrome. Diabetes 1989;38:1165–1174.
10. Dunaif A, Xia J, Book CB, Schenker E, Tang Z. Excessive insulin receptor serine phosphorylation in cultured fibroblasts and in skeletal muscle. A potential mechanism for insulin resistance in the polycystic ovary syndrome. J Clin Invest 1995;96:801–810.
11. Dunaif A, Finegood DT. Beta-cell dysfunction independent of obesity and glucose intolerance in the polycystic ovary syndrome. J Clin Endocrinol Metab 1996;81:942–947.
12. Goodarzi M, Erickson S, Port SC, Jennrich RI, Korenman SG. β-Cell function: a key pathological determinant in polycystic ovary syndrome J Clin Endocrinol Metab 2005;90:310–315.
13. Dunaif A. Insulin resistance and the polycystic ovary syndrome: mechanism and implications for pathogenesis. Endocr Rev 1997;18:774–800.
14. Bjornholm M, Zierath JR. Insulin signal transduction in human skeletal muscle: identifying the defects in Type II diabetes. Biochem Soc Trans 2005;33:354–357.
15. Sorbara LR, Tang Z, Cama A, et al. Absence of insulin receptor gene mutations in three insulin-resistant women with the polycystic ovary syndrome. Metabolism 1994;43:1568–1574.
16. Conway GS, Avey C, Rumsby G. The tyrosine kinase domain of the insulin receptor gene is normal in women with hyperinsulinaemia and polycystic ovary syndrome. Hum Reprod 1994;9: 1681–1683.
17. Talbot JA, Bicknell EJ, Rajkhowa M, Krook A, O'Rahilly S, Clayton RN. Molecular scanning of the insulin receptor gene in women with polycystic ovarian syndrome. J Clin Endocrinol Metab 1996;81: 1979–1983.
18. Rosenbaum D, Haber RS, Dunaif A. Insulin resistance in polycystic ovary syndrome: decreased expression of GLUT-4 glucose transporters in adipocytes. Am J Physiol 1993;264:E197–E202.
19. Ek I, Arner P, Ryden M, et al. A unique defect in the regulation of visceral fat cell lipolysis in the polycystic ovary syndrome as an early link to insulin resistance. Diabetes 2002;51:484–492.
20. Dresner A, Laurent D, Marcucci M, et al. Effects of free fatty acids on glucose transport and IRS-1-associated phosphatidylinositol 3-kinase activity. J Clin Invest 1999;103:253–259.

21. Dunaif A, Wu X, Lee A, Diamanti-Kandarakis E. Defects in insulin receptor signaling in vivo in the polycystic ovary syndrome (PCOS). Am J Physiol Endocrinol Metab 2001;281:E392–E399.
22. Corbould A, Kim YB, Youngren JF, et al. Insulin resistance in the skeletal muscle of women with PCOS involves intrinsic and acquired defects in insulin signaling. Am J Physiol Endocrinol Metab 2005;288:E1047–E1054.
23. Corbould A, Zhao H, Mirzoeva S, Aird F, Dunaif A. Enhanced mitogenic signaling in skeletal muscle of women with polycystic ovary syndrome. Diabetes 2006;55:751–759.

4 Glucose Intolerance in Polycystic Ovary Syndrome

Focus on the β-Cell

David A. Ehrmann, MD

CONTENTS

Summary

Women with polycystic ovary syndrome (PCOS) develop glucose intolerance and diabetes at rates that are among the highest known for women of reproductive age: the prevalence of impaired glucose tolerance is estimated to be between 30 and 40%, whereas that of type 2 diabetes has been placed between 5 and 10%. A number of genetic factors influence the risk for diabetes in PCOS. In addition, several distinct environmental factors are emerging as important influences on predisposition to glucose intolerance in PCOS. Among those proposed are the rate of *in utero* growth and development, as well as exposure to excess androgen concentrations from the maternal circulation. Women with PCOS appear to have an increased risk for developing gestational diabetes mellitus, although this has not been firmly established.

Once defects in insulin secretion develop in the setting of the characteristic insulin resistance of PCOS, glucose intolerance becomes evident. Provocative testing of pancreatic β-cell function may provide insights into the future risk for glucose intolerance among women with PCOS.

Key Words: PCOS; glucose intolerance; diabetes mellitus; gestational diabetes mellitus; β-cell; insulin resistance; insulin secretion.

INTRODUCTION

It is now well established that women with polycystic ovary syndrome (PCOS) are predisposed to develop a number of metabolic abnormalities, including impaired glucose tolerance (IGT) and type 2 diabetes *(1,2)*. In some studies, gestational diabetes mellitus (GDM) has also been observed in women with PCOS with higher than expected frequencies.

From: *Contemporary Endocrinology: Insulin Resistance and Polycystic Ovarian Syndrome: Pathogenesis, Evaluation, and Treatment*
Edited by: E. Diamanti-Kandarakis, J. E. Nestler, D. Panidis, and R. Pasquali © Humana Press Inc., Totowa, NJ

The prevalence of IGT has been estimated to be between 30 and 40%, whereas that of type 2 diabetes has been placed between 5 and 10% (1,2).

PCOS is thought to affect between 5 and 8% (5.7–9.1 million) of reproductive aged women in the United States (3). Based on this estimate and extrapolation of US Census data, approximately three million women with PCOS would be expected to have IGT, whereas approximately one million women with PCOS would have type 2 diabetes.

Although the risk increases with age, it is now well documented that glucose intolerance in PCOS can occur as early as the second decade of life (4–8). In one study of 27 adolescents with PCOS, 8 (30%) were found to have IGT, 1 (4%) had undiagnosed diabetes, and the remaining 18 (66%) had normal glucose tolerance (4). Studies of Arslanian et al. (6) have shown that metabolic precursors to type 2 diabetes (decreased first-phase insulin secretion, decreased glucose disposition index, and increased hepatic glucose production) are evident among obese adolescents with PCOS. Most recently (9), the metabolic syndrome (a precursor and predictor of diabetes) was found to be 4.5 times more likely in adolescents with PCOS compared with age-matched NHANES III girls, even after adjusting for body mass index (BMI; OR 4.5, 95% CI 1.1–17.7; $p = 0.03$).

PCOS and its various phenotypic components, including pancreatic β-cell dysfunction, are thought to be heritable (10–14). Although in rare instances known gene mutations can give rise to the PCOS and its associated metabolic abnormalities (15), PCOS is likely to prove to be a complex, multigenic disorder. Candidate genes that play a role in regulation of the hypothalamic pituitary–ovarian axis, as well as those responsible for defects in insulin secretion and insulin action, have been a focus of linkage and case–control studies. Microarray analyses of target tissues in PCOS (16) have also been used as a means to identify novel candidate genes. These approaches have shown that a number of candidates make a modest contribution to the PCOS.

Relationship of Insulin Secretion to Insulin Action

Glucose intolerance typically develops when defects in insulin secretion are superimposed on a background of insulin resistance (17). Despite the fact that women with PCOS are characteristically insulin resistant, not all develop abnormalities in glucose tolerance. Insulin secretion defects are therefore thought to play an important role in the propensity to develop diabetes in PCOS.

Insulin secretion is most appropriately expressed in relation to the magnitude of ambient insulin resistance. The product of these measures can be quantified (the so-called "disposition index") and related as a percentile to the hyperbolic relationship for these measures established in normal subjects (18). We (12), as well as others (19), have found that a subset of subjects with PCOS has β-cell secretory dysfunction. In absolute terms, women with PCOS had normal first-phase insulin secretion compared with controls. In contrast, when first-phase insulin secretion was analyzed in relation to the degree of insulin resistance, women with PCOS exhibited a significant impairment in β-cell function. This reduction was particularly marked in women with PCOS who had a first-degree relative with type 2 diabetes: the mean disposition index of women with PCOS and a family history of type 2 diabetes was in the 8th percentile, whereas that of women without such a family history was in the 33rd percentile ($p < 0.05$). We have additionally quantified β-cell function in PCOS by examining insulin responses to a graded increase in plasma glucose and by the ability of the β-cell to adjust and respond to induced oscillations in the plasma glucose level *(12)*. Results from both provocative stimuli were consistent: when expressed in relation to the degree of insulin resistance, insulin secretion was impaired in subjects with PCOS who had a family history of type 2 diabetes when compared with controls.

Because these findings were consistent with studies showing a high degree of heritability of β-cell function (particularly when examined in relation to insulin sensitivity) among nondiabetic members of type 2 diabetic kindreds *(20)*, we sought to examine this further. Using the frequently sampled intravenous glucose tolerance test, insulin secretion (AIRg), insulin action (Si), and their product (AIRg × Si) were quantified among women with PCOS (*n* = 33) and their nondiabetic first-degree relatives (*n* = 48) *(21)*. Heritability of these measures was calculated from familial correlations estimated within a genetic model. The sibling correlation for AIRg was highly significant after adjustment for age and BMI, as was the disposition index, a measure of quantifying insulin secretion in relation to insulin sensitivity. This finding was supportive of a heritable component to β-cell dysfunction in families of women with PCOS.

Taken together, these results suggest that the risk imparted by insulin resistance to the development of type 2 diabetes in women with PCOS is enhanced by defects in insulin secretion. Furthermore, a history of type 2 diabetes in a first-degree relative appears to define a subset of subjects with PCOS who have the most profound defects in β-cell function.

Although nearly one-half of women with PCOS will ultimately develop glucose intolerance, most have been able to maintain glucose levels within the normal range at the time of initial clinical presentation *(1,2)*. This has been taken as evidence that their ability to adequately secrete insulin in compensation for the degree of insulin resistance is retained. However, most *(1,22)*, but not all *(23)*, studies have found that the rates of decline in glucose tolerance in PCOS are higher than expected compared with reference populations. This suggests that pancreatic β-cell dysfunction may supervene earlier in the evolution of glucose intolerance in women with PCOS compared to women without PCOS. The basis for this, however, remains unclear.

The development of transient diabetes in previously nondiabetic individuals treated with short-term glucocorticoids (so called "steroid diabetes") has been recognized for many years. The potential of this finding as a predictor for subsequent development of diabetes was first described by Fajans et al. *(24)*, who found that when normal glucose-tolerant individuals with a first-degree relative with diabetes were given small doses of cortisone acetate, 24% had IGT and 19% had diabetes on oral glucose tolerance testing. In contrast, among those without a family history of diabetes, 3% developed IGT and 2% developed diabetes. In addition, an abnormal response to cortisone acetate was predictive of the subsequent development of diabetes over 7 years of follow-up: 35% of those with cortisone-induced glucose intolerance had developed diabetes compared with only 2% of those whose initial response was normal.

Henriksen et al. *(25)* have shown that nondiabetic first-degree relatives of patients with type 2 diabetes with evidence of mild alteration of β-cell function at baseline are unable to enhance their β-cell response to dexamethasone-induced insulin resistance. Specifically, after treatment with dexamethasone (4 mg daily for 5 days), normo-glycemic subjects with or without a first-degree relative with diabetes increased their first-phase insulin secretion to glucose on an intravenous glucose tolerance test. However, the disposition index (AIRg × Si) was significantly lower in the relatives *(25)*.

The predominant mechanism responsible for glucocorticoid-induced glucose intolerance appears to be related to the induction or exacerbation of insulin resistance (26). Insulin-mediated peripheral glucose disposal is markedly impaired at a postinsulin receptor level (27). Both oxidative and nonoxidative pathways of glucose disposal are reduced by glucocorticoids (26), and muscle glycogen synthase activity is reduced (28,29). These alterations in insulin action resemble those observed in type 2 diabetes. Although insulin secretion may be altered by glucocorticoids, this appears to occur only at high doses (30).

We postulated that women with PCOS who had normal glucose tolerance would differ from control women with normal glucose tolerance in their ability to secrete sufficient insulin and maintain normal glucose tolerance after administration of dexamethasone (2 mg orally over 12 hours). In the baseline state (i.e., before the administration of dexamethasone), control women and women with PCOS had normal fasting glucose concentrations (94 ± 2 vs 95 ± 2 mg/dL), as well as similar glucose levels at 2 hours in response to a standard 75-g oral glucose load (120 ± 7 vs 124 ± 5 mg/dL). However, when faced with a reduction in insulin sensitivity induced by the administration of dexamethasone, women with PCOS were significantly less able than control subjects to compensate with adequate insulin secretion. This was evidenced by a relative attenuation in C-peptide levels relative to plasma glucose during the oral glucose tolerance test. These data suggest that short-term, low-dose glucocorticoid treatment augments insulin resistance sufficiently to reveal groups of patients in whom β-cell compensation is inadequate. Thus, glucocorticoid administration may be a useful means by which to determine whether the prevalence or magnitude of defects in insulin secretion differ between women with PCOS and their controls, and likewise, to determine whether such defects are more profound or present more often in a particular subset within a population of women with PCOS.

Maternal–Fetal Factors Influencing Diabetes in PCOS

GDM has been estimated to occur in 2.5–4% of pregnancies in the United States (31), and recent studies suggest that the incidence of GDM is steadily rising (32). GDM is a well-recognized harbinger of subsequent metabolic disturbances for both the mother and offspring. In one study, the risk of developing the metabolic syndrome was 4.4 times higher in women with GDM compared with controls over a period of follow-up lasting 11 years (33). Notably, the lifetime risk of nongestational (usually type 2) frank diabetes in a woman with a prior history of GDM is approx 60–70% (31).

Risk factors for the development of GDM are similar to those for type 2 diabetes in general, and the diabetes associated with PCOS, in particular. These include advanced age, elevated BMI, and a family history of type 2 diabetes, among others. It has been suggested that GDM is evident more often than expected in women with PCOS, and conversely, that PCOS may occur at higher-than-expected rates in women diagnosed with GDM (34–47). This has suggested that PCOS and GDM may be etiologically linked disorders, perhaps through the common elements of defects in insulin secretion and insulin action. Data to support this, however, have been conflicting.

Evidence exists to support the hypothesis that low (48,49) birthweight and/or size for gestational age may lead to insulin resistance, obesity, and type 2 diabetes in later life. The mechanisms underlying these associations are unknown, but alterations in birthweight (reflecting in utero growth/nutritional status) have also been implicated in the pathogenesis of PCOS *per se*, and its associated insulin resistance and glucose intolerance, in some *(50)*, but not all *(34,51)* studies.

Another developmental factor that has been proposed to influence the phenotypic expression of PCOS is *in utero* androgen exposure. In nonhuman primates, fetal exposure to high levels of androgen during early *in utero* development is associated with defects in insulin secretion and action in adult life *(52)*. Prenatally androgenized female rhesus monkeys exhibit glucoregulatory deficits similar to those seen in adult women with PCOS *(53)*. Of interest, the timing of the androgen exposure appears to differentially effect glucose regulation: early androgen exposure has been associated with impaired pancreatic β-cell function, whereas exposure later in gestation appears to primarily alter insulin sensitivity. The extent to which these hormonal factors relate to the pathogenesis of PCOS in the human is not known.

FUTURE AVENUES OF INVESTIGATION

Future investigation into the pathogenesis of alterations in glucose tolerance in PCOS is likely to focus on genetic factors leading to specific defects in insulin secretion and insulin action. Through the identification of genetic markers, it may become possible to characterize those women with PCOS who are at high risk for the development of type 2 diabetes at a time when glucose tolerance is normal. In so doing, specific and targeted interventions may be used to minimize the risk for conversion from normal to abnormal glucose tolerance.

KEY POINTS

- Impaired glucose tolerance and type 2 diabetes occur with higher-than-expected frequency among women with PCOS.
- *In utero* growth retardation and exposure to excess levels of androgens may contribute to the subsequent development of glucose intolerance in PCOS.
- Defects in insulin action and insulin secretion contribute to glucose intolerance in PCOS and are evident as early as the second decade of life.
- Defects in insulin secretion appear to be heritable in PCOS families and may identify those women with PCOS at highest risk for glucose intolerance.
- Provocative testing of β-cell function may identify a subset of women with PCOS at highest risk for future development of impaired glucose tolerance and diabetes.

ACKNOWLEDGMENTS

This work was supported by grants from the National Institutes of Health (M01-RR-00055, DK-41814, AG-11412, HL-075079, and P60-DK20595), a Clinical Research Award (to D.A.E.) from the American Diabetes Association, and a gift from the Blum-Kovler Foundation.

REFERENCES

1. Ehrmann D, Barnes R, Rosenfield R, Cavaghan M, Imperial J. Prevalence of impaired glucose tolerance and diabetes in women with polycystic ovary syndrome. Diabetes Care 1999;22:141–146.
2. Legro R, Kunselman A, Dodson W, Dunaif A. Prevalence and predictors of risk for type 2 diabetes mellitus and impaired glucose tolerance in polycystic ovary syndrome: a prospective, controlled study in 254 affected women. J Clin Endocrinol Metab 1999;84(1):165–169.

3. Knochenhauer E, Key T, Kahsar-Miller M, Waggoner W, Boots L, Azziz R. Prevalence of the polycystic ovary syndrome in unselected black and white women of the southeastern United States: a prospective study. J Clin Endocrinol Metab 1998;83(9):3078–3082.

4. Palmert MR, Gordon CM, Kartashov AI, Legro RS, Emans SJ, Dunaif A. Screening for abnormal glucose tolerance in adolescents with polycystic ovary syndrome. J Clin Endocrinol Metab 2002; 87(3):1017–1023.

5. Lewy VD, Danadian K, Witchel SF, Arslanian S. Early metabolic abnormalities in adolescent girls with polycystic ovarian syndrome. J Pediatr 2001;138(1):38–44.

6. Arslanian SA, Lewy VD, Danadian K. Glucose intolerance in obese adolescents with polycystic ovary syndrome: roles of insulin resistance and beta-cell dysfunction and risk of cardiovascular disease. J Clin Endocrinol Metab 2001;86(1):66–71.

7. Silfen ME, Denburg MR, Manibo AM, et al. Early endocrine, metabolic, and sonographic characteristics of polycystic ovary syndrome (PCOS): comparison between nonobese and obese adolescents. J Clin Endocrinol Metab 2003;88(10):4682–4688.

8. Biro FM. Body morphology and its impact on adolescent and pediatric gynecology, with a special emphasis on polycystic ovary syndrome. Curr Opin Obstet Gynecol 2003;15(5):347–351.

9. Coviello AD, Legro RS, Dunaif A. Adolescent girls with polycystic ovary syndrome have an increased risk of the metabolic syndrome associated with increasing androgen levels independent of obesity and insulin resistance. J Clin Endocrinol Metab 2006;91(2):492–497.

10. Azziz R, Kashar-Miller MD. Family history as a risk factor for the polycystic ovary syndrome. J Pediatr Endocrinol Metab 2000;13(Suppl 5):1303–1306.

11. Urbanek M, Legro R, Driscoll D, et al. Thirty-seven candidate genes for polycystic ovary syndrome: strongest evidence for linkage is with follistatin. Proc Natl Acad Sci USA 1999;96(15):8573–8578.

12. Ehrmann DA, Sturis J, Byrne MM, Karrison T, Rosenfield RL, Polonsky KS. Insulin secretory defects in polycystic ovary syndrome. Relationship to insulin sensitivity and family history of non-insulin-dependent diabetes mellitus. J Clin Invest 1995;96(1):520–527.

13. Legro R, Driscoll D, Strauss J, 3rd, Fox J, Dunaif A. Evidence for a genetic basis for hyperandrogenemia in polycystic ovary syndrome. Proc Natl Acad Sci USA 1998;95(25):14,956–14,960.

14. Kahsar-Miller MD, Nixon C, Boots LR, Go RC, Azziz R. Prevalence of polycystic ovary syndrome (PCOS) in first-degree relatives of patients with PCOS. Fertil Steril 2001;75(1):53–58.

15. Draper N, Walker EA, Bujalska IJ, et al. Mutations in the genes encoding 11beta-hydroxysteroid dehydrogenase type 1 and hexose-6-phosphate dehydrogenase interact to cause cortisone reductase deficiency. Nat Genet 2003;34(4):434–439.

16. Wood JR, Nelson VL, Ho C, et al. The molecular phenotype of polycystic ovary syndrome (PCOS) theca cells and new candidate PCOS genes defined by microarray analysis. J Biol Chem 2003; 278(29):26,380–26,390.

17. Polonsky K, Sturis J, Bell G. Non-insulin-dependent diabetes mellitus—a genetically programmed failure of the beta cell to compensate for insulin resistance. N Engl J Med 1996;334:777–783.

18. Kahn S, Prigeon R, McCulloch D, et al. Quantification of the relationship between insulin sensitivity and B-cell function in human subjects Evidence for a hyperbolic function. Diabetes 1993;42: 1663–1672.

19. Dunaif A, Finegood DT. Beta-cell dysfunction independent of obesity and glucose intolerance in the polycystic ovary syndrome. J Clin Endocrinol Metab 1996;81(3):942–947.

20. Elbein SC, Hasstedt SJ, Wegner K, Kahn SE. Heritability of pancreatic beta-cell function among nondiabetic members of Caucasian familial type 2 diabetic kindreds. J Clin Endocrinol Metab 1999;84(4):1398–1403.

21. Colilla S, Cox NJ, Ehrmann DA. Heritability of insulin secretion and insulin action in women with polycystic ovary syndrome and their first degree relatives. J Clin Endocrinol Metab 2001;86(5): 2027–2031.

22. Norman RJ, Masters L, Milner CR, Wang JX, Davies MJ. Relative risk of conversion from normoglycaemia to impaired glucose tolerance or non-insulin dependent diabetes mellitus in polycystic ovarian syndrome. Hum Reprod 2001;16(9):1995–1998.

23. Legro RS, Gnatuk CL, Kunselman AR, Dunaif A. Changes in glucose tolerance over time in women with polycystic ovary syndrome: a controlled study. J Clin Endocrinol Metab 2005;90(6): 3236–3242.

24. Fajans S, Conn J. An approach to the prediction of diabetes mellitus by modification of the glucose tolerance test with cortisone. Diabetes 1954;3:296–304.

25. Henriksen J, Alford F, Ward G, Beck-Nielsen H. Risk and mechanism of dexamethasone-induced deterioration of glucose tolerance in non-diabetic first-degree relatives of NIDDM patients. Diabetologia 1997;40(12):1439–1448.

26. Tappy L, Randin D, Vollenweider P, et al. Mechanisms of dexamethasone-induced insulin resistance in healthy humans. J Clin Endocrinol Metab 1994;79(4):1063–1069.

27. McMahon M, Gerich J, Rizza R. Effects of glucocorticoids on carbohydrate metabolism. Diabetes Metab Rev 1988;4(1):17–30.

28. Coderre L, Srivastava AK, Chiasson JL. Effect of hypercorticism on regulation of skeletal muscle glycogen metabolism by epinephrine. Am J Physiol 1992;262(4 Pt 1):E434–E439.

29. Coderre L, Srivastava AK, Chiasson JL. Effect of hypercorticism on regulation of skeletal muscle glycogen metabolism by insulin. Am J Physiol 1992;262(4 Pt 1):E427–E433.

30. Matsumoto K, Yamasaki H, Akazawa S, et al. High-dose but not low-dose dexamethasone impairs glucose tolerance by inducing compensatory failure of pancreatic beta-cells in normal men. J Clin Endocrinol Metab 1996;81(7):2621–2626.

31. Beckles GLA, Thompson-Reid PE. Diabetes and Women's Health Across the Life Stages: A Public Health Perspective. Atlanta: U.S. Department of Health and Human Services, Centers for Disease Control and Prevention, National Center for Chronic Disease Prevention and Health Promotion, Division of Diabetes Translation; 2001.

32. Ferrara A, Kahn HS, Quesenberry CP, Riley C, Hedderson MM. An increase in the incidence of gestational diabetes mellitus: northern California, 1991–2000. Obstet Gynecol 2004;103(3):526–533.

33. Verma A, Boney CM, Tucker R, Vohr BR. Insulin resistance syndrome in women with prior history of gestational diabetes mellitus. J Clin Endocrinol Metab 2002;87(7):3227–3235.

34. Laitinen J, Taponen S, Martikainen H, et al. Body size from birth to adulthood as a predictor of self-reported polycystic ovary syndrome symptoms. Int J Obes Relat Metab Disord 2003;27(6): 710–715.

35. Turhan NO, Seckin NC, Aybar F, Inegol I. Assessment of glucose tolerance and pregnancy outcome of polycystic ovary patients. Int J Gynaecol Obstet 2003;81(2):163–168.

36. Bjercke S, Dale PO, Tanbo T, Storeng R, Ertzeid G, Abyholm T. Impact of insulin resistance on pregnancy complications and outcome in women with polycystic ovary syndrome. Gynecol Obstet Invest 2002;54(2):94–98.

37. Sir-Petermann T, Maliqueo M, Angel B, Lara HE, Perez-Bravo F, Recabarren SE. Maternal serum androgens in pregnant women with polycystic ovarian syndrome: possible implications in prenatal androgenization. Hum Reprod 2002;17(10):2573–2579.

38. Kousta E, Cela E, Lawrence N, et al. The prevalence of polycystic ovaries in women with a history of gestational diabetes. Clin Endocrinol (Oxf) 2000;53(4):501–507.

39. Vollenhoven B, Clark S, Kovacs G, Burger H, Healy D. Prevalence of gestational diabetes mellitus in polycystic ovarian syndrome (PCOS) patients pregnant after ovulation induction with gonadotrophins. Aust NZ J Obstet Gynaecol 2000;40(1):54–58.

40. Radon PA, McMahon MJ, Meyer WR. Impaired glucose tolerance in pregnant women with polycystic ovary syndrome. Obstet Gynecol 1999;94(2):194–197.

41. Solomon CG. The epidemiology of polycystic ovary syndrome. Prevalence and associated disease risks. Endocrinol Metab Clin North Am 1999;28(2):247–263.

42. Paradisi G, Fulghesu AM, Ferrazzani S, et al. Endocrino-metabolic features in women with polycystic ovary syndrome during pregnancy. Hum Reprod 1998;13(3):542–546.

43. Lanzone A, Fulghesu AM, Cucinelli F, et al. Preconceptional and gestational evaluation of insulin secretion in patients with polycystic ovary syndrome. Hum Reprod 1996;11(11):2382–2386.

44. Wortsman J, de Angeles S, Futterweit W, Singh KB, Kaufmann RC. Gestational diabetes and neonatal macrosomia in the polycystic ovary syndrome. J Reprod Med 1991;36(9):659–661.

45. Koivunen RM, Juutinen J, Vauhkonen I, Morin-Papunen LC, Ruokonen A, Tapanainen JS. Metabolic and steroidogenic alterations related to increased frequency of polycystic ovaries in women with a history of gestational diabetes. J Clin Endocrinol Metab 2001;86(6):2591–2599.

46. Holte J, Gennarelli G, Wide L, Lithell H, Berne C. High prevalence of polycystic ovaries and associated clinical, endocrine, and metabolic features in women with previous gestational diabetes mellitus. J Clin Endocrinol Metab 1998;83(4):1143–1150.

47. Lanzone A, Caruso A, Di Simone N, De Carolis S, Fulghesu AM, Mancuso S. Polycystic ovary disease. A risk factor for gestational diabetes? J Reprod Med 1995;40(4):312–316.

48. Stocker CJ, Arch JR, Cawthorne MA. Fetal origins of insulin resistance and obesity. Proc Nutr Soc 2005;64(2):143–151.
49. Hofman PL, Regan F, Jackson WE, et al. Premature birth and later insulin resistance. N Engl J Med 2004;351(21):2179–2186.
50. Cresswell JL, Barker DJ, Osmond C, Egger P, Phillips DI, Fraser RB. Fetal growth, length of gestation, and polycystic ovaries in adult life. Lancet 1997;350(9085):1131–1135.
51. Sadrzadeh S, Klip WA, Broekmans FJ, et al. Birth weight and age at menarche in patients with polycystic ovary syndrome or diminished ovarian reserve, in a retrospective cohort. Hum Reprod 2003;18(10):2225–2230.
52. Bruns CM, Baum ST, Colman RJ, et al. Insulin resistance and impaired insulin secretion in prenatally androgenized male rhesus monkeys. J Clin Endocrinol Metab 2004;89(12):6218–6223.
53. Eisner JR, Dumesic DA, Kemnitz JW, Abbott DH. Timing of prenatal androgen excess determines differential impairment in insulin secretion and action in adult female rhesus monkeys. J Clin Endocrinol Metab 2000;85(3):1206–1210.

5 Genes Related to Metabolic Abnormalities or Insulin Resistance in Polycystic Ovary Syndrome

Héctor F. Escobar-Morreale, MD, PhD

CONTENTS

Summary

The familial aggregation of polycystic ovary syndrome (PCOS) suggests that genetic factors are involved in the pathogenesis of this common disorder. Considering that insulin stimulates adrenal and ovarian androgen synthesis, any disorder in which insulin levels are increased facilitates hyperandrogenism and PCOS, especially in women with a primary abnormality in steroidogenesis leading to exaggerated androgen synthesis.

Therefore, several genomic variants related to insulin resistance and hyperinsulinism have been found in association with PCOS influencing glucose homeostasis, but it is unclear whether or not these variants contribute to the hyperandrogenic phenotype of these patients.

In order to reveal the genetic defects that are actually responsible for PCOS, future studies should compare women who, for a similar degree of insulin resistance, present with or without PCOS. Similarly, studies conducted in PCOS patients and non-hyperandrogenic women separately, will provide unbiased evidence of the influence of the genomic variants related to insulin resistance on the metabolic abnormalities frequently found in patients with PCOS and whether or not this influence is specific for PCOS, or is common to every woman irrespectively of her androgenic status.

From: *Contemporary Endocrinology: Insulin Resistance and Polycystic Ovarian Syndrome:
Pathogenesis, Evaluation, and Treatment*
Edited by: E. Diamanti-Kandarakis, J. E. Nestler, D. Panidis, and R. Pasquali © Humana Press Inc., Totowa, NJ

Hopefully, the precise identification of which variants contribute to insulin resistance in PCOS will facilitate the identification of those patients especially predisposed to a favorable response to insulin sensitizers.

Key Words: Insulin; insulin receptor; insulin receptor substrate; insulin-like growth factors; oxidative stress; genomic variants; molecular genetics.

INTRODUCTION

The polycystic ovary syndrome (PCOS) is a common endocrine disorder in women of reproductive age, with an estimated worldwide prevalence of approx 6% *(1–3)*. During the past years it has become evident that PCOS is a complex disorder in terms of etiology and inheritance, and that the phenotype of the affected women might alter through the life cycle and under the influence of various environmental factors *(4)*.

Hyperinsulinemia and insulin resistance are present in a significant proportion of women with PCOS. This chapter reviews whether genomic variants related to insulin synthesis and action, or to other metabolic disorders in which insulin resistance is involved, play a role in the pathogenesis of PCOS. Also, we will formulate several nonmutually exclusive hypotheses in an attempt to explain the origins of these associations, highlighting their possible clinical implications in the management of this common disorder.

EVIDENCE SUGGESTING AN INHERITED COMPONENT IN PCOS AND ITS ASSOCIATED METABOLIC DISORDERS

The major evidence suggesting that there is an inherited component in PCOS is provided by familial aggregation of PCOS cases. Table 1 summarizes most of the studies that reported existence of familial aggregation of PCOS. It should be noted that these studies were hampered from the beginning by the heterogeneity in the populations studied and the criteria used to diagnose PCOS. However, aside from these limitations, it is evident that: (1) PCOS cases are more prevalent in the families of affected women; (2) this familial aggregation does not closely follow any pattern of Mendelian or sex-linked inheritance; and (3) the male equivalent of PCOS has not been clearly identified to date, limiting the resolution of family-based studies of the syndrome.

Recent studies have expanded the familial aggregation of PCOS to the metabolic disorders associated with insulin resistance. The studies conducted by Legro et al. in the late 1990s *(16,17)*, not only demonstrated that PCOS was more frequent in the sisters of patients with PCOS compared to the sisters of nonaffected women, but also that insulin resistance was more prevalent in these women. Specifically, both PCOS (defined by chronic oligomenorrhea and hyperandrogenemia) and hyperandrogenemia without menstrual dysfunction were present in 22 and 24% of the sisters of PCOS women, respectively *(16)*, and insulin resistance was inherited in association with hyperandrogenemia independently of the presence or absence of menstrual dysfunction *(17)*. These results were supported by those of Yildiz et al. *(22)*, who, in addition, found a higher degree of insulin resistance in the brothers of patients with PCOS compared to those of unaffected women.

Furthermore, pancreatic β-cell dysfunction leading to hyperglycemia and disorders of glucose tolerance, is inherited within PCOS families *(23)*, suggesting that predisposition

Table 1
Studies of Familial Aggregation in Functional Hyperandrogenism
and Polycystic Ovary Syndrome

Authors[a]	Phenotype in first-degree relatives	Suggested inheritance
Cooper et al. (5)	Women: Oligomenorrhea and PCO Men: Increased hairiness	Autosomal-dominant with variable penetrance
Wilroy et al., Givens et al. (6–8)	Women: Hyperandrogenism and metabolic disorders Men: Oligospermia and LH hypersecretion	X-linked
Ferriman and Purdie (9)	Women: Infertility, oligomenorrhea Hirsutism.	Not determined
Hague et al. (10)	Women: PCO	Not determined
Lunde et al. (11)	Women: Hyperandrogenic symptoms Men: Premature baldness and increased hairiness	Autosomal-dominant
Carey et al. (12)	Women: PCO Men: Premature baldness	Monogenic
Jahanfar et al. (13,14)	Twin studies: Fasting insulin, androstanediol glucuronide, lipid profile	Poligenic
Norman et al. (15)	Men: Premature baldness, hypertrigly-ceridemia and hyperinsulinemia	Not determined
Legro et al. (16–18)	Women: PCOS (NICHD), hyperandro-genemia, insulin resistance Men: Increased DHEAS	Monogenic
Azziz et al., Kahsar-Miller et al. (19,20)	Women: PCOS (NICHD)	Not determined
Mao et al. (21)	Men: Premature baldness	Not determined
Yildiz et al. (22)	Women: PCOS (NICHD) and insulin resistance Men: Insulin resistance	Not determined

[a]Authors are cited in chronological order.

NICHD, National Institute of Child Health and Human Development criteria for the diagnosis of polycystic ovary syndrome; PCO, polycystic ovaries on ultrasound examination; PCOS, polycystic ovary syndrome; LH, luteinizing hormone.

(Reproduced from ref. 4. Copyright 2005, The Endocrine Society, with permission.)

to type 2 diabetes in patients with PCOS is also determined by genetic factors related to β-cell dysfunction.

Nevertheless, inheritance is not necessarily genetic and this is especially important for a metabolic disorder such as PCOS, in which acquired prenatal and environmental factors may play an important etiological role in certain cases. It is being increasingly accepted that prenatal factors, particularly malnutrition of any origin, exerts a permanent programming of metabolic function leading to a thrifty phenotype characterized by insulin resistance. This may lead to type 2 diabetes, metabolic syndrome, and cardiovascular disease later in life, particularly when the subject is exposed to certain environmental factors such as a high-fat diet and scarce physical activity (24).

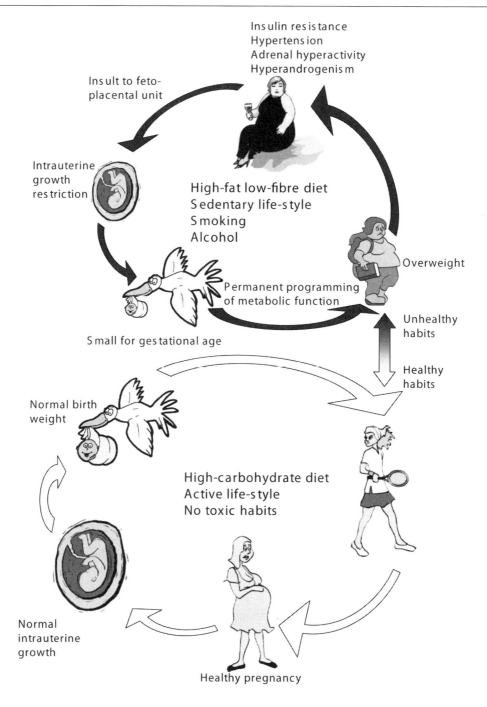

Fig. 1. Intrauterine growth retardation and insulin resistance as an example of non-genetic inheritance, markedly influenced by environmental factors. Insults during pregnancy may result in intrauterine growth retardation, inducing a thrifty phenotype in small for gestational age babies. These women are predisposed to suffer from insulin resistance and may develop hypertension, glucose intolerance, adrenal axis hyperactivity with relative cortisol excess, functional hyperandrogenism and polycystic ovary syndrome later in life, especially if they are exposed to environmental factors such as sedentary lifestyle and a diet rich in saturated fat. These environmental factors

As exemplified in Fig. 1, a female baby small for its gestational age, a condition that could be a result of any *in utero* injury, may turn into an obese girl because of permanent misprogramming of her metabolic function. By reaching fertile age she may develop PCOS, diabetes and hypertension, which might cause further prenatal harm to her offsprings. This prenatal damage may perpetuate the inheritance of these metabolic disorders in her family, without participation of any gene, especially since some environmental factors, such as diet and physical activity, which are heavily dependent on education, contribute to the maintenance of this vicious circle. Such a mechanism is also supported by the studies of Ibáñez et al. in Spaniards *(25–28)*, showing that children born small for gestational age frequently develop premature pubarche and functional hyperandrogenism later in life.

Of note, at least in theory, a change in these environmental conditions that can be achieved through a healthier diet and lifestyle, may break this vicious circle, highlighting the importance of counseling in these families.

Therefore, we would like to conclude this section by emphasizing that although familial aggregation of PCOS and insulin resistant disorders strongly suggest involvement of inherited factors in their pathogenesis, it is by no means proper to assume that all these factors are necessarily genetic, given into consideration that environmental factors related to education are possibly involved and have also a strong familial occurrence.

PATHOPHYSIOLOGY OF PCOS: THE ROLE OF INSULIN RESISTANCE

The primary defect in PCOS appears to be an exaggerated androgen secretion by the ovary and, in some patients, by the adrenal gland *(29)*. This is supported by the series of studies conducted in the past years by McAllister and her group in Hershey, PA. Using primary cultures of ovarian theca cell obtained from women with PCOS and cells from non-hyperandrogenic women as controls, they were able to demonstrate that increased androgen secretion is a stable characteristic of PCOS theca cells, even after four passages of culture, an observation suggesting strongly that this essential defect is intrinsic or primary to these cells and not dependent on environmental factors *(30)*. Further studies demonstrated that most of the enzymes involved in androgen's biosynthetic pathway were overexpressed in these cells *(31)* and some of the mechanisms possibly responsible for these abnormalities *(32–35)*.

This primary tendency toward an augmented androgen synthesis and secretion is triggered by several factors, of which hyperinsulinemia and insulin resistance are, at the time, the best ones studied *(36,37)*. Among others, the mechanism by which insulin stimulates androgen secretion and favors hyperandrogenism includes the increase in secretion and

---

may also cluster in certain families because exercising and diet are heavily influenced by parental habits. The metabolic abnormalities associated with the thrifty phenotype can induce further insult to the pregnancies of small for gestational-age women and the defect might be transmitted to another generation without participation of any genetic abnormality. However, if small for gestational-age babies maintain healthy habits, insulin resistance and its consequences might be avoided and, at least in theory, their fetuses will not be exposed to an unfavorable metabolic milieu during pregnancy, preventing non-genetic inheritance of these conditions. (Modified from ref. *4*. Copyright 2005, The Endocrine Society, with permission. Some images © 2003–2005 www.clipart.com.)

pulsatility of gonadotropins *(38)*; raising the sensitivity of the adrenal androgen secretion to adrenocorticotropic hormone (ACTH) *(39)*; amplification of ovarian androgen secretion in response to luteinizing hormone (LH) stimulation *(40)* and the augmentation of the ovarian and adrenal key enzymes' activity for androgen synthesis, 17α-hydroxylase and 17,20 lyase *(39,41)*. Furthermore, hyperinsulinemia also favors hyperandrogenism by the following indirect mechanisms:

1. Insulin decreases insulin-like growth factor binding protein (IGFBP)-1, thereby increasing insulin-like growth factor-1 availability in target tissues and upregulating the expression of ovarian insulin-like growth factor-1 receptors *(40)*.
2. Insulin favors the development of ovarian cysts and ovarian enlargement, in animal models, acting synergistically with chorionic gonadotropin and LH *(40)*.
3. Insulin decreases hepatic synthesis of sexual hormone-binding globulin (SHBG), leading to an increase in free androgen concentrations in the circulation *(42,43)*.

In conceptual agreement with this favoring role of insulin on hyperandrogenism, any clinical situation in which circulating insulin concentration is amplified should be associated with an increased prevalence of hyperandrogenic disorders, including PCOS. The most common cause for hyperinsulinemia is endogenous hyperinsulinism resulting from insulin resistance *(44)*, and accordingly, increased prevalence of PCOS has been reported in typical insulin resistant disorders, such as type 2 diabetes *(45,46)*, gestational diabetes *(47)*, and morbid obesity *(48)*. In the latter, PCOS may resolve after normalization of insulin sensitivity in response to the sustained and maintained weight loss achieved after bariatric surgery, a remark supporting the important role of insulin resistance and hyperinsulinemia in the PCOS of these women *(48)*. Incidentally, there is also a report of development of PCOS in a premenopausal woman presenting with an insulinoma, in whom PCOS resolved after successful removal of the tumor *(49)*, supporting even further the concept that endogenous hyperinsulinism may result in hyperandrogenism and PCOS.

Additionally, exogenous hyperinsulinism may also induce hyperandrogenism and PCOS. At present, maintenance of a strict metabolic control is the mainstay of long-term therapy of type 1 diabetes, with the ultimate endeavor of avoiding microvascular complications *(50)*. This aim usually requires administration of supraphysiological doses of exogenous insulin, which at least in theory could stimulate androgen secretion by the ovary. Accordingly, we have reported a threefold increase in the prevalence of PCOS and of hyperandrogenic hirsutism in premenopausal women with type 1 diabetes *(51)*, and Codner et al. *(52)* recently found similar results in the Chilean population, confirming that exogenous hyperinsulinism may induce hyperandrogenism is women. Therefore, it appears that current evidence supports the notion that excessive insulin concentrations, irrespectively of its cause, may facilitate the development of hyperandrogenism and PCOS.

However, there is also evidence that insulin resistance and hyperinsulinemia are not universal in patients with PCOS, with an estimated 64% prevalence of these disorders in the syndrome *(53)*. Moreover, a significant proportion of severely insulin-resistant obese women do not develop PCOS *(48)*. Therefore, insulin resistance should be considered as an important contributing factor to the pathogenesis of PCOS in some women, but never as the primary defect leading to this disorder, and the same may apply to the genomic variants related to insulin resistance.

STUDIES OF GENOMIC VARIANTS RELATED
TO INSULIN RESISTANCE IN PCOS

Given the influence of hyperinsulinemia and insulin resistance in the pathogenesis of PCOS, genes related to insulin resistance and its associated disorders, as well as their genomic variants, have been considered as candidate genes for PCOS *(4)*.

Insulin Gene

As previously stated, a primary defect in insulin secretion indicating pancreatic β-cell dysfunction, is associated with the occurrence of diabetes and exhibits a familial constituent *(23,54)*. Most studies related to the possible implication of insulin gene *(INS)* in PCOS focused on a variable number of tandem repeats (VNTR) polymorphism previously described to influence the inheritance of type 1 diabetes *(55)*. This VNTR polymorphism consists in the repeat of 14–15 bp at –596 from the transcription start site *(56)* and, depending on the number of repeats, alleles are classified as I, II, and III, class II alleles being rare in Caucasians.

Waterworth et al. *(57)* suggested a few years ago, using linkage and association studies, that homozygosity for class III alleles was associated with PCOS and serum testosterone levels in Caucasian women of the United Kingdom. This results were initially confirmed by others *(58,59)*, although there were also studies with discrepant results *(60,61)*. Very recently, the authors reporting the initial evidence for association between *INS* VNTR polymorphism and PCOS published a rebuttal based on a series of family-based and case–control studies in British and Finnish population and concluded that "variation at the *INS* VNTR polymorphism has no major role in the development of PCOS" *(62)*.

Insulin Receptor Gene

The frequent finding of insulin resistance in patients with PCOS made the insulin receptor gene *(INSR)*, located at chromosome 19, an obvious candidate gene for earlier genetic studies of PCOS. The whole *INSR* of several patients with PCOS was sequenced but no significant abnormalities were found *(63,64)*. Even when increased phosphorylation of serine residues of the tyrosine kinase domain of the insulin receptor was described both in vitro and in vivo *(65,66)*, no abnormalities were found in this domain of *INSR* *(67)*.

Family-based studies in the United States suggested that PCOS is associated with a genetic marker located relatively close to *INSR*, D19S884 *(68,69)*. However, this association has not been universally confirmed in case–control studies *(70,71)*. Finally, a C/T substitution at the tyrosine kinase domain of *INSR* in exon 17 has been recently found to be associated with PCOS in women from the United States and China *(72,73)*, although its precise role in the pathogenesis of PCOS remains to be elucidated.

Insulin Receptor Substrate 1 and 2 Genes

Insulin receptor substrate 1 *(IRS-1)* and 2 *(IRS-2)* genes mediate the signaling of insulin after its binding with the *INSR* and the autophosphorylation of the latter. Patients with PCOS present with a specific abnormality consisting of a decreased activity of an *IRS-1* phosphatydil-inositol 3 kinase (PI3K), apparently related to increased phosphorylation of Ser312 residues *(74)*.

Several studies have shown that allelic variants of the insulin-receptor substrate genes, *IRS-1* Gly972Arg and *IRS-2* Gly1057Asp, may play a functional role on the abnormalities of glucose metabolism in PCOS *(75–77)*.

Sir-Petermann et al. *(75)* reported that the frequency of Arg972 alleles of the Gly972Arg polymorphism of *IRS-1* was increased in patients with PCOS in the Chilean population. On the contrary, El Mkadem et al. *(76)* did not find any difference between patients with PCOS and controls in the distribution of *IRS-1* Gly972Arg and *IRS-2* Gly1057Asp alleles in Caucasian women of European extraction. However, the following polymorphisms influenced glucose homeostasis:

1. *IRS-1* Arg972 alleles were more prevalent in insulin-resistant compared to noninsulin resistant patients with PCOS or to control subjects *(76)* and carriers of these alleles presented with increased fasting insulin levels and increased insulin resistance measured by homeostasis model assessment (HOMA-IR), compared to subjects homozygous for the wild-type alleles *(76)*.
2. Carriers of *IRS-2* Asp1057 alleles presented with increased 2-hour glucose and insulin levels during an oral glucose tolerance test (OGTT) *(76)*.
3. HOMA-IR was higher in carriers of both *IRS-1* and *IRS-2* variants than in those with *IRS-2* mutations only or those carrying the wild-type alleles *(76)*.

More recently, Ehrmann et al. *(77)* found that nondiabetic subjects carrying one or two Asp1057 alleles of *IRS-2* had significantly lower 2-hour OGTT glucose levels compared to those homozygous for Gly1057 alleles, a study involving 227 nondiabetic white and African-American patients with PCOS *(77)*, in sharp contrast with the results of El Mkadem et al. *(76)*.

Our results in Spaniards *(78)*, confirm that these polymorphism in *IRS-1* and *IRS-2* are equally distributed among patients with PCOS and controls. However, considering control subjects and patients with PCOS as a whole, *IRS-1* Arg972 carriers presented with increased fasting insulin levels and HOMA-IR compared to subjects homozygous for Gly972 alleles, whereas subjects homozygous for the Gly1057 allele of *IRS-2* presented with increased glucose levels during an OGTT compared to carriers of one or two Asp1057 alleles. Therefore, the Gly972Arg in *IRS-1* and Gly1057Asp in *IRS-2* polymorphisms influence glucose homeostasis in premenopausal women, yet this influence is not specific of PCOS.

Insulin-Like Growth Factor System

San Millán et al. *(79)* recently found an association of PCOS with homozygosity for G alleles of the *Apa*I polymorphism in the gene encoding insulin-like growth factor (IGF)-2, but not with a dinucleotide polymorphism in the *IGF-1* gene, a tri-nucleotide polymorphism in the *IGF-1* receptor gene or the ACAA-insertion/deletion polymorphism at the 3′ nontranslated region of the *IGF-2* receptor gene, previously described *(80–82)*.

Considering that IGF-2 stimulates adrenal *(83,84)* and ovarian *(85)* androgen secretion, the increased frequency of homozygosity for these alleles might contribute to hyper-androgenism in some patients with PCOS, assuming that G alleles may increase IGF-2 expression at the ovary, as reported for other tissues: G alleles of the *Apa*I polymorphism in *IGF-2* have been described to increase IGF-2 mRNA in leukocytes compared with A alleles *(86)* and possibly result in increased liver IGF-2 expression and secretion *(87)*.

We also found that, compared to subjects carrying 93-bp alleles, subjects homozygous for 90-bp alleles of a trinucleotide repeat polymorphism in the gene encoding IGF-1 receptor had increased fasting glucose levels and fasting insulin resistance index, but IGF-1 receptor genotypes were not associated with PCOS *(79)*.

Peroxisome Proliferator-Activated Receptor-γ2

Because of the improvement of insulin sensitivity, hyperandrogenism and ovulation in women with PCOS after activation of peroxisome proliferator-activated receptor (PPAR)-γ2 by administrated thiazolidinediones *(88–92)*, the *PPAR-γ2* gene has been extensively studied in PCOS. With the exception of a single report of a marginally significant decrease in the frequency of Ala12 alleles of the Pro12Ala polymorphism in women with polycystic ovaries from Finland *(93)*, no association of this polymorphism has been found either in family-based or case–control PCOS studies *(68,79,94)*. However, this polymorphism appears to be playing just a modifying role on the PCOS phenotype, as it is shown in non-hyperandrogenic subjects. Ala12 alleles of *PPAR-γ2* gene may favor weight gain in obese adults *(95)* and in obese hyperandrogenic girls and adolescents *(96)*. On the other hand, Ala12 alleles preserve insulin sensitivity in Caucasian men *(97)* and Caucasian patients with PCOS *(98–100)*. Therefore, these effects do not appear to be specific for PCOS.

More recently, a silent C to T substitution at position 142 in exon 6 has been explored in patients with PCOS, with T alleles being more frequent in women with PCOS compared to nonhyperandrogenic controls *(94)*. This silent polymorphism is not in linkage disequilibrium with the Pro12Ala polymorphism, yet the possibility of an association with other unknown genomic variants of *PPAR-γ2* gene has not yet been explored *(94)* and its precise functional role remains to be established.

Paraoxonase

Oxidative stress may impair insulin action *(101)*. A higher oxidative stress has been found in patients with PCOS *(102)*, possibly related to a decrease in serum PON1 activity *(103)*. We have recently explored the –108 C/T, Leu55Met, and Gln192Arg polymorphisms in the gene encoding serum PON1 in patients with PCOS and found that homozygosity for T alleles of the –108 C/T polymorphism in *PON1* was more frequent in them compared to nonhyperandrogenic women *(79)*. Accordingly, women homozygous for –108T alleles of *PON1* presented with increased hirsutism scores and androgen concentrations, compared to carriers of –108C alleles *(79)*. Finally, in a logistic regression model, homozygosity for –108T alleles of *PON1* was associated with a 7.1 odds ratio of having PCOS *(79)*.

The possible role of the –108 C/T polymorphism in the insulin resistant phenotype of PCOS is supported by the finding that this polymorphism is responsible of approx 23% of PON1-expression levels in some cell systems, in which –108TT constructs showed reduced PON1 expression compared to –108CC constructs *(104)*.

Regarding the other polymorphisms of the *PON1* gene, homozygosity of Met55 alleles was associated with increased body mass index (BMI) and indexes of insulin resistance, yet the Leu55Met and Gln192Arg polymorphisms were not associated with PCOS *(79)*.

Human Homolog for Sorbin and SH3-Domain-Containing-1 Gene

In addition to studies in adolescents *(105)*, we have recently studied the Thr228Ala polymorphism in adult patients with PCOS. Although no association was found between Thr228Ala alleles with patients with PCOS, carriers of Ala228 alleles of *SORBS1* presented with increased BMI compared to subjects homozygous for Thr228 alleles *(79)*, results in total agreement with a large epidemiological study conducted in Europe *(106)*.

Calpain-10

This enzyme is a cysteine protease that may play a role in insulin secretion and action *(107)*. Several polymorphisms in the gene encoding calpain-10, may increase the risk for diabetes *(108)*, PCOS *(109–111)* and idiopathic hirsutism *(112)* in certain populations, but not in others *(113)*. However, the physiological roles of calpain-10 remain mostly unknown, and the actual importance of these associations remains to be established.

Adiponectin

This is an adipocyte-derived antidiabetic hormone that regulates glucose metabolism favoring insulin sensitivity. Two polymorphisms in the adiponectin gene, 45 T/G and 276 G/T, have been studied in PCOS *(79,114,115)*. It appears that no clear association of neither polymorphism with this syndrome exists *(79,115)*, although these genomic variants might influence insulin resistance and adiposity in patients with PCOS *(115)*.

Genes Encoding for Other Molecules Related to Insulin Resistance and Associated Disorders

No association of PCOS to genomic variants in genes encoding glycogen synthetase *(116)*, resistin *(117,118)*, leptin and its receptor *(119)*, apoprotein E *(120)*, or to variants in the genes of plasma cell differentiation antigen glycoprotein and protein tyrosine phosphatase 1B *(79)* has been reported.

THE ASSOCIATION OF INSULIN RESISTANCE AND PCOS FROM AN EVOLUTIONARY PERSPECTIVE

Aside from the obvious association that arises from the fact that hyperinsulinemia of any cause—including that resulting from insulin resistance—may facilitate androgen excess and PCOS, insulin resistance and PCOS might also have been selected during evolution in concomitance in order to favor survival during times of environmental stress.

During ages the human race has suffered prolonged periods of food shortage, infections and continuous trauma, and gestation and birth were the most common cause of maternal and infant morbidity and mortality. In such an unfriendly environment, hyperandrogenism might favor survival because androgen excess caused an assertive behavior and resulted in a relative infertility in affected women, decreasing birth rate and increasing the interval between pregnancies, thereby favoring both maternal and infant survival. Insulin resistance, on the other hand, favored survival by inducing a thrifty shift of intermediate metabolism to provide the brain with enough glucose for its adequate functioning and also contributed to weight gain and increased fuel storage in fat tissue in the rare periods in which food was available.

Although insulin resistance and PCOS might have favored the survival of our ancestors, nowadays access to food is no more restricted in most Western countries, where we seldom exercise, and our life expectancy has increased markedly because of the improvement of public hygiene and health care. In this favorable, yet actually unexpected in terms of evolution, environment the previously beneficial mechanisms suppose a considerable disadvantage, because hyperandrogenic and insulin resistant genotypes facilitate the development of obesity and metabolic syndrome, leading to atherosclerosis and cardiovascular diseases *(121–123)*. Such a hypothesis might explain the increasing prevalence of the metabolic syndrome and associated disorders, including PCOS, in Westernized countries, providing a unifying evolutionary hypothesis to explain the association of PCOS with insulin resistance (Fig. 2).

CONCLUSIONS

Considering that insulin stimulates ovarian and adrenal androgen synthesis, it is not actually surprising that any clinical situation in which circulating insulin levels are elevated may result in development of hyperandrogenism and PCOS. Accordingly, genomic variants that favor insulin resistance and hyperinsulinism would probably facilitate androgen synthesis, especially in women whose androgen synthesis is primarily exaggerated.

The influence of insulin resistance and its related genomic variants on the development of PCOS is possibly a continuous "gray scale" variable: in one of the extremes, the primary defect in steroidogenesis is severe enough to result in PCOS without the need of the facilitating role of hyperinsulinism, whereas in the other extreme, a mild excess in androgen synthesis is triggered by the concurrent stimulatory effect of insulin resistance and hyperinsulinism. Our recent report that in morbidly obese women, PCOS may actually resolve after normalizing insulin sensitivity in response to the marked and sustained weight loss achieved after bariatric surgery *(48)*, an observation that comes in sharp contrast with the fact that PCOS may also be present in lean insulin-sensitive women, exemplifies the heterogeneity of the contributing factors of this syndrome and especially the wide range of influence of insulin resistance in this disorder.

Therefore, instead of considering the genomic variants related to insulin resistance as the primary genetic mechanisms underlying the development of PCOS, we should study them as important contributors to its full development in predisposed individuals, considering particularly the clinical and therapeutic implications of the association between insulin resistance and PCOS. Hopefully, the exact identification of the variants that contribute to insulin resistance in PCOS will facilitate the identification of those patients that are selectively predisposed to a favorable response to insulin sensitizers, and those in whom, unfortunately, these drugs would elicit no significant clinical response.

FUTURE AVENUES OF INVESTIGATION

In most, if not all, genetic studies conducted to date, PCOS controls and nonaffected women were not controlled for the presence or absence of insulin resistance. Therefore, both PCOS populations and nonhyperandrogenic controls recruited for these studies comprised women with normal insulin sensitivity and others with different degrees of

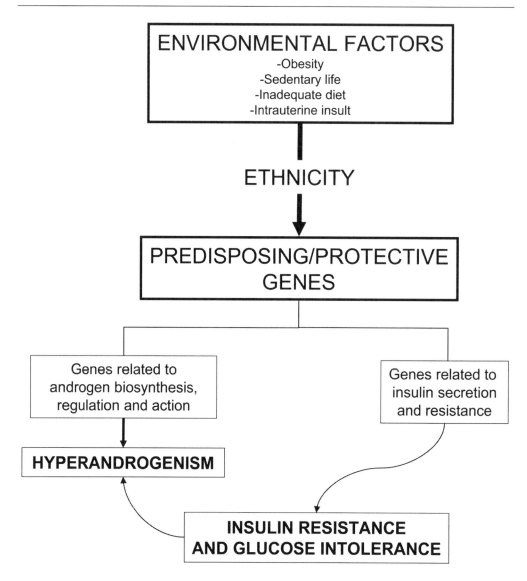

Fig. 2. A unifying hypothesis for the association of hyperandrogenism and insulin resistance. Environmental factors, influenced by ethnicity, act on a delicate balance between predisposing and protective common genetic variants that have been selected during evolution because of previous survival advantage. The genes involved in the pathogenesis of hyperandrogenism may vary depending on the particular environmental and/or ethnic factors that predominate in the different populations studied, providing an explanation for the phenotypic variability of hyperandrogenic disorders. (Modified from ref. *4*. Copyright 2005, The Endocrine Society, with permission.)

insulin resistance. Because hyperinsulinemic women are more likely to develop PCOS, it is not surprising that in many of these studies the PCOS group was more insulin resistant compared to the control group, and that in some cases genomic variants related to insulin resistance were more prevalent in the former. Unfortunately, these variants did not explain why some insulin-resistant women develop PCOS, whereas other, equally insulin-resistant women, do not.

This selection bias has probably played a confounding role in the PCOS genetic studies conducted to date. To find the actual genomic variants that exhibit a causative role in PCOS, future genetic studies should compare women who, for a similar degree of insulin resistance, do or do not present the PCOS. Similarly, the modifying role of the genomic variants related to insulin resistance on the metabolic abnormalities associated with PCOS would require carefully designed studies in which patients with PCOS and nonhyperandrogenic women will be studied separately. Only by doing so will we delimitate the precise influences of these variants to the metabolic profile of these women, and whether these influences are specific in patients with PCOS or not. Finally, given the strong influence of diet alone or in combination with physical activity on these phenotypic variables, every effort should be made to correctly identify these parameters, in order to avoid as much as possible their confounding effect on these studies.

KEY POINTS

- Insulin facilitates adrenal and ovarian androgen synthesis.
- Any disorder, in which insulin levels are increased, facilitates hyperandrogenism and PCOS, especially in women with a primary abnormality in steroidogenesis leading to exaggerated androgen synthesis.
- Therefore, genomic variants related to insulin resistance and hyperinsulinism may be found in association with PCOS and may influence glucose homeostasis, but it is unclear whether these variants contribute to the hyperandrogenic phenotype of these patients or not.
- To find the genetic defects actually responsible for PCOS, future studies should compare women who, for a similar degree of insulin resistance, present with or without PCOS.
- Similarly, studies conducted in patients with PCOS and nonhyperandrogenic women separately, will provide unbiased evidence of the influence of genomic variants related to insulin resistance on the metabolic abnormalities frequently found in patients with PCOS, and whether this influence is specific of PCOS or if it is common to every woman irrespectively of her androgenic status.
- Hopefully, the precise identification of which variants contribute to insulin resistance in PCOS will facilitate identification of those patients that are especially predisposed to a favorable response to insulin sensitizers.

ACKNOWLEDGMENTS

Supported by grants FIS 05/0341 and REDIMET RD 06/0015/0007 from the Fondo de Investigación Sanitaria, Instituto de Salud Carlos III, Spanish Ministry of Health and Consumer Affairs, Spain.

REFERENCES

1. Asunción M, Calvo RM, San Millán JL, Sancho J, Avila S, Escobar-Morreale HF. A prospective study of the prevalence of the polycystic ovary syndrome in unselected Caucasian women from Spain. J Clin Endocrinol Metab 2000;85:2434–2438.
2. Diamanti-Kandarakis E, Kouli CR, Bergiele AT, et al. A survey of the polycystic ovary syndrome in the Greek island of Lesbos: Hormonal and metabolic profile. J Clin Endocrinol Metab 1999;84: 4006–4011.
3. Azziz R, Woods KS, Reyna R, Key TJ, Knochenhauer ES, Yildiz BO. The prevalence and features of the polycystic ovary syndrome in an unselected population. J Clin Endocrinol Metab 2004;89: 2745–2749.

4. Escobar-Morreale HF, Luque-Ramirez M, San Millan JL. The molecular-genetic basis of functional hyperandrogenism and the polycystic ovary syndrome. Endocr Rev 2005;26:251–282.

5. Cooper HE, Spellacy WN, Prem KA, Cohen WD. Hereditary factors in the Stein-Leventhal syndrome. Am J Obstet Gynecol 1968;100:371–387.

6. Wilroy RS Jr., Givens JR, Wiser WL, Coleman SA, Andersen RN, Summitt RL. Hyperthecosis: an inheritable form of polycystic ovarian disease. Birth Defects Orig Artic Ser 1975;11:81–85.

7. Givens JR. Ovarian hyperthecosis. N Engl J Med 1971;285:691.

8. Givens JR. Familial polycystic ovarian disease. Endocrinol Metab Clin North Am 1988;17:771–783.

9. Ferriman D, Purdie AW. The inheritance of polycystic ovarian disease and a possible relationship to premature balding. Clin Endocrinol (Oxf) 1979;11:291–300.

10. Hague WM, Adams J, Reeders ST, Peto TE, Jacobs HS. Familial polycystic ovaries: a genetic disease? Clin Endocrinol (Oxf) 1988;29:593–605.

11. Lunde O, Magnus P, Sandvik L, Hoglo S. Familial clustering in the polycystic ovarian syndrome. Gynecol Obstet Invest 1989;28:23–30.

12. Carey AH, Chan KL, Short F, White D, Williamson R, Franks S. Evidence for a single gene effect causing polycystic ovaries and male pattern baldness. Clin Endocrinol (Oxf) 1993;38:653–658.

13. Jahanfar S, Eden JA, Warren P, Seppala M, Nguyen TV. A twin study of polycystic ovary syndrome. Fertil Steril 1995;63:478–486.

14. Jahanfar S, Eden JA, Nguyen T, Wang XL, Wilcken DE. A twin study of polycystic ovary syndrome and lipids. Gynecol Endocrinol 1997;11:111–117.

15. Norman RJ, Masters S, Hague W. Hyperinsulinemia is common in family members of women with polycystic ovary syndrome. Fertil Steril 1996;66:942–947.

16. Legro RS, Driscoll D, Strauss JF, Fox J, Dunaif A. Evidence for a genetic basis for hyperandrogenemia in polycystic ovary syndrome. Proc Natl Acad Sci USA 1998;95:14,956–14,660.

17. Legro RS, Bentley-Lewis R, Driscoll D, Wang SC, Dunaif A. Insulin resistance in the sisters of women with polycystic ovary syndrome: association with hyperandrogenemia rather than menstrual irregularity. J Clin Endocrinol Metab 2002;87:2128–2133.

18. Legro RS, Kunselman AR, Demers L, Wang SC, Bentley-Lewis R, Dunaif A. Elevated dehydroepiandrosterone sulfate levels as the reproductive phenotype in the brothers of women with polycystic ovary syndrome. J Clin Endocrinol Metab 2002;87:2134–2138.

19. Azziz R, Kashar-Miller MD. Family history as a risk factor for the polycystic ovary syndrome. J Pediatr Endocrinol Metab 2000;13 Suppl 5:1303–1306.

20. Kahsar-Miller MD, Nixon C, Boots LR, Go RC, Azziz R. Prevalence of polycystic ovary syndrome (PCOS) in first-degree relatives of patients with PCOS. Fertil Steril 2001;75:53–58.

21. Mao W, Li M, Zhao Y. Study on parents phenotypes in women with polycystic ovary syndrome. Zhonghua Fu Chan Ke Za Zhi 2000;35:583–585.

22. Yildiz BO, Yarali H, Oguz H, Bayraktar M. Glucose intolerance, insulin resistance, and hyperandrogenemia in first degree relatives of women with polycystic ovary syndrome. J Clin Endocrinol Metab 2003;88:2031–2036.

23. Colilla S, Cox NJ, Ehrmann DA. Heritability of insulin secretion and insulin action in women with polycystic ovary syndrome and their first degree relatives. J Clin Endocrinol Metab 2001;86:2027–2031.

24. Hales CN, Barker DJ, Clark PM, et al. Fetal and infant growth and impaired glucose tolerance at age 64. BMJ 1991;303:1019–1022.

25. Ibanez L, Potau N, Marcos MV, de Zegher F. Exaggerated adrenarche and hyperinsulinism in adolescent girls born small for gestational age. J Clin Endocrinol Metab 1999;84:4739–4741.

26. Ibanez L, Potau N, Enriquez G, de Zegher F. Reduced uterine and ovarian size in adolescent girls born small for gestational age. Pediatr Res 2000;47:575–577.

27. Ibanez L, Potau N, Ferrer A, Rodriguez-Hierro F, Marcos MV, De Zegher F. Anovulation in eumenorrheic, nonobese adolescent girls born small for gestational age: insulin sensitization induces ovulation, increases lean body mass, and reduces abdominal fat excess, dyslipidemia, and subclinical hyperandrogenism. J Clin Endocrinol Metab 2002;87:5702–5705.

28. Ibanez L, Valls C, Miro E, Marcos MV, de Zegher F. Early menarche and subclinical ovarian hyperandrogenism in girls with reduced adult height after low birth weight. J Pediatr Endocrinol Metab 2002;15:431–433.

29. Ehrmann DA. Polycystic ovary syndrome. N Engl J Med 2005;352:1223–1236.

30. Nelson VL, Legro RS, Strauss JF, 3rd, McAllister JM. Augmented androgen production is a stable steroidogenic phenotype of propagated theca cells from polycystic ovaries. Mol Endocrinol 1999;13:946–957.

31. Nelson VL, Qin KN, Rosenfield RL, et al. The biochemical basis for increased testosterone production in theca cells propagated from patients with polycystic ovary syndrome. J Clin Endocrinol Metab 2001;86:5925–5933.

32. Wickenheisser JK, Nelson-DeGrave VL, Quinn PG, McAllister JM. Increased cytochrome P450 17alpha-hydroxylase promoter function in theca cells isolated from patients with polycystic ovary syndrome involves nuclear factor-1. Mol Endocrinol 2004;18:588–605.

33. Wickenheisser JK, Nelson-Degrave VL, McAllister JM. Dysregulation of cytochrome P450 17alpha-hydroxylase messenger ribonucleic acid stability in theca cells isolated from women with polycystic ovary syndrome. J Clin Endocrinol Metab 2005;90:1720–1727.

34. Wood JR, Ho CK, Nelson-Degrave VL, McAllister JM, Strauss JF, 3rd. The molecular signature of polycystic ovary syndrome (PCOS) theca cells defined by gene expression profiling. J Reprod Immunol 2004;63:51–60.

35. Nelson-Degrave VL, Wickenheisser JK, Hendricks KL, et al. Alterations in mitogen-activated protein kinase kinase and extracellular regulated kinase signaling in theca cells contribute to excessive androgen production in polycystic ovary syndrome. Mol Endocrinol 2005;19:379–390.

36. Nestler JE. Obesity, insulin, sex steroids and ovulation. Int J Obes Relat Metab Disord 2000;24: S71–S73.

37. Dunaif A. Insulin resistance and the polycystic ovary syndrome: mechanism and implications for pathogenesis. Endocr Rev 1997;18:774–800.

38. Adashi EY, Hsueh AJ, Yen SS. Insulin enhancement of luteinizing hormone and follicle-stimulating hormone release by cultured pituitary cells. Endocrinology 1981;108:1441–1449.

39. Moghetti P, Castello R, Negri C, et al. Insulin infusion amplifies 17-alpha-hydroxycorticosteroid intermediates response to adrenocorticotropin in hyperandrogenic women—apparent relative impairment of 17,20-lyase activity. J Clin Endocrinol Metab 1996;81:881–886.

40. Poretsky L, Cataldo NA, Rosenwaks Z, Giudice LC. The insulin-related ovarian regulatory system in health and disease. Endocr Rev 1999;20:535–582.

41. Nestler JE, Jakubowicz DJ. Decreases in ovarian cytochrome P450c17 alpha activity and serum free testosterone after reduction of insulin secretion in polycystic ovary syndrome. N Engl J Med 1996; 335:617–623.

42. Nestler JE. Sex hormone-binding globulin: a marker for hyperinsulinemia and/or insulin resistance? J Clin Endocrinol Metab 1993;76:273–274.

43. Nestler JE. Role of hyperinsulinemia in the pathogenesis of the polycystic ovary syndrome, and its clinical implications. Semin Reprod Endocrinol 1997;15:111–122.

44. Reaven GM. Banting Lecture 1988. Role of insulin resistance in human disease. Nutrition 1997; 13:65; discussion 4, 6.

45. Conn JJ, Jacobs HS, Conway GS. The prevalence of polycystic ovaries in women with type 2 diabetes mellitus. Clin Endocrinol (Oxf) 2000;52:81–86.

46. Peppard HR, Marfori J, Iuorno MJ, Nestler JE. Prevalence of polycystic ovary syndrome among premenopausal women with type 2 diabetes. Diabetes Care 2001;24:1050–1052.

47. Holte J, Gennarelli G, Wide L, Lithell H, Berne C. High prevalence of polycystic ovaries and associated clinical, endocrine, and metabolic features in women with previous gestational diabetes mellitus. J Clin Endocrinol Metab 1998;83:1143–1150.

48. Escobar-Morreale HF, Botella-Carretero JI, Alvarez-Blasco F, Sancho J, San Millan JL. The polycystic ovary syndrome associated with morbid obesity may resolve after weight loss induced by bariatric surgery. J Clin Endocrinol Metab 2005;90:6364–6369.

49. Murray RD, Davison RM, Russell RC, Conway GS. Clinical presentation of PCOS following development of an insulinoma: case report. Hum Reprod 2000;15:86–88.

50. The Diabetes Control and Complications Trial Research Group. The effect of intensive treatment of diabetes on the development and progression of long-term complications in insulin-dependent diabetes mellitus. N Engl J Med 1993;329:977.

51. Escobar–Morreale HF, Roldan B, Barrio R, et al. High prevalence of the polycystic ovary syndrome and hirsutism in women with type 1 diabetes mellitus. J Clin Endocrinol Metab 2000;85:4182–4187.

52. Codner E, Soto N, Lopez P, et al. Diagnostic criteria for polycystic ovary syndrome and ovarian morphology in women with type 1 diabetes mellitus. J Clin Endocrinol Metab 2006;91:2250–2256.
53. DeUgarte CM, Bartolucci AA, Azziz R. Prevalence of insulin resistance in the polycystic ovary syndrome using the homeostasis model assessment. Fertil Steril 2005;83:1454–1460.
54. Ehrmann DA, Sturis J, Byrne MM, Karrison T, Rosenfield RL, Polonsky KS. Insulin secretory defects in polycystic ovary syndrome. Relationship to insulin sensitivity and family history of non-insulin-dependent diabetes mellitus. J Clin Invest 1995;96:520–527.
55. Lucassen AM, Julier C, Beressi JP, et al. Susceptibility to insulin dependent diabetes mellitus maps to a 4.1 kb segment of DNA spanning the insulin gene and associated VNTR. Nat Genet 1993;4: 305–310.
56. Bell GI, Selby MJ, Rutter WJ. The highly polymorphic region near the human insulin gene is composed of simple tandemly repeating sequences. Nature 1982;295:31–35.
57. Waterworth DM, Bennett ST, Gharani N, et al. Linkage and association of insulin gene VNTR regulatory polymorphism with polycystic ovary syndrome. Lancet 1997;349:986–990.
58. Michelmore K, Ong K, Mason S, et al. Clinical features in women with polycystic ovaries: relationships to insulin sensitivity, insulin gene VNTR and birth weight. Clin Endocrinol (Oxf) 2001;55: 439–446.
59. Diamanti-Kandarakis E, Bartzis MI, Bergiele AT, Tsianateli TC, Kouli CR. Microsatellite polymorphism (tttta) at −528 base pairs of gene CYP11a influences hyperandrogenemia in patients with polycystic ovary syndrome. Fertil Steril 2000;73:735–741.
60. Calvo RM, Telleria D, Sancho J, San Millan JL, Escobar-Morreale HF. Insulin gene variable number of tandem repeats regulatory polymorphism is not associated with hyperandrogenism in Spanish women. Fertil Steril 2002;77:666–668.
61. Vankova M, Vrbikova J, Hill M, Cinek O, Bendlova B. Association of insulin gene VNTR polymorphism with polycystic ovary syndrome. Ann NY Acad Sci 2002;967:558–565.
62. Powell BL, Haddad L, Bennett A, et al. Analysis of multiple data sets reveals no association between the insulin gene variable number tandem repeat element and polycystic ovary syndrome or related traits. J Clin Endocrinol Metab 2005;90:2988–2993.
63. Sorbara LR, Tang Z, Cama A, et al. Absence of insulin receptor gene mutations in three insulin-resistant women with the polycystic ovary syndrome. Metabolism 1994;43:1568–1574.
64. Talbot JA, Bicknell EJ, Rajkhowa M, Krook A, Orahilly S, Clayton RN. Molecular scanning of the insulin receptor gene in women with polycystic ovarian syndrome. J Clin Endocrinol Metab 1996;81:1979–1983.
65. Dunaif A, Xia J, Book CB, Schenker E, Tang Z. Excessive insulin receptor serine phosphorylation in cultured fibroblasts and in skeletal muscle. A potential mechanism for insulin resistance in the polycystic ovary syndrome. J Clin Invest 1995;96:801–810.
66. Li M, Youngren JF, Dunaif A, et al. Decreased insulin receptor (IR) autophosphorylation in fibroblasts from patients with PCOS: effects of serine kinase inhibitors and IR activators. J Clin Endocrinol Metab 2002;87:4088–4093.
67. Conway GS, Avey C, Rumsby G. The tyrosine kinase domain of the insulin receptor gene is normal in women with hyperinsulinaemia and polycystic ovary syndrome. Hum Reprod 1994;9:1681–1683.
68. Urbanek M, Legro RS, Driscoll DA, et al. Thirty-seven candidate genes for polycystic ovary syndrome: strongest evidence for linkage is with follistatin. Proc Natl Acad Sci USA 1999;96: 8573–8578.
69. Urbanek M, Woodroffe A, Ewens KG, et al. Candidate gene region for polycystic ovary syndrome (PCOS) on chromosome 19p13.2. J Clin Endocrinol Metab 2005;90:6623–6629.
70. Tucci S, Futterweit W, Concepcion ES, et al. Evidence for association of polycystic ovary syndrome in Caucasian women with a marker at the insulin receptor gene locus. J Clin Endocrinol Metab 2001;86:446–449.
71. Villuendas G, Escobar-Morreale HF, Tosi F, Sancho J, Moghetti P, San Millan JL. Association between the D19S884 marker at the insulin receptor gene locus and polycystic ovary syndrome. Fertil Steril 2003;79:219–220.
72. Siegel S, Futterweit W, Davies TF, et al. A C/T single nucleotide polymorphism at the tyrosine kinase domain of the insulin receptor gene is associated with polycystic ovary syndrome. Fertil Steril 2002;78:1240–1243.
73. Chen ZJ, Shi YH, Zhao YR, et al. [Correlation between single nucleotide polymorphism of insulin receptor gene with polycystic ovary syndrome]. Zhonghua Fu Chan Ke Za Zhi 2004;39: 582–585.

74. Corbould A, Kim YB, Youngren JF, et al. Insulin resistance in the skeletal muscle of women with PCOS involves intrinsic and acquired defects in insulin signaling. Am J Physiol Endocrinol Metab 2005;288:E1047–E1054.

75. Sir-Petermann T, Perez-Bravo F, Angel B, Maliqueo M, Calvillan M, Palomino A. G972R polymorphism of IRS-1 in women with polycystic ovary syndrome. Diabetologia 2001;44:1200–1201.

76. El Mkadem SA, Lautier C, Macari F, et al. Role of allelic variants Gly972Arg of IRS-1 and Gly1057Asp of IRS-2 in moderate-to-severe insulin resistance of women with polycystic ovary syndrome. Diabetes 2001;50:2164–2168.

77. Ehrmann DA, Tang X, Yoshiuchi I, Cox NJ, Bell GI. Relationship of insulin receptor substrate-1 and -2 genotypes to phenotypic features of polycystic ovary syndrome. J Clin Endocrinol Metab 2002;87: 4297–4300.

78. Villuendas G, Botella-Carretero JI, Roldan B, Sancho J, Escobar-Morreale HF, San Millan JL. Polymorphisms in the insulin receptor substrate-1 (IRS-1) gene and the insulin receptor substrate-2 (IRS-2) gene influence glucose homeostasis and body mass index in women with polycystic ovary syndrome and non-hyperandrogenic controls. Hum Reprod 2005;20:3184–3191.

79. San Millan JL, Corton M, Villuendas G, Sancho J, Peral B, Escobar-Morreale HF. Association of the polycystic ovary syndrome with genomic variants related to insulin resistance, type 2 diabetes mellitus, and obesity. J Clin Endocrinol Metab 2004;89:2640–2646.

80. Vaessen N, Heutink P, Janssen JA, et al. A polymorphism in the gene for IGF-I: functional properties and risk for type 2 diabetes and myocardial infarction. Diabetes 2001;50:637–642.

81. Meloni R, Fougerousse F, Roudaut C, Beckmann JS. Trinucleotide repeat polymorphism at the human insulin-like growth factor I receptor gene (IGF1R). Nucleic Acids Res 1992;20:1427.

82. Smrzka OW, Fae I, Stoger R, et al. Conservation of a maternal-specific methylation signal at the human IGF2R locus. Hum Mol Genet 1995;4:1945–1952.

83. Mesiano S, Katz SL, Lee JY, Jaffe RB. Insulin-like growth factors augment steroid production and expression of steroidogenic enzymes in human fetal adrenal cortical cells: implications for adrenal androgen regulation. J Clin Endocrinol Metab 1997;82:1390–1396.

84. l'Allemand D, Penhoat A, Lebrethon MC, et al. Insuli-like growth factors enhance steroidogenic enzyme and corticotropin receptor messenger ribonucleic acid levels and corticotropin steroidogenic responsiveness in cultured human adrenocortical cells. J Clin Endocrinol Metab 1996;81:3892–3897.

85. Cara JF. Insulin-like growth factors, insulin-like growth factor binding proteins and ovarian androgen production. Horm Res 1994;42:49–54.

86. Vafiadis P, Bennett ST, Todd JA, Grabs R, Polychronakos C. Divergence between genetic determinants of IGF2 transcription levels in leukocytes and of IDDM2-encoded susceptibility to type 1 diabetes. J Clin Endocrinol Metab 1998;83:2933–2939.

87. O'Dell SD, Miller GJ, Cooper JA, et al. Apal polymorphism in insulin-like growth factor II (IGF2) gene and weight in middle-aged males. Int J Obes Relat Metab Disord 1997;21:822–825.

88. Ghazeeri G, Kutteh WH, Bryer-Ash M, Haas D, Ke RW. Effect of rosiglitazone on spontaneous and clomiphene citrate-induced ovulation in women with polycystic ovary syndrome. Fertil Steril 2003; 79:562–566.

89. Dunaif A, Scott D, Finegood D, Quintana B, Whitcomb R. The insulin-sensitizing agent troglitazone improves metabolic and reproductive abnormalities in the polycystic ovary syndrome. J Clin Endocrinol Metab 1996;81:3299–3306.

90. Azziz R, Ehrmann D, Legro RS, et al. Troglitazone improves ovulation and hirsutism in the polycystic ovary syndrome: a multicenter, double blind, placebo-controlled trial. J Clin Endocrinol Metab 2001;86:1626–1632.

91. Romualdi D, Guido M, Ciampelli M, et al. Selective effects of pioglitazone on insulin and androgen abnormalities in normo- and hyperinsulinaemic obese patients with polycystic ovary syndrome. Hum Reprod 2003;18:1210–1218.

92. Glueck CJ, Moreira A, Goldenberg N, Sieve L, Wang P. Pioglitazone and metformin in obese women with polycystic ovary syndrome not optimally responsive to metformin. Hum Reprod 2003;18: 1618–1625.

93. Korhonen S, Heinonen S, Hiltunen M, et al. Polymorphism in the peroxisome proliferator-activated receptor-gamma gene in women with polycystic ovary syndrome. Hum Reprod 2003;18:540–543.

94. Orio F, Jr., Matarese G, Di Biase S, et al. Exon 6 and 2 peroxisome proliferator-activated receptor-gamma polymorphisms in polycystic ovary syndrome. J Clin Endocrinol Metab 2003;88:5887–5892.

95. Ek J, Urhammer SA, Sorensen TI, Andersen T, Auwerx J, Pedersen O. Homozygosity of the Pro12Ala variant of the peroxisome proliferation-activated receptor-gamma2 (PPAR-gamma2): divergent modulating effects on body mass index in obese and lean Caucasian men. Diabetologia 1999;42:892–895.

96. Witchel SF, White C, Siegel ME, Aston CE. Inconsistent effects of the proline12 → alanine variant of the peroxisome proliferator-activated receptor-gamma2 gene on body mass index in children and adolescent girls. Fertil Steril 2001;76:741–747.

97. Ek J, Andersen G, Urhammer SA, et al. Studies of the Pro12Ala polymorphism of the peroxisome proliferator-activated receptor-gamma2 (PPAR-gamma2) gene in relation to insulin sensitivity among glucose tolerant caucasians. Diabetologia 2001;44:1170–1176.

98. Hara M, Alcoser SY, Qaadir A, Beiswenger KK, Cox NJ, Ehrmann DA. Insulin resistance is attenuated in women with polycystic ovary syndrome with the Pro(12)Ala polymorphism in the PPARgamma gene. J Clin Endocrinol Metab 2002;87:772–775.

99. Tok EC, Aktas A, Ertunc D, Erdal EM, Dilek S. Evaluation of glucose metabolism and reproductive hormones in polycystic ovary syndrome on the basis of peroxisome proliferator-activated receptor (PPAR)-gamma2 Pro12Ala genotype. Hum Reprod 2005;20:1590–1595.

100. Hahn S, Fingerhut A, Khomtsiv U, et al. The peroxisome proliferator activated receptor gamma Pro12Ala polymorphism is associated with a lower hirsutism score and increased insulin sensitivity in women with polycystic ovary syndrome. Clin Endocrinol (Oxf) 2005;62:573–579.

101. Rudich A, Kozlovsky N, Potashnik R, Bashan N. Oxidant stress reduces insulin responsiveness in 3T3-L1 adipocytes. Am J Physiol 1997;272:E935–E940.

102. Fenkci V, Fenkci S, Yilmazer M, Serteser M. Decreased total antioxidant status and increased oxidative stress in women with polycystic ovary syndrome may contribute to the risk of cardiovascular disease. Fertil Steril 2003;80:123–127.

103. Dursun P, Demirtas E, Bayrak A, Yarali H. Decreased serum paraoxonase 1 (PON1) activity: an additional risk factor for atherosclerotic heart disease in patients with PCOS? Hum Reprod 2006;21:104–108.

104. Brophy VH, Jampsa RL, Clendenning JB, McKinstry LA, Jarvik GP, Furlong CE. Effects of 5′ regulatory-region polymorphisms on paraoxonase-gene (PON1) expression. Am J Hum Genet 2001;68:1428–1436.

105. Witchel SF, Trivedi RN, Kammerer C. Frequency of the T228A polymorphism in the SORBS1 gene in children with premature pubarche and in adolescent girls with hyperandrogenism. Fertil Steril 2003;80:128–132.

106. Nieters A, Becker N, Linseisen J. Polymorphisms in candidate obesity genes and their interaction with dietary intake of n-6 polyunsaturated fatty acids affect obesity risk in a sub-sample of the EPIC-Heidelberg cohort. Eur J Nutr 2002;41:210–221.

107. Sreenan SK, Zhou YP, Otani K, et al. Calpains play a role in insulin secretion and action. Diabetes 2001;50:2013–2020.

108. Horikawa Y, Oda N, Cox NJ, et al. Genetic variation in the gene encoding calpain-10 is associated with type 2 diabetes mellitus. Nat Genet 2000;26:163–175.

109. Ehrmann DA, Schwarz PE, Hara M, et al. Relationship of calpain-10 genotype to phenotypic features of polycystic ovary syndrome. J Clin Endocrinol Metab 2002;87:1669–1673.

110. Gonzalez A, Abril E, Roca A, et al. Comment: CAPN10 alleles are associated with polycystic ovary syndrome. J Clin Endocrinol Metab 2002;87:3971–3976.

111. Gonzalez A, Abril E, Roca A, et al. Specific CAPN10 gene haplotypes influence the clinical profile of polycystic ovary patients. J Clin Endocrinol Metab 2003;88:5529–5536.

112. Escobar-Morreale HF, Peral B, Villuendas G, Calvo RM, Sancho J, San Millan JL. Common single nucleotide polymorphisms in intron 3 of the calpain-10 gene influence hirsutism. Fertil Steril 2002;77:581–587.

113. Haddad L, Evans JC, Gharani N, et al. Variation within the type 2 diabetes susceptibility gene calpain-10 and polycystic ovary syndrome. J Clin Endocrinol Metab 2002;87:2606–2610.

114. Panidis D, Kourtis A, Kukuvitis A, et al. Association of the T45G polymorphism in exon 2 of the adiponectin gene with polycystic ovary syndrome: role of Delta4-androstenedione. Hum Reprod 2004;19:1728–1733.

115. Xita N, Georgiou I, Chatzikyriakidou A, et al. Effect of adiponectin gene polymorphisms on circulating adiponectin and insulin resistance indexes in women with polycystic ovary syndrome. Clin Chem 2005;51:416–423.

116. Rajkhowa M, Talbot JA, Jones PW, Clayton RN. Polymorphism of glycogen synthetase gene in polycystic ovary syndrome. Clin Endocrinol (Oxf) 1996;44:85–90.
117. Urbanek M, Du Y, Silander K, et al. Variation in resistin gene promoter not associated with polycystic ovary syndrome. Diabetes 2003;52:214–217.
118. Xita N, Georgiou I, Tsatsoulis A, Kourtis A, Kukuvitis A, Panidis D. A polymorphism in the resistin gene promoter is associated with body mass index in women with polycystic ovary syndrome. Fertil Steril 2004;82:1466–1467.
119. Oksanen L, Tiitinen A, Kaprio J, Koistinen HA, Karonen S, Kontula K. No evidence for mutations of the leptin or leptin receptor genes in women with polycystic ovary syndrome. Mol Hum Reprod 2000;6:873–876.
120. Heinonen S, Korhonen S, Hippelainen M, Hiltunen M, Mannermaa A, Saarikoski S. Apolipoprotein E alleles in women with polycystic ovary syndrome. Fertil Steril 2001;75:878–880.
121. Fernandez-Real JM, Ricart W. Insulin resistance and inflammation in an evolutionary perspective: the contribution of cytokine genotype/phenotype to thriftiness. Diabetologia 1999;42:1367–1374.
122. Eaton SB, Konner M. Paleolithic nutrition. A consideration of its nature and current implications. N Engl J Med 1985;312:283–289.
123. Parsons P. Success in mating: a coordinated approach to fitness through genotypes incorporating genes for stress resistance and heterozygous advantage under stress. Behav Genet 1997;27:75–81.

6 Serine Phosphorylation, Insulin Resistance, and the Regulation of Androgen Synthesis

Andrew A. Bremer, MD, PhD
and Walter L. Miller, MD

CONTENTS

INTRODUCTION
BACKGROUND
FUTURE AVENUES OF INVESTIGATION
KEY POINTS
REFERENCES

Summary

Polycystic ovary syndrome (PCOS) is characterized by hyperandrogenemia and disordered gonadotropin secretion, often associated with insulin resistance. It is likely that PCOS is a group of distinct diseases with similar clinical phenotypes but different pathophysiological mechanisms, rather than being one disease caused by a single molecular defect. The *serine phosphorylation hypothesis* can potentially explain two major features of the syndrome: insulin resistance and hyperandrogenemia. Understanding the cell biology of androgen biosynthesis and insulin action will permit delineating the pathophysiologies of PCOS and may lead to more specific pharmacological therapy.

Key Words: Androgens; steroidogenesis; insulin resistance; ovary; adrenal; 17,20-lyase; 17α-hydroxylase; P450c17; DHEA; androstenedione.

INTRODUCTION

Polycystic ovary syndrome (PCOS), a common cause of menstrual dysfunction, affects approx 4–8% of women during their reproductive years *(1,2)*. PCOS is primarily characterized by oligomenorrhea, hyperandrogenemia, signs of androgen excess, disordered gonadotropin secretion, and obesity, but may also be associated with defects in both insulin action (insulin resistance) and insulin secretion (pancreatic β-cell dysfunction), conferring an increased risk of glucose intolerance, type 2 diabetes, and metabolic

From: *Contemporary Endocrinology: Insulin Resistance and Polycystic Ovarian Syndrome:*
Pathogenesis, Evaluation, and Treatment
Edited by: E. Diamanti-Kandarakis, J. E. Nestler, D. Panidis, and R. Pasquali © Humana Press Inc., Totowa, NJ

syndrome X *(3–5)*. PCOS has also been associated with cardiovascular risk factors *(6)*, although increased morbidity and mortality from coronary artery disease and other vascular disorders in patients with PCOS have been difficult to establish *(7)*.

The extensive heterogeneity and variable phenotypes of PCOS, exemplified by the ongoing debates about the definition of the syndrome, have led to multiple, mutually inconsistent theories of its etiology, including the following *(8)*:

1. A primary defect in insulin action and/or secretion leading to hyperinsulinemia.
2. A primary neuroendocrine defect leading to an exaggerated luteinizing hormone (LH) pulse frequency and amplitude.
3. A primary defect in ovarian/adrenal androgen biosynthesis resulting in hyperandrogenism.

However, no single mechanism appears to account for all forms of the syndrome, suggesting that PCOS is a group of diseases having different pathophysiological mechanisms leading to closely related clinical phenotypes. The *serine phosphorylation hypothesis (9)*, however, may explain insulin resistance and hyperandrogenemia through a single autosomal-dominant mechanism, possibly accounting for one form of PCOS.

BACKGROUND

The Biology of Ovarian/Adrenal Androgen Biosynthesis

THE INITIATION OF STEROID HORMONE SYNTHESIS

The pathways of ovarian and adrenal steroid biosynthesis employ a relatively small number of steroidogenic enzymes, but the variations in their tissue specificity expression and the availability of substrates and cofactors results in the widely varying patterns of steroid production in each steroidogenic tissue *(10)*. Although no cell type expresses all the steroidogenic enzymes, their interrelationships can be seen in the idealized integrated pathway shown in Fig. 1. Cholesterol is the precursor for all steroid hormones. Although the human ovary and adrenal can synthesize cholesterol *de novo* from acetate, most of the cholesterol used for steroid biosynthesis is provided by plasma low-density lipoproteins (LDLs) derived from dietary cholesterol. Adequate amounts of LDL can suppress 3-hydroxy-3-methylglutaryl coenzyme A (HMG-CoA) reductase, the rate-limiting step in cholesterol biosynthesis. Follicle-stimulating hormone (FSH) and LH in the ovary and adrenocorticotropic hormone (ACTH) in the adrenal stimulate production of HMG-CoA reductase and LDL receptor number, and enhanced uptake of LDL cholesterol. Thus, inhibitors of HMG-CoA reductase ("statins") inhibit steroidogenesis in ovarian theca-interstitial cells *(11)*. Steroidogenic cells take up LDL cholesterol esters by receptor-mediated endocytosis and either store them or immediately convert them to free cholesterol for use as substrate for steroidogenesis. The storage vs use of cholesterol esters is controlled by two opposing enzymes: cholesterol synthetase and cholesterol esterase (cholesterol ester hydrolase). LH and ACTH stimulate cholesterol esterase while inhibiting cholesterol synthetase, thus increasing the availability of free cholesterol for steroidogenesis.

QUANTITATIVE REGULATION OF STEROIDOGENESIS

Steroidogenesis is initiated by the conversion of cholesterol to pregnenolone by the cholesterol side chain cleavage enzyme, P450scc *(10)*. Whereas many "peripheral" cell

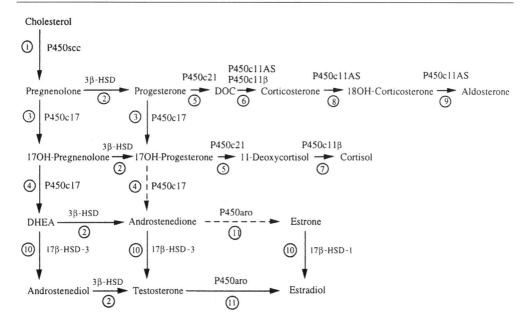

Fig. 1. Integrated view of human steroidogenesis showing adrenal and gonadal pathways. Reaction 1: P450scc converts cholesterol to pregnenolone. Reaction 2: 3β-hydroxysteroid dehydrogenase (HSD) converts Δ^5 steroids (pregnenolone, 17OH-pregnenolone, dehydroepiandrosterone [DHEA], androstenediol) to the corresponding Δ^4 steroids (progesterone, androstenedione, testosterone). Reaction 3: P450c17 catalyzes the 17α-hydroxylation of pregnenolone and progesterone. Reaction 4: The 17,20-lyase activity of P450c17 converts 17OH-pregnenolone to DHEA; the conversion of 17OH-progesterone to androstenedione occurs in cattle and rodents, but human P450c17 cannot catalyze this reaction efficiently. Reaction 5: P450c21 catalyzes the 21-hydroxylation of progesterone and 17OH-progesterone. Reaction 6: Deoxycorticosterone (DOC) can be converted to corticosterone by either P450c11AS (in the adrenal zona glomerulosa) or P450c11β (in the adrenal zona fasciculata). Reaction 7: P450c11β converts 11-deoxycortisol to cortisol. Reactions 8 and 9: P450c11AS catalyzes 18 hydroxylase (reaction 8) and 18 methyl oxidase activities (reaction 9) to produce aldosterone in the adrenal zona glomerulosa. Reaction 10: Two isozymes of 17β-HSD activate sex steroids: 17β-HSD1 produces estradiol and 17β-HSD3 produces androgens. In peripheral tissues 17β-HSD5 has similar activity to 17β-HSD3, and 17β-HSD2 and 4 catalyze the "reverse" reactions to inactivate sex steroids. Reaction 11: P450aro aromatizes C19 androgenic steroids to C18 estrogens.

types (e.g., liver) can modify steroids picked up from the circulation, it is the expression of P450scc that identifies a cell as *steroidogenic*. The quantity of steroid that can be produced by a steroidogenic cell is regulated in two fashions: acute and chronic. Chronic regulation, which determines the net steroidogenic capacity of a cell, is mediated by the transcription of the genes for the cell's steroidogenic enzymes. Among the steroidogenic enzymes, P450scc is by far the slowest and hence is rate-limiting, so that its transcription is the key step. Thus, LH in the ovary and ACTH in the adrenal act through cyclic adenosine monophosphate to increase the transcription of the genes for P450scc and other enzymes, thereby determining the amount of steroidogenic machinery in the cell.

Some steroidogenic cells (e.g., placental syncytiotrophoblasts) make fairly constant amounts of steroid, and hence do not have an acute regulatory mechanism. However, adrenal cells, which must be able to respond to acute stress, and ovarian cells, which must be able to mount an acute estrogenic response to the LH surge, and even Leydig cells, which secrete testosterone episodically, must be able to turn steroidogenesis on and off far more rapidly than can be mediated by the transcriptional control of P450scc. This acute regulation is mediated by the steroidogenic acute regulatory protein (StAR), which facilitates the movement of cholesterol into mitochondria, where it becomes the substrate for P450scc *(12)*. Absence of StAR disrupts fetal and neonatal testicular and adrenal steroidogenesis, but not placental steroidogenesis, causing congenital lipoid adrenal hyperplasia; however, the ovary remains unaffected until it is stimulated at the age of puberty *(13,14)*. Alterations in the expression or activity of StAR have also been implicated in the pathogenesis of PCOS *(15)*, but the clinical relevance of these observations remains uncertain.

QUALITATIVE REGULATION OF STEROIDOGENESIS

The qualitative regulator of steroidogenesis, which determines the class of steroids a cell will produce, is the microsomal enzyme P450c17, which sequentially catalyzes both 17α-hydroxylase activity and 17,20-lyase activity *(16,17)*. In the absence of P450c17, a cell produces C_{21} 17-deoxysteroids, e.g., progesterone in the ovarian granulosa cell or aldosterone in the adrenal glomerulosa cell. If only the 17α-hydroxylase activity is present (e.g., in the adrenal zona fasiculata), C_{21} 17-hydroxysteroids (e.g., cortisol) are produced. If both the 17α-hydroxylase and 17,20-lyase activities are present (e.g., in ovarian theca cells, testicular Leydig cells, or adrenal zona reticularis), C_{19} precursors of sex steroids (e.g., dehydroepiandrosterone [DHEA]) are produced. Alterations in P450c17's expression or activity have been implicated in the etiology of PCOS *(18,19)*. The ratio of 17α-hydroxylase activity to 17,20-lyase activity of P450c17 determines the ratio of C_{21} to C_{19} steroids produced. This ratio varies in different cell types (e.g., adrenal fasiculata vs reticularis) and can be developmentally regulated during human adrenarche. This regulation is mediated posttranslationally by at least three factors *(20)*:

1. The abundance of the electron-donating protein P450 oxidoreductase (POR).
2. The presence of cytochrome b_5.
3. The serine phosphorylation of P450c17.

SEX STEROID BIOSYNTHESIS: FROM DHEA TO ANDROGENS AND ESTROGENS

Essentially all human sex steroids are produced from DHEA. The 17,20-lyase activity of human P450c17 converts 17OH-pregnenolone to DHEA with 30-fold greater efficiency than the conversion of 17OH-progesterone to androstenedione *(21)*, hence human androgen synthesis must proceed through DHEA. By contrast, rodents and cattle can convert 17OH-progesterone directly to androstenedione, highlighting the major differences in the pathways of sex steroid synthesis in various mammals. Sex steroid synthesis is thus initiated by converting DHEA to androstenedione by adrenal or gonadal 3β-hydroxysteroid dehydrogenase type 2 (3β-HSD2). An essentially identical isozyme expressed from a different gene, 3β-hydroxysteroid dehydrogenase type 1 (3β-HSD1), is expressed in placenta, liver, and peripheral tissues *(22,23)*. Deficiencies of 3β-HSD2 are a rare cause of defective androgen synthesis *(24)*. Apparently mild deficiencies of 3β-HSD2 activity have been alleged in some hyperandrogenic women with high serum ratios of DHEA to androstenedione or 17OH-pregnenolone to 17OH-progesterone, but DNA sequencing has shown that these individuals have normal 3β-HSD2 genes *(25)*.

Thus, elevated Δ^5 steroid values from three to seven standard deviations above the mean may be associated with mild hyperandrogenism, but the basis of this phenomenon remains unknown.

Androstenedione can be converted to testosterone by isozymes of 17β-hydroxy-steroid dehydrogenases or to estrone by aromatase (P450aro) (26,27). In the sex steroid target tissues, testosterone may be converted to the biologically more potent androgen dihydrotestosterone (DHT) by 5α-reductase (28), and estrone may be converted to the biologically more potent estrogen estradiol by 17β-hydroxysteroid dehydrogenase type 1 (17β-HSD1) (29). The mechanisms of sex steroid production have been reviewed elsewhere (30).

Circulating Sex Steroids

DHEA sulfate (DHEAS), produced by the sulfation of DHEA by SULT2A1 in the adrenal, is the most abundant steroid in the circulation of adults of reproductive age (31). DHEA, DHEAS, and androstenedione are produced almost exclusively by the adrenal zona reticularis. Adrenal C_{19} steroids, however, do not bind with high affinity to the androgen receptor; hence, they function primarily as precursors that are converted to active androgens or estrogens by isozymes of 17β-HSD and by aromatase in target tissues. Although the adrenal can produce minimal amounts of testosterone, probably through 17β-HSD type 5 (17β-HSD5), it can not synthesize estrogens as it lacks aromatase (P450aro). Sex steroid target tissues express aromatase (mainly in the adipose tissue) (32) and multiple isozymes of 17β-HSD, including 17β-HSD1 (mainly in the ovary, placenta, and breast) (29), 17β-HSD3 (mainly in the testis) (33), and 17β-HSD5 (mainly in the liver and muscle) (34). The breast and other "extraglandular tissue," such as the skin, also express 3β-HSD1 and steroid sulfatase, enzymes that can convert DHEAS to androstenedione (23).

The hyperandrogenism of PCOS is of both ovarian and adrenal origin. When adrenal steroidogenesis is suppressed with dexamethasone, the hyperandrogenism persists, indicating an ovarian source (35,36), and when ovarian steroidogenesis is suppressed with a gonadotropin-releasing hormone (GnRH) agonist, the hyperandrogenism again remains, indicating an adrenal source (37–39). In addition, women with PCOS appear to have steady levels of gonadotropins, as opposed to the cyclical fluctuating levels found in normally ovulating women, resulting in increased ovarian production of testosterone, androstenedione, DHEA, DHEAS, 17α-hydroxyprogesterone, and estrone (40,41). Elevated DHEAS levels have also been reported in brothers of women with PCOS (42), possibly reflecting an underlying defect in steroidogenesis that has been found in the sisters of women with PCOS (43), suggesting a genetic trait.

Hyperinsulinemia and Increased Androgen Biosynthesis

Elevated insulin levels are associated with elevated androgen levels in PCOS (44), and the severity of the hyperinsulinemia directly correlates with the severity of the PCOS (45,46). However, it is unclear whether hyperandrogenism results from the hyperinsulinemia, or the hyperinsulinemia results from hyperandrogenism, or whether hyperinsulinemia and hyperandrogenism are independent variables linked in a noncausal relationship. Most authorities hypothesize that hyperinsulinemia secondary to insulin resistance is the primary factor driving the increased androgen production. Thus, bilateral oophorectomy

(47) and administration of GnRH agonist *(48,49)* or antiandrogenic compounds *(50)*, do not appear to alter the insulin resistance or hyperinsulinemia of PCOS. However, androgen excess may contribute to insulin resistance and hyperinsulinemia. Administration of methyltestosterone to cycling women decreases insulin sensitivity *(51)* and women with congenital adrenal hyperplasia have decreased insulin sensitivity *(52)*. However, endogenous androgens do not cause insulin resistance and hyperinsulinemia in normal men, hence the relationship between hyperandrogenemia and insulin resistance remains unclear.

Disordered insulin action typically precedes the development of hyperandrogenism in PCOS. Thus, insulin may act directly to stimulate androgen secretion alone, and/or augment LH-stimulated androgen secretion from theca cells *(53–55)*. Insulin may also act indirectly to enhance the amplitude of serum LH pulses *(56)*, decrease hepatic production of serum sex hormone-binding globulin (SHBG) *(57)*, and/or decrease insulin-like growth factor binding protein (IGFBP)-1, thus increasing free IGF-1, which also can stimulate theca cell's androgen production *(58,59)*. The hyperinsulinemia of PCOS also appears to contribute to the premature arrest of follicle cell growth seen in affected anovulatory women *(60)*.

Effects of Insulin Sensitizing Agents on Steroidogenesis

PCOS is commonly treated with biguanides and thiazolidinediones. Both classes of drugs are insulin-sensitizing agents that decrease hyperandrogenemia and increase fertility in women with PCOS *(61–65)*. These agents may decrease circulating androgen levels indirectly by lowering insulin levels. Alternatively, they may also decrease circulating androgen levels directly by inhibiting steroidogenic enzymes.

Metformin, a biguanide, improves insulin sensitivity, but its mechanism of action is unclear. It may alleviate glucose toxicity *(66)* or inhibit complex 1 of the mitochondrial respiratory chain *(67)*; at least some of its actions are mediated through activation of adenosine monophosphate-activated protein kinase *(68)*. The principal physiological consequence of metformin treatment is reduction of hepatic gluconeogenesis and hepatic glucose output *(69)*. Furthermore, metformin induces weight loss *(69)*, thus improving insulin sensitivity and decreasing insulin levels. Metformin also lowers circulating androgen levels *(70)* and attenuates the adrenal steroidogenic hyperresponsiveness to ACTH *(71)*, but the mechanism remains unclear. Measurements of serum steroids suggested that metformin inhibits P450c17 *(72–74)*, but direct studies of metformin on human steroidogenic enzymes showed no effects on P450c17 or 3β-HSD2 *(75)*. Thus, the action of metformin to decrease circulating androgens is probably secondary to its reduction of insulin levels.

Thiazolidinediones improve insulin sensitivity as well, probably as ligands of the nuclear peroxisome proliferator-activated receptor γ (PPARγ) *(76,77)*. They also decrease elevated androgen levels in PCOS women, but do not decrease androgens in men, suggesting this action is not on the steroidogenic machinery itself. Although troglitazone, which is no longer used because of hepatotoxicity, can directly inhibit 3β-HSD2 and P450c17 at typical pharmacological concentrations *(75)*, pioglitazone and rosiglitazone exert this effect only at grossly supratherapeutic concentrations, providing evidence that the action of thiazolidinedione drugs to lower serum androgens in women with PCOS is mediated indirectly. Consistent with its direct action on P450c17, troglitazone decreases both basal, insulin-induced, and LH/human chorionic gonadotropin (hCG)-stimulated androsterone production by rat theca–interstitial cells, and progesterone production by human granulosa lutein cells *(78)*; pioglitazone can also reduce adrenal responsiveness to ACTH *(79)*. Pharmacological studies with novel, experimental thiazolidinediones show that different regions of the molecule are involved in PPARγ binding and inhibition of P450c17 and 3β-HSD2 *(80)*. Thus, most data indicate that the thiazolidinediones decrease androgens in patients with PCOS primarily by their ability to improve peripheral insulin sensitivity through PPARγ-mediated pathways, but can also directly inhibit steroidogenic enzymes, whereas metformin has only the former and not the latter action *(75)*.

Mechanisms of Insulin Action and Insulin Resistance

MECHANISMS OF INSULIN ACTION

Insulin acts through the insulin receptor (IR) to stimulate glucose transport, promote storage of carbohydrates and lipids, and regulate cell growth and division *(81)*. IR is a disulfide-linked transmembrane heterotetramer consisting of two identical αβ dimers *(82,83)*. The extracellular α subunit (IRα) contains the ligand-binding domain; the transmembrane β subunit (IRβ) contains an intracellular tyrosine kinase domain *(81)*. Binding of insulin to the IR induces a conformational change in the receptor that activates its tyrosine kinase domain and causes receptor tyrosine autophosphorylation, thus initiating insulin signaling *(84)*.

Endogenous intracellular substrates for the autophosphorylated IR include the insulin receptor substrates (IRS1 through 4), IRS5/DOK4, IRS/DOK5, Gab-1, Cbl, APS and SHC isoforms, and members of the signal regulatory protein (SIRP) family of proteins *(85)*. These proteins bind to the activated IR and undergo tyrosine phosphorylation. IRS-1 and SHC have been studied extensively *(81)*. The phosphorylated tyrosine residues on the IRSs and SHC serve as docking sites for several SH2 domain proteins, including phosphatidylinositol 3-kinase (PI3-K) and the adapter protein Grb2. PI3-K can activate protein kinase B (also known as Akt) and the translocation of GLUT4 to the cell surface, actions involved in the metabolic effects of insulin. The SHC/Grb2 complex can associate with the $p21^{ras}$ nucleotide exchange factor SOS, activating the Ras–mitogen-activated protein (MAP) kinase pathway, actions involved in the mitogenic effects of insulin. Although the mechanisms of signal termination are unclear, they probably involve interactions among various kinases and phosphatases *(84)*; receptor-mediated endocytosis and recycling have also been reported *(86)*.

MECHANISMS OF INSULIN RESISTANCE

Most patients with PCOS have decreased insulin sensitivity, occurring independently of obesity, glucose intolerance, body fat topography, and sex hormone levels *(87)*. PCOS patients do not have structural abnormalities of the IR *(88,89)*, decreases in IR number *(90,91)*, or alterations in insulin-binding affinity *(90,91)*, suggesting a post-receptor mechanism for their insulin resistance. Serine phosphorylation of IRβ inhibits IR tyrosine autophosphorylation but does not inhibit insulin binding, resulting in a form of insulin resistance *(92–95)*. This occurs in a subset of patients with PCOS *(91)*. The mechanism leading to IRβ serine phosphorylation remains undefined, but appears to involve a serine/threonine kinase extrinsic to the receptor *(96)*. Alternatively, an inhibitor of a serine/threonine phosphatase may be involved *(91,97)*.

Insulin resistance in patients with PCOS without IRβ serine phosphorylation may involve other post-receptor defects, possibly involving IRS-1 phosphorylation or PI3-K activation. For example, serine phosphorylation of IRS-1 interferes with its activation by the IR, and thus typically inhibits IRS-1-dependent signaling pathways *(98–100)*. Serine phosphorylation of IRS-1 may also contribute to insulin resistance induced by free fatty acids (FFA) *(101)* and tumor necrosis factor (TNF)-α *(102)*, both of which may be elevated in women with PCOS *(103–105)*. Inflammatory cytokines (e.g., interleukin [IL]-1 and -6) *(106)*, glucosamine *(107)*, and other proteins in the insulin signaling pathways, such as IRS-2 *(108)* and the β isoform of Akt (Akt2) *(109)*, may play a role in insulin resistance, but their potential roles in PCOS are unknown. Plasma membrane glycoprotein PC-1 can also cause insulin resistance, inhibiting IR tyrosine kinase activity through unknown mechanisms *(110)*. Although its gene locus is associated with obesity and an increased risk of glucose intolerance and type 2 diabetes *(111)*, its association with PCOS is unknown.

TISSUE-SELECTIVE IR IN PCOS

The insulin resistance of PCOS appears to be tissue-selective. Insulin resistance has been reported in muscle, adipose tissue, and the liver in patients with PCOS *(87,112)*, but not in the polycystic ovary itself. In fact, insulin increases ovarian androgen production *(113)*. Patients with mutations in both alleles of the IR (leprechaunism) have profound insulin resistance, yet have severe hirsutism and elevated testosterone levels *(114)*, indicating that the action of insulin on the ovary is mediated through a different molecular mechanism. It has been suggested that insulin could act on the ovaries of insulin-resistant individuals through IGF-1 receptors *(113)*. Receptors for IGF-1 (IGF-1R) have the same structure as the IR, and heterodimeric receptors having one IR subunit and one IGF-1R subunit are well described *(113)*. However, antibodies against IGF-1R do not inhibit insulin-stimulated estradiol and progesterone production in cultured granulosa cells from women with PCOS, suggesting that insulin induces ovarian steroidogenesis by activating the IR *(60,115)*. By contrast, insulin-stimulated glycogen synthesis is decreased significantly (with relatively unchanged thymidine incorporation) in fibroblasts from patients with PCOS compared to those of controls *(116)*, suggesting that insulin resistance of PCOS occurs at a postreceptor level affecting the metabolic but not the mitogenic pathways of insulin signaling.

The Serine Phosphorylation Hypothesis

The 17α-hydroxylase and 17,20-lyase activities of P450c17 are catalyzed on a single active site but are differentially regulated during the course of human adrenarche. To explain this unusual enzymology, we considered whether posttranslational modification of P450c17 could alter the ratio of hydroxylase to lyase activity and found that serine phosphorylation of P450c17 dramatically increases its 17,20-lyase activity *(9)*. As it was known that IRβ serine phosphorylation can inhibit IR tyrosine kinase activity *(92–95)*, it was apparent that a single kinase might phosphorylate both the insulin receptor, causing insulin resistance, and P450c17, causing hyperandrogenism *(9)*. A gain-of-function mutation in the hypothetical kinase or in an upstream regulator of the kinase might account for the two cardinal but disparate features of PCOS, hyperandrogenism and insulin resistance, through a single genetic lesion. Furthermore, a gain-of-function mutation would predict dominant inheritance *(9)*. Shortly before this,

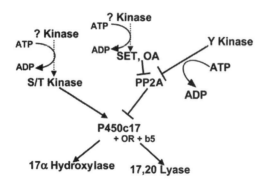

Fig. 2. Regulation of 17,20-lyase activity by reversible phosphorylation of P450c17. Arrows indicate stimulation and blocked lines indicate inhibition. A cyclic adenosine monophosphate-dependent serine/threonine (S/T) kinase stimulates the 17,20-lyase activity of P450c17 and a tyrosine (Y) kinase, and SET and okadaic acid (OA) inhibit PP2A. The natures of the kinases that regulate SET and that presumably regulate Ser/Thr kinases are unknown. (From ref. *125*.)

excess serine phosphorylation of IRβ was reported in a subset of patients with PCOS who have insulin resistance *(91)*, providing evidence for the serine phosphorylation hypothesis from the perspective of IRβ as well as P450c17.

A gain-of-function mutation also suggests that affected patients may have a milder clinical manifestation of the syndrome in earlier life, before the complete phenotype becomes apparent. Indeed, both factors appear to be true, at least in a subset of patients with PCOS. Autosomal-dominant inheritance has been reported in several studies of the genetics of PCOS *(43,117–119)* and clinical data indicate that girls with premature, exaggerated adrenarche are more likely to develop PCOS as adults than girls who undergo normal adrenarche *(59,120–122)*. However, the serine phosphorylation hypothesis remains unproven. A study expressing P450c17 in fibroblasts from patients with PCOS did not show increased 17,20-lyase activity *(123)*. However, these observations are insufficient to reject the hypothesis, as fibroblasts are not steroidogenic and do not normally express large amounts of the POR and cytochrome b_5 needed for maximal lyase activity. Thus, until the kinase(s) responsible for serine phosphorylation of IRβ and P450c17 is (are) characterized, it will not be possible to confirm or reject this hypothesis.

Although the physiological trigger to P450c17 serine phosphorylation remains unknown, IGF-1 may be involved *(9)*, as its serum levels rise and fall in a pattern similar to that of DHEA. Various kinases and phosphatases may also play a role, as proteins activated by phosphorylation usually exist in a state of equilibrium between phosphorylation by a kinase and dephosphorylation by a phosphatase *(124)*. Recent work has shown that protein phosphatase 2A (PP2A) is the physiological agent that dephosphorylates P450c17. PP2A, in turn, is regulated by SET, a phosphoprotein that inhibits PP2A *(125)*. Thus, serine phosphorylation of P450c17 appears to be regulated positively by a kinase pathway and negatively by a phosphatase pathway, both of which probably contain multiple components with several potential sites of regulation by kinases and phosphatases *(see* Fig. 2) *(125)*.

Serine phosphorylation is not the only posttranscriptional mechanism regulating the 17,20-lyase activity of P450c17; this activity is also amplified by the presence of cytochrome b_5, which acts allosterically to promote the association of P450c17 with POR *(21)*. However, cytochrome b_5 has no known effect on insulin action. Serine phosphorylation and the presence of cytochrome b_5 act independently of one another, and each can elicit maximal 17,20-lyase activity *(126)*. The roles of serine phosphorylation and cytochrome b_5 in the normal or PCOS theca cell have not yet been investigated.

Thus, although the serine phosphorylation hypothesis provides a common pathway for hyperandrogenism and insulin resistance, two principal features of some forms of PCOS, it remains an unproven hypothesis until such time as the kinase is cloned and activating mutations are found. Nonetheless, the hypothesis is heuristic and has stimulated further study of the cell biology of PCOS.

FUTURE AVENUES OF INVESTIGATION

Much remain to be learned regarding PCOS and the pathogenesis of its multiple forms. Future areas of investigation include—but are not limited to—the following:

1. Identification of the kinase(s) involved in the serine phosphorylation of P450c17.
2. Identification of the kinase(s) responsible for serine phosphorylation of IRβ.
3. Identification of the upstream factors regulating the activity of this (these) kinase(s).
4. Evaluation of forms of PCOS not accounted for by the serine phosphorylation hypothesis.
5. Development of specific novel therapeutic agents for patients with PCOS based on a more detailed understanding of cell biology.

KEY POINTS

- PCOS is a common cause of menstrual dysfunction and is one of the most frequently encountered endocrine disorders.
- PCOS is probably a group of diseases with different pathophysiological mechanisms, rather than being one disease caused by a single molecular defect.
- Insulin resistance and hyperandrogenism are characteristics of some forms of PCOS.
- The "serine phosphorylation hypothesis" provides a single mechanism for both insulin resistance and hyperandrogenism, implying autosomal-dominant inheritance of a gain-of-function mutation in the responsible kinase.
- Advances in the understanding of the cell biology of PCOS may permit the development of a more specific drug therapy.

REFERENCES

1. Knochenhauer ES, Key TJ, Kahsar-Miller M, Waggoner W, Boots LR, Azziz R. Prevalence of the polycystic ovary syndrome in unselected black and white women of the southeastern United States: a prospective study. J Clin Endocrinol Metab 1998;83:3078–3082.
2. Azziz R, Woods KS, Reyna R, Key TJ, Knochenhauer ES, Yildiz BO. The prevalence and features of the polycystic ovary syndrome in an unselected population. J Clin Endocrinol Metab 2004;89:2745–2749.
3. Dunaif A. Insulin resistance and the polycystic ovary syndrome: mechanism and implications for pathogenesis. Endocr Rev 1997;18:774–800.
4. Sam S, Dunaif A. Polycystic ovary syndrome: syndrome XX. Trends Endocrinol Metab 2003;14: 365–370.
5. Venkatesan AM, Dunaif A, Corbould A. Insulin resistance in polycystic ovary syndrome: progress and paradoxes. Recent Prog Horm Res 2001;56:295–308.

6. Orio F Jr., Palomba S, Spinelli L, et al. The cardiovascular risk of young women with polycystic ovary syndrome: an observational, analytical, prospective case-control study. J Clin Endocrinol Metab 2004;89:3696–3701.

7. Legro RS. Polycystic ovary syndrome and cardiovascular disease: a premature association? Endocr Rev 2003;24:302–312.

8. Tsilchorozidou T, Overton C, Conway GS. The pathophysiology of polycystic ovary syndrome. Clin Endocrinol 2004;60:1–17.

9. Zhang L-H, Rodriguez H, Ohno S, Miller WL. Serine phosphorylation of human P450c17 increases 17,20-lyase activity: implications for adrenarche and the polycystic ovary syndrome. Proc Natl Acad Sci USA 1995;92:10,619–10,623.

10. Miller WL. Molecular biology of steroid hormone synthesis. Endocr Rev 1988;9:295–318.

11. Izquierdo D, Foyouzi N, Kwintkiewicz J, Duleba AJ. Mevastatin inhibits ovarian theca-interstitial cell proliferation and steroidogenesis. Fertil Steril 2004;82 Suppl 3:1193–1197.

12. Miller WL, Strauss JF 3rd. Molecular pathology and mechanism of action of the steroidogenic acute regulatory protein, StAR. J Steroid Biochem Mol Biol 1999;69:131–141.

13. Bose HS, Sugawara T, Strauss JF 3rd, Miller WL. The pathophysiology and genetic of congenital lipoid adrenal hyperplasia. International congenital lipoid adrenal hyperplasia consortium. N Engl J Med 1996;335:1870–1878.

14. Bose HS, Pescovitz OH, Miller WL. Spontaneous feminization in a 46,XX female patient with congenital lipoid adrenal hyperplasia due to a homozygous frameshift mutation in the steroidogenic acute regulatory protein. J Clin Endocrinol Metab 1997;82:1511–1515.

15. Kahsar-Miller MD, Conway-Myers BA, Boots LR, Azziz R. Steroidogenic acute regulatory protein (StAR) in the ovaries of healthy women and those with polycystic ovary syndrome. Am J Obstet Gynecol 2001;185:1381–1387.

16. Nakajin S, Shively JE, Yuan PM, Hall PF. Microsomal cytochrome P-450 from neonatal pig testis: two enzymatic activities (17α-hydroxylase and c17,20-lyase) associated with one protein. Biochemistry 1981;20:4037–4042.

17. Zuber MX, Simpson ER, Waterman MR. Expression of bovine 17α-hydroxylase cytochrome P-450 cDNA in nonsteroidogenic (COS 1) cells. Science 1986;234:1258–1261.

18. Wickenheisser JK, Quinn PG, Nelson VL, Legro RS, Stauss JF 3rd, McAllister JM. Differential activity of the cytochrome P450 17α-hydroxylase and steroidogenic acute regulatory protein gene promoters in normal and polycystic ovary syndrome theca cells. J Clin Endocrinol Metab 2000;85:2304–2311.

19. Jakimiuk AJ, Weitsman SR, Navab A, Magoffin DA. Luteinizing hormone receptor, steroidogenesis acute regulatory protein, and steroidogenic enzyme messenger ribonucleic acids are overexpressed in thecal and granulosa cells from polycystic ovaries. J Clin Endocrinol Metab 2001;86:1318–1323.

20. Miller WL, Auchus RJ, Geller DH. The regulation of 17,20 lyase activity. Steroids 1997;62:133–142.

21. Auchus RJ, Lee TC, Miller WL. Cytochrome b5 augments the 17,20-lyase activity of human P450c17 without direct electron transfer. J Biol Chem 1998;273:3158–3165.

22. Lachance Y, Luu-The V, Labrie C, et al. Characterization of human 3β-hydroxysteroid dehydrogenase/Δ^5-Δ^4-isomerase gene and its expression in mammalian cells. J Biol Chem 1990;265:20,469–20,475.

23. Labrie F, Simard J, Luu-The V, et al. Structure and tissue-specific expression of 3β-hydroxysteroid dehydrogenase/5-ene-4-ene isomerase genes in human and rat classical and peripheral steroidogenic tissues. J Steroid Biochem Mol Biol 1992;41:421–435.

24. Pang S. Congenital adrenal hyperplasia owing to 3β-hydroxysteroid dehydrogenase deficiency. Endocrinol Metab Clin North Am 2001;30:81–99.

25. Carbunaru G, Prasad P, Scoccia B, et al. The hormonal phenotype of nonclassic 3β-hydroxysteroid dehydrogenase (HSD3B) deficiency in hyperandrogenic females is associated with insulin-resistant polycystic ovary syndrome and is not a variant of inherited HSD3B2 deficiency. J Clin Endocrinol Metab 2004;89:783–794.

26. Simpson ER, Mahendroo MS, Means GD, et al. Aromatase cytochrome P450, the enzyme responsible for estrogen biosynthesis. Endocr Rev 1994;15:342–355.

27. Penning TM. Molecular endocrinology of hydroxysteroid dehydrogenases. Endocr Rev 1997;18:281–305.

28. Mahendroo MS, Russell DW. Male and female isoenzymes of steroid 5α-reductase. Rev Reprod 1999;4:179–183.

29. Tremblay Y, Ringler GE, Morel Y, et al. Regulation of the gene for estrogenic 17-ketosteroid reductase lying on chromosome 17cen→q25. J Biol Chem 1989;264:20,458–20,462.

30. Miller WL. Androgen biosynthesis from cholesterol to DHEA. Mol Cell Endocrinol 2002;198:7–14.

31. Orentreich N, Brind JL, Rizer RL, Vogelman JH. Age changes and sex differences in serum dehydroepiandrosterone sulfate concentrations throughout adulthood. J Clin Endocrinol Metab 1984;59:551–555.

32. Simpson ER, Mahendroo MS, Means GD, et al. Aromatase cytochrome P450, the enzyme responsible for estrogen biosynthesis. Endocr Rev 1994;15:342–355.

33. Geissler WM, Davis DL, Wu L, et al. Male pseudohermaphroditism caused by mutations of testicular 17β-hydroxysteroid dehydrogenase 3. Nat Genet 1994;7:34–39.

34. Dufort I, Rheault P, Huang XF, Soucy P, Luu-The V. Characteristics of a highly labile human type 5 17β-hydroxysteroid dehydrogenase. Endocrinology 1999;140:568–574.

35. Lachelin GC, Judd HL, Swanson SC, Hauck ME, Parker DC, Yen SS. Long term effects of nightly dexamethasone administration in patients with polycystic ovarian disease. J Clin Endocrinol Metab 1982;55:768–773.

36. Rittmaster RS, Thompson DL. Effect of leuprolide and dexamethasone on hair growth and hormone levels in hirsute women: the relative importance of the ovary and the adrenal in the pathogenesis of hirsutism. J Clin Endocrinol Metab 1990;70:1096–1102.

37. Hoffman DI, Klove K, Lobo RA. The prevalence and significance of elevated dehydroepiandrosterone sulfate levels in anovulatory women. Fertil Steril 1984;42:76–81.

38. Barnes RB, Rosenfield RL, Burstein S, Ehrmann DA. Pituitary–ovarian responses to nafarelin testing in the polycystic ovary syndrome. N Engl J Med 1989;320:559–565.

39. Ehrmann DA, Rosenfield RL, Barnes RB, Brigell DF, Sheikh Z. Detection of functional ovarian hyperandrogenism in women with androgen excess. N Engl J Med 1992;327:157–162.

40. Heineman MJ, Thomas CM, Doesburg WH, Rolland R. Hormonal characteristics of women with clinical features of the polycystic ovary syndrome. Eur J Obstet Gynecol Reprod Biol 1984;17:263–271.

41. DeVane GW, Czekala NM, Judd HL, Yen SS. Circulating gonadotropins, estrogens, and androgens in polycystic ovarian disease. Am J Obstet Gynecol 1975;121:496–500.

42. Legro RS, Kunselman AR, Demers L, Wang SC, Bentley-Lewis R, Dunaif A. Elevated dehydroepiandrosterone sulfate levels as the reproductive phenotype in the brothers of women with polycystic ovary syndrome. J Clin Endocrinol Metab 2002;87:2134–2138.

43. Legro RS, Driscoll D, Strauss JF 3rd, Fox J, Dunaif A. Evidence for a genetic basis for hyperandrogenism in polycystic ovary syndrome. Proc Natl Acad Sci USA 1998;95:14,956–14,960.

44. Burghen GA, Givens JR, Kitabchi AE. Correlation of hyperandrogenism with hyperinsulinism in polycystic ovarian disease. J Clin Endocrinol Metab 1980;50:113–116.

45. Conway GS, Jacobs HS, Holly JM, Wass JA. Effects of luteinizing hormone, insulin, insulin-like growth factor-I and insulin-like growth factor small binding protein 1 in the polycystic ovary syndrome. Clin Endocrinol 1990;33:593–603.

46. Robinson S, Kiddy D, Gelding SV, et al. The relationship of insulin insensitivity to menstrual pattern in women with hyperandrogenism and polycystic ovaries. Clin Endocrinol 1993;39:351–355.

47. Nagamani M, Van Dinh T, Kelver ME. Hyperinsulinemia in hyperthecosis of the ovaries. Am J Obstet Gynecol 1986;154:384–389.

48. Geffner ME, Kaplan SA, Bersch N, Golde DW, Landaw EM, Chang RJ. Persistence of insulin resistance in polycystic ovarian disease after inhibition of ovarian steroid secretion. Fertil Steril 1986;45:327–333.

49. Dunaif A, Green G, Futterweit W, Dobrjansky A. Suppression of hyperandrogenism does not improve peripheral or hepatic insulin resistance in the polycystic ovary syndrome. J Clin Endocrinol Metab 1990;70:699–704.

50. Diamanti-Kandarakis E, Mitrakou A, Hennes MM, et al. Insulin sensitivity and antiandrogenic therapy in women with polycystic ovary syndrome. Metabolism 1995;44:525–531.

51. Diamond MP, Grainger D, Diamond MC, Sherwin RS, Defronzo RA. Effects of methyltestosterone and insulin secretion and sensitivity in women. J Clin Endocrinol Metab 1998;83:4420–4425.

52. Speiser PW, Serrat J, New MI, Gertner JM. Insulin insensitivity in adrenal hyperplasia due to nonclassical steroid 21-hydroxylase deficiency. J Clin Endocrinol Metab 1992;75:1421–1424.

53. Barbieri RL, Makris A, Ryan KJ. Insulin stimulates androgen accumulation in incubations of human ovarian stroma and theca. Obstet Gynecol 1984;64:73S–80S.

54. Cara JF, Rosenfield RL. Insulin-like growth factor I and insulin potentiate luteinizing hormone-induced androgen synthesis by rat ovarian thecal-interstitial cells. Endocrinology 1988;123:733–739.

55. Hernandez ER, Resnick CE, Holtzclaw WD, Payne DW, Adashi EY. Insulin as a regulator of androgen biosynthesis by cultured rat ovarian cells: cellular mechanism(s) underlying physiological and pharmacological hormonal actions. Endocrinology 1988;122:2034–2043.

56. Nestler JE. Insulin regulation of human ovarian androgens. Hum Reprod 1997;12:53–62.

57. Nestler JE, Powers LP, Matt DW, et al. A direct effect of hyperinsulinemia on serum sex hormone-binding globulin levels in obese women with the polycystic ovary syndrome. J Clin Endocrinol Metab 1991;72:83–89.

58. LeRoith D, McGuinness M, Shemer J, et al. Insulin-like growth factors. Biol Signals 1992;1: 173–181.

59. Ibáñez L, Potau N, Zampolli M, Rique S, Saenger P, Carrascosa A. Hyperinsulinemia and decreased insulin-like growth factor-binding protein-1 are common features in prepubertal and pubertal girls with a history of premature pubarche. J Clin Endocrinol Metab 1997;82:2283–2288.

60. Franks S, Gilling-Smith C, Watson H, Willis D. Insulin action in the normal and polycystic ovary. Endocrinol Metab Clin North Am 1999;28:361–378.

61. Nestler JE, Jakubowicz DJ. Decreases in ovarian cytochrome P450c17α activity and serum free testosterone after reduction of insulin secretion in polycystic ovary syndrome. N Engl J Med 1996; 335:617–623.

62. Nestler JE, Jakubowicz DJ, Evans WS, Pasquali R. Effects of metformin on spontaneous and clomiphene-induced ovulation in the polycystic ovary syndrome. N Engl J Med 1998;338: 1876–1880.

63. Hasegawa I, Murakawa H, Suzuki M, Yamamoto Y, Kurabayashi T, Tanaka K. Effect of troglitazone on endocrine and ovulatory performance in women with insulin resistance-related polycystic ovary syndrome. Fertil Steril 1999;71:323–327.

64. Azziz R, Ehrmann D, Legro RS, et al. Troglitazone improves ovulation and hirsutism in the polycystic ovary syndrome: a multicenter, double blind, placebo-controlled trial. J Clin Endocrinol Metab 2001;86:1626–1632.

65. Azziz R, Ehrmann DA, Legro RS, Fereshetian AG, O'Keefe M, Ghazzi MN, PCOS/Troglitazone Study Group. Troglitazone decreases adrenal androgen levels in women with polycystic ovary syndrome. Fertil Steril 2003;79:932–937.

66. DeFronzo RA, Goodman AM. Efficacy of metformin in patients with non-insulin-dependent diabetes mellitus. The multicenter metformin study group. N Engl J Med 1995;333:541–549.

67. Owen MR, Doran E, Halestrap AP. Evidence that metformin exerts its anti-diabetic effects through inhibition of complex 1 of the mitochondrial respiratory chain. Biochem J 2000;348 Pt 3:607–614.

68. Zhou G, Myers R, Li Y, et al. Role of AMP-activated protein kinase in mechanism of metformin action. J Clin Invest 2001;108:1167–1174.

69. Stumvoll M, Nurjhan N, Perriello G, Dailey G, Gerich JE. Metabolic effects of metformin in non-insulin-dependent diabetes mellitus. N Engl J Med 1995;333:550–554.

70. Vrbikova J, Hill M, Starka L, et al. The effects of long-term metformin treatment on adrenal and ovarian steroidogenesis in women with polycystic ovary syndrome. Eur J Endocrinol 2001;144:619–628.

71. Arslanian SA, Lewy V, Danadian K, Saad R. Metformin therapy in obese adolescents with polycystic ovary syndrome and impaired glucose tolerance: amelioration of exaggerated adrenal response to adrenocorticotropin with reduction of insulinemia/insulin resistance. J Clin Endocrinol Metab 2002;87:1555–1559.

72. la Marca A, Egbe TO, Morgante G, Paglia T, Cianci A, De Leo V. Metformin treatment reduces ovarian cytochrome P-450c17α response to human chorionic gonadotrophin in women with insulin resistance-related polycystic ovary syndrome. Hum Reprod 2000;15:21–23.

73. Attia GR, Rainey WE, Carr BR. Metformin directly inhibits androgen production in human thecal cells. Fertil Steril 2001;76:517–524.

74. Mansfield R, Galea R, Brincat M, Hole D, Mason H. Metformin has direct effects on human ovarian steroidogenesis. Fertil Steril 2003;79:956–962.

75. Arlt W, Auchus RJ, Miller WL. Thiazolidinediones but not metformin directly inhibit the steroidogenic enzymes P450c17 and 3β-hydroxysteroid dehydrogenase. J Biol Chem 2001;276:16,767–16,771.

76. Spiegelman BM. PPAR-gamma: adipogenic regulator and thiazolidinedione receptor. Diabetes 1998;47:507–514.

77. Kersten S, Desvergne B, Wahli W. Roles of PPARs in health and disease. Nature 2000;405:421–424.

78. Mitwally MFM, Witchel SF, Casper RF. Troglitazone: a possible modulator of ovarian steroidogenesis. J Soc Gynecol Investig 2002;9:163–167.

79. Guido M, Romualdi D, Giuliani M, Costantini B, Apa R, Lanzone A. Effect of pioglitazone treatment on the adrenal androgen response to corticotropin in obese patients with polycystic ovary syndrome. Hum Reprod 2004;19:534–539.

80. Arlt W, Neogi P, Gross C, Miller WL. Cinnamic acid based thiazolidinediones inhibit human P450c17 and 3β-hydroxysteroid dehydrogenase and improve insulin sensitivity independent of PPARγ agonist activity. J Mol Endocrinol 2004;32:425–436.

81. Cheatham B, Kahn CR. Insulin action and the insulin signaling network. Endocr Rev 1995;16: 117 142.

82. Ullrich A, Bell JR, Chen EY, et al. Human insulin receptor and its relationship to the tyrosine kinase family of oncogenes. Nature 1985;313:756–761.

83. Goldfine ID. The insulin receptor: molecular biology and transmembrane signaling. Endocr Rev 1987;8:235–255.

84. Saltiel AR. Diverse signaling pathways in the cellular actions of insulin. Am J Physiol 1996; 270(3 Pt 1):E375–E385.

85. Watson RT, Kanzaki M, Pessin JE. Regulated membrane trafficking of the insulin-responsive glucose transporter 4 in adipocytes. Endocr Rev 2004;25:177–204.

86. Kahn CR. The molecular mechanism of insulin action. Annu Rev Med 1985;36:429–451.

87. Dunaif A, Segal KR, Shelley DR, Green G, Dobrjansky A, Licholai T. Evidence for distinctive and intrinsic defects in insulin action in polycystic ovary syndrome. Diabetes 1992;41:1257–1266.

88. Conway GS, Avey C, Rumsby G. The tyrosine kinase domain of the insulin receptor gene is normal in women with hyperinsulinaemia and polycystic ovary syndrome. Hum Reprod 1994;9: 1681–1683.

89. Talbot JA, Bicknell EJ, Rajkhowa M, Krook A, O'Rahilly S, Clayton RN. Molecular scanning of the insulin receptor gene in women with polycystic ovary syndrome. J Clin Endocrinol Metab 1996;81: 1979–1983.

90. Ciaraldi TP, el-Roeiy A, Madar Z, Reichart D, Olefsky JM, Yen SS. Cellular mechanisms of insulin resistance in polycystic ovary syndrome. J Clin Endocrinol Metab 1992;75:577–583.

91. Dunaif A, Xia J, Book C-B, Schenker E, Tang Z. Excessive insulin receptor serine phosphorylation in cultured fibroblasts and in skeletal muscle. A potential mechanism for insulin resistance in the polycystic ovary syndrome. J Clin Invest 1995;96:801–810.

92. Bollage GE, Roth RA, Beaudoin J, Mochly-Rosen D, Doshland DE Jr. Protein kinase C directly phosphorylates the insulin receptor in vitro and reduces its protein-tyrosine kinase activity. Proc Natl Acad Sci USA 1986;83:5822–5824.

93. Stadtmauer L, Rosen OM. Increasing the cAMP content of IM-9 cells alters the phosphorylation state and protein kinase activity of the insulin receptor. J Biol Chem 1986;261:3402–3407.

94. Takayama S, White MF, Kahn CR. Phorbol ester-induced serine phosphorylation of the insulin receptor decreases its tyrosine kinase activity. J Biol Chem 1988;263:3440–3447.

95. Chin JE, Dickens M, Tavare JM, Roth RA. Overexpression of protein kinse C isoenzymes α, βI, γ, and ε in cells overexpressing the insulin receptor. Effects on receptor phosphorylation and signaling. J Biol Chem 1993;268:6338–6347.

96. Li M, Youngren JF, Dunaif A, et al. Decreased insulin receptor (IR) autophosphorylation in fibroblasts from patients with PCOS: effects of serine kinase inhibitors and IR activators. J Clin Endocrinol Metab 2002;87:4088–4093.

97. Guo H, Damuni Z. Autophosphorylation-activated protein kinase phosphorylates and inactivates protein phosphatase 2A. Proc Natl Acad Sci USA 1993;90:2500–2504.

98. Paz K, Hemi R, LeRoith D, et al. A molecular basis for insulin resistance. J Biol Chem 1997;272: 29,911–29,918.

99. Pirola L, Johnston AM, Obberghen EV. Modulation of insulin action. Diabetologia 2004;47: 170–184.

100. Liberman Z, Eldar-Finkelman H. Serine 332 phosphorylation of insulin receptor substrate-1 by glycogen synthase kinase-3 attenuates insulin signaling. J Biol Chem 2005;280:4422–4428.

101. Dresner A, Laurent D, Marcucci M, et al. Effects of free fatty acids on glucose transport and IRS-1-associated phosphatidylinositol 3-kinase activity. J Clin Invest 1999;103:253–259.

102. Hotamisligil GS, Peraldi P, Budavari A, Ellis R, White MF, Speigelman BM. IRS-1-mediated inhibition of insulin receptor tyrosine kinase activity in TNF-α- and obesity-induced insulin resistance. Science 1996;271:665–668.

103. Holte J, Bergh T, Berne C, Lithell H. Serum lipoprotein lipid profile in women with the polycystic ovary syndrome: relation to anthropometric, endocrine and metabolic variables. Clin Endocrinol 1994;41:463–471.

104. Robinson S, Henderson AD, Gelding SV, et al. Dyslipidaemia is associated with insulin resistance in women with polycystic ovaries. Clin Endocrinol 1996;44:277–284.

105. Naz RK, Thurston D, Santoro N. Circulating tumor necrosis factor (TNF)-α in normally cycling women and patients with premature ovarian failure and polycystic ovaries. Am J Reprod Immunol 1995;34:170–175.

106. Spranger J, Kroke A, Mohlig M, et al. Inflammatory cytokines and the risk to develop type 2 diabetes: results of the prospective population-based European Prospective Investigation into Cancer and Nutrition (EPIC)-Potsdam Study. Diabetes 2003;52:812–817.

107. Ciaraldi TP, Carter L, Nikoulina S, Mudaliar S, McClain DA, Henry RR. Glucosamine regulation of glucose metabolism in cultured human skeletal muscle cells: divergent effects on glucose transport/phosphorylation and glycogen synthase in non-diabetic and type 2 diabetic subjects. Endocrinology 1999;140:3971–3980.

108. Previs SF, Withers DJ, Ren JM, White MF, Shulman GI. Contrasting effects of IRS-1 versus IRS-2 gene disruption on carbohydrate and lipid metabolism. J Biol Chem 2000;275:38,990–38,994.

109. Cho H, Mu J, Kim JK, et al. Insulin resistance and a diabetes mellitus-like syndrome in mice lacking the protein kinase Akt2 (PKBβ). Science 2001;292:1728–1731.

110. Maddux BA, Sbraccia P, Kumakura S, et al. Membrane glycoprotein PC-1 and insulin resistance in non-insulin-dependent diabetes mellitus. Nature 1995;373:448–451.

111. Meyre D, Bouatia-Naji N, Tounian A, et al. Variants of ENPP1 are associated with childhood and adult obesity and increase the risk of glucose intolerance and type 2 diabetes. Nat Genet 2005; 37:863–867.

112. Dunaif A, Segal KR, Futterweit W, Dobrjansky A. Profound peripheral insulin resistance, independent of obesity, in polycystic ovary syndrome. Diabetes 1989;38:1165–1174.

113. Poretsky L. On the paradox of insulin-induced hyperandrogenism in insulin-resistant states. Endocr Rev 1991;12:3–13.

114. Taylor SI. Lilly Lecture: molecular mechanisms of insulin resistance. Lessons learned from patients with mutations in the insulin-receptor gene. Diabetes 1992;41:1473–1490.

115. Willis D, Franks S. Insulin action in human granulosa cells from normal and polycystic ovaries is mediated by the insulin receptor and not the type-I insulin-like growth factor receptor. J Clin Endocrinol Metab 1995;80:3788–3790.

116. Book C-B, Dunaif A. Selective insulin resistance in the polycystic ovary syndrome. J Clin Endocrinol Metab 1999;84:3110–3116.

117. Govind A, Obhrai MS, Clayton RN. Polycystic ovaries are inherited as an autosomal dominant trait: analysis of 29 polycystic ovary syndrome and 10 control families. J Clin Endocrinol Metab 1999;84:38–43.

118. Legro RS, Strauss JF 3rd. Molecular progress in infertility: polycystic ovary syndrome. Fertil Steril 2002;78:569–576.

119. Diamanti-Kandarakis E, Piperi C. Genetics of polycystic ovary syndrome: searching for the way out of the labyrinth. Hum Reprod Update 2005;11:631–643.

120. Ibáñez L, Potau N, Virdis R, et al. Postpubertal outcome in girls diagnosed of premature pubarche during childhood: increased frequency of functional ovarian hyperandrogenism. J Clin Endocrinol Metab 1993;76:1599–1603.

121. Oppenheimer E, Linder B, DiMartino-Nardi J. Decreased insulin senstivity in prepubertal girls with premature pubarche and acanthosis nigricans. J Clin Endocrinol Metab 1995;80:614–618.

122. Ibáñez L, Potau N, Virdis R, et al. Hyperinsulinemia in postpubertal girls with a history of premature pubarche and functional ovarian hyperandrogenism. J Clin Endocrinol Metab 1996;81: 1237–1243.

123. Martens JWM, Geller DH, Arlt W, et al. Enzymatic activities of P450c17 stably expressed in fibroblasts from patients with the polycystic ovary syndrome. J Clin Endocrinol Metab 2000; 85:4338–4346.

124. Virshup DM. Protein phosphatase 2A: a panoply of enzymes. Curr Opin Cell Biol 2000;12:180–185.
125. Pandey AV, Mellon SH, Miller WL. Protein phosphatase 2A and phosphoprotein SET regulate androgen production by P450c17. J Biol Chem 2003;278:2837–2844.
126. Pandey AV, Miller WL. Regulation of 17,20 lyase activity by cytochrome b_5 and by serine phosphorylation of P450c17. J Biol Chem 2005;280:13,265–13,271.

7 Adrenarche

The Interrelationship of Androgens/Insulin on the Development of the Metabolic Syndrome/Polycystic Ovary Syndrome

Sharon E. Oberfield, MD, Natasha Leibel, MD, Lauren Antler, BA, Miriam Silfen, MD, Lenore S. Levine, MD, Mary Horlick, MD, Goldy Carbunaru, MD, Ximena Lopez, MD, and Songya Pang, MD

CONTENTS

Summary

The concept that diseases such as the metabolic syndrome (MS) in males and females and polycystic ovary syndrome (PCOS) in females begin in adulthood no longer appears to be accurate. In adults, a major risk factor for development of coronary artery disease and type 2 diabetes is the presence of MS characterized by insulin resistance (IR), glucose intolerance, dyslipidemia, hypertension, and central obesity and, in women, the added feature of PCOS. An uncertain proportion of children with premature adrenarche (PA) appears at risk to develop these adult diseases, but it is not known who among them or when these PA subjects will ultimately manifest these clinical abnormalities. Therefore, the identification in childhood of risk factors or markers of PA for later development of these metabolic and endocrine disorders is of significant importance so that, ultimately, preventative therapy can be used to reduce the associated risk factors or antecedents of adult disease.

Key Words: Adrenarche; insulin resistance; PCOS; metabolic syndrome.

From: *Contemporary Endocrinology: Insulin Resistance and Polycystic Ovarian Syndrome: Pathogenesis, Evaluation, and Treatment*
Edited by: E. Diamanti-Kandarakis, J. E. Nestler, D. Panidis, and R. Pasquali © Humana Press Inc., Totowa, NJ

INTRODUCTION

Premature adrenarche (PA) is a disorder of premature secretion of adrenal androgens in young children (girls < 8 years and boys < 9 years) causing premature androgenic symptoms, including premature development of sexual hair, acne, body odor, and modest acceleration of linear and skeletal growth. The underlying mechanism of PA is unknown. The development of early signs of metabolic syndrome (MS) or of insulin-resistant polycystic ovary syndrome (PCOS) has been described in limited retrospective and prospective studies in children with PA as they mature through adolescence and into early adulthood. However, it is not known who among PA children is at risk of developing these disorders in adulthood. Although reduced insulin sensitivity in some children with PA was noted by our and other relatively small-scale studies, long-term outcome data of subjects with PA who have decreased insulin sensitivity is limited. Further, the preliminary observation suggesting a relationship between hyperinsulinemia of PA and pubertal or postpubertal functional ovarian hyperandrogenism related to PCOS must be verified. Thus, a long-term prospective study of a large cohort of children is essential to better define the childhood risk factor(s) in children with PA for ultimate development of adulthood MS or PCOS.

We will review a number of our studies that allow us to suggest that the risk factor(s) and marker(s) of children with PA associated with development of adulthood MS and PCOS may include the following:

1. Obesity.
2. Hispanic or African American (AA) vs Caucasian.
3. Decreased insulin sensitivity in childhood.
4. The phenotype of excessive adrenal Δ5-steroid secretion.

Better identification in children with PA of the risk factors for the development of adult diseases may ultimately lead to the timely use of therapy to prevent the occurrence of the adult MS and/or PCOS.

Adrenarche

Adrenarche refers to the onset of the production of the C19 steroids dehydro-epiandrosterone (DHEA) and DHEA-sulfate (DHEAS) from the zona reticularis beginning in mid-childhood *(1–3)*. The gradual increase in the amount of DHEA and DHEAS produced by the adrenal cortex provides precursors for the potent androgens testosterone and dihydrotestosterone in peripheral androgen-dependent tissue, and stimulates pubic and axillary hair growth in children of both sexes *(4,5)*. Similar effects of adrenal androgens in apocrine and sebaceous glands cause body odor and acne, respectively. To date, no single regulator for adrenarche has been identified. Adreno-corticotropic hormone (ACTH) exerts only a permissive role in adrenarche. Other suggested regulatory candidates for adrenarche, such as body mass *(6)*, insulin *(7)*, insulin-like growth factor (IGF)-1 *(8)*, or leptin *(9)*, have not been proven to be the sole factor in triggering adrenarche *(10)*. The current understanding of the production of DHEA and DHEAS in adrenarche is that it is the result of the concerted action of CYP11A with StAR *(11,12)*, CYP17 *(13)*, and SULT 2A1 *(11)* in the reticularis cells and the catalytic 17,20-lyase activity of CYP17 by the optimal cofactor protein cytochrome P450 oxidoreductase and B5 levels *(14,15)* in the absence of competing activity of 3β-hydroxysteroid dehydrogenase/Δ5-Δ4 isomerase enzyme *(10,11)*. This ensures metabolism of pregnenolone via the Δ5-steroid pathway to DHEA and DHEAS in the reticularis cells *(10)*.

The rise in adrenal androgens in childhood occurs prior to the increase of gonadal sex steroids *(16)* and is independent of gonadal maturation, leading to true puberty *(17–20)*. Normal female children develop clinical adrenarche at 11.6 ± 1.2 (SD) years *(21,22)* with a range between 8.5 and 13 years *(21–23)*. A recent report indicates that the age of onset of clinical adrenarche in the United States is, on average, 8.8 years in AA girls and 10.5 years in Caucasian girls *(24)*, but the possibility of a bias of adrenarchal age in this report exists because of the inclusion of cases with pathological precocious development *(25–27)*. In male children, clinical adrenarche occurs on average at 11–12.7 years *(28–31)* with a range between 9 and 14 years *(28–30)*, but no racially specific data for adrenarchal age is available for boys.

PREMATURE ADRENARCHE

Overview

PA is a relatively common disorder in children and is defined by the appearance of pubic and/or axillary hair caused by premature adrenal androgen secretion in the absence of breast development in girls before age 8 years, and in the absence of testicular development in boys before age 9 years *(19,20,25–27,32,33)*. The defining age for PA is still somewhat controversial *(25–27,32,34)*. In the majority of children with PA, the etiology of premature adrenal androgen secretion is unknown and is termed *idiopathic PA*. Idiopathic PA occurs in children of both sex, but more frequently in girls than in boys *(19,20,35,36)*. In children with PA, despite premature sexual hair growth and a tendency toward modestly increased growth velocity and skeletal age, true pubertal development and final height are not altered *(19,20,37–39)*. Thus, PA was considered to be a benign childhood aberration for many years *(19,20,35,36,39)*.

The proposed pathogenesis of PA involving altered regulation or phosphorylation of P450C17 *(40,41)*, similar to a postulated mechanism for insulin-resistant PCOS *(40–43)*, is yet to be proven. However, recent studies reported abnormal metabolic and endocrine profiles consistent with MS or pre-PCOS signs in children with PA *(44–53)* and possible MS and PCOS development in pubertal *(45,53,54)* or postpubertal females with a childhood history of PA *(39,54–56)*.

Observations in 24 to 35 post-pubertal females with a childhood history of PA in Northern Spain suggested occurrence of hirsutism, oligomenorrhea, and elevated androgen levels in slightly less than half of the females *(55,56)*. Also, in this study, slightly more than half of the oligomenorrheic females with a history of PA *(55,56)* had higher 17α-hydroxyprogesterone (17-OHP) responses to gonadotrophin releasing hormone (GnRH) analog (GnRHa) stimulation than either the eumenorrheic females with a history of PA or the control females *(55,56)*. This increased ovarian 17-OHP response to GnRHa stimulation was described as "functional ovarian hyperandrogenism" *(55,56)*, similar to the pattern of ovarian hormonal response observed in hyperandrogenic females with PCOS unrelated to PA history *(57,58)*. Anovulatory cycles were increased in postpubertal females with a history of PA and low birth-weight in the same population of Northern Spain *(54)*. These postpubertal Northern Spanish females with a history of PA as a group had a higher mean serum insulin response to oral glucose administration in both the PA females with and without functional ovarian hyperandrogenism *(55)*. In the postpubertal females with PA who had a lower birth-weight, a greater degree of hyperinsulinemia and dyslipidemia was reported *(59)*.

A cross-sectional study of a small group of pubertal females with a history of PA from Northern Spain suggested the occurrence of functional ovarian hyperandrogenism in about half of the females with PA *(45,60)*. However, in all of the reports from the Northern Spain studies *(55,56,59)*, no evaluation was made of obese (OB) vs non-obese (NOB) females with PA for PCOS or MS manifestations *(55,56,59)*. A preliminary report of a small scale study in the United States reported that only OB AA and Caribbean Hispanic adolescent females with a history of childhood obesity and PA were hyperinsulinemic and hyperandrogenic *(52,53)*. In contrast, pubertal females with a history of childhood PA in Finland had no hyperandrogenism *(39)*. These findings indicate a very strong association between PA and the manifestation of MS or PCOS in Northern Spain *(55,56,59)* and the previously studied US populations *(52,59)*, but little association for the same in Finland *(39)*, suggesting an environmental or racial propensity for PA to lead to MS or PCOS.

MS is characterized by glucose intolerance, dyslipidemia, hypertension, abdominal obesity, and insulin resistance (IR) in adults *(61–65)*. PCOS is characterized by clinical and biochemical hyperandrogenism and chronic anovulation with or without morphological changes of polycystic ovaries and is often associated with IR, frequently exacerbated by obesity *(66–70)*. A greater prevalence of MS is seen in women with PCOS *(71–77)*. The health consequences of MS or PCOS are paramount, as patients with these disorders are at risk of type 2 diabetes mellitus and/or cardiovascular disease and stroke *(61–65,75–77)*. Recent evidence indicates that the features of MS and PCOS are increasingly manifested in children and/or adolescents, as childhood obesity is on the rise *(78–85)*. Yet, as previously stated, in lean and obese children with PA, it is uncertain who among them will ultimately develop MS or PCOS as they mature and attain adulthood.

The Role of Obesity

Decreased insulin sensitivity (IS) (i.e., IR) is one of the key components in the pathogenesis of MS *(61–65,71,73,77,78)* and PCOS *(66–77)*. Studies of IS in relatively small groups of PA children by us *(47,48,51)* and other investigators *(44–46,49,50,87)* demonstrate heterogeneous manifestations of decreased IS by various parameters in the same *(47–51)* and differing populations of children with PA children *(47–51,86,87)*. A relatively small group of prepubertal girls with PA from Northern Spain had somewhat higher body mass index (BMI) than control non-PA girls, and had increased mean serum insulin levels and early insulin response to oral glucose administration, but a comparison between OB and NOB PA girls was not made *(45,46)*.

However, limited studies of prepubertal PA girls of Hispanic ethnicity and AA race in the United States *(47–50)* including our studies *(47,48,86)* revealed that almost all OB PA girls had decreased IS and almost all NOB PA girls had greater IS by fasting glucose-to-insulin ratio (FGIR) *(47,48; see* Table 1) or by IS index (S_1) assessment by an intravenous glucose tolbutamide test *(48,49)*. Moreover, IS determined by an oral glucose tolerance test (OGTT) in OB PA girls did not differ from the OB control girls, despite higher androgen levels in PA girls than in the control girls *(47,48)*. These

Table 1
Clinical Characteristics and Measures of Insulin Sensitivity in PA and Non-PA Girls

	Clinical characteristics			Measures of insulin sensitivity					
	Age (yr)	BMI (kg/m^2)	BMI z-score	FGIR	QUICKI	Fasting I (µU/mL)	FIRI	SiM	ISI (comp)
Obese PA IR	7.3*	26.6	5.7	4.2	0.30	26.9	5.6	1.4	8.57
(n = 7)	(0.32)	(2.21)	(0.98)	(0.71)	(0.01)	(6.59)	(1.59)	(0.40)	(1.82)
Non-obese PA IS	6.7	17.9	1.7	13	0.36	7.7	1.4	6.9	26.5
(n = 11)	(0.24)	(0.98)	(0.55)	(1.98)	(0.01)	(0.83)	(0.14)	(1.17)	(3.32)
Control obese	8.4	31.0	6.0	4.7	0.30	34.7	7.5	0.83	7.94
(n = 7)	(0.70)	(1.34)	(0.41)	(1.18)	(0.01)	(13.54)	(2.91)	(0.21)	(2.21)

*Mean
(± SE)
FGIR: fasting glucose to insulin ratio, IR: insulin resistant, IS: insulin sensitive, QUICKI: quantitative IS check index, Fasting I: Fasting Insulin, FIRI: fasting IR index, SiM: adjusted mean measure of IS based on fasting and 120 min insulin and glucose levels, ISI (comp): composite whole body IS index. (Adapted from ref. 47.)

findings suggest that the decreased IS in these PA female children is related to obesity. Further, a preliminary observation suggests that only adolescent females with a history of PA who remain OB from childhood manifest hyperinsulinemia and hyperandrogenism (52,53). However, early evidence of dyslipidemia was present in both groups of girls with PA, including those with IR and those with greater IS, compared with age- and sex-matched national normative data (47). The odds ratio of dyslipidemia was much greater, however, in the obese PA girls with IR than in the NOB PA girls with IS (47; see Table 2). This hypothesis suggests that in children with PA, obesity is a key risk factor for decreased IS and therefore a risk for later development of MS or PCOS, and may compound the dyslipidemia associated with PA (47).

The Role of Ethnicity

The fact that decreased IS in subjects with PA has been predominately observed in Hispanic and AA populations in the United States and in Northern Spanish populations (44–47,49,50,86) and not in other populations suggests that in children with PA, race/ethnicity is an independent risk factor for MS or PCOS development. Race/ethnicity are known to be an independent risk factor for IR PCOS development in women (88–90). Caribbean Hispanic women with PCOS manifest a greater degree of IR than non-Hispanic females with PCOS (88). Lower IS in AA children compared with Caucasian children is well known (91–95), and this difference was suggested to be independent of body and visceral fat (96). Lower IS in Hispanic children has also been suggested to be independent of obesity (97). Most recently, development of MS was assessed in 600 white and black girls by a longitudinal study of BMI, insulin, glucose, homeostasis model assessment, lipids, and blood pressure, as well as waist circumference at ages 9–10 and 18–19 years. Although only one girl of each race had three markers of MS at ages 9–10, 3.5% of AA girls vs 2.3% of Caucasian girls had these symptoms at ages 18–19 years (97).

Table 2
Lipid Levels for PA and Control Obese Girls

	Cholesterol (mg/dL)	LDL (mg/dL)	HDL (mg/dL)	Triglycerides (mg/dL)	Odds ratio ↑ TG, ↓ HDL
OB PA IR	162.3	101	41.9	97.4	14.2, 7.9
(FGIR ≥ 7, n = 7)	(11.74)*	(10.25)	(4.64)	(22.19)	
NOB PA IS	157.6	101.1	42.7	69.0	4.2, 7.4
(FGIR < 7, n = 11)	(7.74)	(5.75)	(2.89)	(8.06)	
Control obese (n = 7)	161.3	105.1	38.9	86.0	
	(10.15)	(8.69)	(2.97)	(11.41)	
National Norm**	163.7	100.4	53.2	60.3	

* mean (± SE); ** The Lipid Research Clinics Population Studies Data Book, Bethesda: *NIH Publication* 80-1527, 1980. (Adapted from ref. *47*.)

Our preliminary data also suggest that the majority of PA children with decreased IS are of Hispanic and AA origin in both girls and boys with PA. In 114 girls with PA (authors' unpublished data), obesity, measured as a BMI z-score greater than 2, was high in all three ethnic/racial groups (56% Hispanic, 68% AA, and 77% in Caucasian groups). However, IR defined by FGIR of less than seven in girls with PA was greater in Hispanic (60%) and AA (50%) girls than in Caucasians (29%). Because of the limited number of subjects, no valid comparison could be made.

In addition, our preliminary pilot long-term prospective study of girls with documented PA suggests a greater occurrence rate of hyperandrogenic symptoms in Hispanic and AA females than in Caucasian females during pubertal maturation and postpuberty (*see* Table 3). We hypothesize that in children with PA, Hispanics and AAs are independent risk factors for the later development of MS or PCOS.

Association With Decreased Insulin Sensitivity

Although decreased IS in children with PA has been presumed to be a risk factor for the future development of metabolic or endocrine disorders, the long-term significance of biochemical evidence of decreased IS in children with PA is yet to be characterized. Long-term follow-up of children with PA who have decreased or normal IS during childhood is limited *(53)*. Although functional ovarian hyperandrogenism or signs of possible PCOS and hyperinsulinemia in pubertal or postpubertal females with childhood history of PA have been documented, these subjects did not have an IS evaluation during childhood *(54–56)*. A study of females with a history of PA and low or normal birth-weight reported increased mean serum insulin levels as a group in childhood, but no outcome data specifically related to decreased vs normal IS during childhood is available *(59)*. Only a preliminary observation suggested that OB hyperandrogenic adolescent females with a history of PA were OB and hyperinsulinemic from childhood *(53)*. Our preliminary studies are too limited at this time to offer conclusions, but of 10 girls with PA proven to be IR by an FGIR of less than seven or S_i less than three by frequently sampled intravenous glucose tolerance test (FSIVGTT), three had hirsutism, and all three girls more than 3 years postmenarache had secondary amenorrhea or oligomenorrhea.

Table 3
Hirsutism and Menstrual Disorders in PA Girls
During Pubertal Maturation and Postmenarche

# of PA girls in true puberty with breast stage > Tanner 2		Hirsutism	Menstrual disorders
Race	Number	(No. and percent)	(postmenarche > 3 yr)
African American	14	8/14* (57%)	2/2 (100%)
Hispanic	4	3/4 (75%)	1/1 (100%)
Caucasian	6	1/6 (16%)	0/0 (0%)
Total	24	12/24 (50%)	3/3 (100%)

*No. of PA / total # PA studied (%).

Association With Excess Δ5-Steroid Secretion

Although children with PA are prematurely exposed to a hyperandrogenic state for age, adrenal androgen levels are generally within the level expected for the stage of pubic hair development (3,16–20). A subset of children with PA, however, manifest progressively increased adrenal Δ5-steroid secretion, including androgens. This has been reported in 9–28% of PA populations (98–104), including our study (101–103).

Twenty-five percent of young women with PCOS who exhibit hirsutism and menstrual disorders also have excessive adrenal Δ5-steroid secretion, which results in adrenal hyperandrogenism (105–109). The phenotype of excess Δ5-steroid secretion, including elevated Δ5-steroid levels (Δ5-17α-hydroxypregnenolone, DHEA, and DHEAS) (98–104), in this subset of children with PA (48,98–104,110) and in women with hirsutism and menstrual disorders (103–108,110–111) was previously misinterpreted as having nonclassic 3β-hydroxysteroid dehydrogenase (3β-HSD) deficiency. The normal type II 3β-HSD gene sequence in children with PA (48,101–103) and in hirsute women with excessive adrenal Δ5-steroid secretion indicates that this condition is not caused by nonclassic 3β-HSD deficiency (48,101). The fact that a significant number of girls with PA (48,100–103,110) and adolescents and young women with hyperandrogenism (48,103–111) exhibit excess adrenal Δ5-steroid secretion indicates that this is a common hormonal phenotype from childhood to adulthood (48,103) (Table 4). The pathogenic mechanism of excess Δ5-steroid secretion in this subset of children with PA and hyperandrogenic females is uncertain. A proposed hypothesis, such as altered phosphorylation of P450 as a mechanism for the excessive adrenal Δ5-steroid secretion, is plausible but not yet proven (40,41).

Our studies in hyperandrogenic females (14–36 years of age) with excessive adrenal Δ5-steroid secretion resulting in adrenal hyperandrogenism revealed marked IR and luteinizing hormone (LH) hypersecretion characteristic of PCOS. IS was investigated by FSIVGTT and OGTT and gonadotropin secretion by GnRH stimulation in hirsute females (HF) with menstrual disorders who exhibited excessive adrenal Δ5-steroid secretion. We compared IS (Table 5) and gonadotropin secretion (Table 6) of these HF to HF with classic PCOS exhibiting normal adrenal Δ5-steroid secretion.

S_1, regardless of normal or high BMI in all six HF with excessive adrenal Δ5-steroids and in all HF with classic PCOS, was significantly lower than S_1 in normal females

Table 4

Clinical and Hormonal Data of Normal Hyperandrogenic Females (HF) With Excessive Adrenal Δ5-Steroid Secretion and HF With Classic PCOS and Normal Adrenal Δ5-Steroid Secretion (Mean ± SE)

Subjects (n)	Age at study (yr)	Age at menarche (yr)	No. of PA by History	Random T (ng/dL)	ACTH stimulated Δ5-steroids (mean ± SE)				
					Δ5-17P (ng/dL)	DHEA (ng/dL)	Δ5-17P/ 17-OHP	Δ5-17P/ F	DHEA/ Δ4-A
Normal females (n = 30)	26 ± 1.3	10–15	0	29 ± 2.1	952 ± 62	1144 ± 68	5.2 ± 0.3	32 ± 2	4.6 ± 0.3
HF with ↑ adrenal Δ5-steroid secretion (n = 6)	18 ± 1.2	9–14	3/6	51 ± 9.3	2464 ± 353	3661 ± 513	32 ± 17	77 ± 14	14 ± 2.4
HF with classic PCOS and normal adrenal Δ5-steroid secretion (n = 9)	23 ± 2.3	11–14	2/9	95 ± 8.6	866 ± 111	1372 ± 185	5.5 ± 1.0	28.6 ± 5	5 ± 0.73

T: Testosterone, Δ5-17P: 17OH Pregnenolone, 17OHP: 17-OH Progesterone, Δ4-A: Androstenedione, Δ5 17P / 17OHP: ng %/ng %, Δ5 17P/F: ng %/μg %, DHEA/Δ4-A: (Adapted from ref. 48.)

Table 5

Insulin Sensitivity in Hyperandrogenic Females (HF) With the Phenotype of Excessive Adrenal Δ5-Steroid Secretion, With Classic PCOS, in Normal and High Body Mass Index Controls

Group (mean ± SE)	Age at study (yr)	BMI: kg/M²	S1 ($\times 10^{-4min}/\mu U/mL$)	IIIns[c] (μU/mL × min)	AUCi (min × μU/mL)	AUCg (min × μU/mL)
NL BMI control females (n = 8–9)	24 ± 3.5	21 ± 0.4	16 ± 5.9	1909 ± 433	4329 ± 969	4650 ± 701
High BMI control females (n = 5)	27 ± 3.2	28 ± 0.6	10.5 ± 6.3	4003 ± 1319	7459 ± 2479	3735 ± 979
HF with phenotype of excess adrenal Δ5-steroids (n = 5–6)	18 ± 1.2	32[b] ± 2.2	0.68[a] ± 0.23	17637[a] ± 5306	27262[a] ± 5981	8773[a] ± 634
HF with classic PCOS (n = 7–8)	23 ± 2.3	34[a] ± 2.1	0.94[a] ± 0.36	14848[a] ± 3078	18352[a] ± 5889	8095 ± 2725

No significant differences in any parameter between HF with ↑ adrenal Δ5-steroid phenotype vs HF with classic PCOS.
[a]p < 0.05 – 0.0001 in the HF compared to each NL ard high BMI controls.
[b]p< 0.05 in the HF compared to only NL BMI controls.
[c]Integrated Incremental Insulin. (Adapted from ref. 48.)

Table 6
Gonadotropin Parameters in Hyperandrogenic Females (HF) With Excessive Adrenal
Δ5-Steroid Secretion, With Classic PCOS, and in Normal and High Body Mass Index Controls

Basal = mean of 4 values	Baseline: mean ± SE			Peak GnRH stimulated: mean ± SE		
	LH (U/mL)	FSH (U/mL)	LH/FSH	LH (U/mL)	FSH (U/mL)	LH/FSH
Control female NL with NL and high BMI ($n = 11$)	3.8 ± 0.46	8.8 ± 1.6	0.48 ± 0.06	15 ± 1.7	12.4 ± 1.9	1.3 ± 0.17
HF with ↑ adrenal Δ5 steroids ($n = 5–6$)	5.2 ± 1.2	4.9 ± 0.44	1.1 ± 0.24[a]	27 ± 5.9[a]	8.4 ± 0.83	3.2 ± 0.6[a]
HF with classic PCOS ($n = 7–8$)	7.2 ± 0.92[a]	4 ± 0.42[b]	17 ± 0.17[a]	36.1 ± 9.4[a]	6.8 ± 1.0[b]	4.7 ± 0.6[b]

[a] $p < 0.05 – 0.0001$ in the HF group to the combined ($n = 11$) normal ($n = 8$) and high ($n = 3$) BMI controls.

[b] $p < 0.05 – 0.0001$ in the HF compared to combined controls.

GnRH stimulation test was performed during the early follicular phase in those with regular menstrual cycle history. (Adapted from ref. *48*.)

with normal or high BMI (Table 5). Integrated incremental insulin (IIIn), irrespective of normal or high BMI in all HF with excessive adrenal Δ5-steroids and in five out of seven HF with classic PCOS, was higher than in normal females with normal or high BMI. There was no significant difference in S_1 or IIIn between the HF with excess adrenal Δ5-steroids and HF with classic PCOS. Insulin area-under-the-curve (AUCinsulin) and glucose area-under-the-curve (AUCglucose) during an OGTT in HF with excessive adrenal Δ5-steroids and in HF with classic PCOS were significantly higher than in the normal females with normal or high BMI. There was no significant difference in AUCinsulin and AUCglucose between HF with excessive adrenal Δ5-steroid secretion and HF with classic PCOS. Our findings of similarly low S_1 and high IIIn and AUCinsulin in HF with excessive adrenal Δ5-steroid secretion and in HF with classic PCOS, irrespective of BMI, suggests the presence of similar degrees of marked IR in both groups of HF females independent of obesity.

The basal LH-to-follicle-stimulating hormone (FSH) ratio and GnRH-stimulated peak LH levels and LH-to-FSH ratio in HF with excess adrenal Δ5-steroids were significantly higher than in normal females and were similar to HF with classic PCOS (Table 6). There were no significant differences in the basal and GnRH-stimulated peak LH and FSH levels and LH-to-FSH ratios between HF with excess adrenal Δ5-steroids and HF with classic PCOS. Marked IR and LH hypersecretion in the HF with excessive adrenal Δ5-steroid secretion causing adrenal hyperandrogenism (and mimicking 3β-HSD-deficiency phenotype) were nearly identical to those of HF with classic PCOS who had excess ovarian androgen secretion. Further, our additional preliminary study of young, NOB adolescent females with PCOS features also demonstrated higher levels of LH and DHEAS than in their OB counterparts (*112*; Table 7).

Additionally, our preliminary study in girls with PA who have excessive adrenal Δ5-steroid secretion revealed a trend of decreased IS compared with AA girls without excessive adrenal Δ5-steroid secretion (*see* Table 6). A positive relationship between increased adrenal Δ5-steroid profile and decreased IS in children with PA *(49)* and a preliminary observation of IR and hyperandrogenism in adolescent females with childhood PA and increased Δ5-steroid levels were also reported by others *(53)*. Our limited follow-up of girls with PA who had excessive adrenal Δ5-steroid secretion showed hyperandrogenism and IR in adolescence. Thus, we hypothesize that the phenotype of excess adrenal Δ5-steroid secretion in girls with PA may be associated with decreased IS and is a risk marker for development of IR PCOS in later life.

Body Composition

The association of visceral adiposity and intramyocellular lipid (IMCL) with IR has been established in adults and OB children and adolescents *(113)*. Women with PCOS also tend to have abdominal adiposity. To date, there are only two published reports of body composition in PA. Sopher et al. *(119)* evaluated lean body components by multiple methods in girls with and without PA, and found greater bone mass by dual energy X-ray absorptiometry (DEXA) in subjects with PA. In this same group of girls, the ratio of DEXA trunk to total fat was significantly greater in the girls with PA compared with controls (unpublished data). Ibanez et al. *(120)* evaluated body composition by DEXA in 67 girls with PA or a history of PA, ages 6–18 years, and 65 controls. The BMI of subjects with PA did not differ from controls, but the girls with PA had significantly greater waist circumference, waist-to-hip ratio, total fat mass, percentage fat mass, and truncal fat mass at each pubertal stage. Truncal fat was found to be significantly related to fasting insulin and free androgen index. DEXA, however, cannot distinguish between subcutaneous and visceral adipose tissue, which are metabolically distinct depots.

The presence of increased trunk fat by DEXA in prepubertal girls with PA compared with BMI-match controls, and its correlation with hyperinsulinism, suggests that there may be an increase in visceral adipose tissue in girls with PA. In addition, as noted previously, increased IMCL, a marker of skeletal IR, has been demonstrated in children who are OB and IR, as well as in thin, young adult offspring of parents with type 2 diabetes *(121)*. We hypothesized that girls with PA would have increased visceral adipose tissue and IMCL, independent of total body adiposity. We also suggested that the pattern of fat distribution and lipid deposition in PA would be an independent predictor of insulin sensitivity and cardiovascular risk factors, and related to alterations in the IGF-1/IGFBP/insulin axis. To test this hypothesis we performed a pilot study to determine abdominal fat depots by magnetic resonance imaging (MRI) and IMCL by magnetic resonance spectroscopy in girls with PA and age- and BMI-matched healthy, prepubertal controls. The study also included an OGTT, lipid profile, and IGF-1 and IGFBP-1 levels on all subjects.

Initial analysis of early subjects demonstrated a significant increase in IMCL deposition in the girls with PA (Table 8; Fig. 1). Volumes of visceral adipose tissue and subcutaneous adipose tissue did not differ between the two groups. Analysis of metabolic parameters is ongoing and may allow for identification of features that are predictive of MS even at a young age.

The clinical and biochemical findings reviewed here strongly suggest that in children with PA, the identification of risk factors or markers for later development of

Table 7
Hormonal Characteristics of Nonobese Patients With PCOS, Obese Patients With PCOS, and Obese Control Females

	LH (mIU/mL)	FSH (mIU/mL)	T (ng/dL)	Free T (pg/mL)[e]	DHT (ng/dL)	Δ4-A (ng/dL)	DHEAS (μg/dL)	SHBG (μg/dL)
Nonobese PCOS (n = 11)	14.9 ± 5.9[a]	6.2 ± 1.5	58.4 ± 20.4	10.9 ± 3.8	17.9 ± 8.5[b]	242.5 ± 46.3[b]	205.3 ± 76.3[a]	0.9 ± 0.4[a]
Obese PCOS (n = 22)	9.5 ± 5.2	5.5 ± 1.6	49.8 ± 18.7	11.5 ± 4.8	9.6 ± 3.4	184.4 ± 52.6	146.1 ± 68.8	0.5 ± 0.2
Obese Controls (n = 15)	3.5 ± 2.3[c]	4.8 ± 2.8	18.4 ± 7.5	3.1 ± 1.4	7.6 ± 3.5	101.7 ± 35.6	92.7 ± 49.9	0.8 ± 0.3[d]

Values are the mean ± SD.

[a] $p < 0.05$ for the nonobese vs. obese PCOS.
[b] $p < 0.01$ for the nonobese vs. obese PCOS.
[c] $P < 0.001$ for obese PCOS vs. obese control.
[d] $p < 0.05$ for obese PCOS vs. obese control.
[e] $n = 21$ for obese PCOS. (Adapted from ref. 112.)

Table 8
Demographics of Study Subjects for MRS Analysis

	Premature adrenarche (n = 4)	Controls (n = 3)
Age (years)	7.7 ± 0.8	8.5 ± 2.0
Ethnicity	3 H, 1 AA	1 A, 1 H, 1 AA
BMI z-score	0.8 ± 0.8	0.4 ± 0.9
%body fat (DXA)	26.1 ± 6.8	26.8 ± 10.1

AA = African-American; H = Hispanic; A = Asian.
Mean ± SD.

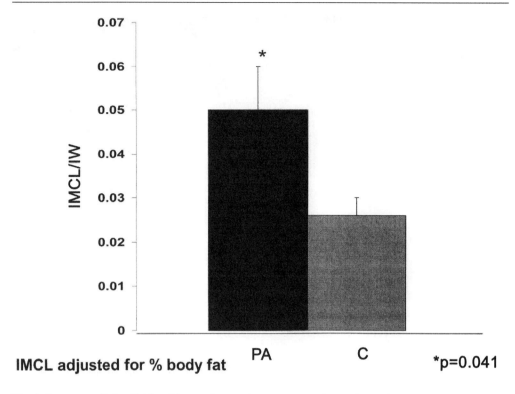

Fig. 1. Intramyocellular lipid and internal water in premature adrenarche and control patients. IMCL, intramyocellular lipid; IW, intramyocellular water.

metabolic and endocrine disorders (MS and PCOS) is of significant importance, and may ultimately point the way to preventative therapy to reduce the development of disease in adulthood.

FUTURE AVENUES

Additional studies are needed to verify the preliminary findings herein and to allow for preventative therapy to reduce the risk factors in PA for developing MS.

KEY POINTS

- Obesity is a key risk factor for decreased IS and, therefore, is a risk for later development of the MS or PCOS, and may compound the dyslipidemia associated with PA.
- In Hispanic and African-American children with PA, race/ethnicity may be an independent risk factor for the later development of MS and PCOS.
- The phenotype of excessive adrenal Δ5-steroid secretion in girls with PA may be associated with decreased IS and is a risk marker for development of insulin-resitant PCOS in later life.
- Preliminary data has demonstrated a significant increase in intramyocellular lipid deposition in girls with PA.

REFERENCES

1. Dhom G. The prepubertal and pubertal growth of the adrenal (adrenarche). Beitr Pathol 1973;150:357–377.
2. Smith MK, Rudd BT, Shirley A, et al. A radioimmunoassay for the estimation of serum dehydro-epiandrosterone sulfate in normal and pathological sera. Clin Chem Acta 1975;65:5–13.
3. dePeretti E, Forest M. Unconjugated dehydroepiandrosterone plasma levels in normal subjects from birth to adolescence in humans: the use of a sensitive radioimmunoassay. J Clin Endocrinol Metab 1976;43:982–991.
4. Hay JB, Hodgins MB. Distribution of androgen metabolizing enzymes in isolated tissue of human forehead and axillary skin. J Endocrinol 1978;79:29–39.
5. Labrie F, Luu-The V, Labrie C, El Alfy M. Intracrinology and the skin. Horm Res 2000;54:218–229.
6. Remer T, Manz F. Role of nutritional status in the regluation of adrenarche. J Clin Endocrinol Metab 1999;84:3936–3944.
7. Guercio G, Rivarola MA, Charler E, Maceiras M, Belgorosky A. Relationship between the growth hormone/insulin like growth factor- I axis, insulin sensitivity and adrenal androgens in normal prepubertal and pubertal girls. J Clin Endocrinol Metab 2003;88:1389–1393.
8. L'Allemand D, Penhoat A, Lebrethon MC, et al. Inuslin like growth factor enhances steroidogenic enzyme and corticotropin receptor messenger ribonucleic acid levels and corticotropin steroidgenic responsiveness in cultured human adrenocortical cells. J Clin Endocrinol Metab 1996;81:3892–3897.
9. Biason-Lauber A, Zachmann M, Schoenle EJ. Effect of Leptin on CYP17 enzymatic activities in human adrenal cells: new insight in the onset of adrenarche. Endocrinology 2000;141:1446–1456.
10. Auchus RJ, Rainey WE. Adrenarche—physiology, biochemistry, and human disease. Clin Endocrinol 2004;60:288–294.
11. Suzuki T, Sasano H, Takeyama J, et al. Developmental changes in steroidogenic enzymes in human postnatal adrenal cortex: immunohistochemical studies. Clin Endocrinol 2000;53:739–747.
12. Stocco DM. The steroidogenic acute regulatory (StAR) protein two years later an update. Endocrine 1997;6:99–109.
13. Miller WL. Early steps in androgen biosynthesis: from cholesterol to DHEA. Bailliere's Clin Endocrinol Metab 1998;12:67–81.
14. Katagiri M, Kagawa N, Waterman MR. The role of cytochrome b5 in the biosynthesis of androgens by human P450c17. Arch Biochem Biophys 1995;317:343–347.
15. Auchus RJ, Lee TC, Miller WL. Cytochrome b5 augments the 17-20 lyse activity of human P450c17 without direct electron transfer. J Biol Chem 1998;273:3158–3165.
16. Korth-Schutz S, Levine LS, New MI. Serum androgens in normal prepubertal and pubertal children with precocious adrenarche. J Clin Endocrinol Metab 1976;42:117–124.
17. Grumbach MM, Richards GE, Conte FA, Kaplan SL. Clinical disorders of adrenal function and puberty: an assessment of the role of the adrenal cortex in normal and abnormal puberty in man and evidence for an ACTH-like pituitary adrenal androgen stimulation hormone. In: James VHT, Serio M, Giusti G, Martini L (eds). *The Endocrine Function of the Human Adrenal Cortex.* Serono Symposium 18. Academic Press, London, 1978; pp. 583–612.
18. Sklar CA, Kaplan SL, Grumbach MM. Evidence for dissociation between adrenarche and gonadarche: studies in patients with idiopathic precocious puberty, gonadal dysgenesis, isolated gonadotropin deficiency, and constitutionally delayed growth and adolescence. J Clin Endocrinol Metab 1980; 51:548–556.
19. Pang S. Premature adrenarche. Pediatr Adol Endocrinol 1984;13:173–184.
20. Pang S. Precocious thelarche and premature adrenarche predictors. Pediatr Ann 1981;10:340–345.
21. Marshall WA, Tanner JM. Variations in patterns of pubertal changes in girls. Arch Dis Child 1969;44: 291–303.
22. Ratcliffe SG, Butler GE, Jones M. Edingburogh study of growth and development of children with sex chromosome abnormalities IV. Birth Defects Original Article Ser 1990;26:1–44.
23. Roche AF, Wellens R, Attie KM, Siervogel RM. The timing of sexual maturation in a group of us white youth. J Pediatr Endocrinol 1995;8:11–18.
24. Herman-Giddens ME, Slora EJ, Wasserman RC, et al. Secondary sexual characteristics and menses in young girls seen in office practice: a study from the pediatric research in office setting network. Pediatrics 1997;99:505–512.

25. Viner R. Splitting hairs: is puberty getting earlier in girls? Arch Dis Child 2002;86:8–10.
26. Bauer A, Francis GL, Merrily P. Review of precocious puberty: part iii premature thelarche and premature adrenarche variations of normal? Endocrinologist 2001;11:196–203.
27. Rosenfield RL, Bachrach LK, Chernausek SD, et al. Current age of onset of puberty. Pediatrics 2000;106:622–623.
28. Preece M, Camerson MA, Donmall MC. The endocrinology of male puberty. In: Borms J, Hauspie RC, Sands A, eds. Human Growth and Development. New York, Plenum, 1984, pp. 23–27.
29. Marshall WA, Tanner JM. Variations in the pattern of pubertal changes in boys. Arch Dis Child 1970;45:13–23.
30. Lee PA. Normal ages of pubertal events among American males and females. J Adolesc Health Care 1980;1:26–29.
31. Biro FM, Lucky AW, Huster GA, Morrisen JA. Pubertal staging in boys. J Pediatr 1995;127:100–102.
32. Midyett LK, Moore WV, Jacobson JD. Are pubertal changes in girls before age 8 benign? Pediatrics 2003;111:47–51.
33. Ibanez L, Dimartino-Nardi J, Potau N, Saenger P. Premature adrenarche– normal variant or forerunner of adult disease? Endocr Rev 2000;21:671–696.
34. Kaplowitz PB, Oberfield SE. Reexamination of the age limit for defining when puberty is precocious in girls in the United States: implications for evaluation and treatment. Drug and Therapeutics Executive Committees of the Lawson Wikins Pediatric Endocrine Society. Pediatrics 1999;104:936–941.
35. Silverman SH, Migeon CJ, Rosenberg E, Wilkins L. Precocious growth of sexual hair without other secondary sexual development: "premature pubarche," a constitutional variation of adolescence. Pediatrics 1952;10:426–432.
36. Sigurjonsdottir TJ, Hayes AS. Premature pubarche. Clin Pediatr (Phila) 1968;7:29–33.
37. Ibanez L, Virdis R, Potau N, et al. Natural history of premature pubarche: an auxological study. J Clin Endocrinol Metab 1992;72:254–257.
38. Ghizzoni L, Milani S. The natural history of premature adrenarche. J Pediatr Endocrinol Metab 2000;13:1247–1251.
39. Pere A, Perheentupa J, Peter M, Voutilainen R. Follow-up of growth and steroids in premature adrenarche. Eur J Pediatr 1995;154:346–352.
40. Zhang LH, Rodriguez H, Ohno S, Miller WL. Serine phosphorylation of human P450c17 increases 17, 20 lyase activity: implications for adrenarche and the polycystic ovary syndrome. Proc Natl Acad Sci USA 1995;92:10,619–10,623.
41. Miller WL. The molecular basis of premature adrenarche and hypothesis. Acta Paediatr Supplement 1999;88:60–66.
42. Dunaif A. Insulin resistance and the polycystic ovary syndrome: mechanisms and implications for pathogenesis. Endocr Rev 1997;18:774–800.
43. Chin CE, Dickens M, Tavare JM, Roth RA. Overexpression of protein kinase c isoenzymes α, $\beta 1$, ν and ε in cells over expressing the inuslin recptor phosphorylation and signaling. J Biol 1993;268:6338–6347.
44. Oppenheimer E, Linder B, DiMartino-Nardi J. Decreased insulin sensitivity in prepubertal girls with premature adrenarche and *Acanthosis nigricans*. J Clin Endocrinol Metab 1995;80:614–618.
45. Ibanez L, Potau N, Zampolli M, Rique S, Saenger P, Carrascosa A. Hyperinsulinemia and decreased insulin-like growth factor-binding protein-1 are common features in prepubertal and pubertal girls with a history of premature pubarche. J Clin Endocrinol Metab 1997;82:2283–2288.
46. Ibanez L, Potau N, Chacon P, Pascual C, Carrascosa A. Hyperinsulinaemia, dyslipaemia and cardio-vascular risk in girls with a history of premature pubarche. Diabetologia 1998;41:1057–1063.
47. Silfen ME, Manibo AM, McMahon DJ, Levine LS, Murphy AR, Oberfield SE. Comparison of simple measures of insulin sensitivity in young girls with premature adrenarche: the fasting glucose to insulin ratio may be a simple and useful measure. J Clin Endocrinol Metab 2001;86:2863–2868.
48. Carbunaru G, Prasad P, Scoccia B, et al. The hormonal phenotype of 3β-hydroxysteroid dehydrogenase (HSD3B) deficiency diagnosed in hyperandrogenic females is associated with insulin resistant polycystic ovary syndrome and is not due to a variant of HSD3B2 deficiency congenital adrenal hyperplasia. J Clin Endocrinol Metab 2004;89:783–794.
49. Vuguin P, Linder B, Rosenfeld RG, Saenger P, DiMartino-Nardi J. The roles of insulin sensitivity, insulin-like growth factor I (IGF-I), and IGF-binding protein-1 and -3 in the hyperandrogenism of African-American and Caribbean Hispanic girls with premature adrenarche. J Clin Endocrinol Metab 1999;84:2037–2042.

50. Vuguin P, Saenger P, DiMartino-Nardi J. Fasting glucose insulin ratio: a useful measure of insulin resistance in girls with premature adrenarche. J Clin Endocrinol Metab 2001;86:4618–4621.
51. Denburg MR, Silfen ME, Manibo AM, et al. Insulin sensitivity and the insulin-like growth factor system in prepubertal boys with premature adrenarche. J Clin Endocrinol Metab 2002;87:5604–5609.
52. DiMartino-Nardi J. Premature adrenarche: findings in prepubertal African-American and Caribbean-Hispanic Girls. Acta Paediatr Supplement 1999;88:67–72.
53. DiMartino-Nardi J. Pre- and postpubertal findings in premature adrenarche. J Clin Endocrinol Metab 2000;13:1265–1269.
54. Ibanez L, de Zegher F, Potau N. Anovulation after precocious pubarche: early markers and time course in adolescence. J Clin Endocrinol Metab 1999;84:2691–2695.
55. Ibanez L, Potau N, Zampolli M, et al. Hyperinsulinemia in postpubertal girls with a history of premature pubarche and functional ovarian hyperandrogenism. J Clin Endocrinol Metab 1996;81:1237–1243.
56. Ibanez L, Potau N, Virdis R, et al. Postpubertal outcome in girls diagnosed of premature pubarche during childhood: increased frequency of functional ovarian hyperandrogenism. J Clin Endocrinol Metab 1993;76:1599–1603.
57. Ehrmann DA, Rosenfield RL, Barnes RB, Brigell DF, Sheikh Z. Detection of functional ovarian hyperandrogenism in women with androgen excess. N Engl J Med 1992;327:157–162.
58. Barnes RB, Rosenfield R, Burstein S, Ehrmann DA. Pituitary-ovarian response to nafarelin testing in the polycystic ovary syndrome. N Engl J Med 1989;320:559–565.
59. Ibanez L, Valls C, Potau N, Marcos MV, de Zegher F. Polycystic ovary syndrome after precocious pubarche: ontogeny of the low-birthweight effect. Clin Endocrinol 2001;55:667–672.
60. Ibanez L, Potau N, Zampolli M, Street ME, Carrascosa A. Girls diagnosed with premature pubarche show an exaggerated ovarian androgen synthesis from the early stages of puberty: evidence from gonadotropin-releasing hormone agonist testing. Fertil Steril 1997;67:845–855.
61. Reaven GM. Banting lecture 1988. Role of insulin resistance in human disease. Diabetes 1988;37:1595–1607.
62. National Institute of Health. Third Report of the National Cholesterol Education Program Expert Panel on Detection, Evaluation, and Treatment of High Lipid Cholesterol in Adults (Adult Treatment Panel III) Executive Summary, Bethesda MD. National Institute of Health, National Heart, Lung and Blood Institute, 2001.
63. Scott CL. Diagnosis, prevention, and intervention for the metabolic syndrome. Am J Cardiol 2003;92:35i–42i.
64. Brunzell JD, Ayyobi AF. Dyslipidemia in the metabolic syndrome and type 2 diabetes mellitus. Am J Med 2003;115:24S–28S.
65. Gonzalez MA, Selwyn AP. Endothelial function, inflammation and prognosis in cardiovascular disease. Am J Med 2003;115:99S–106S.
66. The Rotterdam ESHRE/ASRM-Sponsored PCOS Consensus Workshop Group. Revised 2003 consensus on diagnostic criteria and long-term health risks related to polycystic ovary syndrome. Fertil Steril 2004;81:19–25.
67. Hart R, Hickey M, Franks S. Definitions, prevalence and symptoms of polycystic ovaries and polycystic ovary syndrome. Best Pract Res Clin Obstet Gynecol 2004;18:671–683.
68. Balen A, Michelmore K. What is polycystic ovary syndrome? Are national views important? Hum Reprod 2002;17:2219–2227.
69. Homburg R. What is polycystic ovary syndrome? A proposal for a consensus on the definition and diagnosis of polycystic ovarian syndrome. Hum Reprod 2002;17:2495–2499.
70. Azziz R. PCOS: a diagnostic challenge. Reprod Biomed Online 2004;8:644–648.
71. Legro RS, Kunselman AR, Dodson WC, Dunaif A. Prevalence and predictors of risk for type 2 diabetes mellitus and impaired glucose tolerance in polycystic ovary syndrome: a prospective, controlled study in 254 affected women. J Clin Endocrinol Metab 1999;84:165–169.
72. Sam S, Dunaif A. Polycystic ovary syndrome: Syndrome XX? Trends Endocrinol Metab 2003;14:365–370.
73. Apridonidze T, Essah PA, Iuorno MJ, Nestler JE. Prevalance and characteristics of the metabolic syndrome in women with polycystic ovary syndrome. J Clin Endocrinol Metab 2005;90:1929–1935.
74. Fleming R, Hopkinson ZE, Wallace AM, Greer IA, Sattar N. Ovarian function and metabolic factors in women with oligomenorrhea treated with metformin in a randomized, double-blind, placebo-controlled trial. J Clin Endocrinol Metab 2002;87:569–574.

75. Talbott EO, Guzick DS, Sutton-Tyrrell K, et al. Evidence for association between polycystic ovary syndrome and premature carotid atherosclerosis in middle-aged women. Arterioscler Thromb Vasc Biol 2000;20:2414–2421.

76. Christian RC, Dumesic DA, Behrenbeck T, Oberg AL, Sheedy PF, Fitzpatrick LA. Prevalance and predictors of coronary artery calcification in women with polycystic ovary syndrome. J Clin Endocrinol Metab 2003;88:2562–2568.

77. Dereli D, Ozgen G, Buyukkececi F, Guney E, Yilmaz C. Platelet dysfunction in lean women with polycystic ovary syndrome and association with insulin sensitivity. J Clin Endocrinol Metab 2003; 88:2263–2268.

78. Weiss R, Dziura J, Burgert TS, et al. Obesity and the metabolic syndrome in children and adolescents. N Engl J Med 2004;350:2362–2374.

79. Duncan GE, Li SM, Zhou XH. Prevalence and trends of a metabolic syndrome phenotype among US adolescents, 1999–2000. Diabetes Care 2004;27:2438–2443.

80. Cook S, Weitzman M, Auinger P, Nguyen M, Dietz WH. Prevalence of metabolic syndrome phenotype in adolescents: findings from the third National Health and Nutrition Examination Survey. 1988–1994. Arch Pediatr Adolesc Med 2003;157:821–827.

81. Fagot-Campagna A, Pettitt D, Engelgau MM, et al. Type 2 diabetes among North American children and adolescents: an epidemiologic review and a public health perspective. J Pediatr 2000;136:664–672.

82. Raitakari OT, Porkka KVK, Ronnemaa T, et al. The role of insulin in clustering of serum lipids and blood pressure in children and adolescents: the cardiovascular risk in young Finns study. Diabetologia 1995;38:1042–1050.

83. Bao W, Srinivasan SR, Berenson GS. Persistent elevation of plasma insulin levels is associated with increased cardiovascular risk in children and young adults. The Bogalusa Heart Study. Circulation 1996;93:54–59.

84. Arslanian SA, Witchel SF. Polycystic ovary syndrome in adolescents: is there an epidemic? Curr Opin Endocrinol Diabetes 2002;9:32–42.

85. Arslanian S, Suprasongsin C. Insulin sensitivity, lipids, and body composition in childhood: is "syndrome X" present? J Clin Endocrinol Metab 1996;81:1058–1062.

86. Silfen ME, Manibo AM, Ferin M, McMahon DJ, Levine LS, Oberfield SE. Elevated free IGF-I levels in prepubertal hispanic girls with premature adrenarche: relationship with hyperandrogenism and insulin sensitivity. J Clin Endocrinol Metab 2002;87:398–403.

87. Potau N, Ibanez L, Rique S, Sanchez-Ufarte C, de Zegher F. Pronounced adrenarche and precocious pubarche in boys. Horm Res 1999;51:238–241.

88. Dunaif A, Sorbara L, Delson R, Green G. Ethnicity and polycystic ovary syndrome are associated with independent and additive decreases in insulin action in Caribbean-Hispanic women. Diabetes 1993;42:1462–1468.

89. Norman RJ, Mahabeer S, Masters S. Ethnic differences in insulin and glucose response to glucose between white and Indian women with polycystic ovary syndrome. Fertil Steril 1995;63:58–62.

90. Carmina E, Koyama T, Chang L, Stanczyk FZ, Lobo RA. Does ethnicity influence the prevalence of adrenal hyperandrogenism and insulin resistance in polycystic ovary syndrome? Am J Obstet Gynecol 1992;167:1807–1812.

91. Gungor N, Saad R, Janosky J, Arslanian S. Validation of surrogate estimates of insulin sensitivity and insulin secretion in children and adolescents. J Pediatr 2004;144:47–55.

92. Arslanian S, Suprasongsin C, Janosky JE. Insulin secretion and sensitivity in black versus while prepubertal healthy children. J Clin Endocrinol Metab 1997;82:1923–1927.

93. Schuster DP, Kien CL, Osei K. Differential impact of obesity on glucose metabolism in black and white american adolescents. Am J Med Sci 1998;316:361–367.

94. Goran MI, Gower BA. Longitudinal study on pubertal insulin resistance. Diabetes 2001;50:2444–2450.

95. Uwaifo GI, Nguyen TT, Keil MF, et al. Differences in insulin secretion and sensitivity of Caucasian and African American prepubertal children. J Pediatr 2002;140:673–680.

96. Goran MI, Bergman RN, Cruz ML, Watanabe R. Insulin resistance and associated compensatory responses in African-American and Hispanic children. Diabetes Care 2002;25:2184–2190.

97. Morrison J, Friedman LA, Harlan WR, et al. Development of the metabolic syndrome in black and white adolescent girls: a longitudinal assessment. Pediatrics 2005;116:1178–1182.

98. Likitmaskul S, Cowell CT, Donaghue K, et al. "Exaggerated adrenarche" in children presenting with premature adrenarche. Clin Endocrinol (Oxf) 1995;42:265–272.

99. Banerjee S, Raghavan S, Wasserman EJ, Linder BL, Saenger P, DiMartino-Nardi J. Hormonal findings in African-American and Caribbean Hispanic girls with premature adrenarche: implications for polycystic ovarian syndrome. Pediatrics 1998;102:E36.

100. Temeck JW, Pang SY, Nelson C, New MI. Genetic defects of steroidogenesis in premature pubarche. J Clin Endocrinol Metab 1987;64:609–617.

101. Chang YT, Zhang L, Alkaddour HS, et al. Absence of molecular defect in the type II 3β–hydroxysteroid dehydrogenase (3β-HSD) gene in premature pubarche children and hirsuit female patients with moderately decreased adrenal 3β-HSD activity. Pediatr Res 1995;37:820–824.

102. Sakkal-Alkaddour H, Zhang L, Yang X, et al. Studies of 3β-hydroxysteroid dehydrogenase genes in infants and children manifesting premature pubarche and increased ACTH stimulated Δ5 steroid levels. J Clin Endocrinol Metab 1996;81:3961–3965.

103. Lutfallah C, Wang W, Mason JI, et al. Newly proposed hormonal criteria via genotypic proof for the type II 3β-hydroxysteroid dehydrogenase deficiency. J Clin Endocrinol Metab 2002;87:2611–2622.

104. Zerah M, Rheaume E, Mani P, et al. No evidence of mutations in the genes for type I and type II 3β-hydroxysteroid Dehydrogenase (3β-HSD) in nonclassical 3β-HSD deficiency. J Clin Endocrinol Metab 1994;79:1811–1817.

105. Lobo RA, Goebelsmann U. Evidence for reduced 3β-ol-hydroxysteroid dehydrogenase activity in some hirsute women thought to have polycystic ovary syndrome. J Clin Endocrinol Metab 1981;53:394–400.

106. Pang SY, Lerner A, Stoner E, et al. Late-onset adrenal steroid 3β-hydroxysteroid dehydrogenase deficiency. A cause of hirsutism in pubertal and postpubertal women. J Clin Endocrinol Metab 1985;60:428–439.

107. Siegel SF, Finegold DN, Lanes R, Lee PA. ACTH stimulation tests and plasma dehydroepiandrosterone sulfate levels in women with hirsutism. N Engl J Med 1990;323:849–854.

108. Eldar-Geva I, Hurwitz A, Becsei P, Palti A, Milwidsky A, Rosler A. Secondary biosynthetic defects in women with late-onset congenital adrenal hyperplasia. N Engl J Med 1990;323:855–863.

109. Moran C, Azziz R. The role of the adrenal cortex in polycystic ovary syndrome. Obstet Gynecol 2001;28:63–75.

110. Hawkins LA, Chasalow FI, Blethen SL. The role of adrenocorticotropin testing in evaluating girls with premature adrenarche and hirsutism/oligomenorrhea. J Clin Endocrinol Metab 1992;74:248–253.

111. Gibson M, Lackritz R, Schiff I, Tulchinsky D. Abnormal adrenal responses to adrenocorticotropic hormone in hyperandrogenic women. Fertil Steril 1980;33:43–48.

112. Silfen ME, Denburg MR, Manibo AM, et al. Early endocrine, metabolic, and sonographic characteristics of polycystic ovary syndrome (PCOS): comparison between nonobese and obese adolescents. J Clin Endocrinol Metab 2003;88(10):4682–4688.

113. Despres JP. Abdominal obesity as important component of insulin-resistance syndrome. Nutrition 1993;9:452–459.

114. Sinha R, Dufour S, Petersen KF, et al. Assessment of skeletal muscle triglyceride content by ^{1}H nuclear magnetic resonance spectroscopy in lean and obese adolescents. Diabetes 2002;51:1022–1027.

115. Bacha F, Saad R, Gungor N, Janosky J, Arslanian SA. Obesity, regional fat distribution, and syndrome X in obese black versus obese white adolescents: race differential in diabetogenic and atherogenic risk factors. J Clin Endocrinol Metab 2003;88:2534–2540.

116. Weiss R, Dufour S, Taksali SE, et al. Prediabetes in youth: a syndrome of impaired glucose tolerance, severe insulin resistance, and altered myocellular and abdominal fat partitioning. Lancet 2003;362:951–957.

117. Machann J, Haring H, Schick F, Stumvoll M. Intramyocellular lipids and insulin resistance. Diabetes Obes Metab 2004;6:239–248.

118. Weiss R, Taksali SE, Dufour S, et al. The "obese insulin-sensitive" adolescent: importance of adiponectin and lipid partitioning. J Clin Endocrinol Metab 2005;90:3731–3737.

119. Sopher AB, Thornton JC, Silfen ME, et al. Prepubertal girls with premature adrenarche have greater bone mineral content and density than controls. J Clin Endocrinol Metab 2001;86:5269–5272.

120. Ibanez L, Ong K, de Zegher F, Marcos MV, del Rio L, Dunger DB. Fat distribution in non-obese girls with and without precocious pubarche: central adiposity related to insulinemia and androgenemia from prepuberty to postmenarche. Clin Endocrinol (Oxf) 2002;58:372–379.

121. Petersen KF, Dufour S, Befroy D, Garcia R, Shulman GI. Impaired mitochondrial activity in the insulin-resistant offspring of patients with type 2 diabetes. N Eng J Med 2004;350:664–671.

8 Involvement of the Endocannabinoid System in Metabolism and Fertility

Potential Implication in the Polycystic Ovary Syndrome

Uberto Pagotto, MD, PhD,
Alessandra Gambineri, MD,
Valentina Vicennati, MD,
and Renato Pasquali, MD

CONTENTS

Summary

    Obesity, and in particular the visceral type, is one of the most relevant phenotypic characteristics of a large percentage of patients with the polycystic ovary syndrome (PCOS). Although adjustments to nutritional lifestyle and an increase in physical activity remain the milestones of the therapy to lose weight, it is evident from the exponential increase in the number of obese subjects in Western countries that these two approaches alone are no longer able to limit this progression.

From: *Contemporary Endocrinology: Insulin Resistance and Polycystic Ovarian Syndrome:*
Pathogenesis, Evaluation, and Treatment
Edited by: E. Diamanti-Kandarakis, J. E. Nestler, D. Panidis, and R. Pasquali © Humana Press Inc., Totowa, NJ

This alarming phenomenon occurs in spite of the great efforts made over the last 10 years to shed light on the pathogenetic mechanisms inducing obesity. No substantial progress has, however, been achieved so far and many inconclusive hopes have been generated in the field of pharmaco-therapeutics to tackle obesity.

Among the several targets exploited in recent years, the endocannabinoid system nowadays constitutes the most promising and the most intriguing one proposed so far. On one hand this chapter is aimed at providing an overview on the role of the endocannabinoid system in the physiology of metabolism and fertility, whereas on the other a further aim is to summarize how the system also controls food intake and energy balance by acting at both cerebral and peripheral level. Finally, a brief summary of the results obtained with the first clinical trials in obese patients will also be included to discuss the potential application of cannabinoid receptor type 1 blockers in the treatment of not only obesity but also of the PCOS.

Key Words: Polycystic ovary syndrome; cannabinoid receptor type 1; cannabinoid type 1 receptor antagonist; rimonabant; Δ^9-tetrahydrocannabinol.

HISTORY OF THE ENDOCANNABINOID SYSTEM

Although ancient medical traditions of eastern origin included *Cannabis sativa* as therapy for various diseases, no in-depth research on cannabinoids was performed to prove its putative mechanism of action on a scientific basis until 40 years ago *(1)*. Only after the identification of the most important psychoactive component from hemp, Δ^9-tetrahydrocannabinol (THC) *(2)*, did the research on cannabinoids receive a new impulse in understanding the mechanisms of action of marijuana. However, when the binding site of THC was identified first as the cannabinoid type 1 receptor (CB1) *(3)* and afterward as type 2 (CB2) *(4)*, both G-protein coupled recep-tors, it became logical to carry on with the studies searching for putative endogenous ligands. The identification of these substances, named endocannabinoids, completed the circle. The endogenous ligands, the endocannabinoids, the enzymatic machinery for their synthesis, and degradation and the specific CB1 and CB2 receptors thus made up the so-called endocannabinoid system (*see* reviews in refs. *5–7*). Endocannabinoids are derivatives of arachidonic acid and they belong to a family composed of an increasing number of compounds, the most studied so far being arachidonoyl ethanolamide, named anandamide (AEA) *(8)*, and 2-arachidonoyl glycerol (2-AG) *(9,10)*.

An interesting aspect of the endocannabinoid system is its activity "on demand," meaning that the system can be activated with a closely regulated spatial and temporal selectivity: only "when" and "where" it is needed *(5,6)*. This property poses an important distinction that should be taken into account when the physiological functions of the endocannabinoid system are compared to the pharmacological actions of exogenous cannabinoid receptor compounds, which lack such selectivity.

The original distinction between CB1 and CB2 receptors as the "brain type" for the first and the "peripheral" one for the second does not, in our opinion, hold true anymore. In fact, the original definition was initially proposed taking into account the first anatomical mapping distribution that described CB1 receptor expression eminently in the central nervous system (including cortical regions, several parts of basal ganglia, thalamic nuclei, cerebellar cortex, brainstem nuclei, and hypothalamus) *(11)* and the CB2 receptors preferentially at the level of immune cells *(11)*. According to this distribution, most of the studies were aimed at identifying the mode of action of endocannabinoids at these sites, contributing to disregard the effects of endocannabinoids at peripheral levels for CB1 receptor and at cellular levels other than immune cells for CB2. Recent views attribute both CB receptors with a broader spectrum of action than in the past and it is no longer surprising to note that endocannabinoids are believed to modulate physiological functions not always connected with the neural activity for CB1 receptors and the immune activity for CB2 receptors. In fact, CB1 receptor expression has been found to be more ubiquitous than originally thought, according to its presence in peripheral organs such as the pituitary, thyroid, adrenal glands, testis, sperms, ovary, oviduct muscularis, uterus, adipose tissue, skeletal muscles, pancreas, hepatocytes, vascular endothelial cells, gastrointestinal tract, in particular in the fundus of the stomach, and in vagal nerve ends innervating the gastrointestinal tract (*see* review in ref. *12*). Conversely, CB2 is also present in cells of the central nervous system and in peripheral cells such as keratinocytes, osteoclasts, the pancreas, and neural cells (*see* review in ref. *12*).

PHYSIOLOGY OF THE ENDOCANNABINOID SYSTEM

An astonishing amount of data has recently been accumulated, providing increasingly deeper insights regarding the biological roles of the endocannabinoid system. A huge contribution in this context has been provided by tools such as the generation of an increasing number of synthetic compounds acting as specific CB receptor agonists or antagonists (*see* review in ref. *7*) and by the animal models in which CB receptors were genetically ablated. In general, it can be summarized that the endocannabinoid system is involved in different physiological functions, many of which are related to the stress-recovery systems and to the maintenance of homeostatic balance *(13)*. Among other functions, the endocannabinoid system is involved in neuroprotection, modulating nociception, regulating motor activity, and controlling certain phases of memory processing. In addition, the endocannabinoid system contributes to modulate the immune and inflammatory responses. It also influences the cardiovascular and the respiratory systems by controlling heart rate, blood pressure and bronchial functions. Finally, yet importantly, endocannabinoids are known to exert important anti-proliferative actions (*see* reviews in refs. *5–7*).

However, very recent lines of evidence showed that endocannabinoid signalling may, in the presence of certain diseases, represent on one hand a self-defense of the body to counteract the pathological processes, and on the other hand, when pathologically over-activated, the system may represent one of the causative factors underlying the disease or its symptoms *(7)*. Such fluctuations may be pharmacologically modulated by the CB1 receptor agonists when high levels of endocannabinoids are believed to be required or by the CB1 receptor antagonists when the system needs to reach normalization from a pathological state of over-activation. In this sense, cannabis or some of its derivatives have been therapeutically used to inhibit pain, knowing that they were able to produce nociception either via CB1 or via CB2 receptor activity *(7)*. The same holds true after the synthesis of the first specific CB1 receptor antagonist, rimonabant, generated in the lab of Sanofi-Synthelabo in 1994 *(14)*. In this case, the putative therapeutical applications of CB1 receptor antagonists were hypothesized for various diseases in which the endocannabinoid system was believed to be over activated.

ENDOCANNABINOIDS MODULATE ENERGY METABOLISM
THROUGH CB1 RECEPTOR ACTIVATION

Since ancient times it has been reported that marijuana, in whatever way it is administered, increases appetite, particularly for palatable food *(1)*. After the identification of THC as the main principle in marijuana, a huge number of reports have documented the ability of this compound to promote food intake. Since the discovery of specific cannabinoid receptors and the synthesis of selective antagonists, the increase in food intake caused by THC could be linked exclusively to CB1 receptor activation *(15)*. In a similar way, endocannabinoids were also reported to play an orexigenic role when administered either systemically or into the ventromedial hypothalamus, and, as for the exogenous cannabinoids, this effect could be attributed to a stimulation of CB1 receptors *(15)*. As mentioned before, the prominent anatomical localization of CB1 receptors in the mesolimbic and the hypothalamic areas were suggestive of their involvement in both the hedonic and homeostatic control of eating *(15)*. However, in the last 2 years new findings have clearly highlighted the ability of endocannabinoids to deeply modulate the metabolic processes not only at central but also at peripheral level. Recent results obtained by several independent labs shed light on the peripheral mode of action of the endocannabinoid system. Indeed, after the first demonstration of the presence and the functional role of the CB1 receptor on the adipocytes *(16,17)*, it is now becoming clear that endocannabinoids are able to interact with all the organs involved in the control of metabolic functions. Therefore, we can conclude that CB1 receptor antagonists may act as antiobesity drugs by a dual mechanism of action that initially targets neuronal sites controlling food intake and thereafter peripheral organs involved in energy storage and expenditure *(12)*. Intriguingly, all the organs involved in the metabolic processes are sites of action of endocannabinoids *(12)*. In fact, at the white adipocyte level, we found that CB1 receptors are stimulators of lipogenesis *(16)*. Their activation enhances lipoprotein lipase activity and this effect can be specifically blocked by rimonabant, a CB1 receptor antagonist *(16)*. Others authors have shown that CB1 receptors are predominantly expressed in mature adipocytes rather than in pre-adipocytes in both humans and rodents *(17,18)*, meaning that the putative role of the CB1 receptor is not related to the adipocyte processes of differentiation but likely associated with some metabolic function of these cells. More importantly, rimonabant has been shown to induce adiponectin release from adipocytes in vitro *(17)*. Adiponectin is a circulating adipokine secreted by adipose tissue, playing a key regulatory role in fat and glucose metabolism (*see* review in ref. *19*). This protein exhibits anti-atherogenic and anti-diabetic properties. It is associated with increased insulin sensitivity, and in the liver adiponectin decreases hepatic glucose production and regulates free fatty acid metabolism, via suppression of lipogenesis and activation of free fatty acid oxidation (*see* review in ref. *19*). A recent advancement is represented by a study by Jbilo et al. who showed that 40 days of rimonabant treatment reversed the alterations in gene expression obtained by a prolonged high-fat diet *(20)*. In detail, they found that the reduction of adipose mass favored by CB1 receptor antagonist treatment was induced by a series of events such as: (1) enhanced lipolysis through the induction of enzymes of the β-oxidation and tricarboxylic acid cycle *(20)*, (2) an increase in energy expenditure through futile cycle stimulation, and (3) an improvement in the regulation of glucose homeostasis as demonstrated by the stimulation of glucose-transporter 4, a key-player in glucose metabolism *(20)*. Together with adipose tissue, the liver seems to be another key-organ to explain the action of endocannabinoids at peripheral levels *(21)*. In fact, CB1 receptors are expressed in hepatocytes and when activated by endocannabinoids a stimulation of *de novo* lipogenesis has been shown to occur. Moreover, a prolonged high-fat diet in mice increases hepatic levels of anandamide and induces an upregulation of CB1 receptor expression that may in turn promote the development of steatosis *(21)*. Importantly, CB1–/– mice are resistant to the development of hepatic steatosis *(21)*. CB1 receptor and endocannabinoids are also highly expressed in the gastrointestinal tract neurons. In the small intestine, starvation induces a sevenfold increase in AEA release and this effect is reversed on refeeding *(22)*. CB1 receptors are also present in skeletal muscles *(12)* and in the endocrine pancreas *(23)*, although at present little is known about their role in these organs.

In conclusion, the endocannabinoid system may target a large variety of peripheral organs while modulating metabolic processes; the detailed characterization of each individual contribution and the reciprocal interactions among the organs is mandatory in future studies approaching this issue.

ROLE OF EXOGENOUS AND ENDOGENOUS CANNABINOIDS ON THE HYPOTHALAMIC-PITUITARY-OVARY AXIS

Among the various actions attributed to exogenous and endogenous cannabinoids at the endocrine axes, those at the level of the hypothalamic–pituitary–ovary (HPO) axis together with those at the HPO axis represent the most extensively studied so far. As is evident, the first anedoctal reports to study the interaction of cannabinoids with HPO were made by the observation of changes in reproductive functions by using cannabis derivatives. As for the studies regarding food intake, exogenous cannabinoids did not always give consistent data when administered, as a result of the well-known problems related to the variability of the dosages, the purity of the extracts, and the routes of administration. However, in general terms, we can unify the whole body of the data summarizing the concept that cannabinoids exert a potent negative effects on reproduction in both sexes and this finding has been confirmed in various species *(24)*. Moreover, most of the evidence seems to confirm that the primary negative effects are ascribed to a hypothalamic action, although some of these downregulating influences may be mediated directly at the level of the pituitary and the ovary.

By suppressing the secretory pulse of luteinizing hormone (LH) *(25–27)*, cannabinoids have been shown to downregulate blood LH levels *(28–31)*. Administration of gonadotropins or GnRH can restore ovulation or LH release, respectively, even in the presence of high levels of THC *(25,26)*, confirming the relevant role of the cannabinoids at the hypothalamic levels. Importantly, tolerance to the antireproductive effect seems to develop after a few chronic treatment cycles *(32)*.

The common notion is that cannabinoids indirectly modify GnRH secretion by negatively modulating the activity of neurotransmitters known to facilitate GnRH secretion, such as norepinephrine and glutamate, and by stimulating those modulators known to downregulate GnRH secretion, such as dopamine, GABA, opioids, and CRH (*see* review in ref. *33*). However, a recent finding demonstrated that the immortalized hypothalamic GnRH neurons contain a complete and functional endocannabinoid system, and that by perifusion experiments a cannabinoid agonist completely disrupts pulsatile secretion of GnRH *(27)*.

Although cannabinoids are able to modulate the HPO axis, it is not yet known how, where and under what circumstances the endocannabinoids are produced to do so. It has been demonstrated that AEA fluctuates during the ovarian cycle in both the hypothalamus and pituitary *(28)*, thus influencing hormonal secretion and sexual behavior through CB1 receptor activation *(34)*. Furthermore, considerable endocannabinoid production was found in the ovary, in particular at the time of ovulation, making it possible to hypothesize that the endocannabinoids may help to regulate follicular maturation and development of the ovary *(35)*. However, an excess of cannabinoids may conversely impair regular ovulation, not only acting at hypothalamic level but also directly affecting ovarian granulosa layers *(36)*.

The endocannabinoid system also displays an important role during early pregnancy and in modulating embryo–uterine interactions. The uterus contains the highest level of AEA detected so far in mammalian tissues *(37)*. Starting from this observation and from the finding of high levels of CB1 receptor expression in preimplantation embryos *(38)*, it has been speculated that high levels of AEA may adversely affect embryo development and implantation *(39)*, whereas low levels of AEA promote embryonic growth and differentiation *(40)*. It is known that AEA is degraded by a specific enzyme fatty acid amide hydrolase (FAAH) *(41)*; interestingly this protein represents a crucial enzymatic checkpoint in the control of reproduction. In fact, an inverse correlation was described between levels of FAAH activity in maternal peripheral blood mononuclear cells and spontaneous miscarriage in women *(42)*. In addition, FAAH activity is lower, and consequently AEA higher, in patients who fail to achieve pregnancy during in vitro fertilization-embryo transfer in comparison to patients who become pregnant *(43)*. Furthermore, AEA levels in the mouse uterus are inversely related to uterine receptivity for implantation, being higher with uterine refractoriness to blastocyst implantation *(37)* and lower at implantation sites *(44)*. In conclusion, we can say that high levels of maternal AEA are detrimental to early placental and fetal development. It has recently been demonstrated that FAAH activity is under the strict regulation of several hormones, such as progesterone, leptin, and FSH, very well known modulators of fertility *(40)*.

Although an increased endocannabinoid tone is detrimental for fertility, a failure or a blockade of the endocannabinoid signaling may also induce important changes in this function. In fact, it has recently been shown that an impairment in endocannabinoid signaling leads to retention of a large number of embryos in the mouse oviduct, leading to pregnancy failure. This is because of a profound impairment of coordinated oviductal smooth muscle contraction and relaxation *(45)*. The authors propose that their findings may have strong implications for ectopic pregnancy in women because one major cause of tubal pregnancy is embryo retention in the fallopian tube *(45)*. Consistently, both endogenous and exogenous cannabinoids exert a CB1 receptor-mediated relaxant effect, not only on the oviductal smooth muscle but also on the human pregnant myometrium, highlighting a possible role of endocannabinoids during human parturition and pregnancy *(40)*. In fact, pregnancy seems to be also closely controlled by the endocannabinoid system *(46)*.

In summary, all the steps starting with gonadotropin pulsatility up to pregnancy seem to be closely modulated by endocannabinoids, reinforcing the concept that the endocannabinoid system should not only be considered as a central neuromodulator, but as a physiological actor in a wider scenario.

CANNABINOID TYPE 1 ANTAGONISTS AS A NEW PHARMACOLOGICAL FRONTIER IN TACKLING OBESITY

A recent series of reports identified a close association between the formation of a state of obesity with a simultaneous over-activation of the endocannabinoid system expressed as an overproduction of endocannabinoids or an over-expression of CB1 receptors. In fact, there is now evidence that the CB1 receptor is over-expressed in tissues derived from obese animals when compared to lean controls such as the liver *(21)*, the skeletal muscles *(12)*, and the adipose tissue *(17)*. Nothing is at present known in humans, with the exception of human white adipose tissue in which, at variance to mice, this finding has not been confirmed *(18)*.

An increased production of endocannabinoids has been proposed in hepatocytes *(21)*, adipocytes, and pancreatic cells *(47)* derived from fat mice in comparison to lean controls. Intriguingly, increased levels of plasma endocannabinoids have been found in obese postmenopausal women when compared to lean controls *(18)*.

A recent study has begun to shed light on the mechanism leading to a hyperactivation of the endocannabinoid tone in obesity demonstrating that a missense polymorphism exists in a population of obese subjects, predictive of a substitution of threonine for a highly conserved proline residue (P129T) in the sequence of the FAAH, the enzyme that quickly degrades anandamide after its action *(48)*. Patients with this polymorphism have approximately half the enzymatic activity and this physiologic reduction of function may influence the clearance of endocannabinoids, leading to a sustained and possibly pathological tone as found in animal models *(48)*.

As previously mentioned, the discovery of rimonabant not only made it possible to understand many aspects of the endocannabinoid system but it also very soon appeared to be a promising tool for various diseases in which a pathological increased endocannabinoid tone was presumed to occur. As regards the overactivation of the endocannabinoid tone, the most promising data concerning the use of rimonabant in humans are emerging from the clinical trials on tackling obesity.

In fact, a phase III trial named RIO (rimonabant in obesity) was initiated few years ago including more than 6600 obese or overweight patients with or without concomitant comorbidities *(49)*. This study consisted of four different clinical trials. Two of them named RIO-Europe and RIO-North America recruited obese or overweight patients with or without comorbidities who were treated for 2 years with 5 or 20 mg rimonabant vs placebo. Obviously, the pharmacological treatment was always associated with a hypocaloric diet of 600 Kcal subtracted from the basal metabolic rate for all subjects recruited in the four trials. The patients were also encouraged to increase their physical activity. The other two trials were named RIO-Lipids and RIO-Diabetes and were set up in order to investigate the improvement of specific comorbidity factors associated with obesity such as hyperlipidemia and diabetes, respectively, after rimonabant treatment.

The primary goal of the four RIO studies was body weight reduction, which was associated in the RIO-North America trial with the prevention of weight regain after rerandomization (second year) and in the RIO-Europe trial with the assessment of weight loss by using the same dosages after 2 years of treatment. The secondary endpoints of all four studies were also similar, as represented by the number of weight responders and the changes in waist circumference. Secondary measures also included changes from baseline in levels of high-density lipoprotein cholesterol, triglycerides, glucose, and insulin during an oral glucose-tolerance test and the prevalence of the metabolic syndrome as defined by the criteria of the National Cholesterol Education Program's Adult Treatment Program III (NCEP-ATP III) (50).

Two studies out of four have been published up to now: the RIO-Europe *ad interim* analysis of the first year (51) and the RIO-Lipids study (52). Importantly, the results provided by both trials were very similar in both primary and secondary endpoints and this result highlights the relevance of the studies. To simplify, only the data concerning the 20 mg rimonabant treatment will be mentioned when compared to placebo because the treatment with 5 mg rimonabant often did not provide statistically significant changes.

In the RIO-Europe study, the weight reduction in the 20 mg treatment group of patients was similar in both studies (–8.6 kg) compared to the –3.6 kg detected in the placebo treated group in the RIO-Europe and –2.3 kg in the RIO-Lipids study (51,52); the reduction in waist circumference was also similar –9 cm in both groups of rimonabant-treated patients vs 3–4 cm in the placebo groups (51,52). The pattern of weight loss showed a sustained profile for up to 36–40 weeks, followed by a plateau phase in both trials. The proportion of those who had a weight loss equal to or greater than 10% in the 20-mg treatment group was 39% in the RIO-Europe study and 32% in the RIO-Lipids study when compared to 12.4 and 7.2% in the placebo group of the two studies, respectively (51,52).

A significant improvement of the lipidic profile was detected in both studies with an increase of HDL-cholesterol and a decrease of triglyceride concentrations in patients treated with 20 mg rimonabant. Importantly, glucose and insulin areas under the curve after an oral glucose tolerance test decreased significantly in the group receiving 20 mg of rimonabant in both studies. The RIO-Lipids study also examined the variation of leptin and adiponectin, both hormones being implicated in the regulation of metabolic functions. Plasma leptin levels decreased significantly in the group receiving 20 mg rimonabant vs placebo, whereas plasma adiponectin significantly increased when compared to placebo in the group treated with 20 mg rimonabant (52). Interestingly, by means of logistic regression models and/or ANCOVA using weight loss as a covariate in the RIO-Europe study it was found that nearly half the changes in HDL-cholesterol and triglycerides were independent of weight loss, as reflected by the last weight measurement (51,52). Similarly, 57% of the increase in adiponectin levels observed in the RIO-Lipids group receiving 20 mg of rimonabant could not be attributable to weight loss (52). These effects partially independent of weight loss are very important, because they confirmed in humans what has been hypothesized in animals, i.e., that CB1 receptor antagonist drugs may directly target peripheral metabolic functions more than a pure anorexigenic drug (16,53–55).

Finally, the prevalence of the metabolic syndrome in the patients before and after 1 year of treatment was analyzed in the RIO-Lipids study. Interestingly, at baseline 54% of the patients met the criteria for the syndrome, whereas the prevalence fell to 25.8% in the 20-mg rimonabant group vs 41% in the placebo group (52).

Great care is taken with regard to the issues of safety and tolerability of any new drug tackling obesity proposed for clinical praxis. Both RIO studies showed a slightly higher rimonabant-treatment adverse or serious adverse event number when compared with placebo. The most common events occurring more frequently with 20 mg rimonabant were nausea, vomiting, diarrhea, dizziness, depression, and anxiety. However, they were for the most part mild to moderate in intensity and considered to be transient, based on the occurrence mainly during the first months of the studies (51,52).

THE PCOS AS A POTENTIAL FUTURE TARGET FOR CB1 RECEPTOR ANTAGONIST THERAPY

The promising data of the two previously mentioned RIO studies need to be substantiated by the results of the other two ongoing clinical trials with rimonabant still to be published and to be definitively confirmed by the data obtained by future trials in which specific questions will be asked and hopefully solved. Importantly, as hypothesized in studies in animals, rimonabant seems to work not only as an anorectic drug but also, and even more importantly, as a positive modulator of crucial metabolic steps at peripheral level inducing an improvement of the lipidic and glycemic profiles partially independent of body weight loss. Rimonabant and related upcoming CB1 receptor antagonist drugs may therefore be proposed not only for tackling visceral obesity but also for dealing with the variety of alterations related to the pathological fat increase in abdominal depots. In this sense, the PCOS represents a unique model in which CB1 receptor antagonists may exhibit a powerful dual effect. On one hand, in the case of the PCOS associated with obesity this class of drugs may offer the opportunity to associate a relevant improvement of insulin resistance, which is one of the most important features of the syndrome, with an important effect on body weight, whereas the improvement in the lipid profile and the increase in adiponectin may correct metabolic alterations frequently associated with the syndrome. In addition, the deleterious effects of exogenous and endogenous cannabinoids on the HPO axis at various levels may be corrected by the addition of a drug believed to normalize the overactivation of the system. In this context, we can speculate that a disturbance of the GnRH pulse, usually present in PCOS patients, may be normalized by adding CB1 receptor antagonists to dietary counseling and change of life style.

Time will tell whether rimonabant and other drugs of the same class may become suitable for the treatment of PCOS patients.

FUTURE AVENUES OF INVESTIGATION

The data from the studies in animals and in humans with Rimonabant, the first CB1 antagonist tested in clinical trials, will presumably help us to better tackle obesity and related metabolic diseases. Moreover, the entry of this class of drugs on the market may allow us to begin considering the possibility of individually targeting the therapeutic strategies according to phenotype characteristics and to the pathophysiological mechanisms inducing obesity. Obese PCOS patients may represent an ideal target population for the CB1 antagonist treatment. In fact, rimonabant and other drugs of the same class may improve insulin resistance by reducing body weight and by a direct effect at the level of key-organs involved in metabolic processes. Moreover, the improvement in the lipid profile and the increase in adiponectin may also contribute to correct the metabolic alterations frequently associated with the syndrome. In addition, the putative effect of CB1 antagonists may normalize the overactivation of the endocannabinoid system on the HPO. In such context one can realistically hypothesize that PCOS may become an ideal target for the action of CB1 antagonists. Future trials on these patients are mandatory to solve this issue.

KEY POINTS

- The EC system is a general stress-recovery system and is overall "silent;" among other functions it becomes transiently activated to stimulate food intake.
- In obesity the endocannabinoid system is pathologically overactivated.
- CB1 antagonists on top of the anorectic action exert a positive peripheral role on crucial metabolic steps inducing an improvement of several metabolic parameters partially independently of body weight loss.
- All the steps starting with gonadotropin pulsatility up to pregnancy seem to be closely modulated by endocannabinoids, reinforcing the concept that the endocannabinoid system should not only be considered as a central neuromodulator, but as a physiological actor in a wider scenario.
- In obese PCOS CB1 antagonists may offer the opportunity to associate a relevant improvement of insulin resistance with an important effect on body weight, while the improvement in the lipid profile and the increase in adiponectin may correct metabolic alterations frequently associated with the syndrome.
- The deleterious effects of cannabinoids on the HPO axis at various levels may be corrected by the addition of CB1 antagonists believed to normalize the overactivation of the system. In this context, we can speculate that a disturbance of the GnRH pulse, usually present in PCOS patients, may be normalized by adding CB1 receptor antagonists to dietary counseling and change of life style.

REFERENCES

1. Peters H, Nahas GG. A brief history of four millennia (B.C. 2000-A.D. 1974). In: Nahas GG, Sutin K, Harvey D, Agurel S, ed. Marihuana and Medicine. Totowa, NJ: Humana Press Inc., 1999, pp. 3–7.
2. Gaoni Y, Mechoulam R. Isolation, structure and partial synthesis of an active constituent of hashish. J Am Chem Soc 1964;86:1646–1647.
3. Matsuda LA, Lolait SJ, Brownstein MJ, Young AC, Bonner TI. Structure of a cannabinoid receptor and functional expression of the cloned cDNA. Nature 1990;346:561–564.
4. Munro S, Thomas KL, Abu-Shaar M. Molecular characterization of a peripheral receptor for cannabinoids. Nature 1993;365:61–65.
5. Piomelli D. The molecular logic of endocannabinoid signalling. Nat Rev Neurosci 2003;4:873–884.
6. De Petrocellis L, Cascio MG, Di Marzo V. The endocannabinoid system: a general view and latest additions. Br J Pharmacol 2004;141:765–774.
7. Di Marzo V, Bifulco M, De Petrocellis L. The endocannabinoid system and its therapeutic exploitation. Nat Rev Drug Discov 2004;3:771–784.

8. Devane WA, Hanus L, Breuer A, et al. Isolation and structure of a brain constituent that binds to the cannabinoid receptor. Science 1992;258:1946–1949.
9. Mechoulam R, Ben-Shabat S, Hanus L, et al. Identification of an endogenous 2-monoglyceride, present in canine gut, that binds to cannabinoid receptors. Biochem Pharmacol 1995;50:83–90.
10. Sugiura T, Kondo S, Sukagawa A, et al. 2-Arachidonoylglycerol: a possible endogenous cannabinoid receptor ligand in brain. Biochem Biophys Res Commun 1995;215:89–97.
11. Howlett AC, Barth F, Bonner TI, et al. International Union of Pharmacology. XXVII. Classification of cannabinoid receptors. Pharmacol Rev 2002;54:161–202.
12. Pagotto U, Marsicano G, Cota D, Lutz B, Pasquali R. The emerging role of the endocannabinoid system in endocrine regulation and energy balance. Endocr Rev 2006;27:73–100.
13. Di Marzo V, Melck D, Bisogno T, De Petrocellis L. Endocannabinoids: endogenous cannabinoid receptor ligands with neuromodulatory action. Trends Neurosci 1998;21:521–528.
14. Rinaldi-Carmona M, Barth F, Heaulme M, et al. SR141716A, a potent and selective antagonist of the brain cannabinoid receptor. FEBS Lett 1994;350:240–244.
15. Cota D, Marsicano G, Lutz B, et al. Endogenous cannabinoid system as a modulator of food intake. Int J Obes Relat Metab Disord 2003;27:289–301.
16. Cota D, Marsicano G, Tschop M, et al. The endogenous cannabinoid system affects energy balance via central orexigenic drive and peripheral lipogenesis. J Clin Invest 2003;112:423–431.
17. Bensaid M, Gary-Bobo M, Esclangon A, et al. The cannabinoid CB1 receptor antagonist SR141716 increases Acrp30 mRNA expression in adipose tissue of obese fa/fa rats and in cultured adipocyte cells. Mol Pharmacol 2003;63:908–914.
18. Engeli S, Bohnke J, Feldpausch M, et al. Activation of the peripheral endocannabinoid system in human obesity Diabetes 2005;54:2838–2843.
19. Chandran M, Phillips SA, Ciaraldi T, Henry RR. Adiponectin: more than just another fat cell hormone? Diabetes Care 2003;26:2442–2450.
20. Jbilo O, Ravinet-Trillou C, Arnone M, et al. The CB1 receptor antagonist rimonabant reverses the diet-induced obesity phenotype through the regulation of lipolysis and energy balance FASEB J 2005;19:1567–1569.
21. Osei-Hyiaman D, DePetrillo M, Pacher P, et al. Endocannabinoid activation at hepatic CB1 receptors stimulates fatty acid synthesis and contributes to diet-induced obesity. J Clin Invest 2005;115:1298–1305.
22. Gomez R, Navarro M, Ferrer B, et al. A peripheral mechanism for CB1 cannabinoid receptor-dependent modulation of feeding. J Neurosci 2002;22:9612–9617.
23. Juan-Picò P, Fuentes E, Bermùdez-Silva FJ, et al. Cannabinoid receptors regulate Ca^{2+} signals and insulin secretion in pancreatic b-cells. Cell Calcium 2006;39:155–162.
24. Bloch E, Thysen B, Morrill GA, Gardner E, Fugimoto G. Effects of cannabinoids on reproduction and development. Vitam Horm 1978;36:203–259.
25. Tyrey L. Δ^9-tetrahydrocannabinol suppression of episodic luteinizing hormone secretion in the ovariectomized rat. Endocrinology 1978;102:1808–1814.
26. Smith CG, Smith MT, Besch NF, Smith RG, Asch RH. Effect of Δ^9-tetrahydrocannabinol (THC) on female reproductive function. Adv Biosci 1978;22:449–467.
27. Gammon CM, Freeman M Jr, Xie W, Petersen S, Wetsel WC. Regulation of gonadotropin-releasing hormone secretion by cannabinoids Endocrinology 2005;146:4491–4499.
28. Gonzalez S, Bisogno T, Wenger T, et al. Sex steroid influence on cannabinoid CB1 receptor mRNA and endocannabinoid levels in the anterior pituitary gland. Biochem Biophys Res Commun 2000;270:260–266.
29. Murphy LL, Steger RW, Smith MS, Bartke A. Effects of Δ^9-tetrahydrocannabinol, cannabinol and cannabidiol, alone and in combinations, on luteinizing hormone and prolactin release and on hypothalamic neurotransmitters in the male rat. Neuroendocrinology 1990;52:316–321.
30. Wenger T, Toth BE, Martin BR. Effects of anandamide (endogen cannabinoid) on anterior pituitary hormone secretion in adult ovariectomized rats. Life Sci 1995;56:2057–2063.
31. Besch NF, Smith CG, Besch PK, Kaufman RH. The effect of marihuana (Δ^9-tetrahydrocannabinol) on the secretion of luteinizing hormone in the ovariectomized rhesus monkey. Am J Obstet Gynecol 1977;128:635–642.
32. Smith CG, Almirez RG, Berenberg J, Asch RH. Tolerance develops to the disruptive effects of D^9-tetrahydrocannabinol on primate menstrual cycle. Science 1983;219:1453–1455.

33. Murphy LL, Munoz RM, Adrian BA, Villanua MA. Function of cannabinoid receptors in the neuroendocrine regulation of hormone secretion. Neurobiol Dis 1998;5:432–446.

34. Stella N. How might cannabinoids influence sexual behavior? Proc Natl Acad Sci USA 2001;98: 793–795.

35. Schuel H, Burkman LJ, Lippes J, et al. N-Acylethanolamines in human reproductive fluids. Chem Phys Lipids 2002;121:211–227.

36. Treinen KA, Sneeden JL, Heindel JJ. Specific inhibition of FSH-stimulated cAMP accumulation by Δ^9-tetrahydrocannabinol in cultured rat granulosa cells. Toxicol Appl Pharmacol 1993;118:53–57.

37. Schmid PC, Paria BC, Krebsbach RJ, Schmid HH, Dey SK. Changes in anandamide levels in mouse uterus are associated with uterine receptivity for embryo implantation. Proc Natl Acad Sci USA 1997;94:4188–4192.

38. Paria BC, Das SK, Dey SK. The preimplantation mouse embryo is a target for cannabinoid ligand-receptor signaling. Proc Natl Acad Sci USA 1995;92:9460–9464.

39. Paria BC, Ma W, Andrenyak DM, et al. Effects of cannabinoids on preimplantation mouse embryo development and implantation are mediated by brain-type cannabinoid receptors. Biol Reprod 1998;58:1490–1495.

40. Maccarrone M, Finazzi-Agro A. Anandamide hydrolase: a guardian angel of human reproduction? Trends Pharmacol Sci 2004;25:353–357.

41. Giang DK, Cravatt BF. Molecular characterization of human and mouse fatty acid amide hydrolases. Proc Natl Acad Sci USA 1997;94:2238–2242.

42. Maccarrone M, Valensise H, Bari M, Lazzarin N, Romanini C, Finazzi-Agro A. Relation between decreased anandamide hydrolase concentrations in human lymphocytes and miscarriage. Lancet 2000;355:1326–1329.

43. Maccarrone M, Falciglia K, Di Rienzo M, Finazzi-Agro A. Endocannabinoids, hormone-cytokine networks and human fertility. Prostaglandins Leukot Essent Fatty Acids 2002;66:309–317.

44. Paria BC, Dey SK. Ligand-receptor signaling with endocannabinoids in preimplantation embryo development and implantation. Chem Phys Lipids 2000;108:211–220.

45. Wang H, Guo Y, Wang D, et al. Aberrant cannabinoid signaling impairs oviductal transport of embryos. Nat Med 2004;10:1074–1080.

46. Helliwell RJ, Chamley LW, Blake-Palmer K, et al. Characterization of the endocannabinoid system in early human pregnancy. J Clin Endocrinol Metab 2004;89:5168–5174.

47. Matias I, Gonthier MP, Orlando P, et al. Regulation, function and dysregulation of endocannabinoids in models of adipose and β-pancreatic cells and in obesity and hyperglicemia. J Clin Endocrinol Metab 2006;91:3171–3180.

48. Sipe JC, Waalen J, Gerber A, Beutler E. Overweight and obesity associated with a missense polymorphism in fatty acid amide hydrolase (FAAH). Int J Obes Relat Metab Disord 2005;29:755–759.

49. Fernandez JR, Allison DB. Rimonabant Sanofi-Synthelabo. Curr Opin Investig Drugs 2004;5:430–435.

50. Third Report of the National Cholesterol Educational Program (NCEP) expert panel on detection, evaluation, and treatment of high blood cholesterol in adults (Adult Treatment Panel III) final report. Circulation 2002;106:3143–3421.

51. Van Gaal LF, Rissanen AM, Scheen AJ, Ziegler O, Rossner S, RIO-Europe Study Group. Effects of the cannabinoid-1 receptor blocker rimonabant on weight reduction and cardiovascular risk factors in overweight patients: 1-year experience from the RIO-Europe study. Lancet 2005;365:1389–1397.

52. Despres JP, Golay A, Sjostrom L, Rimonabant in Obesity-Lipids Study Group. Effects of rimonabant on metabolic risk factors in overweight patients with dyslipidemia. N Engl J Med 2005;353:2121–2134.

53. Ravinet-Trillou C, Arnone M, Delgorge C, et al. Anti-obesity effect of SR141716, a CB1 receptor antagonist, in diet-induced obese mice. Am J Physiol Regul Integr Comp Physiol 2003;284:R345–R353.

54. Ravinet-Trillou C, Delgorge C, Menet C, Arnone M, Soubrié P. CB1 cannabinoid receptor knockout in mice leads to leanness, resistance to diet-induced obesity and enhanced leptin sensitivity. Int J Obes Relat Metab Disord 2004;28:640–648.

55. Hildebrandt AL, Kelly-Sullivan DM, Black SC. Antiobesity effects of chronic cannabinoid CB1 receptor antagonist treatment in diet-induced obese mice. Eur J Pharmacol 2003;462:125–132.

9 Diet and Lifestyle Factors in the Etiology and Management of Polycystic Ovary Syndrome

R. J. Norman, BSc, BND *and L. J. Moran,* BSc, MBCHB, MD, FRACOG, FRACP

Contents

Summary

Conditions of overweight and obesity contribute to reproductive dysfunction. Appropriate dietary strategies and exercise can reverse these disorders. This chapter covers the causes and consequences of lifestyle disorders in polycystic ovary syndrome and relevant interventions.

Key Words: Diet; lifestyle; polycystic ovary syndrome; weight loss.

INTRODUCTION

Polycystic ovary syndrome (PCOS) is thought to arise from a combination of familial and environmental factors that interact to cause the characteristic menstrual and metabolic disturbances. It is our contention that alteration of the environmental components of this condition is fundamental to the management of the condition, and that pharmaceutical treatment (including clomiphene citrate, gonadotrophins, and insulin-sensitizing agents) should only be used after adequate counseling and action relating to lifestyle alterations. Attention to weight loss, altered diet, and exercise are important aspects to discuss with the patient, as well as stopping smoking and improving psychological attitudes. Because of the importance of overweight in the majority of women with this condition, much of this chapter will concentrate on obesity in PCOS.

From: *Contemporary Endocrinology: Insulin Resistance and Polycystic Ovarian Syndrome: Pathogenesis, Evaluation, and Treatment*
Edited by: E. Diamanti-Kandarakis, J. E. Nestler, D. Panidis, and R. Pasquali © Humana Press Inc., Totowa, NJ

MATERIALS AND METHODS

Obesity and Disease

Obesity is a costly and increasingly prevalent condition in Western society. In the United States, 50% of the population are overweight, with women (34%), blacks (49%), and Hispanics (47%) showing the highest rates of obesity. In Australia, 40% of the population are overweight or obese according to recent Australian Bureau of Statistics data. The prevalence of overweight/obesity increases in Australian women as they age, with 34% of all women between 20 and 69 years of age having a body mass index (BMI) higher than 25 kg/m^2 and 12% with a BMI higher than 30 kg/m^2. In the Repromed Centre at the University of Adelaide, 40% of women have a BMI higher than 25 kg/m^2 and 20% a BMI greater than 30 kg/m^2 based on more than 5000 patients presenting between 1991 and 1997.

Obesity is associated in women with an increased risk of diabetes mellitus, osteoarthritis, cardiovascular disease, sleep apnea, breast and uterine cancer, and reproductive disorders. Although women have increased body fat as an essential requirement for reproductive efficiency in pregnancy *(1,2)*, fat in excess of the normal can lead to menstrual abnormality, infertility, miscarriage, and difficulties in performing assisted reproduction (Table 1). Observational and theoretical considerations indicate that body weight has an inverted "U" effect on reproduction, whereby low and high body mass contributes to infertility, menstrual disorders, and poor reproductive outcome *(3)*.

The most commonly used index of obesity is the BMI (weight in kg/height in m^2), which correlates reasonably well with body fat, although at height extremes there is less association. Total body fat has been assessed by physical methods (such as skinfold thickness, underwater weighing, DEXA densitometry, magnetic resonance imaging, and infrared spectroscopy) *(4)*. The distribution of fat is also thought to be important and can be assessed by these methods, although the waist-to-hip ratio (WHR) or, simply, the waist circumference is the easiest clinical method. The reproductive literature is largely based on weight or BMI, with little data available on body composition or distribution. However, the general medical literature does contain evidence that even peripheral (non-central) obesity is highly significant in poor health outcomes, and the absence of information on fat distribution relating to reproductive factors may not be essential to an understanding of the importance of obesity.

Women have greater fat reserves than men but fat distribution is more likely to be peripheral (gynecoid) than abdominal (android). Obese and overweight women are overrepresented in gynecological and reproductive medicine clinics. BMI ranges are usually defined as follows: underweight (<19 kg/m^2), normal weight (19.1–24.9 kg/m^2), overweight (25–29.9 kg/m^2), and obese (≥30 kg/m^2). Central or peripheral obesity is usually divided at WHRs of 0.82–0.85.

Metabolic Activity of Fat Tissue

Adipose tissue is an important site of active steroid production and metabolism *(5)*. It is able to convert androgens to estrogens (aromatase activity) and estradiol to estrone and dehydroepiandrosterone to androstenediol (17β-HSD activity). Aromatase is found in bone, the hypothalamus, liver, muscle, kidney, and adipose tissue in the breast, abdomen, omentum, and marrow. Within adipose tissue, aromatase activity has been identified in

Table 1
Impact of Obesity on Reproduction

Condition	Associated risks
Menstration	↑ risk of menstrual dysfunction: amenorrhea, oligomenorrhea and menorrhagia
Infertility	↑ risk of ovulatory and anovulatory infertility: anovulation, poor response to fertility drugs
Miscarriage	↑ risk of miscarriage, spontaneously and after infertility treatment
Glucose intolerance	↑ risk of impaired glucose tolerance and type 2 diabetes mellitus
Infertility treatment	↑ requirement for clomiphene citrate/gonadotrophin ovulation induction. ↓ success rate for IVF/ICSI/GIFT pregnancies
Pregnancy	↑ prevalence of pregnancy-induced hypertension, gestational diabetes, Cesarean section, and Down's syndrome

GIFT, gamete intrafallopian transfer; ICSI, intracytoplasmic sperm injection; IVF, in vitro fertilization.

the cells of peri-adipocyte fibrovascular stroma and may be different between various depots of adipose tissue. Although in "simple" obesity, blood levels of androgens do not appear to differ from nonobese controls, production and clearance rates are significantly different (5). Abdominal fat distribution also significantly influences androgen and estrogen metabolism. In hyperandrogenic obesity, such as PCOS, increased production rates of androgens are associated with menstrual irregularities. The amount of androstenedione converted to estrone varies depending on the total body weight with women in the following groups showing conversion rates in brackets: 49–63 kg, (1.0%) 63.1–91 kg, (1.5%), >91 kg, (2.3%). Other mechanisms that influence the adipose tissue as an endocrine organ are the metabolism of estrogens to 2 hydroxy estrogen (relatively inactive) or to 16 hydroxylated estrogen (active in obesity), the storage of steroid hormones in fat, the effects of adiposity on insulin secretion from the pancreas and hence the levels of sex hormone-binding globulin (SHBG).

Leptin, the product of the *ob* gene, is a protein produced in fat cells that signals the magnitude of the energy stores to the brain and has significant effects on the reproductive system of rodents. Absence of the full-length *ob* gene, or its receptor, leads to obesity and reproductive dysfunction. Replacement of leptin in *ob/ob* mice restores fertility. Administration of recombinant leptin to rodents induces puberty earlier than in control animals indicating important effects, directly or indirectly, on ovarian function. Zachow and Magoffin (6) have shown that leptin directly affects insulin-like growth factor-induced estradiol production in the rodent ovary in the presence of follicle-stimulating hormone.

Initial reports suggested that leptin was increased in a significant proportion of women with anovulation, specifically with PCOS. Subsequently, this has not been confirmed (7), and leptin does not alter in women who are put on insulin-sensitizing agents, such as troglitazone (8) or gonadotrophin-reducing drugs, such as the oral contraceptive pill (9). Therefore, the true role of leptin in influencing ovarian function remains unclear. This hormone may have an affect on ovarian function directly via actions on the ovary or, alternatively, through the hypothalmic–pituitary–ovarian axis.

Whereas the exact role of leptin remains unclear in PCOS, current techniques for intervention by weight loss or drugs have little impact on concentrations of leptin other than by reduction of body fat. Other hormones, such as adiponectin and resistin, are produced by cells associated with fat tissue and may play a role in metabolism in PCOS. The authors and others have also shown that appetite regulation may be disturbed in PCOS, and that this may be regulated through a gut hormone named ghrelin *(10)*.

Obesity, PCOS, and Menstruation

The original description of what is now known as PCOS associated obesity and anovulation with infertility. Classical studies by Mitchell and Rogers *(11)* and Hartz et al. *(12)* confirmed these findings in much larger groups of women. The former group reported that obesity was present at a four-times higher rate in women with menstrual disturbances than in women with normal cycles. Forty-five percent of amenorrheic women were obese, whereas only 9–13% of women with normal periods were overweight. Hartz et al. *(12)* studied 26,638 women by questionnaire and noted that anovulation was strongly associated with obesity. Grossly obese women had a rate of menstrual disorders 3.1 times more frequent than women in the normal weight range. In their study, teenage obesity was positively correlated with menstrual irregularity later in life, and obesity was correlated with abnormal and long cycles, heavy flow, and hirsutism. This study was however selective in that volunteers were recruited from a weight-control organization, data was self–reported, and only one-third of all subjects were suitable for analysis. Lake et al. *(13)* studied nearly 5800 women who were born in 1958 and seen at ages 7, 11, 16, 23, and 33 years. Obesity in childhood and the early 20s increased the risk of menstrual problems (OR 1.75 and 1.59, respectively). Women who were overweight at 23 years (BMI 23.9–28.6 kg/m^2) were 1.32 times more likely and if obese (>28.6 kg/m^2) 1.75 times more likely to have menstrual disorders. Interestingly, in view of the association between overweight and early menarche, girls with menarche at 9, 10, or 11 were more likely to have menstrual problems at 16.5 years (OR 1.45 for mild and 1.94 for severe menstrual abnormality), but this was not reflected at age 33 years. Balen et al. *(14)* in London have also shown a close relationship between weight and menstrual disorders. Of 1741 subjects with PCOS, 70% had menstrual disturbances and only 22% had normal menstrual function if their BMI was higher than 30 kg/m^2. Similar results were reported by Kiddy et al. *(15)*: obese subjects with PCOS had an 88% chance of menstrual disturbance compared with 72% in nonobese subjects with PCOS.

It is likely that obesity and overweight do contribute to a significant proportion of menstrual dysfunction. There is little in the literature to separate predisposing or associated features, such as PCOS from so-called "simple" obesity, although there are suggestions that women with polycystic ovaries suffer more from weight-related menstrual dysfunction than those with normal ovaries *(12)*.

Obesity, PCOS, and Infertility

Many multiparous women are obese and, indeed, most obese women are able to get pregnant readily. Initial study of the literature suggests that several excellent investigators have not been able to confirm the adverse effect of weight on reproductive performance. The Oxford Family Planning Study *(16)* did not show any relationship between conception rates and weight or BMI in women stopping contraception, but those women were a selected group of largely parous subjects. Similar criticism applies to a well-conducted prospective study on fecundity in volunteer women who were followed for 6 months to examine the effect of environmental agents on reproduction.

Hartz et al. *(12)* found in a very large study that obesity in the teenage years was more common among married women who never became pregnant than for married women who did become pregnant. In the Nurses' Health Study, which examined 2527 married, infertile nurses, the risk of ovulatory infertility increased from a RR of 1.3, (1.2–1.6) in the group with a BMI as low as 24 kg/m^2 to a rate of 2.7 (2.0–3.7) in women with a BMI higher than 32 kg/m^2 *(17)*. In the same year, Grodstein et al. *(18)* showed that anovulatory infertility in 1880 infertile women and 4023 controls was higher in those with a BMI of more than 26.9 kg/m^2 (RR 3.1, 2.2–4.4) with a smaller non-significant risk of 1.2 (0.8–1.9) in those with a BMI of 25–26.9 kg/m^2. This indicates that even high normal to slightly overweight levels may have an effect on fertility.

Lake et al. *(13)* studied a cohort of women born in 1958 and followed up at 7, 11, 16, 23, and 33 years. They showed that weight during childhood did not predict subsequent fecundity, but weight at 23 years did predict fecundity if the woman was obese (OR 0.69, 0.56–0.87). Results relating BMI at 33 years of age were weaker but consistent with those for 23 years of age. Obese women at 23 years of age were less likely to become pregnant within 12 months than women of normal weight (infertility rates = obese, 33.6% vs normal weight, 18.6%). Zaadstra et al. *(19)* found that the upper quartile of BMI (33.1 kg/m^2) in a group of apparently normal women who were undergoing donor insemination had a reduced chance of pregnancy (OR 0.43). This was a particularly significant study because few of the women required medication to stimulate ovulation. Balen et al. *(14)* in the United Kingdom also found that obese women had higher infertility rates. In 204 North American women studied by Green et al. *(20)* there was a reduced fertility rate among women with more than 20% of ideal body weight (OR 2.1), but this did not apply to women who had previously been pregnant.

The literature is therefore quite clear in associating increased body mass with a higher incidence of infertility. Most of the studies do not clearly classify women as having PCOS or normal ovaries, but a large percentage of the obese female population are likely to have this condition.

Obesity, PCOS, and Miscarriage

Weight excess is associated with an increased risk of miscarriage. In a study of more than 13,000 women seeking their first spontaneous pregnancy *(21)*, 11% of women with a BMI of 19–24.9 kg/m^2, 14% with a BMI of 25–27.9 kg/m^2, and 15% of those with a BMI higher than 28 kg/m^2 miscarried (OR 1, 1.26, and 1.37, respectively). Women weighing more than 82 kg are more likely to miscarry than thinner women after ovulation induction *(22)* (OR 2.7 for 82–95 kg and 3.4 for >95 kg), whereas even a mild increase in BMI (25–28 kg/m^2) leads to a significant risk of pregnancy loss (OR 1.37, 1.18–1.60) in some series *(21,23)* but not in others *(24)*. It has been generally claimed that women with PCOS are more likely to miscarry than those without PCOS. This has been attributed, at least in part, to higher luteinzing hormone (LH) concentrations in PCOS that may lead to impaired oocyte and embryo quality.

Obesity, PCOS, and Pregnancy

Since the 1940s, there have been many articles on the effect of obesity on pregnancy and obstetric outcome. Some of the American studies detail results on massively obese women, indicating much higher health risks and increased costs to the health system. Studies from Europe *(25)* confirm that high pre-pregnancy weight is associated with an increased risk in pregnancy of hypertension, toxemia, gestational diabetes, urinary infection, macrosomia, Cesarean section, increased hospitalization, and cost. Despite this, overall neonatal outcome appears to be satisfactory.

Obesity, PCOS, and Glucose Intolerance

There is abundant evidence associating increasing BMI with diabetes mellitus. Subjects with PCOS have a substantial added risk of glucose intolerance. In a study from Adelaide, 18% of all women with BMI higher than 30 kg/m^2 in their 20s and 30s had impairment of glucose metabolism, whereas 15% of women with PCOS who had normal glucose tolerance when initially studied showed conversion to impaired glucose tolerance or frank diabetes when restudied 5–7 years later *(26)*. Conway et al. *(27)* showed that 8% of lean and 11% of obese women with PCOS had abnormal glucose tolerance. In a recent prospective study, we have shown that women with PCOS convert from initially normal glucose tolerance to impaired glucose tolerance or diabetes mellitus at a rate of approx 3% per year. Almost all of this change can be associated with increasing obesity, and prevention of weight gain would be expected to be beneficial in the minimization of abnormal glucose tolerance.

There is controversial evidence that women with PCOS are more likely to exhibit gestational diabetes when pregnant, and that many women with glucose intolerance in pregnancy have features of PCOS. This makes it even more important that potential complications from PCOS should be sorted out before embarking on treatment to induce pregnancy.

Obesity, PCOS, and Response to Infertility Treatment

Most studies show conclusive evidence that increasing BMI is associated with an increased requirement for clomiphene citrate. In several of these, large doses of clomiphene (up to 200 mg per day) were required to ensure ovulation in the heaviest women. If this drug is considered to have some association with ovarian cancer, it is probably undesirable for so much to be used per cycle of treatment. There does not, however, appear to be an association of body weight with poor conception rates in cycles of oral anti-estrogens. In a study of 2841 cycles of clomiphene citrate, there was no association between body weight and pregnancy rate *(28)*, as previously suggested by Friedman and Kim *(29)*. Doses of gonadotrophins required to induce ovulation are also higher in anovulatory women and those requiring ovarian stimulation for any reason *(24)*.

Recently, we have shown that the procedure of intrauterine insemination with gonadotrophins in women with normal menstrual cycles and unexplained infertility gives similar pregnancy rates up to BMI of 30 kg/m^2 *(30)*. Although women with a

BMI higher than 35 kg/m^2 have a lower pregnancy result, paradoxically this treatment was statistically more successful in women with BMIs between 30 an 34.9 kg/m^2, suggesting a subtle endocrine abnormality in this group of women.

The data relating to in vitro fertilization (IVF) and other assisted reproduction is less certain. Although Clark et al. *(31)* found a poor success rate in IVF pregnancies for the very obese, other studies have not shown any difference for women with moderate to severe obesity *(32)*. However, more recent studies from our group *(33)* and others confirm the negative association between IVF outcome and weight status.

Fat Distribution, PCOS, and Reproduction

Obesity can be central or peripheral in distribution, and there is a lot of data suggesting different hormonal and metabolic responses depending on the distribution of fat. Women with central fat have high levels of LH, androstenedione, estrone, insulin, triglycerides, very low-density lipoproteins and apolipoprotein B, and lower levels of high-density lipoprotein *(23,34)*. Gynecological effects of central adiposity are also significant. Zaadstra et al. *(19)* showed that a high WHR (central adiposity) was associated with a markedly lower conception rate in a donor insemination program. The Iowa Women's Health Study also indicated that high WHR was associated with more menstrual abnormalities and higher prevalence of infertility *(35)*. Norman et al. *(34,36)* showed that high WHR was associated with greater disturbance in reproductive hormones, particularly insulin, in PCOS as subsequently confirmed by others *(37)*. Reproductive response to diet and infertility treatment is likely to be closely related to central fat, as indicated by the data by Clark et al. *(31,38)*.

Effect of Weight Loss on Menstruation and Infertility

There were several reports in the 1950s that indicated that weight loss induces menstrual regulation in a proportion of women with obesity and anovulation. Later Bates and Whitworth *(39)* were the first to show a reduction in plasma androgens with dieting and associated return of menstrual cycles. These endocrine and clinical observations have been confirmed by several studies including those by Pasquali et al. *(4,40)*. Kiddy et al. *(41,42)* and Pettigrew *(23)* revisited dietary manipulation of subjects with obesity and PCOS, showing that strict calorie restriction with a subsequent 5% or greater weight loss led to changes in insulin, IGF, SHBG, and menstruation. Menstrual regularity and hirsutism improved, with some spontaneous pregnancies resulting. Since then, there have been several studies confirming that weight loss improves clinical and biochemical parameters that are disordered because of weight problems *(31,38,40,37)*. All the previously described studies, although showing the principle that dietary control leads to favorable reproductive outcomes, fail to address the issue of long-term compliance in a clinical situation. The exceptions are the work published by us in Adelaide who have shown how menstrual regularity and pregnancy can be restored by exercise and dietary advice without an emphasis on low calories *(31,38)* and that from Italy *(43)*. More than 90% of obese, oligomenorrhoeic women showed a dramatic improvement in menstrual patterns, with a higher spontaneous conception rate and a lower miscarriage rate than before treatment. Even women with causes of infertility not related to anovulation (such as tubal blockage or a male partner with oligospermia) showed dramatic improvements in assisted reproduction pregnancies. Weight loss into the normal range is not required for a good clinical response, indicating that weight loss *per se* was not the main reason for success. Mitchell and Rogers in 1953 *(11)* had previously made the observation that "the onset of menses frequently precedes any marked loss of weight and occurs so soon after the start of the therapeutic regimen that the absolute degree of obesity cannot be the only factor involved." The Italian group has shown that weight loss-inducing diets with or without metformin can induce substantial clinical and metabolic changes *(43)*.

Several studies have reported that surgically induced weight loss (gastrojejunal anastomosis and gastric stapling) are successful in restoring menstruation and pregnancy, but these operations may have significant morbidity and very poor neonatal outcome. However, in one of these studies, the miscarriage rate was substantially reduced after the operation when compared with that before the operation *(44)*.

Weight Loss and Exercise Programs in Lifestyle Modification

We have previously described how dietary and exercise programs, specifically a 6-month group program with weekly meetings, achieved sustained weight loss and alteration of reproduction function (Tables 3 and 4). Having become frustrated by the lack of results when individual dietary advice was given by a dietician or medical practitioner, Clark pioneered the unique concept (at least in gynecology) of lifestyle modification within groups of overweight women seeking to achieve a pregnancy. Women were encouraged to agree to join a group for 6 months, during which they understood they would not be given any fertility treatment. At the first meeting, they were encouraged to bring their partners, who were given the information about the group approach, and subsequent meetings were held every week for about 2 hours. At these meetings, exercise and dietary advice were combined with other activities, such as fashion information for the overweight, supermarket trips, and medical information on the pathophysiology of PCOS. The exercise component lasted approx 1 hour with gentle exercises, such as stepping and walking, and was conducted by a keep-fit instructor who appreciated the problem of the overweight person. This was followed by a group session in which a lecture, seminar, or discussion concentrated on subjects of interest to the women. Initially, a dietician gave advice on healthy eating patterns without seeking to prescribe a low-calorie diet. No attempt was made to induce massive caloric reduction and slow weight loss was the preferred option. Initially, many of the women expected diet sheets and advice similar to those obtained from commercial weight-loss companies, but in time they realized that sustained weight loss can only be achieved by a life-long alteration in eating patterns and not by crash diets.

Weight and fat redistribution is the first obvious sign before weight loss in this program. Menstrual regularity can be induced without any weight loss, provided the dietary retraining and exercise is taken seriously. Even 2–5% weight change can be effective in restoring ovulation. In our first paper *(31)* we studied anovulatory women with PCOS, 12 of 13 ovulated by the end of 6 months and the majority became pregnant within 1 year, most spontaneously. In a subsequent report *(38)*, we extended this success rate to all women with obesity who had a range of infertility conditions and showed the efficacy of this approach. In most of the women, weight loss has been sustained and it is likely that long-term health benefits will result. Our philosophy is that alteration of lifestyle, particularly weight, will lead to short-, medium-, and long-term benefits.

Table 2
Compensatory Changes in the Macronutrient Composition of Various Diets

Diet description	Fat (% kj)	Carbohydrate (% kj)	Protein (% kj)	Alcohol (% kj)
Average	34	49	14	3
Low-fat, high-carbohydrate, low-protein	30	55	15	–
Very low-fat, very high-carbohydrate	15	70	15	–
Moderate-protein, moderate-carbohydrate	30	40	30	–
Moderate-protein, very low-carbohydrate	55	15	30	–

Menstruation can be restored, fertility promoted naturally or by assisted reproduction with better results, the risks of diabetes mellitus, cardiovascular disease and hyperlipidemia ameliorated, and the musculoskeletal and metabolic side-effects reduced. Retraining of diet and exercise patterns can have life-long benefits and alter health outcomes significantly.

What Diet for PCOS?

A low-fat, moderate protein, and high-carbohydrate intake diet (30:15:55%) with a restricted caloric input is the standard recommended diet in most countries. Concomitant exercise is essential for weight maintenance and contributes to reducing stress and improves the sense of well-being. Weight loss is maintained more effectively and compliance is increased when an *ad libitum* low-fat high-carbohydrate dietary pattern is followed over longer periods of time compared with fixed-energy diets *(45)*. There has also been increased community interest in a dietary protocol advocating a moderate increase in protein (to approx 30% of total energy intake) and concomitant reduction in dietary carbohydrates *(46)* (Table 2). Furthermore, altering the type of carbohydrate to produce a lower glycemic response (low glycemic index [GI]) is also proposed to improve satiety and metabolic parameters *(47)* (Fig. 1).

High-protein diets range from the medically acceptable 30% protein, 40% carbohydrate, 30% fat, to the Atkins-type diet, which is much higher in protein (50%) and is high in fat. High-protein diets are more likely to reduce *ad libitum* intake, increase subjective satiety, and decrease hunger compared with high-carbohydrate diets *(46,48)*. Weight loss may be more substantial with these approaches in the short-term but is no better in other diets in the longer-term. The evidence for improved insulin sensitivity with high-protein diets is debateable and metabolic improvements are not better in PCOS when caloric intake is matched for low-protein diets *(49)*. Indeed, there is some concern that metabolic changes and cardiovascular risk may increase with high-protein diets, particularly with large amounts of red meat. Overall it appears as if dietary composition is not a key component of diets for PCOS, provided caloric intake is reduced substantially. Ultimately, weight loss will result from a decrease in energy intake or increase in energy expenditure, and this should be the key approach.

The potentially detrimental effects of a high-carbohydrate diet might also be minimized through modifying the source of the dietary carbohydrate, achieved practically through changing the GI of the carbohydrate. The GI is a classification index of carbohydrate foods based on postprandial glucose response and is defined as the incremental

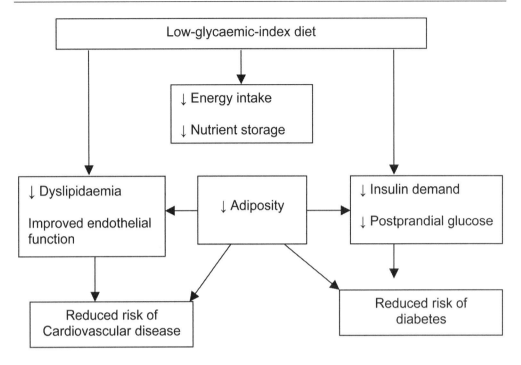

Fig. 1. Pathways by which a low glycemic index might be of benefit.

area-under-the-blood glucose curve produced by a standard amount of carbohydrates in a food relative to the incremental area produced by the same amount of carbohydrate from a standard source *(50)*. Claims have been made that low-GI foods reduce postprandial insulin demand and thereby reduce hyperinsulinemia *(57)*. There are no studies in the role of GI and diets for women with PCOS.

Dietary Intervention and Insulin-Sensitizing Agents

Metformin alone or with clomiphene citrate is effective in increasing ovulation rates and pregnancy. Some studies have also suggested that metformin helps with weight loss *(8)*. In a randomized, controlled trial of diet with or without metformin, insulin-sensitizing drugs were better than placebo in women with PCOS with respect to loss of weight, reduction in visceral fat, waist circumference, and testosterone. There was no differential effect on glucose or insulin levels. Other studies have not confirmed these observations when comparing metformin and placebo use *(52)*. Other glitazones are of no value in weight loss, although they are effective in restoring ovulation.

Reasons for Weight-Related Menstrual Problems

Infertile, anovulatory obese women have higher plasma androgens, insulin, and LH concentrations and lower SHBG levels when compared with normal weight women or obese subjects with regular periods. It is possible that the increased estrogen production from peripheral tissues leads to a disorder of the hypothalamic–pituitary–ovarian axis. Insulin resistance is common in anovulatory women and together with reduced hepatic clearance of insulin and increased sensitivity of the β-cells to secretory stimuli is

Table 3
The Fertility Fitness Program

- Information about role of weight and body composition in reproductive disorders
- Agreement to seek lifestyle changes for at least 6 months
- Group meeting with partners to explain the course
- Weekly meetings for 2–2.5 hours with women
- Gentle aerobic exercises for 1 hour (walking, stepping, and so on)
- Lecture/seminar for 1 hour (good eating—nutrition/alcohol/smoking/caffeine, psychological aspects, medical information, and so on)
- Put into practice for next 6 months
- If return of periods, pregnancy, and others, no further medical treatment
- If disorder persists after 6 months, offer appropriate medical treatment

Table adapted from ref. *64*.

thought to be the major cause of hyperinsulinemia. Insulin in turn can induce androgen secretion from an ovary that is polycystic or genetically prone to excess androgen production. Current hypotheses suggest that hyperinsulinemia is a result of genetic or environmentally induced insulin resistance from peripheral tissues and this leads to increased androgen production from ovaries that are not resistant to the action of insulin. Reduction of hyperinsulinemia should lead to reduction of hyperandrogenemia and restoration of reproduction function. This hypothesis is clearly supported by the experimental observations by a number of investigators.

We have followed women participating in a weight loss program and have shown that return of ovulation coincides with a reduction in insulin resistance and a fall in central adiposity. In a group of anovulatory subjects who returned to ovulation with exercise and dietary restraint, waist circumference, central fat, LH, and insulin fell more than in those who remained anovulatory throughout. In a less-extensive previous study, we had shown that fasting insulin was significantly reduced by weight loss in anovulatory women who became ovulatory *(31)*. Although there is convincing evidence that insulin sensitivity can be restored in overweight women with PCOS who lose weight *(53,55)*, first-phase insulin release remains significantly abnormal indicating an underlying problem in pancreatic secretion in these subjects. Other investigators have disputed this observation. The return to ovulation associated with a reduction in insulin reinforces studies with insulin-sensitizing agents, such as troglitazone, where improved insulin sensitivity without weight loss promotes ovulation and fertility *(56,57)*.

LH pulse frequency and amplitude does not appear to alter during weight loss in obese subjects *(58)*, although absolute values of LH do decrease significantly in responders to diet as judged by ovulation.

Other factors involved may include androgens, hypothalmic endorphins, and leptin, all of which are increased in anovulatory, overweight women. Although leptin is increased in obese subjects with PCOS, there is no increase over obesity not associated with PCOS, and the return of ovulation is not associated with a reduction in leptin concentrations prior to return of periods.

Depression is frequent in women with PCOS and infertility as shown by assessments performed in women from Adelaide. Participation in the program was associated with an improvement in well-being and psychological parameters that may indicate restoration

Table 4
Lifestyle Modification Suggested for Treatment of Polycystic
Ovary Syndrome in Overweight Women

- Moderate exercise ($\geq$30 min/day)
- Dietary modification (fat $\leq$30% daily intake, $\downarrow$ saturated and trans fat and glycemic load, $\uparrow$ fiber and polyunsaturated fat)
- For weight loss, establishing an energy deficit of 500–1000 kcal/day
- Reduction of psychosocial stressors
- Cessation of smoking
- Moderate alcohol consumption
- Moderate caffeine consumption
- Group interaction/intervention to provide support and assist implementing changes

Table adapted from ref. *65*.

of reproductive potential is closely tied in with psychological changes *(59,60)*. These may have an effect through the endorphin system and other neurotransmitters in the hypothalamic–pituitary axis.

Smoking

Many women with PCOS choose to smoke in response to stress or the desire to prevent further weight gain. Our experience shows that 40% of women in our unit who have PCOS are also smokers. There is convincing data that, apart from the well-known health hazards of smoking with respect to the cardiovascular and respiratory system, there are effects on reduction of fertility potential.

Studies show that the time to conception is increased by 30% for smokers and there is a two- to threefold increased risk of failing to conceive after 1 year of attempting pregnancy. Augood et al. *(61)* have recently published a systematic review and meta-analysis of the effects of smoking on fertility and concluded that the risk of infertility in smokers vs non-smokers was 1.60 (95% confidence interval 1.34–1.91). Women who subsequently went through a cycle of assisted reproduction were found to have an OR of 0.66 (0.49–0.88) for pregnancies per number of attempts in smokers vs non-smokers. This does not appear to be attributable to smoking in the male partner, where the time to conception was not increased in male smokers when their partner's smoking status is taken into consideration.

Maternal smoking does not appear to affect the risk of spontaneous abortion but may alter the rate of abnormal placentation, abruptio placentae, and perinatal death after ante-partum bleeding *(62)*. Growth of the fetus is definitely altered by smoking, with birth weight reduced by an average of 200 g. There is a dose–response effect where birth weight decreases as the number of cigarettes smoked increases. Perinatal mortality rates are increased by about 30% because of excesses in low birth weight, prematurity, and abnormal placentation.

All women with PCOS who are trying to become pregnant should be strongly advised to reduce or eliminate their smoking habit prior to therapeutic attempts at inducing ovulation with drugs. Although this may require considerable effort, including

Table 5
NIH Clinical Guidelines for Long-Term Treatment of Overweight and Obesity

- Sensible diet and changed eating habits for long term
- Effective physical activity program sustainable long term
- Behavior modification, reduction of stress, well-being
- Combination of dietary and behavioral therapy and increased physical activity
- Social support by physician, family, spouse, and peers
- Smoking cessation and reduction in alcohol consumption
- Avoidance of "crash diets" and short-term weight loss
- Minor roles for drugs involved in weight loss
- Avoidance of aggressive surgical approaches for majority
- Adaptation of weight-loss programs to meet individual needs
- Long-term observation, monitoring, and encouraging of patients who have successfully lost weight

the use of nicotine patches and hypnotherapy, the end results are well justified in terms of improved pregnancy rates, perinatal mortality, and health outcomes.

Stress Reduction

Several studies have shown that women with PCOS are more likely to have a poor quality-of-life assessment, have eating disorders, and poor self-image (63). Intervention by counseling and reassurance lead to improvement in these parameters and should be part of any program.

CONCLUSIONS

Although the attending doctor may be tempted or pressured to use fertility drugs for subjects with PCOS, lifestyle changes are critically important in these women, not only for successful management but also for long-term health. Overall recommendations are shown in the Table 5.

FUTURE AVENUES OF INVESTIGATION

1. Determine the exact role of insulin-sensitizing agents in lifestyle modification.
2. Dissecting respective roles of diet and exercise in lifestyle modification.
3. Understanding the role of low-GI diets.
4. Developing lifestyle programs that work, both in the short and long term.

KEY POINTS

- Obesity is increasing and has significant effects on reproduction.
- Weight loss has been shown to lead to improvements of reproductive function.
- Dietary management is critical and is based on low-calorie diets.
- It does not seem to matter whether you use a high-protein or high-carbohydrate diet.
- Insulin-sensitizing agents may assist lifestyle modification.

REFERENCES

1. Frisch RE. Fatness, menarche, and female fertility. Perspect Biol 1985;28:611–633.
2. Frisch RE. Body fat, menarche, fitness and fertility. Human Reprod 1987;2:521–533.

3. Correa H, Jacoby J. Nutrition and fertility: some iconoclastic results. Am J Clin Nutr 1978;31:1431–1436.
4. Pasquali R, Casimirri F, Colella P, Melchionda N. Body fat distribution and weight loss in obese women [letter]. Am J Clin Nutr 1989;49:185–187.
5. Pasquali R, Casimirri F. The impact of obesity on hyperandrogenism and polycystic ovary syndrome in premenopausal women. Clin Endocrinol (Oxf) 1993;39:1–16.
6. Zachow RJ, Magoffin DA. Direct intraovarian effects of leptin: impairment of the synergistic action of insulin-like growth factor-I on follicle-stimulating hormone-dependent estradiol-17 beta production by rat ovarian granulosa cells. Endocrinology 1997;138:847–850.
7. Chapman IM, Wittert GA, Norman RJ. Circulating leptin concentrations in polycystic ovary syndrome: relation to anthropometric and metabolic parameters. Clin Endocrinol (Oxf) 1997;46:175–181.
8. Mantzoros CS, Dunaif A, Flier JS. Leptin concentrations in the polycystic ovary syndrome [see comments]. J Clin Endocrinol Metab 1997;82:1687–1691.
9. Nader S, Riad Gabriel MG, Saad MF. The effect of a desogestrel-containing oral contraceptive on glucose tolerance and leptin concentrations in hyperandrogenic women. J Clin Endocrinol Metab 1997;82:3074–3077.
10. Moran LJ, Clifton PM, Wittert GA, et al. Ghrelin and measures of satiety are altered in polycystic ovary syndrome but not differentially affected by diet composition. J Clin Endocrinol Metab 2004; 89:3337–3344.
11. Mitchell GW, Rogers J. The influence of weight reduction on amenorrhea in obese women. N Engl J Med 1953;249:835–837.
12. Hartz AJ, Barboriak PN, Wong A, Katayama KP, Rimm A. The association of obesity with infertility and related menstrual abnormalities in women. Int J Obes 1979;3:57–73.
13. Lake JK, Power C, Cole TJ. Women's reproductive health: the role of body mass index in early and adult life. Int J Obes Relat Metab Disord 1997;21:432–438.
14. Balen AH, Conway GS, Kaltsas G, et al. Polycystic ovary syndrome: the spectrum of the disorder in 1741 patients. Human Reprod 1995;10:2107–2111.
15. Kiddy DS, Sharp PS, White DM, et al. Differences in clinical and endocrine features between obese and non-obese subjects with polycystic ovary syndrome: an analysis of 263 consecutive cases. Clin Endocrinol (Oxf) 1990;32:213–220.
16. Howe G, Westhoff C, Vessey M, Yeates D. Effects of age, cigarette smoking, and other factors on fertility: findings in a large prospective study. Br Med J (Clin Res Ed) 1985;290:1697–1700.
17. Rich Edwards JW, Goldman MB, Willett WC, et al. Adolescent body mass index and infertility caused by ovulatory disorder. Am J Obstet Gynecol 1994;171:171–177.
18. Grodstein F, Goldman MB, Cramer DW. Body mass index and ovulatory infertility. Epidemiology 1994;5:247–250.
19. Zaadstra BM, Seidell JC, Van Noord PA, et al. Fat and female fecundity: prospective study of effect of body fat distribution on conception rates [see comments]. BMJ 1993;306:484–487.
20. Green BB, Weiss NS, Daling JR. Risk of ovulatory infertility in relation to body weight. Fertil Steril 1988;50:721–726.
21. Hamilton-Fairley D, Kiddy D, Watson H, Paterson C, Franks S. Association of moderate obesity with a poor pregnancy outcome in women with polycystic ovary syndrome treated with low dose gonadotrophin. Br J Obstet Gynaecol 1992;99:128–131.
22. Bohrer M, Kemmann E. Risk factors for spontaneous abortion in menotropin-treated women. Fertil Steril 1987;48:571–575.
23. Pettigrew R, Hamilton Fairley D. Obesity and female reproductive function. PMID 1997;53:341–358.
24. McClure N, McQuinn B, McDonald J, Kovacs GT, Healy DL, Burger HG. Body weight, body mass index, and age: predictors of menotropin dose and cycle outcome in polycystic ovarian syndrome? Fertil Steril 1992;58:622–624.
25. Galtier Dereure F, Montpeyroux F, Boulot P, Bringer J, Jaffiol C. Weight excess before pregnancy: complications and cost. Int J Obes Relat Metab Disord 1995;19:443–448.
26. Wang JX, Norman RJ. Risk factors for the deterioration of glucose metabolism in polycystic ovary syndrome. Reprod Biomed Online 2004;9:201–204.
27. Conway GS, Agrawal R, Betteridge DJ, Jacobs H. Risk factors for coronary artery disease in lean and obese women with the polycystic ovary syndrome. Clin Endocrinol (Oxf) 1992;37:119–125.

28. Dickey RP, Taylor SN, Curole DN, Rye PH, Lu PY, Pyrzak R. Relationship of clomiphene dose and patient weight to successful treatment. Human Reprod 1997;12:449–453.
29. Friedman CI, Kim MH. Obesity and its effect on reproductive function. Clin Obstet Gynecol 1985; 28:645–663.
30. Fuh KW, Wang X, Tai A, Wong I, Norman RJ. Intrauterine insemination: effect of the temporal relationship between the LH surge, hCG administration and insemination on pregnancy rates. Hum Reprod 1997;12:2162–2166.
31. Clark AM, Ledger W, Galletly C, et al. Weight loss results in significant improvement in pregnancy and ovulation rates in anovulatory obese women. Human Reprod 1995;10:2705–2712.
32. Lewis CG, Warnes GM, Wang XJ, Matthews CD. Failure of body mass index or body weight to influence markedly the response to ovarian hyperstimulation in normal cycling women. Fertil Steril 1990;53: 1097–1099.
33. Wang JX, Davies MJ, Norman RJ. Obesity increases the risk of spontaneous abortion during infertility treatment. Obes Res 2002;10:551–554.
34. Norman RJ, Masters SC, Hague W, Beng C, Pannall P, Wang JX. Metabolic approaches to the sub-classification of polycystic ovary syndrome. Fertil Steril 1995;63:329–335.
35. Kaye SA, Folsom AR, Prineas RJ, Potter JD, Gapstur SM. The association of body fat distribution with lifestyle and reproductive factors in a population study of postmenopausal women. Int J Obes 1990;14:583–591.
36. Norman RJ, Hague WM, Masters SC, Wang XJ. Subjects with polycystic ovaries without hyperandrogenaemia exhibit similar disturbances in insulin and lipid profiles as those with polycystic ovary syndrome. Hum Reprod 1995;10:2258–2261.
37. Hollmann M, Runnebaum B, Gerhard I. Impact of waist-hip-ratio and body-mass-index on hormonal and metabolic parameters in young, obese women. Int J Obes Relat Metab Disord 1997;21:476–483.
38. Clark AM, Thornley B, Tomlinson L, Galletley C, Norman RJ. Weight loss in obese infertile women results in improvement in reproductive outcome for all forms of fertility treatment. Hum Reprod 1998;13:1502–1505.
39. Bates GW, Whitworth NS. Effect of body weight reduction on plasma androgens in obese, infertile women. Fertil Steril 1982;38:406–409.
40. Pasquali R, Antenucci D, Casimirri F, et al. Clinical and hormonal characteristics of obese amenorrheic hyperandrogenic women before and after weight loss. J Clin Endocrinol Metab 1989;68: 173–179.
41. Kiddy DS, Hamilton Fairley D, Seppala M, et al. Diet-induced changes in sex hormone binding globulin and free testosterone in women with normal or polycystic ovaries; correlation with serum insulin and insulin-like growth factor-I. Clin Endocrinol (Oxf) 1989;31:757–763.
42. Kiddy DS, Hamilton Fairley D, Bush A, et al. Improvement in endocrine and ovarian function during dietary treatment of obese women with polycystic ovary syndrome. Clin Endocrinol (Oxf) 1992;36: 105–111.
43. Pasquali R, Gambineri A, Biscotti D, et al. Effect of long-term treatment with metformin added to hypocaloric diet on body composition, fat distribution, and androgen and insulin levels in abdominally obese women with and without the polycystic ovary syndrome. J Clin Endocrinol Metab 2000; 53:2767–2774.
44. Bilenka B, Ben Shlomo I, Cozacov C, Gold CH, Zohar S. Fertility, miscarriage and pregnancy after vertical banded gastroplasty operation for morbid obesity. Acta Obstet Gynecol Scand Acta Obstetrica Gynecologica Scandinavia 1995;74:42–44.
45. Toubro S, Astrup A. Randomised comparison of diets for maintaining obese subjects' weight after major weight loss: ad lib, low fat, high carbohydrate diet vs fixed energy intake. BMJ 1997;314:29–34.
46. Skov AR, Toubro S, Ronn B, Holm L, Astrup A. Randomized trial on protein vs carbohydrate in ad libitum reduced fat diet for the treatment of obesity. Int J Obes Relat Metab Disord 1999;23:528–536.
47. Ludwig DS. Dietary glycemic index and obesity. J Nutr 2000;130:280S–283S.
48. Johnston CS, Tionn SL, Swan PD. High-protein, low-fat diets are effective for weight loss and favourably alter biomarkers in healthy adults. J Nutr 2004;134:586–591.
49. Moran LJ, Noakes M, Clifton PM, Tomlinson L, Norman RJ. Dietary composition in restoring reproductive and metabolic physiology in polycystic ovary syndrome. J Clin Endocrinol Metab 2003;88: 812–819.

50. Wolever TM, Jenkins DJ, Jenkins AL, Josse RG. The glycemic index: methodology and clinical implications. Am J Clin Nutr 1991;54:846–854.
51. Jarvi AE, Karlstrom BE, Granfeldt YE, Bjork JE, Asp NG, Vessby BO. Improved glycemic control and lipid profile and normalized fibrinolytic activity on a low-glycemic index diet in type 2 diabetic patients. Diabetes Care 1999;22:10–18.
52. Acbay O, Gundogdu S. Can metformin reduce insulin resistance in polycystic ovary syndrome? Fertil Steril 1996;65:946–949.
53. Holte J, Bergh T, Berne C, Berglund L, Lithell H. Enhanced early insulin response to glucose in relation to insulin resistance in women with polycystic ovary syndrome and normal glucose tolerance. J Clin Endocrinol Metab 1994;78:1052–1058.
54. Holte J, Bergh T, Berne C, Wide L, Lithell H. Restored insulin sensitivity but persistently increased early insulin secretion after weight loss in obese women with polycystic ovary syndrome. J Clin Endocrinol Metab 1995;80:2586–2593.
55. Holte J. Disturbances in insulin secretion and sensitivity in women with the polycystic ovary syndrome. Baillieres. J Clin Endocrinol Metab 1996;10:221–247.
56. Dunaif A, Scott D, Finegood D, Quintana B, Whitcomb R. The insulin-sensitizing agent troglitazone improves metabolic and reproductive abnormalities in the polycystic ovary syndrome. J Clin Endocrinol Metab 1996;81:3299–3306.
57. Ehrmann DA, Schneider DJ, Sobel BE, et al. Troglitazone improves defects in insulin action, insulin secretion, ovarian steroidogenesis, and fibrinolysis in women with polycystic ovary syndrome. J Clin Endocrinol Metab 1997;82:2108–2116.
58. Guzick DS, Wing R, Smith D, Berga SL, Winters SJ. Endocrine consequences of weight loss in obese, hyperandrogenic, anovulatory women. Fertil Steril 1994;61:598–604.
59. Galletly C, Clark A, Tomlinson L, Blaney F. A group program for obese, infertile women: weight loss and improved psychological health. J Psychosom Obstet Gynaecol 1996;17:125–128.
60. Galletly C, Clark A, Tomlinson L, Blaney F. Improved pregnancy rates for obese, infertile women following a group treatment program. An open pilot study. Gen Hosp Psychiatry 1996;18:192–195.
61. Augood C, Duckitt K, Templeton A. Smoking and female infertility: a systematic review and meta-analysis. Hum Reprod 1998;13:532–539.
62. Werler MM. Teratogen update: smoking and reproductive outcomes. Teratology 1997;55:382–388.
63. Jahanfer S, Eden JA, Nguyent TV. Bulimia nervosa and polycystic ovary syndrome. Gynecol Endocrinol 1995;9:113–117.
64. Norman RJ, Clark AM. Lifestyle factors in the aetiology and management of polycystic ovary syndrome. In: Kovacs GT, ed, Polycystic Ovary Syndrome. Cambridge: Cambridge University Press, 2000, pp. 98–116.
65. Norman RJ, Davies MJ, Lord J, Moran LJ. The role of lifestyle modification in polycystic ovary syndrome. Trends Endocrinol Metab 2002;13:251–257.

II EVALUATION OF PCOS

10 Clinical Evaluation of Polycystic Ovary Syndrome

Ann E. Taylor, MD

CONTENTS

Summary

The goals of the clinical evaluation of women with possible polycystic ovary syndrome (PCOS) include: (1) making the proper diagnosis (excluding other more serious diagnoses); (2) determining whether to screen for associated health complications of PCOS in the patient and/or her family members; (3) determining the appropriate current treatment; and (4) discussing a long-term management plan for the patient.

The clinical evaluation begins with a complete medical history and physical examination. Although the evaluation will naturally focus on those areas of greatest concern to the patient, the clinician must remember the myriad associated health abnormalities that can occur with PCOS and has a responsibility to evaluate all the health impacts of the condition on the patient, whether or not intervention is currently requested or required.

Key Words: Polycystic ovary syndrome; polycystic ovaries; hyperandrogenemia; hirsutism; acne; menstrual dysfunction; infertility; clinical evaluation; history; physical examination.

INTRODUCTION

The goals of the clinical evaluation of women with possible polycystic ovary syndrome (PCOS) include:

From: *Contemporary Endocrinology: Insulin Resistance and Polycystic Ovarian Syndrome: Pathogenesis, Evaluation, and Treatment*
Edited by: E. Diamanti-Kandarakis, J. E. Nestler, D. Panidis, and R. Pasquali © Humana Press Inc., Totowa, NJ

1. Make the proper diagnosis (excluding other more serious diagnoses).
2. Determine whether to screen for associated health complications of PCOS in the patient and/or her family members.
3. Determine the appropriate current treatment.
4. Discuss a long-term management plan for the patient.

The clinical evaluation begins with a complete medical history and physical examination. Although the evaluation will naturally focus on those areas of greatest concern to the patient, the clinician must remember the myriad associated health abnormalities that can occur with PCOS and has a responsibility to evaluate all the health impacts of the condition on the patient, whether or not intervention is currently requested or required.

Although diagnostic criteria for PCOS for research studies have been proposed, it is important to remember that individual patients who may not meet strict criteria may still benefit from some of the same interventions. The revised consensus criteria proposed at Rotterdam in 2003 require two of the following three conditions to make the diagnosis *(1)*:

1. Oligo- or anovulation.
2. Clinical and/or biochemical signs of hyperandrogenism.
3. Polycystic ovaries.

Thus, for women complaining of hyperandrogenic symptoms such as acne or hirsutism, an understanding of their menstrual history and metabolic profile is required, whereas for those women complaining of infertility or menstrual problems, an evaluation of hyperandrogenic symptoms and metabolic status is required. In addition, other causes of hyperandrogenism and menstrual irregularity, such as congenital adrenal hyperplasia, androgen-secreting tumors, and hyperprolactinemia, must be excluded.

HISTORY

The history naturally begins with the symptoms that are causing most concern to the patient. However, a complete medical history should cover each of the following areas.

Menstrual Irregularity

There are many different types of menstrual dysfunction observed in women with PCOS. The menstrual irregularity of PCOS typically manifests in the peripubertal period. Affected women may have a normal or slightly delayed menarche followed by irregular cycles. Other women may apparently have regular cycles at first and subsequently develop menstrual irregularity in association with weight gain. The menstrual pattern may be one of oligomenorrhea (typically defined as fewer than six or nine menstrual periods in a year) or amenorrhea (no menstrual periods for three or more consecutive months). In addition to menstrual irregularity, menstrual periods that do occur are often anovulatory, and may be associated with dysfunctional bleeding. Some women with PCOS have prolonged amenorrhea associated with endometrial atrophy. Elevated endogenous androgen levels appear to cause endometrial atrophy in a subset of patients. Although the mechanism is not fully elucidated, many obese women with PCOS resume more regular menstrual cycles after relatively small amounts of weight loss. Finally, women with PCOS are at increased risk of endometrial hyperplasia and even endometrial cancer, owing to the unopposed estrogenic stimulation of the endometrium *(2)*.

An evaluation of menstrual function should include age of menarche, current menstrual status (frequency of periods, number per year), pregnancies, oral contraceptive use (why, when, for how long, which pills, response), and presence of symptoms of ovulation or of premenstrual symptoms (ovulatory pain, premenstrual discomfort, breast tenderness). Prior oral contraceptive use may have masked or delayed the recognition of menstrual dysfunction or hyperandrogenic symptoms. Although not all patients have a peri-pubertal onset of irregular menses, the sudden onset of menstrual dysfunction should raise the consideration of other etiologies. The presence of amenorrhea is not uncommon as the manifestation of menstrual dysfunction in PCOS. All women with menstrual dysfunction, and especially those with prolonged amenorrhea, should have a complete evaluation to include consideration of etiologies including pregnancy, weight- and exercise-related causes, hyperprolactinemia, thyroid dysfunction, and ovarian failure.

The management of women with recurrent irregular bleeding requires great clinical judgment to help distinguish between hormonal (anovulation) and anatomical (endometrial hyperplasia and cancer) causes of the bleeding. Pelvic ultrasonography can be a useful tool to evaluate the risk of anatomical causes (*see* Ultrasonography) whereas endometrial protection (induction of regular menses with oral contraceptives or intermittent progestin) will help prevent the clinical symptoms and therefore the need for continued evaluation.

Some women with hyperandrogenic symptoms appear to have regular menstrual cycles. Thus, the evaluation of the hyperandrogenic woman with regular cycles should include at least one or two assessments to document ovulation (*see* Ultrasonography).

Infertility

Infertility was included in the original description of PCOS by Stein and Leventhal *(3)*. Infertility related to PCOS is typically not difficult to diagnose because of the associated menstrual irregularity and anovulation. The primary cause of infertility is irregular ovulation, leading to a reduced number of ovulations and unpredictable timing, and relative infertility. In addition to anovulation, other factors appear to be important because women with PCOS have, in comparison to women with hypothalamic amenorrhea, a reduced rate of conception relative to the rate of ovulation after therapy with clomiphene citrate and exogenous gonadotropins. Many studies have also described an increased rate of early pregnancy loss in PCOS, the mechanism of which is poorly understood *(4)*.

Some women do not receive the diagnosis of PCOS until they are being evaluated for infertility. In such patients, two key principles must be remembered. First, the presence of PCOS does not rule out other abnormalities, so that male factor infertility and tubal patency still must be assessed. Second, if the patient is at risk for metabolic defects, these must be screened for and treated as appropriate, to minimize pregnancy complications related to diabetes in particular. Finally, women with polycystic ovaries on ultrasound may be more likely to hyperstimulate in response to ovulation inducing medications.

Hyperandrogenic Symptoms

Hyperandrogenism is the second defining characteristic of PCOS. Most women with PCOS have both clinical and biochemical evidence of hyperandrogenism. The major clinical manifestations of hyperandrogenism include hirsutism, acne, and male pattern balding or alopecia. In rare instances, increased muscle mass, deepening of the voice, or clitoromegaly may occur, but these findings are suggestive of virilizing androgen levels and should prompt a search for an underlying neoplasm (of the ovary or adrenal gland).

The history of all skin problems should be assessed, including hirsutism, acne, hair loss, and other skin problems. The age at onset, the rate of progression, and any change with any treatment or with fluctuations in weight should be determined. Progressive worsening of hirsutism, a later age of onset, or rapid rate of progression suggest the possibility of ovarian or adrenal tumor, but could be caused by responses to previous treatments or changes in weight.

By history, acne is typically the first manifestation of hyperandrogenism, in the teenage years. Terminal hair growth is age dependent, and may not be apparent until the early 20s after several years of exposure to excess androgens. Male pattern hair loss tends to present even later, in the later 20s and beyond.

Hirsutism is defined as excess terminal (thick, pigmented) body hair in a male distribution, and is commonly noted on the upper lip, chin, around the nipples (periareolar), and along the linea alba of the lower abdomen. The history of hirsutism should include such information as time of onset, site of onset, progression, treatments used, and nature of the hirsutism relative to other family members.

The typical acne lesions include blackheads, whiteheads, and inflammatory lesions, in increasing order of severity. Similar to the history of hirsutism, the history of acne should include the time of onset, site of onset, progression, changes in response to acne or other therapies, and nature of the acne relative to other family members.

The main diagnostic question is how best to identify the small number of women who have other causes for the clinical constellation of findings similar to those seen in PCOS. Several findings in the history may raise the level of suspicion for one of the rare causes of hyperandrogenic symptoms:

1. Abrupt onset, short duration (typically less than 1 year), or sudden progressive worsening.
2. Onset of clinical symptoms in the third decade of life or later, rather than near puberty.
3. Symptoms or signs of virilization, including frontal balding, severe pustular acne, clitoromegaly, increased muscle mass, or deepening of voice.

Additional Components Related to the Health Assessment of Women With PCOS

WEIGHT PROBLEMS

From the earliest depictions of hyperandrogenic women, obesity has been a prominently recognized clinical feature. Thus, some clinicians mistakenly fail to consider the PCOS diagnosis in lean women. However, several recent population based studies of PCOS indicate that obesity is not a universal feature, with 50–70% of women with menstrual dysfunction and evidence of hyperandrogenism not being obese. Compared with age-matched population rates of obesity, there may be a maximum of a twofold relative risk of obesity if a woman has PCOS vs not. Typical patient series showing higher rates of obesity likely reflect diagnosis and referral biases. It is important to make clinicians aware of the health implications of PCOS even in lean subjects.

DIABETES MELLITUS TYPE 2

Because women with PCOS have an increased risk of insulin resistance and type 2 diabetes, it is important to assess the specific risk factors in each patient. In addition to weight, which is a major factor that increases the risk of diabetes, a history of glucose intolerance during pregnancy also increases the risk of later diabetes. The risk of type 2 diabetes in increased especially in women with a first degree relative with type 2 diabetes *(5,6)*. In a study of 122 obese women with PCOS, 45% had either impaired glucose tolerance (35%) or type 2 diabetes mellitus (10%) by age 40 *(5)*. The women with diabetes had a 2.6-fold higher prevalence of first-degree relatives with type 2 diabetes. In a subset of 25 women who underwent repeat oral glucose tolerance testing after a mean of 34 months, 40% had a deterioration in glucose tolerance.

SLEEP APNEA

Two studies have shown a dramatic increased risk of obstructive sleep apnea in women with PCOS (ninefold odds ratio by questionnaire *[7]*, eightfold by overnight polysomnography *[8]*). Thus, women with PCOS should be questioned about signs and symptoms of sleep apnea. Such symptoms include habitual snoring, nocturnal restlessness, and daytime sleepiness.

POSSIBLE PREDISPOSITION TO NONALCOHOLIC STEATOHEPATITIS

The prevalence of nonalcoholic steatohepatitis (NASH) may be increased in women with PCOS *(9)*. It appears reasonable to inquire about symptoms and risk factors for liver disease, including family history and alcohol ingestion.

POSSIBLE PREDISPOSITION TO CORONARY HEART DISEASE

Many studies have suggested that women with PCOS have an increased number of risk factors for coronary heart disease, including obesity and type 2 diabetes *(10,11)*. Whether the actual rate of cardiovascular events is increased, relative to body weight and glucose control or not, has not yet been determined *(12–15)*. In this setting, it seems prudent to include in the history a review of the family history of heart disease, including age of onset, gender, and specific conditions of family members with heart disease or strokes, and symptoms of chest pain, TIAs and claudication in older women with PCOS.

METABOLIC SYNDROME

The prevalence of the metabolic syndrome appears to be very high in women with PCOS. In one retrospective study, 43% of PCOS patients had the metabolic syndrome, roughly twofold higher than that of age-matched women in the general population *(16)*. In a second study, the prevalence of metabolic syndrome in women with PCOS was approx 47% compared to 4% in age-matched (but not weight-matched) controls with regular menses and no hirsutism *(17)*.

MOOD AND QUALITY OF LIFE

Several recent studies have evaluated the quality of life in women with PCOS and have begun to document the adverse psychological and health impacts of this condition.

Completion of a proposed quality of life instrument by 100 women with PCOS indicated five factors that were relevant to them, including emotions, body hair, weight, infertility, and menstrual problems *(18)*. In a small study of 50 patients with PCOS and 50 controls, women with PCOS had a significant reduction in quality of life as measured by psychological disturbances in the dimensions for obsessive-compulsive, interpersonal sensitivity, depression, anxiety, aggression, and psychoticism *(19)*. However, they had a lower degree of life satisfaction for health, self, and sex evaluated by life satisfaction questionnaire scales *(19)*. Most of the differences were not affected by correction for body weight *(19)*. This early data suggests that the management of PCOS should also include an understanding of the life impact and questions about depression and anxiety.

Another aspect of PCOS that may impact quality of life for patients is the costs of their diagnosis and management. A recent study used epidemiologic data and general cost estimates in the United States to estimate the total annual cost of evaluating and providing care to reproductive aged women that PCOS in the United States was $4.36 billion, 2.1% for the initial evaluation, 31% for hormonally treating menstrual dysfunction/abnormal uterine bleeding, 12.2% for providing infertility care, 40.5% for PCOS-associated diabetes, and 14.2% for treating hirsutism *(20)*. Because not all of these costs may be accepted by third party payors, the management of the patient with PCOS may be optimized if the clinician understands the economic burden of PCOS for each individual.

Family History

Several studies have documented an increased risk of PCOS in sisters and daughters of women with PCOS, so the family history provides an opportunity to identify new cases of PCOS. Hirsutism, acne, menstrual irregularity, infertility, early cardiovascular disease, and obesity are all potential indicators of a familial tendency toward the PCOS. A family history of infertility and/or hirsutism may also indicate disorders such as non-classic congenital adrenal hyperplasia, a disorder particularly common in Ashkenazi Jewish women *(21)*. The presence of symptoms that are very different from that of other family members may increase the level of concern for a more pathologic explanation for the menstrual defects or the androgenic symptoms.

The family history is also an opportunity to quantify the family history of other cardiovascular risk factors, including diabetes mellitus, overweight, and hyperlipidemia. A family history of early heart disease might lower the threshold for treatment of cardiovascular risk factors. Because women with defects in the *21OH* gene must have two defective alleles to have clinically relevant symptoms, it is unlikely that the diagnosis of CAH would be uncovered by review of the family history, although membership in a high-risk ethnic group such as Ashkenazi Jews or Yupik Eskimos would increase the clinical suspicion.

Past Medical History

A complete list of past and current medical diagnoses may contribute to the diagnosis and management of PCOS symptoms, and may impact the choice of therapies. Knowledge of prior cancer would lead the clinician to inquire about radiation or chemotherapy, that could impact hair growth and menstrual function. Prior ovarian surgery, for cysts, tumors, bleeding, or infection, could impact current hormonal and menstrual status. Prior records of an abdominal procedure may provide information as to the appearance of the uterus and/or ovaries. However, a history of ovarian cyst removal is not sufficient to make the diagnosis of PCOS.

Even if not used for the specific treatment of PCOS, a complete history of prior therapies must be documented, including topical treatments for acne and hirsutism that are likely to influence the appearance of the skin over time. In some cases, it may be apparent that the symptoms of PCOS just became evident because a woman has recently discontinued oral contraceptive pills that masked the symptoms. At the other extreme, new onset androgenic symptoms could also be explained by the recent use of topical testosterone creams for the treatment of low libido or vulvar dermopathies. The medication list may also reveal prior treated conditions that the patient had not recognized might be related to variability in their menstrual cycles or weight profiles. Finally, acne is known to be caused by certain medications, including azathioprine, barbiturates, corticosteroids, cyclosporine, disulfiram, halogens, iodides, isoniazid, lithium, phenytoin, psoralens, thiourea, and vitamins B2, B6, and B12 *(22,26)*.

Finally, a list of all cosmetic therapies is necessary for the interpretation of physical findings. Specifically, topical and other treatments of hirsutism and acne will influence the clinical manifestations of these conditions.

PHYSICAL EXAMINATION

General

It is important to assess weight at baseline and to regularly monitor weight in women with PCOS, because the incidence of obesity appears to be increased and because obesity increases the risk of other metabolic disorders. Similarly, blood pressure, as an independent cardiovascular risk factor, should be monitored at each visit. Waist circumference may add additional information as to the cardiovascular risk profile for individual women. In addition, the pattern of body fat distribution (truncal obesity, a buffalo hump, and supraclavicular fat) may suggest the presence of Cushing's syndrome

Skin

Hirsutism is defined as excess terminal (thick pigmented) body hair in a male distribution, and is commonly noted on the upper lip, chin, periareolar, in the midsternum, and along the linea alba of the lower abdomen. There is substantial ethnic variability in hirsutism; Asian women, for example, often have a lesser degree of hirsutism *(3)*. Another important source of variability is prior therapy, which needs to be documented. The most common scoring system, the modified Ferriman-Gallway score *(23)*, is a reasonable way for the individual clinician to assess hair growth at baseline, and monitor response to therapy. However, the between observer variability of this score is large *(24)*. Hirsutism should be distinguished from hypertrichosis, the excessive growth of androgen-independent hair which is vellus, prominent in non-sexual areas, and most commonly familial or caused by systemic disorders (hypothyroidism, anorexia nervosa, malnutrition, porphyria, and dermatomyositis) or medications (phenytoin, penicillamine, diazoxide, minoxidil, or cyclosporine).

The typical acne lesions include blackheads, whiteheads, and inflammatory lesions, in increasing order of severity. Residual scarring and hyperpigmentation are possible even after acne is inactive. Some acne scoring systems focus on the severity of the lesions, whereas others focus on the number and location of the lesions. The best method for the baseline evaluation and monitoring of therapy in women with PCOS has not been determined.

An evaluation of hair thinning should be performed as objectively as possible. This can be difficult without prior examinations of the subject and without knowing typical hair patterns in her family members. For women with hair loss, it may be helpful to record baseline and response to therapy using a descriptive scoring system, such as that of Ludwig (25) proposed for use in women. For clinical trials of treatment of hair loss, much more extensive methods may be used, including pulling and weighing hairs in a defined region, standardized photographs, and assessing hair density in defined regions of the scalp.

Other skin findings that should be sought include seborrhea, acanthosis nigricans (may indicate insulin resistance), and striae, thin skin, or bruising, which suggest possible Cushing's syndrome.

Reproductive System Examination

A complete reproductive system examination should be conducted at the time of diagnosis and in follow up examinations as appropriate to the initial findings and progression of symptoms. The breast exam should include a specific assessment of atrophy (potential evidence of significant hyperandrogenemia), and galactorrhea, as well as the mandatory assessment for pathologic masses. The abdominal examination should include assessment of hepatic size (to evaluate possible hepatic enlargement as a result of steatosis), as well as palpation for adrenal and pelvic masses. The external genitalia should be examined for evidence of clitoromegaly, which would prompt a search for androgen-producing neoplasms. One study demonstrated that the normal clitoris in adult women is less than 35 mm^2 (length × width) (26). The examination should also verify that the internal genitalia (vagina, uterus, and ovaries) are present. Otherwise, an evaluation for other rare causes of amenorrhea and hyperandrogenism (ex testicular feminization) must be considered.

LABORATORY EVALUATION

Androgens

Depending upon which androgens are measured, up to 90% of PCOS women will have an elevated serum androgen concentration (27). The excess androgens can be derived from the ovary, the adrenal cortex, or both. Serum androgens fall with age in normal women, and appear to also fall with age in women with PCOS (28). After age 47, androgen levels remained stable, although they were high compared with a group of control women. The persistent, although reduced hyperandrogenemia in older women with PCOS has been suggested as a factor contributing to the increased risk of cardio-vascular disease and endometrial cancer that has been observed.

An elevation in free testosterone is the most sensitive test to establish the presence of hyperandrogenemia. This is because elevated insulin levels (a frequent concomitant of PCOS) and elevated androgen levels both act to inhibit hepatic production of sex hormone-binding globulin (SHBG), thus both low SHBG and increased testosterone production combine to result in elevated free testosterone levels. However, it is critical that an appropriate measurement of free testosterone be performed. If an equilibrium dialysis method is not available, the clinician should measure total testosterone and SHBG and calculate the free testosterone, rather than relying on an indirect assay method that is notoriously unreliable (29).

Total testosterone (but not free testosterone) levels have been validated to evaluate the risk of androgen-secreting ovarian or adrenal tumors. Women with tumors typically have serum testosterone concentrations greater than 150 ng/dL (30) and those with adrenal tumors usually have serum dehydroepiandrosterone sulfate concentrations higher than 800 µg/dL. Their serum LH concentrations are low.

Other Biochemical Findings

Other biochemical findings that are often, but not universally present, may include:

1. Elevation in serum luteinizing hormone (LH) concentrations. The likelihood of finding an elevation in serum LH is dependent upon the timing of the sample relative to the last menstrual period, the ovarian activity, the use of oral contraceptive pills, and the frequency of LH-sampling given the pulsatile nature of its secretion (31). Because it does not influence the treatment or the diagnosis, measurement of LH is not required for the routine evaluation of a women with suspected PCOS. The serum concentration of follicle stimulating hormone (FSH) may be normal or low in PCOS, leading to an elevated LH/FSH ratio compared with normally cycling, early follicular phase young control women.
2. Normal serum estradiol and increased serum estrone concentrations. Again, these values do not influence treatment or diagnosis and their measurement is not required for the routine evaluation. However, the demonstration of a normal, rather than reduced, estradiol level can be reassuring to the subset of PCOS patients who have amenorrhea and are worried about their bone density.
3. 17-OH progesterone: testing for late onset congenital adrenal hyperplasia (CYP21A2 deficiency) should be considered in women with an early onset of hirsutism (including those with premature adrenarche), hyperkalemia, a family history of congenital adrenal hyperplasia, women planning pregnancy with a man at high risk for carrying CAH genes, or a strong desire to know a specific etiologic diagnosis.

A morning value of 17 hydroxyprogesterone greater than 200 ng/dL in the early follicular phase strongly suggests the diagnosis of adrenal hyperplasma, which may be confirmed by a high dose (250 mcg) ACTH stimulation test. Most patients with 21 hydroxylase deficiency have values exceeding 1500 ng/dL after ACTH stimulation (32,33).

If performed without adrenal stimulation, the blood sample must be obtained in the early morning to take advantage of the fact that endogenous ACTH levels are highest at that time as a result of the diurnal variation in its secretion. Measurement after ACTH is given is slightly more cumbersome, but the results obtained in this manner are highly reproducible and can be compared to published nomograms (15,33).

Testing for Cushing's Syndrome

Screening for Cushing's syndrome may be considered in hyperandrogenic women with symptoms and signs of cortisol excess, such as obesity, hypertension, striae, that suggest the presence of Cushing's syndrome. Screening tests include a 24-hour urine collection for cortisol or an overnight dexamethasone suppression test.

Other Tests

1. Diabetes: if women with PCOS are older, obese, or have a family history of type 2 diabetes, screening for diabetes is recommended. Unfortunately, a fasting glucose does not appear to be a sensitive test in women with PCOS, so an oral glucose tolerance test should be performed, with acquisition of a glucose level 2 hours after the 75-g glucose load *(5,34)*.

2. Lipid panel: several studies have demonstrated more lipid abnormalities in women with PCOS than in age and weight matched normal women *(35)*. Occasional monitoring of fasting lipids is prudent. Although other cardiovascular risk factors have been associated with PCOS, to date, no studies have demonstrated that identification of these factors modifies treatment of that treatment of these factors improves outcomes, so this author does not support their measurement.

Summary of Tests

Diagnosis: total testosterone or free testosterone (most commonly assessed by measuring total testosterone and SHBG and calculating the free amount), FSH, serum progesterone (if need to document anovulation), prolactin, TSH.

Health management: glucose level measured 2 hours after an oral load (75 g) or a mixed meal, especially if overweight or a family history of diabetes, fasting lipid profile occasionally.

ULTRASONOGRAPHY

Pelvic ultrasonography may assist in the diagnosis and management of women with PCOS but is not required for making the diagnosis. A well-performed ultrasound can screen for some ovarian androgen secreting tumors, and evaluate the endometrium, in addition to identifying the classic morphologic appearance of polycystic ovaries. Suspicious findings include large cysts, solid masses, and complex cysts that do not resolve spontaneously in 2–4 weeks. However, the sensitivity and specificity of ultrasonography for the diagnosis of ovarian tumors in hyperandrogenic women has not been determined. Small hilus-cell tumors of the ovary that produce large amounts of testosterone may not be seen by ultrasonography or even at the time of surgery.

The definition of polycystic ovaries by ultrasound has changed as the ultrasonography methodology has improved. The original definition of Adams required the presence of eight or more small (2–8 mm) follicles in a single plane, in each ovary, that are typically peripherally arrayed *(36)*. The typical appearance also includes increased stroma. More recently, the criteria have been revised. The current criteria considered to have sufficient specificity and sensitivity to define PCO are the presence of 12 or more follicles (2–9 mm) in each whole ovary and/or increased ovarian volume (>10 mL; calculated using the formula 0.5 × length × width × thickness) *(37)*. It was suggested that follicle distribution and an increase in stromal echogenicity and volume be eliminated as diagnostic criteria. Many patients need to be reassured that the name PCOS refers to the tiny follicles, not to large, cystic, and painful ovaries.

This morphology can be visible by either transvaginal or transabdominal techniques, but may be difficult to discern transabdominally, especially in the patient with large amounts of abdominal fat. However, transabdominal scans may be preferred in young and/or sexually inactive subjects.

Although 80–100% of women with the PCOS do have polycystic ovaries, so do many women with idiopathic hirsutism or other disorders causing androgen excess. For example, 92% of women with idiopathic hirsutism *(36)*, 87% with oligomenorrhea *(36)*, 82% of premenopausal women with type 2 diabetes mellitus *(38)*, 82% of women with congenital adrenal hyperplasia *(39)*, 26% of women with amenorrhea *(36)*, 40% of women with a history of gestational diabetes mellitus *(40)*, and at least 23% of women who considered themselves normal and reported regular menstrual cycles *(41,42)* have been reported to have polycystic ovarian morphology by ultrasound.

DIFFERENTIAL DIAGNOSIS

The diagnosis of PCOS is often a diagnosis of exclusion. Other causes of hyperandrogenism include hyperprolactinemia, drugs (danazol and androgenic progestins), nonclassic congenital adrenal hyperplasia, and tumors, including those of the pituitary (Cushing's syndrome, prolactinoma), ovary, and adrenal gland.

The differential diagnosis of acne includes acne rosacea (which generally responds to antibiotic therapy and is not a typical feature of PCOS), acne fulminans (which is most common in adolescent males and is associated with fever, arthalgias, and leukocytosis), the SAPHO syndrome (which is defined as synovitis, acne, pustulosis, hyperostosis, and osteitis and requires referral for systemic therapy).

Other causes of menstrual dysfunction need to be considered, including pregnancy, ovarian failure, outflow track obstruction, and hypothalamic amenorrhea, in the proper clinical context.

FUTURE AVENUES OF INVESTIGATION

1. International standardization and validation of physical examination assessments of hirsutism, acne, and hair loss, with establishment of normative values for different ethnic groups.
2. Identification of those health risk factors for which treatment is determined to provide health benefit.

KEY POINTS

- Evaluation requires complete medical and family history and careful objective physical examination with standardized record keeping to monitor response to therapy.
- Evaluation focuses not only on patient concerns, but also on long-term health assessment of the patient.

REFERENCES

1. The Rotterdam ESHRE/ASRM-Sponsored PCOS Consensus Workshop Group. Revised 2003 consensus on diagnostic criteria and long-term health risks related to polycystic ovary syndrome. Fert Steril 2004;81:19–25.

2. Hardiman P, Pillay OC, Atiomo W. Polycystic ovary syndrome and endometrial carcinoma. Lancet 2003;361:1810.

3. Stein I, Leventhal M. Amenorrhea associated with bilateral polycystic ovaries. Am J Obstet Gynecol 1935;29:181.

4. Balen AH, Tan SL, MacDougall J, Jacobs HS. Miscarriage rates following in-vitro fertilization are increased in women with polycystic ovaries and reduced by pituitary desensitization with buserelin. Hum Reprod 1993;8:959–964.

5. Ehrmann DA, Barnes RB, Rosenfield RL, Cavaghan MK. Prevalence of impaired glucose tolerance and diabetes in women with polycystic ovary syndrome. Diabetes Care 1999;22:141–146.

6. Ehrmann DA, Sturis J, Byrne MM, Karrison T, Rosenfield RL, Polonsky KS. Insulin secretory defects in polycystic ovary syndrome. Relationship to insulin secretion and family history of non-insulin-dependent diabetes mellitus. J Clin Invest 1995;96:520–527.

7. Vgontzas AN, Legro RS, Bixler EO, Grayev A, Kales A, Chrousos GP. Polycystic ovary syndrome is associated with obstructive sleep apnea and daytime sleepiness: role of insulin resistance. J Clin Endocrinol Metab 2001;86:517–520.

8. Fogel RB, Malhotra A, Pillar G, Pittman SD. Increased prevalence of obstructive sleep apnea syndrome in obese women with polycystic ovary syndrome. J Clin Endocrinol Metab 2001;86: 1175–1180.

9. Schwimmer JB, Khorram O, Chiu V, Schwimmer WB. Abnormal aminotransferase activity in women with polycystic ovary syndrome. Fertil Steril 2005;83:494–497.

10. Conway GS, Agrawal R, Betteridge DJ, Jacobs HS. Risk factors for coronary artery disease in lean and obese women with the polycystic ovary syndrome. Clin Endocrinol (Oxf) 1992;37:119–125.

11. Talbott E, Clerici A, Berga SL, et al. Adverse lipid and coronary heart disease risk profiles in young women with polycystic ovary syndrome: results of a case-control study. J Clin Epidemiol 1998;51: 415–422.

12. Talbott EO, Guzick DS, Sutton-Tyrrell K, et al. Evidence for association between polycystic ovary syndrome and premature carotid atherosclerosis in middle-aged women. Arterioscler Thromb Vasc Biol 2000;20:2414–2421.

13. Wild S, Pierpoint T, McKeigue P, Jacobs H. Cardiovascular disease in women with polycystic ovary syndrome at long-term follow-up: a retrospective cohort study. Clin Endocrinol (Oxf) 2000;52:595–600.

14. Pierpoint T, McKeigue PM, Isaacs AJ, Wild SH, Jacobs HS. Mortality of women with polycystic ovary syndrome at long-term follow-up. J Clin Epidemiol 1998;51:581–586.

15. Solomon CG, Hu FB, Dunaif A, et al. Menstrual cycle irregularity and risk for future cardiovascular disease. J Clin Endocrinol Metab 2002;87:2013–2017.

16. Apridonidze T, Essah PA, Iuorno MJ, Nestler JE. Prevalence and characteristics of the metabolic syndrome in women with polycystic ovary syndrome. J Clin Endocrinol Metab 2005;90:1929–1935.

17. Dokras A, Bochner M, Hollinrake E, Markham S, Vanvoorhis B, Jagasia DH. Screening women with polycystic ovary syndrome for metabolic syndrome. Obstet Gynecol 2005;106:131–137.

18. Cronin L, Guyatt G, Griffith EW, et al. Development of a health-related quality-of-life questionnaire (PCOSQ) for women with polycystic ovary syndrome (PCOS). J Clin Endocrinol Metab 1998;83:1976–1987.

19. Elsenbruch S, Hahn S, Kowalsky D, et al. Quality of life, psychosocial well-being, and sexual satisfaction in women with polycystic ovary syndrome. J Clin Endocrinol Metab 2003;88:5801–5807.

20. Azziz R, Marin C, Hoq L, Badamgarav E, Song P. Health care-related economic burden of the polycystic ovary syndrome during the reproductive life span. J Clin Endocrinol Metab 2005;90: 4650–4658.

21. Speiser PW. Congenital adrenal hyperplasia owing to 21-hydroxylase deficiency. Endocrinol Metab Clin North Am 2001;30:31–59.

22. Goldstein SM, Wintroub BU. Adverse Cutaneous Reactions to Medication: A Physician's Guide. New York: CoMedica Inc., 1994.

23. Ferriman D, Gallwey J. Clinical assessment of body hair growth in women. J Clin Endocrinol Metab 1961;21:1440–1447.

24. Wild RA, Vesely S, Beebe L, Whitsett T, Owen W. Ferriman Gallwey self-scoring I: performance assessment in women with polycystic ovary syndrome. J Clin Endocrinol Metab 2005;90:4112–4114.

25. Ludwig E. Classification of the types of androgenetic alopecia (common baldness) occurring in the female sex. Br J Dermatology 1977;97:247–254.

26. Tagatz GE, Kopher RA, Nagel TC, Okagaki T. The clitoral index: a bioassay of androgenic stimulation, Obstet Gynecol 1979;54:562–564.

27. DeVane GW, Czekala NM, Judd HL, Yen SS. Circulating gonadotropins, estrogens, and androgens in polycystic ovarian disease. Am J Obstet Gynecol 1975;121:496–500.

28. Winters SJ, Talbott E, Guzick DS, Zborowski J, McHugh KP. Serum testosterone levels decrease in middle age in women with the polycystic ovary syndrome. Fertil Steril 2000;73:724–729.

29. Miller KK, Rosner W, Lee H. Measurement of free testosterone in normal women and women with androgen deficiency: comparison of methods. J Clin Endocrinol Metab 2004;89:525–533.

30. Derksen J, Nagesser SK, Meinders AE, Haak HR, van de Velde CJ. Identification of virilizing adrenal tumors in hirsute women. N Engl J Med 1994;331:968–973.

31. Taylor AE, McCourt B, Martin KA, et al. Determinants of abnormal gonadotropin secretion in clinically defined women with polycystic ovary syndrome. J Clin Endocrinol Metab 1997;82:2248–2256.

32. Azziz R, Dewailly D, Owerbach D. Clinical review 56: nonclassic adrenal hyperplasia: current concepts. J Clin Endocrinol Metab 1994;78:810–815.

33. New MI, Lorenzen F, Lerner AJ, et al. Genotyping steroid 21-hydroxylase deficiency: Hormonal reference data. J Clin Endocrinol Metab 1983;57:320–326.

34. Legro RS, Kunselman AR, Dodson WC, Dunaif A. Prevalence and predictors of risk for type 2 diabetes mellitus and impaired glucose tolerance in polycystic ovary syndrome: a prospective, controlled study in 254 affected women. J Clin Endocrinol Metab 1999;84:165–169.

35. Legro RS, Kunselman AR, Dunaif A. Prevalence and predictors of dyslipidemia in women with polycystic ovary syndrome. Am J Med 2001;111:607–613.

36. Adams J, Polson DW, Franks S. Prevalence of polycystic ovaries in women with anovulation and idiopathic hirsutism. BMJ 1986;293:355–359.

37. Balen AH, Laven JS, Tan SL, Dewailly D. Ultrasound assessment of the polycystic ovary: international consensus definitions. Hum Reprod Update 2003;9:505–514.

38. Conn JJ, Jacobs HS, Conway GS. The prevalence of polycystic ovaries in women with type 2 diabetes mellitus. Clin Endocrinol (Oxf) 2000;52:81–86.

39. Hague WM, Adams J, Rodda C, et al. The prevalence of polycystic ovaries in patients with congenital adrenal hyperplasia and their close relatives. Clin Endocrinol 1990;33:501–510.

40. Koivunen RM, Juutinen J, Vauhkonen I, Morin-Papunen LC, Ruokonen A, Tapanainen JS. Metabolic and steroidogenic alterations related to increased frequency of polycystic ovaries in women with a history of gestational diabetes. J Clin Endocrinol Metab 2001;86:2591–2599.

41. Polson DW, Adams J, Wadsworth J, Franks S. Polycystic ovaries a common finding in normal women. Lancet 1988;1:870–872.

42. Adams JM, Taylor AE, Crowley WF Jr. Hall JE. Polycystic ovarian morphology with regular ovulatory cycles: insights into the pathophysiology of polycystic ovarian syndrome. J Clin Endocrinol Metab 2004;89:4343–4350.

11 Evaluation for Insulin Resistance and Comorbidities Related to Insulin Resistance in Polycystic Ovary Syndrome

Ricardo Azziz, MD, MPH, MBA

CONTENTS

Summary

Patients with polycystic ovary syndrome (PCOS) often have coexisting insulin resistance (IR), glucose intolerance or diabetes, and metabolic syndrome. For larger epidemiological studies, detection of IR may be accomplished using surrogate measures, such as the homeostatic model assessment or the quantitative insulin-sensitivity check index. Alternatively, research studies of IR, particularly those involving a smaller number of subjects, should strive to utilize the clamp, the frequently sampled intravenous glucose tolerance test, the insulin suppression test, or oral glucose tolerance test techniques. Clinically, in PCOS the standard 2-hour oral glucose tolerance test, measuring both insulin and glucose, yields the highest amount of information for a reasonable cost and risk, providing an assessment of both the degrees of hyperinsulinemia and glucose tolerance. However, considering the current variability in insulin assays, each laboratory should set its own normal range and establish a method for periodically reevaluating the acceptability of their results. Up to 25% of nonobese patients and 50% of obese patients with PCOS will have features consistent with the metabolic syndrome. Detection of the metabolic syndrome will include obtaining a thorough medical history, waist and hip circumferences, blood pressure measures, calculation of the body mass index, a lipid profile, and either serum-fasting glucose levels or, preferably, the glucose response to a standard OGTT.

Key Words: PCOS; insulin resistance; dyslipidemia; metabolic syndrome; diabetes.

From: *Contemporary Endocrinology: Insulin Resistance and Polycystic Ovarian Syndrome:
Pathogenesis, Evaluation, and Treatment*
Edited by: E. Diamanti-Kandarakis, J. E. Nestler, D. Panidis, and R. Pasquali © Humana Press Inc., Totowa, NJ

INTRODUCTION

As discussed in Chapters 1 and 2, 50–70% of patients with the polycystic ovary syndrome (PCOS) demonstrate insulin resistance (IR) and secondary hyperinsulinism *(1,2)*, and the prevalence of the metabolic syndrome is increased compared with age- and weight-matched controls *(3–5)*. Consequently, the rate of type 2 diabetes mellitus (DM) *(6–8)*, and possibly cardiovascular disease (CVD) *(9)*, is increased in PCOS. Effective methods of screening and early detection of these morbidities will be imperative in the management of the patient with PCOS. The following subheadings discuss methods of diagnosing IR, glucose intolerance and type 2 DM, and the metabolic syndrome in these women; alternatively, the detection and diagnosis of established CVD is beyond the scope of this chapter.

DETECTING INSULIN RESISTANCE IN PCOS

The definition of IR varies, with the American Diabetes Association (ADA) defining it as an impaired metabolic response to either exogenous or endogenous insulin *(10)*, whereas some investigators define it as a common pathological state in which target cells fail to respond to ordinary levels of circulating insulin *(11)*. Even without a common definition, IR appears to affect 10–25% of the general population, and the risk increases with obesity *(12)*. Detectable IR occurs in 50–70% of patients with PCOS *(1,2)* and, because β-cell function is frequently partially or totally conserved *(2)*, most of these women also demonstrate secondary hyperinsulinism. Detection of IR is clinically important because it is an independent risk factor for type 2 DM and CVD.

There are two general approaches to determining insulin sensitivity. The first are those direct and dynamic measures requiring an intervention (e.g., intravenous administration of glucose and insulin) that can be used to estimate the ability of insulin to dispose of glucose. Second, other methods estimate insulin action through surrogate measures utilizing the fasting values of glucose and insulin *(13)*, or the insulin, C-peptide, or glucose responses to a physiological glucose load (e.g., oral glucose tolerance test [OGTT]). These two approaches to measuring insulin sensitivity and hyperinsulinemia will be discussed in more detail in the following subheadings.

Direct Measurements of Assessing Insulin Action In Vivo

GLUCOSE CLAMP

The *glucose clamp technique* is presumed to be the most accurate test available for the measurement of insulin action in vivo *(14)*. During this test, a constant intravenous infusion of insulin is given at a rate designed to maintain a preselected steady-state insulin level, while simultaneously maintaining or "clamping" the plasma glucose concentration at the normal fasting level (the hyperinsulinemic–euglycemic clamp) by using variable intravenous glucose (or dextrose) infusion. It is assumed that at a steady state (when both the amount of glucose being infused and the circulating glucose levels are stable) endogenous glucose production is fully suppressed and the amount of total glucose being shunted intracellularly by the insulin (i.e., peripheral tissue insulin sensitivity or insulin-mediated glucose disposal) equals the glucose infusion rate. This measurement is expressed as a value termed the *insulin sensitivity index* (ISI or M value). Combining the clamp with tracer studies using radiolabeled glucose also allows for a determination of hepatic glucose uptake (i.e., hepatic insulin sensitivity). On occasion, a clamp achieving supraphysiological levels of glucose (i.e., hyperglycemic clamp) is used to simultaneously obtain measurements of peripheral insulin sensitivity, β-cell sensitivity, and glucose effectiveness (or noninsulin-mediated glucose uptake) *(15)*.

FREQUENTLY SAMPLED INTRAVENOUS GLUCOSE TOLERANCE TEST

Intravenous glucose tolerance tests have also been used to assess the degree of insulin sensitivity in vivo *(16)*. Generally, a computer-generated mathematic analysis of the glucose–insulin dynamics observed during a frequently sampled intravenous glucose tolerance test (FS-IVGTT), the so-called the minimal model (MINMOD), is used to calculate a number of parameters estimating insulin sensitivity *(16,17)*. The FS-IVGTT usually requires 11–34 blood samples taken over 3 hours, and the test is frequently modified by intravenously infusing tolbutamide (a sulfonylurea medication that stimulates insulin secretion), or more commonly insulin itself, during the early part of the study. A modified FS-IVGTT requires a smaller insulin response than the standard protocol to achieve the same precision in assessing insulin sensitivity *(18)*.

The FS-IVGTT is generally easier and less invasive to perform than the clamp and does not require a continuous glucose infusion. The FS-IVGTT also allows for the determination of insulin-dependent and insulin-independent (i.e., glucose effectiveness) glucose utilization *(16)*, but does not distinguish between peripheral and hepatic glucose utilization as the clamp can. Another problem generally associated with this technique is that it is based on the assumption that there is a constant hepatic extraction (clearance) of insulin during the test, which may not always be the case.

INSULIN SUPPRESSION TEST

Pei et al. *(19)* described a modified insulin suppression test (IST) useful for measuring insulin-mediated glucose disposal. During this test, glucose values are not measured at all times during the test as they are for the clamp or the FS-IVGTT; the operator sets fixed-rate infusions of insulin and glucose, but the plasma glucose is not clamped at a certain value. In the insulin-sensitive patient, the steady-state plasma glucose (SSPG) levels decrease with time, whereas in the insulin-resistant patient SSPG increases. Because the glucose infusion rate remains constant without requiring frequent adjustments, this test is less labor-intensive than the clamp or FS-IVGTT and does not require extensive operator skills. Nonetheless, to date, the IST has been utilized in a limited fashion.

INSULIN TOLERANCE TEST

The insulin tolerance test (ITT) consists of the administration of an intravenous bolus of regular insulin (0.1 IU/kg), measuring glucose before and at frequent intervals after the injection of insulin for up to 20 minutes. The test is terminated by the intravenous injection of a 50% dextrose solution. The rate of decline of glucose (i.e., plasma glucose disappearance rate) during the test is calculated (K_{ITT}), generally using the glucose values between the 3- and 15-minute time points when the decline is generally more linear. The K_{ITT} value is taken as a measure of insulin action. Published K_{ITT} values range from 0.026 to 0.085 mmol/L/minute for subjects with a body mass index (BMI) of less than 30 kg/m^2, to 0.012–0.017 mmol/L/minute for subjects with a BMI higher than 30 kg/m^2 *(20)*. The ITT correlates well with the results of euglycemic and hyperglycemic glucose clamp studies *(20,21)*. However, a substantial number of patients become hypoglycemic prior to the end of the test, and there is a potential risk for of serious morbidity secondary to this.

FREQUENTLY SAMPLED ORAL GLUCOSE TOLERANCE TEST

During the frequently sampled oral glucose tolerance test (FS-OGTT), as for the regular OGTT, 75 g of glucose or dextrose in a flavored drink is administered orally to the patient and consumed at an even rate more than 5 minutes. Measurements are obtained several times before and after the ingestion of the glucose solution for up to 3 hours afterward *(22–24)*. For example, samples for glucose and insulin measurements can be obtained at –10 and 0 minutes before and 15, 30, 60, 90, 120, 150, and 180 minutes after glucose ingestion, although specific protocols vary. One of the many measures frequently calculated is the integrated insulin response assessed by calculating the insulin area-under-the-curve *(25)*, although other measures have been proposed *(22–24)*. The FS-OGTT has been found to be more physiological, simpler, and less invasive to perform than the FS-IVGTT and can yield results that correlate well with more complex measures *(26)*. The measurement of C-peptides (a byproduct of insulin synthesis) may also allow investigators to estimate insulin secretion and clearance rates.

Surrogate Estimates

The surrogate approach to assessing IR uses either the fasting measurements determined at the basal state or the insulin values obtained during a standard OGTT. The major benefit to utilizing fasting measurements, as opposed to using methods of directly assessing insulin action, is to provide clinicians and researchers with more rapid and less invasive methods of evaluating individual patients or larger populations. This form of measurement also requires less time and skill so that less experienced personnel can be utilized to gather the data from human subjects.

FASTING INSULIN LEVEL

The fasting insulin value is a simple test to perform and one that can be obtained with relative ease. In a study by Yeni-Komshian et al. *(25)*, fasting plasma insulin concentrations were significantly correlated with insulin action estimated by the SSPG, although it accounted for only one-third of the variability in estimated glucose disposal. In the author's experience, normal basal levels generally range from 3 to 30 μIU/mL. However, on an individual basis, fasting insulin levels may be normal in up to 40% of patients with PCOS who have hyperinsulinemia diagnosed by the OGTT. Overall, fasting insulin measures should only be used qualitatively, not quantitatively.

GLUCOSE-TO-INSULIN RATIO

The glucose-to-insulin ratio (GIR; insulin in μIU/mL and glucose in mg/dL) has been used as a measure of insulin sensitivity. In a small study by Legro et al. *(1)*, obese patients with a fasting GIR of less than 4.5 were generally insulin-resistant. However, this method has recently fallen out of favor because its calculation is felt to not be physiological, its exact value varies widely, and the use of this ratio has not been fully validated in non-obese patients *(27)*.

HOMEOSTATIC MODEL ASSESSMENT

The homeostatic model assessment (HOMA) calculation uses fasting plasma glucose and insulin concentrations to estimate insulin resistance (HOMA-IR) and percent β-cell function (HOMA-β-cell) using a mathematical model *(28)*.

$$\text{HOMA - IR} = \frac{(\text{Glucose in mmol / L})* \times \text{Insulin in } \mu\text{IU / mL}}{22.5}$$

$$\text{HOMA-}\beta\text{-cell} = \frac{20 \times \text{Insulin in } \mu\text{IU/mL}}{(\text{Glucose in mmol/L}) - 3.5}$$

An ideal, normal-weight individual aged younger than 35 years old has a HOMA-IR of 1.0 and a β-cell function of 100%. This test has been well correlated to insulin-mediated glucose disposal assessed by the glucose clamp technique *(28)*, although less so in patients with PCOS *(29)*. The HOMA is most appropriate for large epidemiological studies. Recently, a more complicated, albeit purportedly more accurate, HOMA calculation was described and was termed the "HOMA2" *(30)*. The calculation of the HOMA2 requires a computer, and easy-to-use programs can be downloaded (http://www.dtu.ox.ac.uk/index.html?maindoc=/homa/).

QUANTITATIVE INSULIN SENSITIVITY CHECK INDEX

The quantitative insulin sensitivity check index (QUICKI) is another measurement of insulin sensitivity that utilizes fasting insulin and fasting glucose values *(31,32)*:

$$\text{QUICKI} = 1/ [\log (\text{insulin in } \mu\text{IU/mL}) + \log (\text{glucose in mg/dL})]$$

This test has been well correlated to measure insulin-moderated glucose disposal assessed by the glucose clamp technique, especially in those patients with type 2 DM and/or those who are obese *(31)*. Although calculated using different units of glucose, QUICKI is basically the log of the inverse of HOMA (*see* Fig. 1). Consequently, both QUICKI and the log of HOMA-IR behave the same, and as predictors of outcome, they are interchangeable. Like the HOMA-IR estimate, the QUICKI measure does not appear to correlate well with the results of clamp studies in women with PCOS *(29)*.

STANDARD ORAL GLUCOSE TOLERANCE TEST

Clinically, a 2-hour OGTT administering 75 g of oral glucose is frequently used to determine the presence of glucose intolerance and hyperinsulinemia. Samples for glucose and insulin measurements are generally obtained at 0 minutes before and 60 and 120 minutes after glucose ingestion. Measurement of peak stimulated insulin levels can be used to estimate the degree of hyperinsulinemia and, by inference, obtain a qualitative assessment of the degree of IR. However, it should be noted that the normal range of insulin values during a standard OGTT vary widely, in part because of the variability in value assay results (*see* following subheading).

In our experience, peak insulin levels during an OGTT are normally less than 75–100 μIU/mL. In general, insulin levels between of 100 and 150 μIU/mL denote mild IR/hyperinsulinemia; values of 150–300 μIU/mL denote moderate

---

*To convert to glucose levels in mmol/L, multiply glucose in mg/dL by 0.05551.

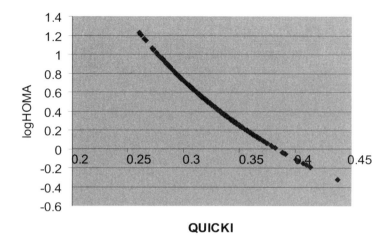

Fig. 1. Both the quantitative insulin-sensitivity check index (QUICKI) and homeostatic model assessment insulin resistance (HOMA-IR) measure the same parameter of insulin resistance. Using 490 fasting insulin and glucose levels obtained from the Mexican-American Coronary Artery Disease study we note that QUICKI and the log of HOMA-IR are linearly related. (Data courtesy of Drs. Mark Goodarzi and Willa A. Hsueh.)

IR/ hyperinsulinemia; and levels of greater than 300 µIU/mL are indicative of severe IR/ hyperinsulinemia.

Measuring Insulin: Caveats and Limitations

Accurate measurement of insulin is critical to the assessment of IR and hyperinsulinism. The measurement of insulin is most commonly conducted using radioimmunoassay or enzyme-linked immunoabsorbent assays. Unfortunately, the plasma insulin values obtained may vary greatly from one laboratory to the next. In 1996, the ADA convened a task force to study the possible standardization of the insulin assay (33). As part of the work of this task force, insulin measurements were conducted on identical samples by several competent laboratories, and little agreement in the values of insulin obtained was noted, even when the same assays were used. The task force therefore recommended that each laboratory (and investigator) examine all available assays and determine which one is most acceptable for their laboratory. They also recommended that laboratories compare their results with other laboratories and periodically reevaluate their assays. It is critical that clinicians and investigators alike discuss with their laboratory the quality of the insulin assays being used and the methods used to establish the "normal" range. Finally, the task force suggested a three-step process for the assessment and certification of insulin assays (Table 1).

Summary on Methods of Assessing IR in PCOS

Direct measures of insulin action include the euglycemic or hyperglycemic clamp, FS-IVGTT, IST, ITT, and FS-OGTT, whereas surrogate measures include the fasting insulin levels, GIR, HOMA, QUICKI, and the insulin levels during a standard OGTT. Direct techniques are generally considered more accurate, but they are expensive, laborious, potentially dangerous, and require well-trained individuals to complete the study. The fasting indexes and the insulin levels during a standard OGTT are less difficult to obtain than direct measurements and have adequate correlation with the results of

Table 1
A Three-Step Process for the Assessment and Certification of Insulin Assays

Parameter	Definition
Precision	Measure of the reproducibility of the analytical method
Accuracy	Comparing results of the in-house standard with a gold standard
Recovery	The ability of an analytical test to accurately measure throughout the working range of the calibration curve
Specificity	The ability to measure the desired analyte in the presence of other similar components in a complex matrix
Linearity	Ability of the analytical method to provide measurements that are directly proportional to the concentration the analyte in the sample
LOD/LLOQ	The LOD is the lowest measurable concentration that is statistically different from zero. The LLOQ is the lower limit of quantitation or the lowest concentration that can be determined with an acceptable degree of accuracy and precision

Modified from ref. *33*.

more invasive studies. They are also more readily applicable to large epidemiological studies *(34)*.

DETECTING IMPAIRED GLUCOSE INTOLERANCE AND TYPE 2 DM IN PCOS

The risk of impaired glucose tolerance (IGT) and type 2 DM is increased five- to sevenfold in PCOS *(6–8)* (Fig. 2). Although many patients can be diagnosed as having frank type 2 DM by a fasting glucose of greater than 126 mg/dL *(35)*, patients with PCOS frequently require an OGTT to diagnose more subtle forms of diabetes or IGT *(7)*. In addition to allowing the detection of hyperinsulinemia, the performance of a standard OGTT has the additional advantage of diagnosing patients with IGT or type 2 DM. Using the glucose levels during the OGTT, according to the World Health Organization 1985 criteria, type 2 DM is diagnosed if the 2-hour glucose during the OGTT is ≥200 mg/dL and IGT is diagnosed by a fasting plasma glucose of less than 140 mg/dL *and* a 2-hour glucose level during the OGTT of between 140 and 199 mg/dL *(36)*. It should be noted that these diagnoses require that the abnormal results be confirmed.

DETECTING DYSLIPIDEMIA IN PCOS

It is still unclear whether the prevalence of dyslipidemia is grossly increased in PCOS. In a study of 195 women with PCOS and 62 controls, Legro et al. reported that the prevalence of borderline-high total cholesterol (≥200 mg/dL) was higher among patients with PCOS than controls (48 vs 22%, respectively), although the prevalence of abnormally low HDL-cholesterol (<35 mg/dL) was similar in both groups (48 vs 45%, respectively) *(37)*. In another study of 398 women with PCOS screened for inclusion in a trial evaluating the benefits of troglitazone, Legro et al. reported on the prevalence of abnormal baseline lipid levels as defined by the National Cholesterol Education Program guidelines *(38)*. They observed that 8.8% had a total cholesterol of ≥240 mg/dL, 8.5% had an LDL-cholesterol of ≥160 mg/dL, 15% had an HDL-cholesterol

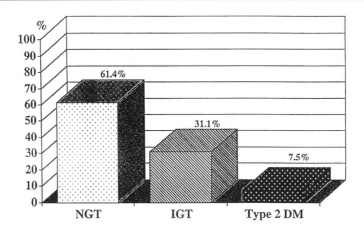

Fig. 2. Prevalence of glucose intolerance diagnosed by a 2-hour, 75-g glucose tolerance test, using WHO 1985 criteria, in 254 women with polycystic ovary syndrome. NGT, normal glucose tolerance; IGT, impaired glucose tolerance; Type 2 DM, type 2 diabetes mellitus. (Reprinted with permission from ref. *7*.)

less than 35 mg/dL, and 2.5% had trilgycerides of ≥400 mg/dL. However, the prevalence of abnormally high total cholesterol levels in this population was similar to, and the prevalence of low HDL-cholesterol levels was actually less than, that observed among women aged 20–39 years in the NHANES IIII survey (i.e., 7.6 and 25.6%, respectively) *(39)*.

Overall, it remains unclear whether women with PCOS, at least of reproductive age, have a higher prevalence of dyslipidemia compared with matched controls or the general population. Nonetheless, because dyslipidemia is an important predictor of CVD and forms part of the criteria for detecting the metabolic syndrome (*see* Diagnosing the Metabolic Syndrome in PCOS), it is recommended that, at a minimum, a complete lipid profile be evaluated at the initial evaluation, regardless of age, and periodically thereafter.

DIAGNOSING THE METABOLIC SYNDROME IN PCOS

The metabolic syndrome (i.e., syndrome X, IR syndrome, dysmetabolic syndrome) is defined as a constellation of signs and features that predict an increased risk of CVD *(40)*. Principle features variably include abdominal obesity, atherogenic dyslipidemia, raised blood pressure, IR, glucose intolerance, and a proinflammatory and prothrombotic state *(41)*. Up to six different definitions of the metabolic syndrome currently exist *(41–46)*, although the most frequently used is that based on the Third Report of the National Cholesterol Education Program (NCEP) Expert Panel on Detection, Evaluation, and Treatment of High Blood Cholesterol in Adults, resulting in the Adult Treatment Panel III, or ATP III *(43)*. Specifically, the NCEP defines the metabolic syndrome as the presence of at least three of the following five features:

1. Abdominal obesity (waist circumference >88 cm).
2. Serum triglycerides ≥150 mg/dL.
3. Serum HDL-cholesterol less than 50 mg/dL.

4. Blood pressure ≥130/85.
5. Serum fasting glucose ≥110 mg/dL.

At least in the United States, small studies suggest that approx 50% of women with PCOS demonstrate evidence of the metabolic syndrome, as defined by modified ATP III criteria *(3,4)*. Abdominal obesity is an important feature of the metabolic syndrome, and as women with PCOS are frequently obese, most of these patients will already have at least one of the features of the metabolic syndrome. Furthermore, in PCOS obesity is associated with greater degrees of IR and dyslipidemia, increasing the probability that these patients will exhibit the metabolic syndrome.

Alternatively, it is less clear that non-obese women with PCOS are at increased risk for the metabolic syndrome. In one study of 106 patients with PCOS, the prevalence of the metabolic syndrome was not increased in those women whose BMI was less than 25 kg/m^2 and younger than 30 years old; nonetheless, patients with a BMI higher than 25 kg/m^2 and/or who were 30 years of age or older had a higher prevalence of the metabolic syndrome compared with age-matched controls *(4)*. The importance of obesity and possibly diet on the prevalence of metabolic syndrome is further highlighted by the relatively low prevalences of the metabolic syndrome observed in non-US patients with PCOS *(47,48)*, compared with those patients residing in the United States *(3–5)*. In general, women with PCOS who live in the United States are significantly more obese than their non-US counterparts *(49)*.

We should note that the prevalence of the metabolic syndrome in PCOS is, at least in part, a matter of definition. Some definitions, such as that of the NCEP-ATP III, primarily target the detection of dyslipidemia as early evidence of cardiovascular CVD, whereas that of the WHO aims to identify individuals who are primarily IR by first identifying those with evidence of glucose intolerance. For example, Vural and colleagues evaluated 43 women with PCOS and 43 age-matched controls in Turkey *(48)*. Using the WHO criteria, 11.6% of women with PCOS were diagnosed as having the metabolic syndrome, significantly greater than controls (0%). Alternatively, if the ATP III criteria were used, only 2.3% of patients with PCOS were affected with the metabolic syndrome, a nonsignificant difference from controls.

Screening for the metabolic syndrome can be performed by obtaining the following measures:

1. Waist circumference (>88 cm) or waist-to-hip ratio (>0.85).
2. BMI based on actual height and weight (>30 kg/m^2).
3. Blood pressure (or a history of hypertension on treatment).
4. Lipid profile, including serum total glucose and HDL-cholesterol.
5. Serum fasting glucose or preferably glucose response to a standard OGTT (or a history of diabetes on treatment).

The value of routinely obtaining markers of inflammation (e.g., C-reactive protein [CRP]) or hypercoagulability (e.g., plasminogen activator inhibitor [PAI]-1) in PCOS is unclear.

Finally, the prevalence of the metabolic syndrome increases with age; nonetheless, 24 and 47% of patients aged less than 30 years or 30–39 years of age, respectively, had metabolic syndrome at least in one report *(3)*. These data clearly denote the importance of screening all women with PCOS for the metabolic syndrome, regardless of age.

CONCLUSIONS

Patients with PCOS often have coexisting IR, glucose intolerance or DM, and metabolic syndrome. For large epidemiological studies, detection of IR may be accomplished using the HOMA-IR or the QUICKI measures. Alternatively, research studies of IR, particularly those involving a smaller number of subjects, should strive to utilize the clamp, FS-IVGTT, IST, or FS-OGTT techniques. Clinically, in PCOS, the standard 2-hour OGTT measuring both insulin and glucose may yield the highest amount of information for a reasonable cost and risk, providing an assessment of both hyperinsulinemia and glucose tolerance. Considering the current variability in insulin assays, each laboratory should set its own normal range and establish a method for periodically reevaluating the acceptability of their results. Up to 25% of non-obese and 50% of obese patients with PCOS will have features consistent with the metabolic syndrome. Detection of the metabolic syndrome will include obtaining a thorough medical history, waist and hip circumferences, blood pressure measures, calculation of the BMI, a lipid profile, and either a serum fasting glucose levels or, preferably, the glucose response to a standard OGTT. Screening should be initiated at the time of the initial diagnosis, regardless of age, and repeated periodically thereafter.

FUTURE AVENUES OF INVESTIGATION

More precise assessments of the prevalence of IR in PCOS and its relationship with other phenotypic features of the disorder, with environmental factors such as diet, and with the ethnicity or geographic location of the population are still required. Likewise, careful prospective studies evaluating the cost-effectiveness of the various measures assessing the risk of metabolic syndrome and CVD, including the age at which such screening should be initiated and the frequency at which it should be repeated. Finally, future studies are needed to better define the value of routinely performing a standard OGTT for detecting hyperinsulinism and glucose intolerance in PCOS and the normal ranges of insulin during the test.

KEY POINTS

- IR affects 50–70% of patients with PCOS.
- The risk of impaired glucose tolerance and diabetes is increased five- to sevenfold in patients with PCOS.
- For larger epidemiological research studies, detection of IR may be accomplished using surrogate measures, such as the HOMA-IR or the QUICKI measures.
- For research studies involving a smaller number of subjects, the clamp, FSIVGTT, IST, or FSOGTT techniques should be used.
- Clinically, the standard 2-hour OGTT, measuring both insulin and glucose, provides an assessment of both the degree of hyperinsulinism and the presence of impaired glucose tolerance or diabetes mellitus.
- Considering the current variability in insulin assays, each laboratory should set its own normal range and establish a method for periodically reevaluating the acceptability of their results.

- Although it is unclear whether the prevalence of dyslipidemia is increased in PCOS, up to 25% of non-obese and 50% of obese patients with PCOS will have features consistent with the metabolic syndrome.
- Detection of the metabolic syndrome will include obtaining a thorough medical history, waist and hip circumferences, blood pressure measures, calculation of the body mass index, a lipid profile, and either a serum fasting glucose levels or, preferably, the glucose response to a standard OGTT.

REFERENCES

1. Legro R, Finegood D, Dunaif A. A fasting glucose to insulin ratio is a useful measure of insulin sensitivity in women with polycystic ovary syndrome. J Clin Endocrinol Metab 1998;83: 2694–2698.
2. DeUgarte CM, Bartolucci AA, Azziz R. Prevalence of insulin resistance in the polycystic ovary syndrome using the homeostasis model assessment. Fertil Steril 2005;83:1454–1460.
3. Dokras A, Bochner M, Hollinrake E, Markham S, Vanvoorhis B, Jagasia DH. Screening women with polycystic ovary syndrome for metabolic syndrome. Obstet Gynecol 2005;106:131–137.
4. Apridonidze T, Essah PA, Iuorno MJ, Nestler JE. Prevalence and characteristics of the metabolic syndrome in women with polycystic ovary syndrome. Obstet Gynecol Surv 2005;60:589–591.
5. Sam S, Legro RS, Bentley-Lewis R, Dunaif A. Dyslipidemia and metabolic syndrome in the sisters of women with polycystic ovary syndrome. J Clin Endocrinol Metab 2005;90:4797–4802.
6. Ehrmann DA, Barnes RB, Rosenfield RL, Cavaghan MK, Imperial J. Prevalence of impaired glucose tolerance and diabetes in women with polycystic ovary syndrome. Diabetes Care 1999; 22:141–146.
7. Legro RS, Kunselman AR, Dodson WC, Dunaif A. Prevalence and predictors of risk for type 2 diabetes mellitus and impaired glucose tolerance in polycystic ovary syndrome: a prospective, controlled study in 254 affected women. J Clin Endocrinol Metab 1999;84:165–169.
8. Ehrmann DA, Kasza K, Azziz R, Legro RS, Ghazzi MN. PCOS/Troglitazone Study Group. Effects of race and family history of type 2 diabetes on metabolic status of women with polycystic ovary syndrome. J Clin Endocrinol Metab 2005;90:66–71.
9. Legro RS. Polycystic ovary syndrome and cardiovascular disease: a premature association? Endocr Rev 2003;24:302–312.
10. American Diabetes Association. Consensus development conference on insulin resistance. Diabetes Care 2001;24:588–597.
11. Le Roith D, Zick Y. Recent advances in our understanding of insulin action and insulin resistance. Diabetes Care 2001;24:588–597.
12. Karter AJ, Mayer-Davis EJ, Selby JV, et al. Insulin sensitivity and abdominal obesity in African-American, Hispanic, and non-Hispanic white men and women. The Insulin Resistance and Atherosclerosis Study. Diabetes 1996;45:1547–1555.
13. Radziuk J. Insulin sensitivity and its measurement: structural commonalities among the methods. J Clin Endocrinol Metab 2000;85:4426–4433.
14. Ferrannini E, Mari A. How to measure insulin sensitivity. J Hypertens 1998;16:895–906.
15. Elahi D. In praise of the hyperglycemic clamp. A method for assessment of beta-cell sensitivity and insulin resistance. Diabetes Care 1996;19:278–286.
16. Folcy JE, Chen YD, Lardinois CK, Hollenbeck CB, Liu GC, Reaven GM. Estimates of in vivo insulin action in humans: comparison of the insulin clamp and the minimal model techniques. Horm Metab Res 1985;17:406–409.
17. Bergman RN. Lilly lecture 1989. Toward physiological understanding of glucose tolerance. Minimal-model approach. Diabetes 1989;38:1512–1527.
18. Yang YJ, Youn JH, Bergman RN. Modified protocols improve insulin sensitivity estimation using the minimal model. Am J Physiol 1987;253:E595–E602.
19. Pei D, Jones CN, Bhargava R, Chen YD, Reaven GM. Evaluation of octreotide to assess insulin-mediated glucose disposal by the insulin suppression test. Diabetologia 1994;37:843–845.
20. Akinmokun A, Selby PL, Ramaiya K, Alberti KG. The short insulin tolerance test for determination of insulin sensitivity: a comparison with the euglycaemic clamp. Diabet Med 1992;9: 432–437.

21. Bonora E, Moghetti P, Zancanaro C, et al. Estimates of in vivo insulin action in man: comparison of insulin tolerance tests with euglycemic and hyperglycemic glucose clamp studies. J Clin Endocrinol Metab 1989;68:374–378.

22. Matsuda M, DeFronzo RA. Insulin sensitivity indices obtained from oral glucose tolerance testing: comparison with the euglycemic insulin clamp. Diabetes Care 1999;22:1462–1470.

23. Breda E, Cavaghan MK, Toffolo G, Polonsky KS, Cobelli C. Oral glucose tolerance test minimal model indexes of beta-cell function and insulin sensitivity. Diabetes 2001;50:150–158.

24. Penesova A, Radikova Z. Comparison of insulin sensitivity indices calculated from standard 3-sampled and frequently sampled oral glucose tolerance test. Endocr Regul 2004;38:167–171.

25. Yeni-Komshian H, Carantoni M, Abbasi F, Reaven GM. Relationship between several surrogate estimates of insulin resistance and quantification of insulin-mediated glucose disposal in 490 healthy nondiabetic volunteers. Diabetes Care 2000;23:171–175.

26. Hollenbeck CB, Chen N, Chen Y-DI, Reaven GM. Relationship between the plasma insulin response to oral glucose and insulin-stimulated glucose utilization in normal subjects. Diabetes 1984;33:460–463.

27. Quon MJ. Editorial: limitations of the fasting glucose to insulin ratio as an index of insulin sensitivity. J Clin Endocrinol Metab 2001;86:4615–4617.

28. Matthews DR, Hosker JP, Rudenski AS, Naylor BA, Treacher DF, Turner RC. Homeostasis model assessment: insulin resistance and beta-cell function from fasting plasma glucose and insulin concentrations in man. Diabetologia 1985;28:412–419.

29. Diamanti-Kandarakis E, Kouli C, Alexandraki K, Spina G. Failure of mathematical indices to accurately assess insulin resistance in lean, overweight, or obese women with polycystic ovary syndrome. J Clin Endocrinol Metab 2004;89:1273–1276.

30. Levy JC, Matthews DR, Hermans MP. Correct homeostasis model assessment (HOMA) evaluation uses the computer program. Diabetes Care 1998;21:2191–2192.

31. Katz A, Nambi SS, Mather K, et al. Quantitative insulin sensitivity check index: a simple accurate method for assessing insulin sensitivity in humans. J Clin Endocrinol Metab 2000;85:2402–2410.

32. Rabassa-Lhoret R, Bastard JP, Jan V, et al. Modified Quantitative Insulin Sensitivity Check Index is better correlated to hyperinsulinemic glucose clamp than other fasting-based index of insulin sensitivity in different insulin-resistant states. J Clin Endocrinol Metab 2003;88:4917–4923.

33. Robbins DC, Andersen L, Bowsher R, Chance R, Dineson B, Frank B. Report of the American Diabetes Association's task force on standardization of the insulin assay. Diabetes 1996;45:242–256.

34. Radikova Z. Assessment of insulin sensitivity/resistance in epidemiological studies. Endocr Regul 2003;37:189–194.

35. Report of the Expert Committee on the Diagnosis and Classification of Diabetes Mellitus. Diabetes Care 1997;20:1183–1197.

36. World Health Organization. Diabetes Mellitus: Report of a WHO Study Group. Geneva: WHO, 1985; Technical Report Series 727.

37. Legro RS, Kunselman AR, Dunaif A. Prevalence and predictors of dyslipidemia in women with polycystic ovary syndrome. Am J Med 2001;111:607–613.

38. Legro RS, Azziz R, Ehrmann D, et al. Minimal response of circulating lipids in women with polycystic ovary syndrome to improvement in insulin sensitivity with troglitazone. J Clin Endocrinol Metab 2003;88:5137–5144.

39. Brown CD, Higgins M, Donato KA, et al. Body mass index and the prevalence of hypertension and dyslipidemia. Obes Res 2000;8:605–619.

40. Hu G, Qiao Q, Tuomilehto J, Balkau B, Borch-Johnsen K, Pyorala K. Prevalence of the metabolic syndrome and its relation to all-cause and cardiovascular mortality in nondiabetic European men and women. Arch Intern Med 2004;164:1066–1076.

41. Grundy SM, Brewer HB Jr, Cleeman JI, Smith SC Jr, Lenfant C. National Heart, Lung, and Blood Institute, American Heart Association: definition of metabolic syndrome: report of the National Heart, Lung, and Blood Institute/American Heart Association conference on scientific issues related to definition. Circulation 2004;109:433–438.

42. World Health Organization: Definition, Diagnosis, and Classification of Diabetes Mellitus and its Complications: Report of a WHO Consultation. Geneva, WHO, 1999.

43. Expert Panel on the Detection, Evaluation, and Treatment of High Blood Cholesterol in Adults: executive summary of the Third Report of the National Cholesterol Education Program (NCEP) Expert Panel on Detection, Evaluation, and Treatment of High Blood Cholesterol in Adults (Adult Treatment Panel III). JAMA 2001;285:2486–2497.

44. Balkau B, Charles MA, Drivsholm T, et al. Frequency of the WHO metabolic syndrome in European cohorts, and an alternative definition of an insulin resistance syndrome. Diabetes Metab 2002;28:364–376.

45. Einhorn D, Reaven GM, Cobin RH, et al. American College of Endocrinology position statement on the insulin resistance syndrome. Endocr Pract 2003;9:237–252.

46. Kahn R, Buse J, Ferrannini E, Stern M. The metabolic syndrome: time for a critical appraisal: joint statement from the American Diabetes Association and the European Association for the Study of Diabetes. Diabetes Care 2005;28:2289–2304.

47. Vrbikova J, Vondra K, Cibula D, et al. Metabolic syndrome in young Czech women with polycystic ovary syndrome. Hum Reprod 2005;20:3328–3332.

48. Vural B, Caliskan E, Turkoz E, Kilic T, Demirci A. Evaluation of metabolic syndrome frequency and premature carotid atherosclerosis in young women with polycystic ovary syndrome. Hum Reprod 2005;20:2409–2413.

49. Carmina E, Legro RS, Stamets K, Lowell J, Lobo RA. Difference in body weight between American and Italian women with polycystic ovary syndrome: influence of the diet. Hum Reprod 2003;18: 2289–2293.

12 Hormonal and Biochemical Evaluation of Polycystic Ovary Syndrome

Bulent O. Yildiz, MD

CONTENTS

Summary

Polycystic ovary syndrome (PCOS) is a common and complex disorder characterized by endocrine, metabolic, and reproductive disturbances. Both the clinical and laboratory features of the syndrome are remarkably heterogeneous and may change even in a single patient over time. Laboratory investigations are used in PCOS mainly for the determination of biochemical hyperandrogenemia and ovulatory dysfunction. These tests are also helpful for the exclusion of other related androgen excess disorders. Measurement of serum-free testosterone levels by sensitive methods or calculation of free androgen index, in addition to measurement of dehydroepiandrosterone sulfate, are used for the determination of hyperandrogenism. Serum levels of luteinizing hormone or the luteinizing hormone/follicle stimulating hormone ratio are not recommended for the routine evaluation of PCOS, whereas luteal-phase progesterone measurements might be helpful to confirm ovulatory function in hyperandrogenic patients with apparently regular menses. Initial work-up of a patient with PCOS includes, at a minimum, thyroid-stimulating hormone, prolactin, and basal or stimulated 17(OH) progesterone levels to exclude thyroid dysfunction, hyperprolactinemia, and nonclassical congenital adrenal hyperplasia, respectively. If other rare disorders with similar clinical presentations are suspected, further hormonal and biochemical evaluation would be necessary.

Key Words: Hyperandrogenism; hyperandrogenemia; androgens; ovulation.

INTRODUCTION

In 1935, Stein and Leventhal *(1)* reported their findings on seven cases with infertility, amenorrhea, and bilateral enlarged polycystic ovaries. Three of these patients were obese and five were hirsute. This original description of the polycystic ovary syndrome

From: *Contemporary Endocrinology: Insulin Resistance and Polycystic Ovarian Syndrome: Pathogenesis, Evaluation, and Treatment*
Edited by: E. Diamanti-Kandarakis, J. E. Nestler, D. Panidis, and R. Pasquali © Humana Press Inc., Totowa, NJ

(PCOS) by these investigators did not include any hormonal or biochemical measurement. However, development of the radioimmunoassay (RIA) in 1967 by Berson and Yalow *(2)* enabled investigators to measure hormone concentrations at very small levels, and changed the course of research in PCOS, as in several other fields of science. Numerous studies over the next two decades reported hormonal alterations using the RIA technique in PCOS, and provided a better understanding of the pathophysiology of the syndrome. An expert meeting held in 1990 and sponsored by the National Institute of Child Health and Human Development (NICHD) suggested that the diagnostic criteria for PCOS should include both clinical and/or biochemical hyperandrogenism and chronic anovulation after exclusion of other known androgen excess disorders *(3)*. In 2003, another expert meeting held in Rotterdam and sponsored by the European Society for the Human Reproduction and Embryology (ESHRE) and the American Society for Reproductive Medicine (ASRM) expanded this definition by adding the criterion of polycystic ovaries (PCO) on ultrasound to the diagnostic criteria *(4,5)*.

Hormonal and biochemical abnormalities in PCOS include high serum androgen levels, low sex hormone-binding globulin (SHBG), inappropriate gonadotropin secretion, acyclic estrogen production, hyperinsulinemia/insulin resistance, and lipid/lipoprotein alterations. Like the symptoms of the syndrome, there is considerable heterogeneity in laboratory measurements among women with PCOS, and biochemical phenotype could change over time even in a single patient. Here, we briefly review the hormonal and biochemical assessment in PCOS.

BACKGROUND

Hormonal and biochemical evaluation should be performed at the initial visit of a patient with PCOS (Table 1). This evaluation may include the following:

1. Determination of androgen levels in the circulation.
2. Measurement of gonadotropins.
3. Biochemical confirmation of ovulatory dysfunction.
4. Biochemical tests for the exclusion of other related disorders.
5. Tests for insulin resistance (*see* Chapter 30).
6. Measurement of lipid/lipoprotein levels (*see* Chapter 7).

It is important to emphasize that most of the pharmacological agents used in the treatment of PCOS, particularly oral contraceptive pills, may affect hormonal values, making interpretation difficult. For example, patients should be off medication at least for 3 months to get a true androgen value.

Hyperandrogenism

Clinical manifestations of hyperandrogenism, including hirsutism, acne, and androgenic alopecia, can be observed in the absence of biochemical hyperandrogenemia. When serum androgen levels are apparently normal, it is likely that androgenic skin and hair changes result from increased local tissue sensitivity to circulating androgens and/or ethnic differences in phenotypic expression of peripheral androgen excess signs. Alternatively, biochemical hyperandrogenemia may present in some patients with PCOS, particularly in Asian women, without obvious peripheral manifestations of hyperandrogenism. Thus, evaluation of PCOS includes determination of clinical and/or biochemical androgen excess.

There is a wide variability of circulating androgens in women, and it is critical to note that there is no clear distinction between normal and abnormal in interpreting androgen levels. Nevertheless, evaluation of excessive androgen production is usually performed by the measurement of androgenic hormones in the circulation. These hormones include testosterone (T), androstenedione (A4), dehydroepiandrosterone (DHEA), and its sulfate form (DHEAS) *(6)* (Table 1).

A Synopsis of the Androgen Physiology in Women

Androgens are produced by both the ovaries and the adrenal gland. All androgens are synthesized from a steroid substrate pregnenolone, which is derived from cholesterol. The regulation of androgen secretion involves stimulation of the adrenal gland and the ovaries by adrenocorticotropic hormone (ACTH) and luteinizing hormone (LH), respectively, together with intraglandular paracrine and autocrine mechanisms. The adrenal gland preferentially secretes weak androgens DHEA and DHEAS in large amounts, which may be converted to A4 and then to T. The adrenal gland contributes 100% of DHEAS, 90% of DHEA, 50% of A4, and 25% of T in the reproductive-aged women. The ovary secretes androgenic steroids primarily in the form A4, and contributes about 50% of circulating A4, 25% of T, and 10% of DHEA. The remaining 50% of circulating T is produced from the peripheral conversion of the weaker androgens A4 and DHEAS. Much of the extraglandular conversion of T takes place in the liver and the skin.

Whereas DHEA and DHEAS are carried in circulation loosely bound to albumin, approx 75% of total T is bound to SHBG and about 23% is weakly bound to albumin. Free T (fT) constitutes less than 2% of the circulating T. Free and weakly bound T is called bioavailable T. We should bear in mind that changes in the SHBG levels with disease or drugs may influence the interpretation of total T levels.

Once formed, T is either converted to estradiol (E2) by the enzyme aromatase, or it is metabolized to its active product dihydrotestosterone (DHT) by 5α-reductase in androgen-sensitive tissues. DHT is responsible for most of the T's activity at the tissue level.

Normative ranges for androgens may differ depending on age and body mass index (BMI). Circulating levels of both total and fT *(7)*, and DHEAS decline with age. There is a paucity of normative androgen data for adolescents and elderly women. However, it is well-known that normal menopausal androgen levels are lower than those produced during the reproductive years. Obesity, particularly the abdominal type, could increase formation of T from A4, and decrease SHBG levels resulting in increased free androgen index in obese women *(8)*.

Testosterone

The majority of the circulating T is formed from A4 in the liver and androgen-sensitive tissues such asthe skin. Total T levels are routinely measured by RIA using highly specific antibodies, without the need for extraction or chromatography. However, decreased (e.g., in androgen excess or obesity) or increased (e.g., with the use of oral contraceptive pills) SHBG levels may influence total T levels. Thus, measurement of the free and albumin-bound (bioavailable) forms of T is necessary for the proper interpretation of elevated total T levels. Recommended methods for the measurement of fT are equilibrium dialysis and ammonium sulfate precipitation *(9)*. Alternatively, free androgen index can be calculated from the measurement of total T and SHBG (100 × total T/SHBG). Currently available commercial assays for the measurement of fT appear to have limited value for the evaluation of androgen excess in women *(10)*.

Table 1
Suggested Biochemical Testing in PCOS

Determination of hyperandrogenemia
T, fT, SHBG, free androgen index
DHEAS, A4
Gonadotropins
LH, LH/FSH ratio
Ovulatory dysfunction
D20-22 progesterone
Exclusion of other related disorders
Thyroid-stimulating hormone
Prolactin
Basal or stimulated 17(OH)P
FSH, E2

See text for abbreviations.

A specific DHT metabolite, 3α-androstanediol glucuronide (3α-diol G), has been proposed as an index of 5α-reductase activity within the pilosebaceous unit of the skin *(11)*, especially when hirsutism is not associated with biochemical hyperandrogenemia of either an ovarian or adrenal source. However, routine measurement of this metabolite in PCOS is not recommended.

DEHYDROEPIANDROSTERONE AND ITS SULFATE FORM

DHEAS is the major androgenic steroid secreted by the adrenal gland. More than 90% of DHEA is sulfated before secretion from the adrenal gland. DHEAS is determined directly in serum or plasma by RIA with the use of highly specific antibodies.

The circulating levels of DHEAS are age-related. Young children have low levels, whereas increased levels are observed with adrenarche and puberty. Maximal DHEAS levels are achieved during the second decade of life, and the concentration of DHEAS remains fairly constant in any given healthy woman or patient with PCOS over long periods of time during reproductive years *(12)*, with a decline occurring in the elderly, particularly after the age of 70 *(13)*.

Between 20 and 30% of patients with PCOS show increased DHEAS levels, whereas a few patients may have "isolated" elevations in DHEAS. Thus, measurement of DHEAS could be of limited value in the hormonal evaluation of women with PCOS.

ANDROSTENEDIONE

A4 levels reflecting both ovarian and adrenal androgenic steroid production are measured by RIA. Highly specific antibodies for A4 allow for its direct measurement in serum or plasma without the need for extraction or chromatography. However, normative and clinical data for A4 is lacking and there is little data available regarding the value of A4 in evaluation of androgen excess in women. Thus, measurement of this androgenic steroid is not recommended for the routine assessment of women with PCOS.

Gonadotropins

PCOS is associated with an inappropriate gonadotropin secretion. The frequency of pulsatile gonadotropin-releasing hormone (GnRH) secretion appears to be increased in the syndrome. Serum LH levels were found to be elevated in patients with PCOS primarily because of increased LH pulse amplitude and frequency, whereas FSH levels were comparable to healthy women *(14–16)*. Therefore, an elevated LH/FSH ratio of 2–3/1 is commonly used to indicate abnormal gonadotropin secretion in PCOS. Increased serum LH concentrations and an elevated LH/FSH ratio may be observed in 40–60% and up to 95% of patients, respectively *(17,18)*. However, LH measurements may be influenced by the pulsatile nature of secretion of this hormone, the temporal relation to ovulation, by BMI and percentage of body fat, and the variable and imprecise nature of the assays used. Currently, LH levels or LH/FSH ratio are not included in the diagnostic criteria of PCOS. Measurement of LH levels could be taken as a secondary parameter, particularly in lean patients.

Tests of Ovulatory Dysfunction

Chronic anovulation in PCOS usually presents as oligomenorrhea, amenorrhea, or dysfunctional uterine bleeding. Some women with PCOS have regular cycles at first and experience menstrual irregularity in association with weight gain. Up to 20% of patients with PCOS report regular vaginal bleeding, and ovulatory dysfunction could be confirmed in these patients by obtaining a luteal phase progesterone level on D20–22 (i.e., 20–22 days after the start of menstruation) with or without basal body temperature monitoring. Progesterone secreted by the corpus luteum reaches a peak in the midluteal phase of the ovulatory menstrual cycle approx 7 days prior to menses. Ovulatory dysfunction may be evidenced by a luteal phase progesterone level less than 3–5 ng/mL in a patient with eumenorrhea.

Biochemical Tests for Exclusion of Other Related Disorders

Biochemical tests are helpful in PCOS to exclude other disorders with similar clinical presentation, including thyroid dysfunction, hyperprolactinemia, nonclassical congenital adrenal hyperplasia (NCAH), androgen-secreting neoplasms, HAIRAN syndrome, Cushing's syndrome, and acromegaly (Table 1).

Thyroid-stimulating hormone levels may be considered to identify thyroid dysfunction. However, routine measurement of TSH levels appears to have limited value because the prevalence of thyroid disorders in women with PCOS is similar to that of the general population of reproductive-aged women.

Prolactin levels should be measured in the evaluation of hyperandrogenic patients to exclude hyperprolactinemia. High prolactin levels may have gonadotropin-like effects on androgen production and must be considered in the differential diagnosis of PCOS. Prolactin levels are usually normal or slightly elevated in up to 30% of the patients with PCOS *(19)*. However, persistent elevation of serum prolactin levels would require imaging studies to rule out a pituitary adenoma. Moreover, patients with prolactinomas may have ovaries that appear to be polycystic on ultrasound *(20)*.

Depending on ethnicity, between 1 and 10% of hyperandrogenic women will have NCAH *(21)*. The most common form of NCAH is a deficiency in the activity of 21-hydroxylase (21-OH). The precursors to 21-OH, specifically 17(OH)P and A4, accumulate in excesses that result in hirsutism, oligo-anovulation, and often PCO. NCAH is clinically indistinguishable from PCOS. Moreover, the levels of DHEAS are not any higher than in other hyperandrogenic women. Thus, the diagnosis of NCAH is based on either baseline or stimulated 17(OH)P measurements. 17(OH)P levels are obtained in the morning and during follicular phase. The cutoff value for basal measurements is 2–3 ng/dL. If baseline values are higher than the cutoff, an ACTH stimulation test should be performed for the diagnosis *(21)*. For this test, 250 µg of 1-24 ACTH is injected intravenously, and 17(OH)P levels are measured at 30 and 60 minutes. The diagnosis of 21-OH-deficient NCAH is made biochemically if the stimulated levels are higher than 10 ng/mL and this diagnosis could be confirmed by genotyping of CYP21. Other uncommon causes of NCAH include deficiencies of 11α-hydroxylase and 3β-hydroxysteroid dehydrogenase. These forms are very rare and screening for them is not suggested in every patient with PCOS. Nevertheless, prevalence of these disorders among different ethnicities should always be considered when patients from high-risk populations are evaluated.

Clinical features are usually helpful in making the diagnosis of androgen-producing tumors. These tumors are relatively rare and usually originate from the adrenal gland and the ovary. The onset of these tumors is usually sudden and they may rapidly lead to virilization and masculinization. Although clinical presentation is the most sensitive indicator of an androgen-producing tumor, particular attention should be given to occasional cases of slowly evolving tumors. Biochemical tests would be required in these patients. Adrenal tumors can be suspected when serum DHEAS levels are higher than 7000 ng/mL, whereas circulating T levels higher than 200–300 ng/dL should raise the suspicion of ovarian tumors. In cases of high clinical and biochemical suspicion of an adrenal or ovarian androgen-producing tumor, imaging studies and venous sampling could be of value in identifying the tumor.

Clinical stigmata of severe insulin resistance, such as acanthosis nigricans, may require measurement of insulin resistance. Up to 4% of hyperandrogenic women will have HAIRAN syndrome. These patients generally have extremely high levels of circulating insulin (usually >80 µU/mL in the fasting state and/or 500 µU/mL during an oral glucose tolerance test) *(22)*.

Biochemical tests for Cushing's syndrome or acromegaly would be necessary only if clinical features are suggestive for these disorders. Measurement of 24-hour urinary free cortisol levels or low-dose dexamethasone suppression test is performed to exclude Cushing's syndrome, whereas growth hormone, insulin-like growth factor 1 measurements, and growth hormone suppression test are needed for the diagnosis of acromegaly.

Serum FSH and E2 levels are measured in women with ovulatory dysfunction to exclude hypogonadotropic hypogonadism characterized by low FSH, low E2, or premature ovarian failure characterized by high FSH or low E2 levels. These hormones are usually in the normal range in patients with PCOS because the syndrome appears to be a part of World Health Organization (WHO) type 2 normoestrogenic anovulation.

Finally, hirsute patients who have regular ovulatory cycles will be diagnosed with idiopathic hirsutism. Most of these women will have normal circulating androgen levels and increased 5α-reductase activity in the skin and hair follicle that might lead to hirsutism despite normal serum androgen levels. However, it turns out that many of these patients have hyperandrogenemia that may not be detectable with routine clinical androgen assays.

CONCLUSIONS

It is becoming increasingly apparent that the laboratory evaluation of PCOS is of extreme value both for the clinical investigator and the practicing physician. Overall, hormonal and biochemical assessment is helpful in PCOS both for the confirmation of hyperandrogenism and ovulatory disfunction and for the exclusion of other related androgen excess disorders. Although specific guidelines do not exist, it might also be helpful in PCOS to gather hormonal and biochemical information to make clinical decisions regarding treatment. At a minimum, initial laboratory work-up of a patient with PCOS may include measuring fT, DHEAS, prolactin, and 17(OH)P levels. In a hirsute patient with apparently regular menses, luteal phase progesterone level would be useful to confirm ovulatory function.

FUTURE AVENUES OF INVESTIGATION

More research is required to determine the biological importance of various androgens and other associated biochemical abnormalities in PCOS. Clinical relevance of gonadotropin abnormalities needs further clarification in future studies. Large, well-characterized population studies are needed to determine normative ranges for circulating androgens. These studies should take into account age and BMI. Biochemical intermediary phenotypes potentially representing the mild forms of PCOS should be studied prospectively. These studies might ultimately provide insight into the issues of proper identification and, perhaps, follow-up of patients with PCOS.

KEY POINTS

- Hormonal and biochemical investigations are useful to determine hyperandrogenism and ovulatory dysfunction. These tests are also required to exclude other androgen excess disorders.
- Evaluation of biochemical hyperandrogenemia includes the measurement of free T by sensitive methods or calculation of free androgen index by measurement of total T and sex hormone-binding globulin. Serum sulfated dehydroepiandrosterone levels could be obtained in the assessment, whereas routine measurement of androstenedione levels is not recommended.
- Routine measurement of LH or LH/follicle stimulating hormone ratio is not recommended in polycystic ovary syndrome.
- Luteal phase progesterone levels might be helpful to confirm ovulatory function in patients with apparently regular menses.
- Thyroid-stimulating hormone, prolactin, and basal or stimulated 17(OH)P levels are required to exclude thyroid dysfunction, hyperprolactinemia, and nonclassical congenital adrenal hyperplasia, respectively. If clinical findings are highly suggestive of other rare disorders with similar clinical presentation, further biochemical testing might be needed.

REFERENCES

1. Stein IF, Leventhal, ML. Amenorrhea associated with bilateral polycystic ovaries. Am J Obstet Gynecol 1935;29:181–191.
2. Berson SA, Yalow RS. Radioimmunoassays of peptide hormones in plasma. N Engl J Med 1967; 277:640–647.

3. Zawadzki JK, Dunaif A. Diagnostic criteria for polycystic ovary syndrome. In: Dunaif A, Givens J, Haseltine F, Merriam GR, eds. Polycystic Ovary Syndrome. Boston, MA: Blackwell Scientific Publications, 1992, pp.377–384.

4. Rotterdam ESHRE/ASRM-sponsored PCOS Consensus Workshop Group. Revised 2003 consensus on diagnostic criteria and long-term health risks related to polycystic ovary syndrome. Fertil Steril 2004;81:19–25.

5. Rotterdam ESHRE/ASRM-sponsored PCOS Consensus Workshop Group. Revised 2003 consensus on diagnostic criteria and long-term health risks related to polycystic ovary syndrome (PCOS). Hum Reprod 2004;19:41–47.

6. Robinson S, Rodin DA, Deacon A, Wheeler MJ, Clayton RN. Which hormone tests for the diagnosis of polycystic ovary syndrome? Br J Obstet Gynaecol 1992;99:232–238.

7. Zumoff B, Strain GW, Miller LK, Rosner W. Twenty-four-hour mean plasma testosterone concentration declines with age in normal premenopausal women. J Clin Endocrinol Metab 1995;80: 1429–1430.

8. Gambineri A, Pelusi C, Vicennati V, Pagotto U, Pasquali R. Obesity and the polycystic ovary syndrome. Int J Obes Relat Metab Disord 2002;26:883–896.

9. Vermeulen A, Verdonck L, Kaufman JM. A critical evaluation of simple methods for the estimation of free testosterone in serum. J Clin Endocrinol Metab 1999;84:3666–3672.

10. Rosner W. Errors in the measurement of plasma free testosterone. J Clin Endocrinol Metab 1997;82:2014–2015.

11. Horton R, Hawks D, Lobo R. 3 alpha, 17 beta-androstanediol glucuronide in plasma. A marker of androgen action in idiopathic hirsutism. J Clin Invest 1982;69:1203–1206.

12. Yildiz BO, Woods KS, Stanczyk F, Bartolucci A, Azziz R. Stability of adrenocortical steroidogenesis over time in healthy women and women with polycystic ovary syndrome. J Clin Endocrinol Metab 2004;89:5558–5562.

13. Orentreich N, Brind JL, Rizer RL, Vogelman JH. Age changes and sex differences in serum dehydroepiandrosterone sulfate concentrations throughout adulthood. J Clin Endocrinol Metab 1984;59: 551–555.

14. Kazer RR, Kessel B, Yen SS. Circulating luteinizing hormone pulse frequency in women with polycystic ovary syndrome. J Clin Endocrinol Metab 1987;65:233–236.

15. Burger CW, Korsen T, van Kessel H, van Dop PA, Caron FJ, Schoemaker J. Pulsatile luteinizing hormone patterns in the follicular phase of the menstrual cycle, polycystic ovarian disease (PCOD) and non-PCOD secondary amenorrhea. J Clin Endocrinol Metab 1985;61:1126–1132.

16. Marshall JC, Eagleson CA. Neuroendocrine aspects of polycystic ovary syndrome. Endocrinol Metab Clin North Am 1999;28:295–324.

17. Laven JS, Imani B, Eijkemans MJ, Fauser BC. New approach to polycystic ovary syndrome and other forms of anovulatory infertility. Obstet Gynecol Surv 2002;57:755–767.

18. Taylor AE, McCourt B, Martin KA, et al. Determinants of abnormal gonadotropin secretion in clinically defined women with polycystic ovary syndrome. J Clin Endocrinol Metab 1997;82:2248–2256.

19. Luciano AA, Chapler FK, Sherman BM. Hyperprolactinemia in polycystic ovary syndrome. Fertil Steril 1984;41:719–725.

20. Franks S. Polycystic ovary syndrome. N Engl J Med 1995;333:853–861.

21. Azziz R, Dewailly D, Owerbach D. Clinical review 56: nonclassic adrenal hyperplasia: current concepts. J Clin Endocrinol Metab 1994;78:810–815.

22. Azziz R. The hyperandrogenic-insulin-resistant acanthosis nigricans syndrome: therapeutic response. Fertil Steril 1994;61:570–572.

13 Imaging Studies in Polycystic Ovary Syndrome

Sophie Jonard, MD, Yann Robert, MD,
Yves Ardaens, MD, and Didier Dewailly, MD

CONTENTS

Summary

The need for a calibrated imaging of polycystic ovaries (PCO) is now stronger than ever since the recent consensus conference held in Rotterdam, May 1–3, 2003. However, imaging PCO is not an easy procedure and it requires a thorough technical and medical background. The two-dimensional ultrasonography remains the standard for imaging PCO and the current consensus definition of PCO determined at the joint American Society for Reproductive Medicine/European Society of Human Reproduction and Embryology (ASRM/ESHRE) consensus meeting on polycystic ovary syndrome rests on this technique: either 12 or more follicles measuring 2–9 mm in diameter and/or increased ovarian volume (>10 cm^3). The other techniques, such as Doppler, three-dimensional, and magnetic resonance imaging, can help with the diagnosis, but are only second-line techniques.

Key Words: Polycystic ovary; ultrasonography; follicle; stroma; diagnosis; doppler; MRI.

INTRODUCTION

In the wake of the consensus conference held in Rotterdam in 2003, the need for calibrated imaging of polycystic ovaries (PCO) is stronger than ever. Indeed, the subjective criteria that were proposed 20 years ago and were still used until recently by the vast majority of authors are now being replaced by a stringent definition using objective criteria *(1,2)*.

From: *Contemporary Endocrinology: Insulin Resistance and Polycystic Ovarian Syndrome: Pathogenesis, Evaluation, and Treatment*
Edited by: E. Diamanti-Kandarakis, J. E. Nestler, D. Panidis, and R. Pasquali © Humana Press Inc., Totowa, NJ

Imaging PCO is not an easy procedure. It requires a thorough technical and medical background. The goal of this chapter is to provide the reader with the main issues ensuring a well-controlled imaging for the diagnosis of PCO. The two-dimensional (2D) ultrasonography (U/S) will be first and extensively addressed because it remains the standard for imaging PCO. Other techniques, such as Doppler, three-dimensional (3D), and magnetic resonance imaging (MRI) will be described more briefly.

2D U/S

Technical Aspects and Recommendations

The transabdominal route should always be the first step of pelvic sonographic examination, followed by the transvaginal route, except in virgin or refusing patients. Of course, a full bladder is required for visualization of the ovaries. However, one should be cautious that an overfilled bladder can compress the ovaries, yielding a falsely increased length. The main advantage of this route is that it offers a panoramic view of the pelvic cavity. Therefore, it allows excluding associated uterine or ovarian abnormalities with an abdominal development. Indeed, lesions with cranial growth could be missed when using the transvaginal approach exclusively.

With the transvaginal route, high-frequency probes (>6 MHz) with a better spatial resolution but less examination depth can be used because the ovaries are close to the vagina and/or the uterus, and because the presence of fatty tissue is usually less disturbing (except when very abundant). With this technique, not only are the size and the shape of ovaries visible, but so are their internal structure, namely, the follicles and stroma. It is now possible to get pictures that have a definition close to anatomical cuts. However, the evaluation of the ovarian size via the transvaginal approach is difficult. To be the most accurate, it requires meticulously choosing the picture where the ovary appears the longest and the widest. This picture must then be frozen. Two means can be proposed for calculating the ovarian area: either fitting an ellipse to the ovary with the area given by the machine, or outlining the ovary by hand with automatic calculation of the outlined area. This last technique must be preferred in cases of non-ellipsoid ovaries, as sometimes observed. The volume is the most complete approach. Traditionally, it can be estimated after the measurement of the length, width, and thickness using the classical formula for a prolate ellipsoid: $L \times W \times T \times 0.523$ *(3–5)*. However, the ovaries have to be studied in three orthogonal planes, a condition that is not always respected. The 3D U/S is an attractive alternative for the accurate assessment of ovarian volume, but this technique is not commonly available *(see 3D Ultrasound)*.

In order to count the total number of "cysts" (in fact, follicles) and to evaluate their size and position, each ovary should be scanned in longitudinal and/or transversal cross-sections from the inner to outer margins.

The Consensual Definition of PCO

According to the literature review dealing with all available imaging systems and the discussion at the joint ASRM/ESHRE consensus meeting on PCOS held in Rotterdam, May 1–3, 2003, the current consensus definition of PCO is the following: *either 12 or more follicles measuring 2–9 mm in diameter and/or increased ovarian volume (>10 cm³)*.

The priority was given to the ovarian volume and to the follicle number because both have the advantage of being physical entities that can be measured in real-time conditions and because both are still considered the key and consistent features of PCO.

INCREASED OVARIAN VOLUME

Many studies have reported an increased mean ovarian volume in series of patients with polycystic ovary syndrome (PCOS) *(4,6,7,16,17)*. However, the upper normal limit of the ovarian volume suffers from some variability in the literature (from 8 to 15.6 cm^3). Such variability may be explained by the following:

- The small number of controls in some studies; and/or
- Differences in inclusion or exclusion criteria for control women; and/or
- Operator-dependent technical reasons. It is difficult indeed to obtain strictly longitudinal ovarian cuts, which is an absolute condition for accurate measures of the ovarian axis (length, width, thickness).

The consensual volume threshold to discriminate a normal ovary from a PCO is 10 cm^3 *(1)*. It has been empirically retained by the expert panel for the Rotterdam consensus as being the best compromise between the most complete studies *(6,7)*. Indeed, no study published so far has used an appropriate statistical appraisal of sensitivity and specificity of the volume threshold. This prompted us to recently revisit this issue through a prospective study including 154 women with PCOS compared with 57 women with normal ovaries. The receiver operating characteristic (ROC) curves indicated that a threshold of 10 cm^3 yielded a good specificity (98.2%) but a bad sensitivity (39%). Setting the threshold at 7 cm^3 offered the best compromise between specificity (94.7%) and sensitivity (68.8%) *(8)*. Thus, in our opinion, the threshold at 10 cm^3 should be lowered in order to increase the sensitivity of the PCO definition.

INCREASED FOLLICLE NUMBER

The polyfollicular pattern (i.e., excessive number of small echoless regions <10 mm in diameter) is strongly suggestive because it is in perfect reminiscence with the label of the syndrome (i.e., "polycystic"). It is now broadly accepted that most of these cysts are in fact healthy oocyte-containing follicles and are not atretic.

The consensus definition for a PCO is one that contains 12 or more follicles of 2–9 mm in diameter. Again, the expert panel for the Rotterdam consensus considered this threshold as being the best compromise between the most complete studies, including the one in which we compared 214 patients with PCOS with 112 women with normal ovaries *(9)*. By ROC analysis, a follicle number per ovary (FNPO) of 12 or more follicles of 2–9 in mm diameter yielded the best compromise between sensitivity (75%) and specificity (99%) for the diagnosis of PCO.

The Rotterdam consensus did not address the difficult issue of the presence of multifollicular ovaries (MFO) in situations other than PCOS. Again, the terminology might be better annotated as multifollicular rather than multicystic. There is no consensual definition for MFO, although these have been described as ovaries in which there are multiple (≥6) follicles, usually 4–10 mm in diameter, with normal stromal echogenicity *(4)*. No histological data about MFO are available. MFO are characteristically seen during puberty and in women recovering from hypothalamic amenorrhea—both situations being associated with follicular growth without consistent recruitment of a dominant follicle *(10,11)*. Although the clinical pictures are theoretically different, there may be some overlap, however, resulting in the confusion between PCO and MFO by inexperienced ultrasonographers. This stresses the need for considering carefully the other clinical and/or biological components of the consensual definition for PCOS. We recently revisited the ovarian follicular pattern in a group of women with hypothalamic amenorrhea. About one-third had a FNPO higher than 12 (unpublished personal data). Because they were anovulatory or oligo-ovulatory, they could be considered as having PCOS if one applied the Rotterdam definition too inflexibly! This might be true in some patients whom we do believe had PCOS whose clinical and biological expression had been modified by the chronically suppressed luteinizing hormone (LH) levels caused by their secondary hypothalamic dysfunction *(12)*. In the others, however, such an overlap in the FNPO emphasizes the need for a wise and careful utilization of the Rotterdam criteria, as well as for considering other ultrasound criteria for PCO in difficult situations.

Other Criteria and Other Definitions

EXTERNAL MORPHOLOGICAL SIGNS OF PCO

At its beginning in the 1970s, the weak resolution of U/S abdominal probes allowed the exclusive detection of the external morphological ovarian features that were used as the first criteria defining PCO:

- The length, the upper limit of which is 4 cm, is the simplest criterion, but this uni-dimensional approach may lead to false-positive results when a full bladder compresses the ovary (with the transabdominal route), or false-negative results when the ovaries are spheric, with a relatively short length.
- Because of the increased ovarian size and the normal uterine width, the uterine width/ovarian length (U/O) ratio is decreased (<1) in PCO.
- PCO often display a spherical shape, in contrast to normal ovaries, which are ellipsoid. This morphological change can be evaluated by the sphericity index (ovarian width/ovarian length), which is higher than 0.7 in PCO.

These parameters are less used nowadays because of their poor sensitivity *(13)*.

THE OVARIAN AREA

It is less used than the volume and was not retained in the consensus definition but, in our recent study revisiting the ovarian volume *(8)*, the diagnostic value of the ovarian area (assessed by the ROC curves) was slightly better than the ovarian volume (sensitivity: 77.6%, specificity: 94.7% for a threshold at 5 cm^2/ovary). We also observed that the measured ovarian area (by outlining the ovary by hand or by fitting an ellipse to the ovary) was more informative than the calculated ovarian area (by using the formula for an ellipse: length × width × $\pi/4$). Indeed, ovaries are not strictly ellipsoid and this can explain why the diagnostic value of the former was better than the latter. We previously reported that the sum of the area of both ovaries was less than 11 cm^2 in a large group of normal women *(14,15)*, but a threshold at 10 cm^2 seems to offer the best compromise between sensitivity and specificity. Beyond this threshold, the diagnosis of PCO can be suggested.

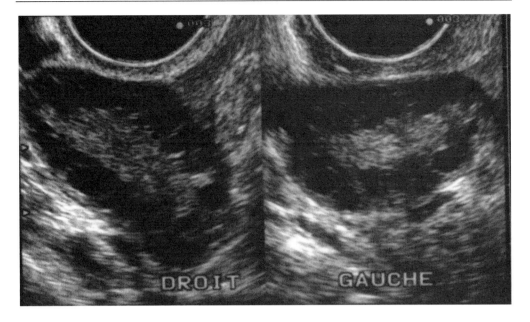

Fig. 1. Polycystic ovary (B mode). The ovarian outlined areas (9.7 cm^2 at right and 8.9 cm^2 at left) are increased. The follicle number, with a diameter between 2 and 9 mm, is more than 12. The small follicles display a typical peripheral pattern around the hyperechoic stroma.

THE INCREASED STROMA

Stromal hypertrophy is characterized by an increased component of the ovarian central part, which seems to be rather hyperechoic (Fig. 1). In our *(13,14)* and in others' opinions *(16)*, the stromal hypertrophy and hyperechogenicity help to distinguish between PCO and MFO because these features are specific for the former. However, the estimation of hyperechogenicity is considered highly subjective, mainly because it depends on the settings of the ultrasound machine. Likewise, in the absence of a precise quantification, the stromal hypertrophy is also a subjective sign.

For standardizing the assessment of stromal hypertrophy, we designed a computerized quantification of ovarian stroma, allowing selective calculation of the stromal area by subtraction of the cyst area from the total ovarian area on a longitudinal ovarian cut *(14,15)*. By this means, we were able to set the upper normal limit of the stromal area (i.e., 95th percentile of a large control group of 48 normal women) at 380 mm^2 per ovary. However, providing a precise outlining of the ovarian shape on a strictly longitudinal cut of the ovaries, the diagnostic value of the total ovarian equaled the one of stromal area because both were highly correlated.

Fulghesu et al. *(17)* proposed the ovarian stroma/total area ratio as a good criterion for the diagnosis of PCOS. The ovarian stromal area was evaluated by outlining with the caliper the peripheral profile of the stroma, identified by a central area slightly hyperechoic with respect to the other ovarian area. However, this evaluation seems to be difficult to reproduce in routine practice.

Stromal echogenicity has been described in a semi-quantitative manner with a score for normal (1), moderately increased (2), or frankly increased (3) *(18)*. In this study, the total follicle number of both ovaries combined correlated significantly with stromal echogenicity. Echogenicity has been quantified by Al-Took et al. *(19)* as the sum of the product of each intensity level (ranging from 0 to 63 on the scanner), and the number of pixels for that intensity level divided by the total number of pixels in the measured area. Buckett et al. *(20)* used this same formula, but no difference of the stromal echogenicity was found between women with PCOS and women with normal ovaries. The conclusion is that the subjective impression of increased stromal echogenicity is the result of both increased stromal volume alongside reduced echogenicity of the multiple follicles.

In summary, ovarian volume or area correlates well with ovarian function and is both more easily and reliably measured in routine practice than ovarian stroma. Thus, to define the polycystic ovary, neither qualitative nor quantitative assessment of the ovarian stroma is required.

FOLLICLE DISTRIBUTION

In PCO, the follicle distribution is predominantly peripheral, with typically an echoless peripheral array, as initially described by Adams et al. *(4)* (Fig. 1). For some authors *(21)*, younger patients more often display this peripheral distribution, whereas a more generalized pattern, with small cysts in the central part of the ovary, is noticed in older women. At the Rotterdam meeting, this subjective criterion was judged to be too inconstant and subjective to be retained for the consensus definition of PCO *(1)*.

OTHER TECHNIQUES FOR IMAGING PCO

3D Ultrasound

To avoid the difficulties and pitfalls in outlining or measuring the ovarian shape, the 3D U/S has been proposed as a dedicated volumic probe or a manual survey of the ovary *(22–24)*. From the stored data, the scanned ovarian volume is displayed on the screen in three adjustable orthogonal planes, allowing the three dimensions and, subsequently, the volume to be more accurately evaluated. In a study of Kyei-Mensah et al. *(25)*, three groups of patients were defined:

1. Those with normal ovaries.
2. Those with asymptomatic PCO.
3. Those with PCOS.

The ovarian and stromal volumes were similar in groups 2 and 3 and both were greater than group 1. Stromal volume was positively correlated with serum androstenedione concentrations in group 3 only. The mean total volume of the follicles was similar in all groups, indicating that increased stromal volume is the main cause of ovarian enlargement in PCO.

Nardo et al. *(26)* found good correlations between 2D and 3D ultrasound measurements of ovarian volume and polycystic ovary morphology. However, in this prospective study, total ovarian volume, ovarian stromal volume, follicular volume, and follicle number did not correlate with testosterone concentration.

Because 3D ultrasound requires expensive equipment, intensive training, and a long time for storage and data analysis, its superiority over 2D ultrasound to image PCO in clinical practice is not evident.

Doppler U/S

The assessment of uterine arteries will not be addressed in this chapter exclusively devoted to PCO imaging. Color (or power) Doppler allows detection of the vascularization network within the ovarian stroma. Power Doppler is more sensitive to the slow flows and shows more vascular signals within the ovaries, but it does not discriminate between arteries and veins. Moreover, the sensitivity of the machines differs from one to another. The Pulsed Doppler focuses on the hilum or internal ovarian arteries and offers a more objective approach. Because of the slow flows, the pulse repetition frequency (PRF) is at a minimum (400 Hz) with the lowest frequency filter (50 Hz).

The study of the ovarian vascularization by these techniques is still highly subjective. The blood flow is more frequently visualized in PCOS (88%) than in normal patients (50%) in early follicular phase and seems to be increased (27). No significant difference was found between obese and lean women with PCO, but the stroma was less vascularized in patients displaying a general cystic pattern than in those with peripherical cysts. In the latter, the Pulsatility Index (PI) values were significantly lower and inversely correlated to the follicle-stimulating hormone (FSH)/LH ratio (28). In another study (29), the Resistive Index (RI) and PI were significantly lower in PCOS (RI = 0.55 + 0.01 and PI = 0.89 + 0.04) than in normal patients (RI = 0.78 + 0.06 and PI = 1.87 + 0.38) and the peak systolic velocity was greater in PCOS (11.9 + 3.2) than in normal women (9.6 + 2.1). No correlation was found with the number of follicles and the ovarian volume, but there was a positive correlation between LH levels and increased peak systolic velocity. In the Zaidi et al. (30) study, no significant difference in PI values was found between the normal and PCOS groups, whereas the ovarian flow, as reflected by the peak sytolic velocity, was increased in the former. Some data indicate that Doppler blood flow may have some value in predicting the risk for ovarian hyperstimulation during gonadotropin therapy (31). Increased stromal blood flow has also been suggested as a more relevant predictor of ovarian response to hormonal stimulation than parameters, such as ovarian or stromal volume (20,32).

To summarize, the increased stroma component in PCO seems to be accompanied by an increased peak systolic velocity and a decreased PI at the ovarian Doppler study. However, in all studies, values in patients with PCO overlapped widely those of the normal patients. No data support so far any diagnostic usefulness of Doppler in PCO.

Magnetic Resonance Imaging

Data about MRI for PCO are still scarce in the literature (33–35). This technique allows a multiplanar approach of the pelvic cavity, which helps to localize the ovaries. Imaging quality is improved by the use of pelvic-dedicated phased-array coil receiver. The most useful planes are the transversal and coronal views. The T2-weighted sequence suits the best to the ovarian morphology. With this sequence, the follicular fluid displays an hypersignal (white), and the solid component (stroma) displays a low signal (black). T1-weighted sequences offer less information, but the Gadolium injection allows studying the stromal vascularization. The fat saturation technique increases the contrast obtained after the medium uptake by the vascularized areas.

The external signs of PCO (see External Morphological Signs of PCO) are easy to analyze on MRI transversal sections. In addition, the T2-weighted sequence displays the excessive number of follicles, but their detection and numbering is less easy than with

U/S because of the poor spatial resolution of MRI, unless high magnetic fields are used (1–1.5 Tesla). As with U/S, the stromal hypertrophy remains a subjective observation, although obvious in many cases. After Gadolinium injection, there is a high uptake by the stroma, suggesting that it is highly vascularized in PCO.

In most cases in practice, MRI does not afford more information than U/S for imaging PCO *(34)*. It is only helpful in difficult situations, such as a severe hyperandrogenism, when U/S is not possible or not contributive (virgin or obese patients, respectively). Its main role is to exclude a virilizing ovarian tumor, which should be suspected when the ovarian volume is not symetrical and/or when there is a circumscribed signal abnormality, either before or after Gadolinium injection. PCO associated with an ovarian tumor might be a pitfall.

CONCLUSIONS AND FUTURE AVENUES OF INVESTIGATION

The U/S study of PCO has now left its era of artistic haziness. It must be viewed as a diagnostic tool that requires the same quality control as a biological one, such as the plasma LH assay. This supposes that its results are expressed as quantitative variables rather than purely descriptive data. Last, it can be used by the clinician only if the ultrasonographer is sufficiently trained and his/her results are reproducible. Through its sensitivity (providing that sufficient specificity is guaranteed), U/S has widened the clinical spectrum of PCOS, and this has led to a reduction in the number of cases diagnosed with "idiopathic hirsutism" and "idiopathic anovulation."

The establishment of an international consensus definition for PCO was essential. However, one should keep in mind that the endovaginal U/S is an improving technique and becomes more and more accurate with time. Therefore, the thresholds of the currently used criteria are prone to change and new criteria defining PCO will probably appear in the future. Sooner or later, some new consensus shall probably be needed.

KEY POINTS

- The 2D U/S is the standard for imaging PCO.
- The transabdominal route should always be the first step of pelvic sonographic examination, followed by the transvaginal route (excepte in virgin or refusing patients), which offers a better spatial resolution.
- The current consensus definition of PCO determined at the joint ASRM/ESHRE consensus meeting on PCOS is the following: either 12 or more follicles measuring 2–9 mm in diameter and/or increased ovarian volume (>10 cm^3) at U/S.
- The other techniques such as Doppler, 3D, and MRI can help with the diagnosis, but are only second-line techniques.

REFERENCES

1. Balen AH, Laven JSE, Tan SL, Dewailly D. Ultrasound assessment of the polycystic ovary: international consensus definitions. Human Reproduction Update 2003;9:505–514.
2. The Rotterdam ESHRE/ASRM-sponsored PCOS consensus workshop group. Revised 2003 consensus on diagnostic criteria and long-term health risks related to polycystic ovary syndrome (PCOS). Hum Reprod 2004;19:41–47.
3. Sample WF, Lippe BM, Gyepes MT. Grey-scale ultrasonography of the normal female pelvis. Radiology 1977;125:477–483.

4. Adams JM, Polson DW, Abulwadi N, et al. Multifollicular ovaries: clinical and endocrine features and response to pulsatile gonadotropin-releasing hormone. Lancet 1985;2:1375–1378.

5. Orsini LF, Venturoli S, Lorusso R. Ultrasonic findings in polycystic ovarian disease. Fertil Steril 1985;43:709–714.

6. Yeh HC, Futterweit W, Thornton JC. Polycystic ovarian disease: US features in 104 patients. Radiology 1987;163:111–116.

7. Van Santbrink EJP, Hop WC, Fauser BCJM. Classification of normogonadotropic infertility: polycystic ovaries diagnosed by ultrasound versus endocrine characteristics of polycystic ovary syndrome. Fertil Steril 1997;67:452–458.

8. Jonard S, Robert Y, Dewailly D. Revisiting the ovarian volume as a diagnostic criterion for polycystic ovaries. Hum Reprod 2005;20:2893–2898.

9. Jonard S, Robert Y, Cortet-Rudelli C, Pigny P, Decanter C, Dewailly D. Ultrasound examination of polycystic ovaries: is it worth counting the follicles? Hum Reprod 2003;18:598–603.

10. Venturoli S, Porcu E, Fabbri R, Paradisi R, Orsini LF, Flamigni C. Ovaries and menstrual cycles in adolescence. Gynecol Obstet Invest 1983;17:219–223.

11. Stanhope R, Adams J, Jacobs HS, Brook CG. Ovarian ultrasound assessment in normal children, idiopathic precocious puberty, and during low dose pulsatile gonadotrophin releasing hormone treatment of hypogonadotrophic hypogonadism. Arch Dis Child 1985;60:116–119.

12. Reyss AC, Merlen E, Demerle C, Dewailly D. Revelation of a polymicrocystic ovary syndrome after one month's treatment by pulsatile GnRH in a patient presenting with functional hypothalamic amenorrhea. Gynecol Obstet Fertil 2003;31:1039–1042.

13. Ardaens Y, Robert Y, Lemaitre L, Fossati P, Dewailly D. Polycystic ovarian disease: contribution of vaginal endosonography and reassessment of ultrasonic diagnosis. Fertil Steril 1991;55:1062–1068.

14. Dewailly D., Robert Y, Helin I, et al. Ovarian stromal hypertrophy in hyperandrogenic women. Clin Endocrinol 1994;41:557–562.

15. Robert Y, Dubrulle F, Gaillandre G, et al. Ultrasound assessment of ovarian stroma hypertrophy in hyperandrogenism and ovulation disorders: visual analysis versus computerized quantification. Fertil Steril 1995;64:307–312.

16. Pache TD, Wladimiroff JW, Hop WCJ, Fauser BCJM. How to descriminate between normal and polycystic ovaries: transvaginal US study. Radiology 1992;183:421–423.

17. Fulghesu AM, Ciampelli M, Belosi C, Apa R, Pavone V, Lanzone A. A new ultrasound criterion for the diagnosis of polycystic ovary syndrome: the ovarian stroma/total area ratio. Fertil Steril 2001;76:326–331.

18. Pache TD, Hop WC, Wladimiroff JW, Schipper J, Fauser BCJM. Transvaginal sonography and abnormal ovarian appearance in menstrual cycle disturbances. Ultrasound Med Biol 1991;17:589–593.

19. Al-Took S, Watkin K, Tulandi T, Tan SL. Ovarian stromal echogenicity in women with clomiphene citrate-sensitive and clomiphene citrate-resistant polycystic ovary syndrome. Fertil Steril 1999;71:952–954.

20. Buckett WM, Bouzayen R, Watkin KL, Tulandi T, Tan SL. Ovarian stromal echogenicity in women with normal and polycystic ovaries. Hum Reprod 1999;14:618–621.

21. Battaglia C, Artini PG, Salvatori M, et al. Ultrasonographic pattern of polycystic ovaries: color Doppler and hormonal correlations. Ultrasound Gynaecol Obstet 1998;11:332–336.

22. Wu M-H, Tang H-H, Hsu C-C, Wang S-T, Huang K-E. The role of three-dimensional ultrasonographic imaging in ovarian measurement. Fertil Steril 1998;69:1152–1155.

23. Kyei-Mensah A, Maconochie N, Zaidi J, Pittrof R, Campbell S, Tan SL. Transvaginal three-dimensional ultrasound: accuracy of ovarian follicular volume measurements. Fertil Steril 1996;65:371–376.

24. Kyei-Mensah A, Zaidi J, Campbell S. Ultrasound diagnosis of polycystic ovary syndrome. Bailliere's Clin Endocrinol Metab 1996;10:249–262.

25. Kyei-Mensah A, Tan SL, Zaidi J, Jacobs HS. Relationship of ovarian stromal volume to serum androgen concentrations in patients with polycystic ovary syndrome. Hum Reprod 1998;13:1437–1441.

26. Nardo LG, Buckett WM, Khullar V. Determination of the best-fitting ultrasound formulaic method for ovarian volume measurement in women with polycystic ovary syndrome. Fertil Steril 2003;79:632–633.

27. Battaglia C, Artini PG, Genazzani AD, et al. Color Doppler analysis in lean and obese women with polycystic ovaries. Ultrasound Gynaecol Obstet 1996;7:342–346.

28. Battaglia C, Genazzani AD, Salvatori M, et al. Doppler, ultrasonographic and endocrinological environment with regard to the number of small subcapsular follicles in polycystic ovary syndrome. Gynecol Endocrinol 1999;13:123–129.
29. Aleem FA, Predanic MP. Transvaginal color Doppler determination of the ovarian and uterine blood flow characteristics in polycystic ovary disease. Fertil Steril 1996;65:510–516.
30. Zaidi J, Campbell S, Pittrof R, et al. Ovarian stromal blood flow in women with polycystic ovaries: a possible new marker for diagnosis? Human Reprod 1995;10:1992–1996.
31. Agrawal R, Conway G, Sladkevicius P, et al. Serum vascular endothelial growth factor and Doppler blood flow velocities in in vitro fertilization: relevance to ovarian hyperstimulation syndrome and polycystic ovaries. Fertil Steril 1998;70:651–658.
32. Engmann L, Sladkevicius P, Agrawal LR, Bekir JS, Campbell S, Tan SL. Value of ovarian stromal blood flow velocity measurement after pituitary suppression in the prediction of ovarian responsiveness and outcome of in vitro fertilization treatment. Fertil Steril 1999;71: 22–29.
33. Maubon A, Courtieu C, Vivens F, et al. Magnetic resonance imaging of normal and polycystic ovaries. Preliminary results. Ann NY Acad Sci 1993;687:224–229.
34. Kimura I, Togashi K, Kawakami S, et al. Polycystic ovaries: implications of diagnosis with MR imaging. Radiology 1996;201:549–552.
35. Woodward PJ, Gilfeather M. Magnetic resonance imaging of the female pelvis. Semin Ultrasound CT MRI 1998;19:90–103.

III

LONG-TERM RISKS OF PCOS: ASSOCIATION WITH INSULIN RESISTANCE

14 Glucose Intolerance

Vincenzo Toscano, MD

CONTENTS

Summary

Polycystic ovary syndrome (PCOS) affects 5–8% of reproductive-age women. Patients with PCOS present with signs and symptoms that are very heterogeneous and variable over time. The symptoms of the PCOS usually begin around menarche, but onset after puberty may also occur as a result of environmental modifiers such as weight gain. The consequences of the PCOS, not adequately treated, extend beyond the reproductive axis; in fact, women with the disorder are at substantial risk for the development of metabolic and cardiovascular abnormalities similar to those observed in the metabolic syndrome. This finding is not surprising, considering both PCOS and the metabolic syndrome share insulin resistance as a central pathogenetic problem. PCOS might thus be regarded as a sex-specific form of the metabolic syndrome. Thirty to 40% of obese women with PCOS who are of reproductive age have impaired glucose tolerance, and 10% have type 2 diabetes. These prevalence rates are the highest known among women of similar age. Most women with PCOS are able to compensate fully for their insulin resistance, thus, maintaining a normal glucose tolerance, but a substantial proportion have a disordered and insufficient β-cell response to meals or a glucose challenge and develop hyperglycemia.

Key Words: PCOS; insulin resistance; glucose intolerance; type 2 diabetes; hyperandrogenism.

INTRODUCTION

Polycystic ovary syndrome (PCOS) affects 5–8% of reproductive-age women. Patients with PCOS present with signs and symptoms that are very heterogeneous and

From: *Contemporary Endocrinology: Insulin Resistance and Polycystic Ovarian Syndrome:
Pathogenesis, Evaluation, and Treatment*
Edited by: E. Diamanti-Kandarakis, J. E. Nestler, D. Panidis, and R. Pasquali © Humana Press Inc., Totowa, NJ

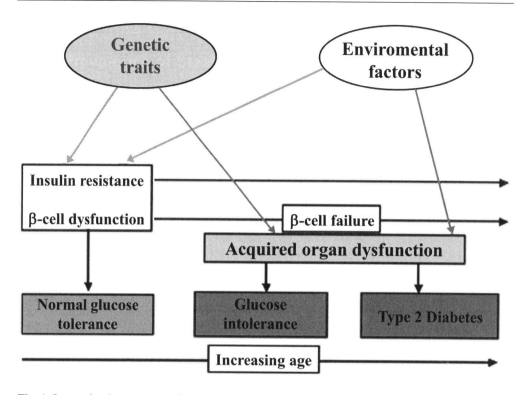

Fig. 1. Interaction between genetic traits and environmental factors in type 2 diabetes development.

variable over time. Moreover, a precise and uniform definition of the syndrome has been not defined. An international workshop *(1)* in 2003 proposed that the syndrome can be diagnosed after the exclusion of other medical conditions that cause irregular menstrual cycles and androgen excess like NC-CAH, androgen-secreting tumors, Cushing syndrome, and hyperprolactinemia, and the determination that at least two of the following are present: oligoovulation or anovulation (clinically manifested as oligomenorrhea or amenorrhea), elevated levels of circulating androgens (hyperandrogenemia) or clinical manifestations of androgen excess (hyperandrogenism), and polycystic ovaries as defined by ultrasonography *(2)*.

A large proportion of women with PCOS are overweight, many are obese, and some showed an extreme fat excess *(3)*. Although obesity itself is not considered the initiating event in the development of the syndrome, excess fat can exacerbate associated reproductive and metabolic clinical features.

The symptoms of PCOS usually begin around menarche *(4)*, but onset after puberty may also occur as a result of environmental modifiers, such as weight gain. Premature pubarche, the result of early secretion of adrenal steroids, may be a harbinger of the syndrome during prepuberty *(5)*. In addition, an aberrant intrauterine environment has been implicated in the condition's pathogenesis, particularly for its metabolic components *(6–9)*. This data is not confirmed by other studies *(10)*.

The consequences of PCOS extend beyond the reproductive axis; in fact, women with the disorder are at substantial risk for the development of metabolic and cardiovascular abnormalities similar to those observed in the metabolic syndrome *(11)*. This finding is not surprising, considering that both PCOS and the metabolic syndrome share insulin resistance as a central pathogenetic mechanism. PCOS might thus be regarded as a sex-specific form of the metabolic syndrome *(12,13)*.

Thirty to 40% of obese women with PCOS at reproductive age have impaired glucose tolerance (IGT), and 10% have type 2 diabetes *(3,14)*. These prevalence rates are the highest known among women of similar age *(15)*. An enhanced rate of deterioration in glucose tolerance is also evident in longitudinal studies carried out in PCOS *(3,16)*.

Dunaif et al. *(17–19)* have indicated in several studies that women with PCOS are more insulin resistant than controls matched for body mass index (BMI), fat-free body mass, and body-fat distribution. A defect in the insulin-signaling pathway appears to be present in both the adipocyte and skeletal muscle, the primary target tissues of insulin action *(18,19)*.

Insulin resistance alone cannot fully account for the predisposition to development of IGT and type 2 diabetes among patients with PCOS. In insulin-resistant patients with normal glucose tolerance, insulin secretion is sufficient for the degree of insulin action impairment; when the pancreatic β-cell is no longer able to compensate for this defect, glucose tolerance begins to deteriorate *(20,21)*.

Most women with PCOS are able to compensate fully for their insulin resistance, but a substantial proportion (particularly those with first-degree relatives with type 2 diabetes) have a disordered and insufficient β-cell response to meals or a glucose challenge *(22–26)*. Before the development of frank glucose intolerance, defects in insulin secretion may be revealed only in circumstances that augment insulin resistance, as in pregnancy *(27)* or after glucocorticoid administration *(25)*.

GENETIC PREDISPOSITION

Evidence suggests a genetic basis for PCOS *(28)*. Different approaches have been used in the attempt to define a mode of inheritance, but very confusing results were obtained. This may be due, at least in part, to the heterogeneity in the disease phenotype and in criteria by which PCOS is defined. The metabolic aspects of the disease, even if considered in the papers finalized to define diagnostic criteria, have never been considered essential features for the diagnosis.

Genetic factors clearly contribute in the development of glucose intolerance and type 2 diabetes in patients who do not have PCOS, and several gene mutations and/or polymorphisms have been described, leading to the consideration of type 2 diabetes a polygenic disorder. In this model, the extent to which any single gene defect may contribute to the predisposition to glucose intolerance and type 2 diabetes is highly variable. Also, it is generally assumed that there may be great genetic variability in different families and ethnic groups.

Analogously, PCOS, in which several candidate genes have been proposed, can be regarded as a polygenic disorder. Several data have been collected from clinical and gene expression studies to focus the attention on metabolic pathways, which, when perturbated, may affect either ovarian and adrenal steroidogenesis or insulin secretion and action.

Members of the PCOS family have been demonstrated to be at an increased risk to develop glucose intolerance and type 2 diabetes. In 2003, Yildiz et al. *(29)* reported that the first-degree relatives of women with PCOS had an increased prevalence of glucose intolerance and insulin resistance. The prevalence rates for glucose intolerance and diabetes were 30 and 16% in the mothers and 31 and 27% in the fathers, which is almost three times the reported prevalence in the general population of the same race and age. In the same study, analyses of glucose tolerant family members showed that mothers and sisters of women with PCOS have insulin resistance. This finding confirms the results of the preliminary study by Norman et al. *(30)*, which reported that hyper-insulinemia may be highly prevalent in family members of patients with PCOS. This is relevant, as insulin resistance and hyperinsulinemia are common antecedents of glucose intolerance and type 2 diabetes *(31,32)*.

The risk for patients with PCOS to develop metabolic abnormalities is highly impacted by race and first-degree history of glucose intolerance. Ehrmann et al. *(33)* reported that in these women the prevalence of IGT and type 2 diabetes was 23 and 4%, respectively. In this study, black women with PCOS had higher insulin levels and were more insulin-resistant than white women with PCOS. These differences remained statistically significant even after taking the family history of diabetes into account.

The same authors found that 44% of women with PCOS who had diabetes and 39% of those with glucose intolerance had a first-degree relative with type 2 diabetes. In contrast, significantly fewer (21%) women with PCOS who had normal glucose tolerance had a diabetic first-degree relative. In the same paper, nondiabetic subjects with PCOS who had a positive family history of diabetes had significantly higher levels of hemoglobin A1c, as well as higher glucose and insulin levels during an oral glucose tolerance test (OGTT). These findings are consistent with the hypothesis that impairment of insulin action and insulin secretion is hereditary in PCOS families *(34,35)*. Interestingly, in nondiabetic patients with PCOS, although the mean BMI was nearly identical in subjects with positive or negative family history for diabetes (36.8 ± 0.8 vs 35.9 ± 0.5 kg/m^2), the proportion of body fat distributed to the upper body/abdomen was significantly greater in those having a positive family history, as reflected in a higher waist-to-hip ratio (WHR; 0.90 ± 0.01 vs 0.87 ± 0.01). An increased WHR has been consistently correlated with insulin resistance and the risk for development of diabetes in several studies *(36)*. Indeed, women with positive family history for type 2 diabetes were more insulin resistant, as reflected in a significantly higher homeostasis model assessment for insulin resistance (HOMA-IR) (6.6 ± 0.6 vs 4.9 ± 0.3).

Several lines of evidence support a role for the insulin receptor substrates, IRS1 and IRS2, in the pathogenesis of type 2 diabetes *(37)* and PCOS *(38)*. IRS1 is present in a variety of insulin-responsive tissues and is a key molecule in the insulin signal transduction. Polymorphism in the human IRS1 Gly to Arg at codon 972 has been reported to be increased in type 2 diabetes *(39)* and has been associated with an impairment in insulin secretion *(40,41)* and insulin action *(42,43)*.

In PCOS, several polymorphisms of IRS1 and IRS2 have been described *(38,44)*. El Mkadem et al. *(38)* have reported that the polymorphism Gly972Arg of IRS1 and Gly1057Asp of IRS2 are significantly more frequent in patients with PCOS than in controls. These polymorphisms may be associated with altered fasting insulin and 2 hours of insulin on oral glucose tolerance testing. Twenty-four percent of carriers of the Gly1057Asp of IRS2 showed IGT. However, Florez et al., in a study carried out in 9000 subjects, failed to confirm the association of the IRS1 G972R polymorphism with type 2 diabetes *(45)*.

Wu et al. *(46)* have demonstrated that in the granulosa cell of the ovaries from patients with PCOS, immunohistochemical staining for IRS1 was decreased, whereas in the theca interna cells, immunohistochemical staining for IRS2 was increased when compared with normal ovulatory women. The meaning of this finding in relation to ovarian steroid production, however, is not clear and needs further study.

Microarray experiments or proteomic studies in the next 10 years will probably give precise answers to all these open problems, identifying the genes responsible for the different clinical aspects of PCOS, probably allowing us to distinguish different subsets of patients within the heterogeneous group of women with PCOS.

ENVIROMENTAL FACTORS

An important concept is that the diabetes genotype causes only a predisposition for glucose intolerance. Whether one develops the diabetes phenotype depends on environmental factors, some obvious in how they act, others less so. For instance, the Nurses Health Survey showed positive associations between obesity and lack of physical activity in the development of type 2 diabetes (as expected), but also protection by not smoking and moderate alcohol intake *(47)*. Many studies have shown an association between TV watching, high-calorie diets, and lack of physical activity with risk of diabetes, i.e., our modern lifestyle. These predisposing factors share an ability to negatively impact the glucose homeostasis system through worsening of insulin resistance or impaired β-cell function. Superimposing these factors onto a genetically compromised glucose homeostasis system raises the risk of progressing to hyperglycemia. It is the rapid emergence of these disadvantageous environmental factors that is causing the worldwide diabetes epidemic. This concept of environmental changes promoting diabetes was highlighted many years ago by the occurrence of populations rarely experiencing type 2 diabetes before moving from a nomadic or farm existence to urban environments. This change was followed by an explosion of diabetes, which is typically associated with severe obesity. This was the case of Pima Indians in the Southwest United States, Saharan nomadic tribes, Australian Aborigines, and many others. Particularly dramatic were studies that showed reversal of the diabetes when they returned to their prior way of life *(48)*. A recent example of this is the rapidly rising incidence of type 2 diabetes in China and India. As people moved in China from the country to cities, there was an increased incidence of diabetes from 0.1 to 0.2% for rural farmers to more than 5% for city dwellers. Perhaps the scariest example of this is children in the United States, where the obesity statistics worsen yearly. As many as 20% of US children are now obese, and they are developing all of the elements of the metabolic syndrome—insulin resistance, hypertension, hyperlipidemia, and glucose intolerance *(49)*. An obvious conclusion is that a manipulation of lifestyle provides an opportunity to reverse the diabetes trend. Actually, we cannot change our genetic make-up, but we can alter environmental factors. Indeed, many studies have shown that diet and exercise slow the onset of diabetes in people with glucose intolerance *(50–52)*. Also, low-glycemic-index diets have been shown to promote weight loss, as well as having several metabolic benefits in subjects with type 2 diabetes *(53)*.

The difficulty, of course, is trying to get people to change their habits. In subjects without PCOS, lifestyle modifications have also proved more efficacious than pharmacological intervention in reducing the risk of developing type 2 diabetes. The Diabetes Prevention Program compared lifestyle intervention (a low-fat diet and 150 minutes exercise per week) to metformin (850 mg twice a day) and a placebo in overweight ($n = 3234$) subjects with IGT. This lifestyle intervention reduced the risk of developing diabetes by 58%, whereas metformin reduced the risk by 31% *(54)*. It is important to note that the lifestyle intervention was modest, involving an approx 7% weight loss and 20 minutes of brisk walking daily. It is apparent that a strong emphasis needs to be placed on lifestyle modification in the management of the long-term health risks of PCOS *(55)*.

However, Tang *(56)* was unable to demonstrate an improvement in insulin sensitivity in extremely obese patients with PCOS, demonstrating that metformin and lifestyle modifications have reduced effects in massive obesity.

In a pilot randomized study on the effect of metformin therapy and lifestyle modification on ovulation and androgen concentrations in women with PCOS, treated for 48 weeks, Hoeger *(57)* reported that glucose metabolism either improved or did not change in subjects completing the treatment arms, whereas a deterioration of glucose status occurred in two subjects in the placebo group. This is consistent with the results of the Diabetes Prevention Trial *(54)*. Therefore, weight loss through lifestyle modification should be a primary treatment aim for PCOS, with pharmacological intervention as an additional option.

No studies exist in patients with PCOS having as a final outcome the prevention of glucose intolerance or type 2 diabetes using lifestyle modifications. The majority of the studies in these women have, as a main outcome, the fertility induction or menstrual cycle and androgen plasma levels regulation.

In PCOS patients weight loss reduces hyperinsulinemia and hyperandrogenism. In the study by Kiddy et al. *(58)*, about 40% of obese women with PCOS (mean BMI ~34 kg/m^2) who lost more than 5% of initial body weight with caloric restriction achieved spontaneous pregnancy. A more recent trial compared the effects of an energy-restricted diet (~1400 kcal/day) through either a low- or high-protein diet in 28 obese (mean BMI ~37 kg/m^2) subjects with PCOS over 12 weeks. Sixty subjects were also advised to increase exercise to a minimum of three times weekly, though no information was reported as to the actual duration and/or intensity achieved. Average weight loss was 7.5% (with abdominal fat decreasing 12.5%), and 3 of the 20 subjects actively trying to conceive did so (two in the high-protein and one in the low-protein group) for a rate of 15%. Thus, lifestyle modification needs to be stressed also in the treatment of infertility. A 3–6 month trial of aggressive lifestyle modification may be a prudent first step before considering an insulin sensitizer.

Very recently, Escobar Morreale et al. *(59)* have demonstrated that PCOS is a frequent finding in women with morbid obesity and may resolve either in terms of ovulation restoration or in terms of clinical and biochemical hyperandrogenism disappearance after weight loss induced by bariatric surgery.

GLUCOSE INTOLERANCE DEVELOPMENT:
RATE OF CONVERSION AND RISK PREDICTORS

Studies in American and Asian subjects, and more recently in a cohort of Mediterranean women, have shown that, as compared with the general population, women with PCOS have an increased risk for glucose intolerance and type 2 diabetes *(3,13,60,61)*. The connection between PCOS and glucose intolerance is further emphasized by the high prevalence of polycystic ovaries found on ultrasonography in premenopausal women with type 2 diabetes *(62)* and in those with previous gestational diabetes *(63)*.

In the Ehrman study *(3)*, in which the 2-hour glucose level during the OGTT was measured in 122 women with PCOS, glucose tolerance was normal in 67 (55%) of these subjects, whereas 43 (35%) had IGT and 12 (10%) type 2 diabetes. When fasting glucose levels were analyzed, 104 (85%) women had a normal fasting glucose (<110 mg/dL), 11 (9%) had impaired fasting glucose (110–126 mg/dL), and 7 (6%) were diabetic (>126 mg/dL). For the entire cohort, the mean age at presentation was 25.5 ± 0.7 years (range 13.5 to 40). Although the women with type 2 diabetes tended to be slightly older (mean age 29 ± 2 years), difference in age was not significantly different between groups. The women with type 2 diabetes differed from those with normal glucose tolerance in that they had a 2.6-fold higher prevalence of first-degree relatives with type 2 diabetes (83 vs 31%; $p < 0.01$) and were significantly more obese (BMI 41.0 ± 2.4 vs 33.4 ± 1.1 kg/m^2; $p < 0.01$), underlining the fact that advancing age, family history of glucose intolerance or diabetes, and severe obesity represent important risk factors. Of the 25 women in the follow-up group with normal glucose tolerance at baseline, followed over 25.7 months with a range of 6 to 60, 11 (44%) had normal glucose tolerance at their initial study. Of these 11, 5 (45%) maintained normal glucose tolerance at follow-up. Six (55%) women experienced deterioration in glucose tolerance: five converted to IGT and one to type 2 diabetes. The incidence rate for conversion to glucose intolerance or type 2 diabetes from normal was six cases in 17.75 person-years of follow-up (i.e., 338 cases per 1000 person-years of observation). Those women whose glucose tolerance deteriorated were slightly more severely obese (BMI 44.6 ± 3.5 vs 40.4 ± 4.4 kg/m^2), but were of similar age (27.0 ± 2.6 vs 26.1 ± 4.1 years) to those with stable glucose tolerance. The presence of a family history of type 2 diabetes was not more prevalent among those whose glucose tolerance deteriorated. Among the 14 women with glucose intolerance at baseline, 3 (21%) reverted to normal glucose tolerance at the time of their second OGTT, 7 (50%) had persistent glucose intolerance, and 4 (29%) progressed to type 2 diabetes, with an incidence rate for conversion from glucose intolerance to type 2 diabetes of 4 cases in 10.75 person-years of follow-up (i.e., 372 cases per 1000 person-years of observation). Those who converted to type 2 diabetes from glucose intolerance were significantly more obese at the time of the second OGTT when compared with those who did not progress (BMI 44.9 ± 2.3 vs 36.2 ± 1.3 kg/m^2; $p = 0.005$). There was no significant age difference between those who did and those who did not progress. A family history of type 2 diabetes was present in all four women who developed type 2 diabetes, as compared with the 6 of 10 who maintained or improved their level of glucose tolerance, although this difference did not reach statistical significance.

Another longitudinal study by Norman et al. *(15)* evaluated the frequency of change of glucose intolerance and type 2 diabetes over an average period of 6.2 years, (range

4 to 8.6 yr) in 67 women with PCOS. Of the women who were normoglycemic at baseline, 9% had developed IGT and 8% type 2 diabetes, with an annualized incidence rate of 2.2%. Of those with IGT at baseline, 54% converted to type 2 diabetes, with an annualized incidence rate of 8.7%, 15% showed normal glucose tolerance at follow-up, and 31% remained in the same category as at baseline. Patients converting to glucose intolerance or type 2 diabetes have significantly greater BMI, waist circumference, and WHR, as compared with those who remained normoglycemic.

The overall rate of conversion to type 2 diabetes in the Norman's study *(15)* was lower as compared with data from Ehrmann et al. *(3)*, probably because of a different selection of the cases at baseline. The data from Norman *(15)* confirmed that obesity is a strong predictor of deterioration in glucose metabolism. Obese women with PCOS had a 10-fold increase in their risk of suffering from glucose intolerance or type 2 diabetes as compared with normal-weight women with PCOS. Overweight women with PCOS who had BMI ranging between 25 and 30 kg/m^2 still had an approx sevenfold increase *(15)*.

In a study carried out by Legro et al. *(13)* in 254 women with PCOS the prevalence for IGT was 30.0% and for type 2 diabetes was 7.3% in the urban, ethnically diverse population of Mt. Sinai, and it was 31.9% for IGT and 7.6% for diabetes in the rural, predominantly non-Hispanic white population of Pennsylvania State University. Also in this study, nonobese women with PCOS showed glucose intolerance (10.3% IGT; 1.5% type 2 diabetes). The prevalence rates of glucose intolerance in PCOS (31.1% IGT; 7.5% undiagnosed diabetes) were substantially higher than in a large population-based study (Second National Health and Nutrition Survey) *(64)* of US women of similar age (7.8% glucose intolerance; 1.0% undiagnosed diabetes). The prevalence rate of glucose intolerance was also higher than in reproductive-age, Latino women with a history of gestational diabetes mellitus (26%) *(65)*. The prevalence rates of glucose intolerance and type 2 diabetes were well above those reported among US Hispanic and African-American women of similar age *(66)* and are comparable to those reported by Ehrmann et al., who found similar prevalence rates in an ethnically mixed PCOS population from the Chicago area. These observations suggest that, in young women, PCOS is a more important risk factor for glucose intolerance than race or ethnicity. Obesity and age, however, substantially increase the risk for glucose intolerance and diabetes in young, nonobese women with PCOS.

In a recent study, Legro et al. *(67)* showed that glucose tolerance, as categorized by WHO criteria, tended to worsen over time in women with PCOS. Moreover, there was a nearly twofold increase in the rates of conversion for subjects with PCOS and baseline normal glucose tolerance compared with a reference population, although this change did not reach statistical significance because of the limited sample size. There was also a significant chance for reversion to normal glucose tolerance in the women with PCOS and IGT. These counteracting trends led to little net effect on glucose tolerance categories and little change in mean glucose levels at any time point in the OGTT at follow-up in women with PCOS. Women with PCOS continued to maintain normal fasting glucose levels as evidenced by the lack of change in the fasting glucose levels at follow-up and the minimal conversion rate based on the fasting American Diabetes Association criteria (5%). The annualized incidence rate of conversion to type 2 diabetes was 2% per year both for the PCOS and control populations.

In a Weerakiet's study *(60)*, carried out on 79 Asian women with PCOS, the prevalence of glucose intolerance and type 2 diabetes was 22.8 and 15.2%, respectively, according to the 1985 WHO criteria. The prevalence of type 2 diabetes was higher in this report than in studies from Legro and Ehrmann. However, when the overall glucose intolerance was considered, the rate was similar. The incidence rate of progression from IGT to type 2 diabetes was 372 cases per 1000 person-years and from normal glucose tolerance to IGT and type 2 diabetes was 338 cases per 1000 person-years. These findings suggest that the women with PCOS having either normal glucose tolerance or glucose intolerance should be closely followed up. However, there is no recommendation on the optimal interval for OGTT testing of these women. Like in other ethnic groups, a positive family history of diabetes and obesity are significant predictors of altered glucose tolerance in the Asian population.

The study performed in the Mediterranean area by Gambineri et al. *(61)* in 2004 found that 2.5% of 121 women with PCOS had type 2 diabetes and 15.7% had glucose intolerance. This prevalence rate was significantly higher than that described in the general population of similar age *(64)*, but lower than that reported in previous studies from the United States *(3,13)* and Asia *(60)*. Different selection criteria of the patients enrolled, and possibly behavioral aspects, may explain these differences: in this study, patients with PCOS were younger than those investigated in the other studies, supporting the concept that glucose tolerance tends to worsen with increasing age *(64)*. Moreover, body weight was lower in the cohort from Italy, strongly supporting, once again, the role of obesity as a fundamental prerequisite for the development of glucose intolerance. The young age of the cohort from the Mediterranean area reinforces the concept that glucose intolerance states in women with PCOS tend to appear earlier in life than expected *(3,13,60)*. Of particular interest in the study of Gambineri is the identification of two early markers of the development of glucose intolerance in women with PCOS. The first was represented by the presence of lower birth weight in the glucose intolerance group with respect to the two normally tolerant groups, confirming the association of this feature with insulin resistance and susceptibility to developing type 2 diabetes *(68)*. The second factor was the earlier menarchal age found in women with PCOS with glucose intolerance in comparison with those with normal glucose tolerance. These data are in line with those observed in a different group of patients, where a precocious pubarche was related to hyperinsulinemia and low birth weight *(69)*.

Taken together, all these studies demonstrated that glucose intolerance is more frequent in PCOS population than in age- and weight-matched populations of women without PCOS, with small differences with regards to ethnicity or dietary composition. The conversion rate from normal to altered glucose tolerance and type 2 diabetes is accelerated in patients with PCOS, at least if left untreated. Glucose intolerance in PCOS appears earlier than expected in life. Obesity, strictly correlated with insulin resistance, represents the major predictor for the conversion from normal to altered glucose tolerance in almost all the studies currently available. Other predictors may be represented by low birth weight and precocious menarche, even if these markers were evaluated only in the study carried out in the Mediterranean area.

Why do patients with PCOS show these differences with respect to general population? One contributing factor to the glucose intolerance of PCOS may be related to the elevated androgen concentrations. It is now well recognized that a dynamic interaction exists between hyperinsulinemia and hyperandrogenemia. Most evidence favors insulin resistance and the compensatory hyperinsulinemia as the predominant, perhaps primary, defect in PCOS *(17)*. Hyperinsulinemia appears to synergize with pituitary gonadotropins to stimulate ovarian theca cell and adrenal ACTH-induced androgen production, which in turn, exacerbates the insulin resistance.

The finding that women with PCOS and glucose intolerance have significantly higher levels of both total and free testosterone when compared with those with normal glucose tolerance *(3)* can be interpreted to indicate that hyperandrogenemia *per se* contributes to the development of glucose intolerance. According to Holte *(70)*, androgens may provide a basis for increased muscular strength, selecting more insulin-resistant fibers, worsening insulin sensitivity, and hyperinsulinemia and leading to a vicious circle.

ACQUIRED ORGAN DYSFUNCTION: INSULIN RESISTANCE AND β-CELL DERANGEMENT

One of the most controversial topics within the field of glucose intolerance and type 2 diabetes is represented by the roles of insulin resistance and β-cell dysfunction in this disorder. Both defects were frequently present when people with glucose intolerance or type 2 diabetes were investigated. Attempts to delve earlier into the course of the disease by studying persons at high risk who were still normoglycemic—high-risk ethnic groups such as Pima Indians, those whose parents both had type 2 diabetes, and women who previously had gestational diabetes—often reported that insulin resistance, but not β-cell dysfunction, was an early finding *(71)*, suggesting that insulin resistance was the initial (and thus dominant) defect in this condition.

However, whereas there are reliable procedures to evaluate insulin action, the assessment of β-cell function is much more complex. The insulin response to a meal normally occurs in a biphasic pattern, and the amount of insulin released is dependent on the prevailing glucose value. As glucose tolerance moves from normal to minimally impaired, the insulin secretion that occurs within the first 30 minutes of eating (first phase) becomes markedly attenuated, resulting in an elevated prandial rise in glycemia, i.e., the physiological definition of glucose intolerance. It is this postprandial hyperglycemia that causes the insulin secretion after the first 30 minutes (second phase) to be higher as a compensatory response. The early studies typically assessed β-cell function by measuring the insulin value before and 2 hours after a meal. Consequently, it was concluded that, based on the 2-hour insulin value being higher than normal, in the early stages of type 2 diabetes, there was no β-cell dysfunction, just insulin resistance that was assumed to be responsible for the supernormal 2-hour insulin value.

More informative were large cross-sectional and natural history studies in terms of the relative importance of β-cell dysfunction vs insulin resistance in this disorder. They confirmed the findings of the earlier studies that insulin resistance occurs early in the disease, typically when glucose values are still within the normal glucose tolerance range. The reasons are multifactorial—related to genetic abnormalities that affect insulin sensitivity and several lifestyle factors, such as obesity, lack of exercise, high-fat diets, aging, and so on. Thereafter, however, insulin resistance does not change much. Thus, it is not the worsening of insulin resistance that causes blood glucose values to go from normal to IGT and to diabetes, but rather worsening of β-cell function.

Whereas prior studies had shown that insulin resistance occurs before the prediabetes stage of the disease, it is now clear from more recent studies *(72–75)* that β-cell dysfunction also precedes any measured defect in glucose tolerance. The natural history studies of type 2 diabetes reported a biphasic pattern of rise barely above normal, but still within the normal glucose tolerance range, showing that subjects with 2-hour OGTT glucose values of 101–120 mg/dL, well below the glucose intolerance 2-hour cutoff of 140 mg/dL, had 60% lowered mealtime insulin responses than those with 2-hour glucose values less than 100 mg/dL. In other words, there must be defective β-cell function for blood glucose values to rise even minimally above normal because of the extraordinary precision of a healthy glucose homeostasis system at maintaining normoglycemia.

The majority of the authors agrees that obese women with PCOS are generally insulin-resistant. Controversy remains for the prevalence and the mechanisms of insulin resistance in lean patients with PCOS patients. There are some studies that suggest that increased central adiposity may be responsible for the defects in insulin action of these women *(76,77)*, and this could also be important in subjects with a normal BMI. Many of the conflicting data can be explained by different diagnostic criteria for PCOS and by the inclusion of both lean and obese women in the studies. Anovulation and hyperandrogenism seems to be strongly associated with insulin resistance *(78–80)*. Women with a regular ovulatory menstrual cycle, even with hyperandrogenism or with PCO detected by ovarian ultrasound *(79,80)*, do not seem to be constantly insulin-resistant.

In the presence of peripheral insulin resistance, pancreatic β-cell insulin secretion increases in a compensatory fashion. Glucose intolerance and type 2 diabetes develop when the compensatory increase in insulin levels is no longer sufficient to maintain euglycemia *(81,82)*.

In very elegant studies, Erhmann et al. *(83,84)* demonstrated that β-cell dysfunction in PCOS is demonstrable by reduced insulin secretory responses either to boluses or graded infusions of intravenous glucose when expressed relative to the degree of insulin resistance and by the impairment in the ability to entrain endogenous insulin secretion with glucose. These defects are also much more pronounced in women with PCOS who have a first-degree relative with type 2 diabetes, suggesting that several mechanisms might explain why such women are at particularly high risk to develop glucose intolerance.

In 1996, Dunaif et al. *(25)* showed that both obese and nonobese women with PCOS have β-cell dysfunction as well as insulin resistance. However, this was not associated with glucose intolerance in the majority of women with PCOS. The findings in nonobese women with PCOS were particularly interesting because these women had evidence of inadequate insulin secretion in the absence of confounding variables, such as increased WHR, glucose intolerance, or a family history of type 2 or gestational diabetes mellitus *(85)*. In a paper published in 2004, Erhmann et al. *(86)* showed that, after dexamethasone, control subjects averaged a 9% increase (to 131 ± 12 mg/dL) in 2-hour OGTT glucose levels, whereas women with PCOS had a significantly greater 26% increase (to 155 ± 6 mg/dL). The C-peptide-to-glucose ratios during the OGTT increased by 44% in control subjects and by only 15% in PCOS subjects. These results suggested that the accelerated conversion from normal to glucose intolerance and from glucose intolerance to frank diabetes in PCOS may result, at least in part, from a relative attenuation in the response of the pancreatic β-cell to the demand placed on it by factors, like corticosteroids, exacerbating insulin resistance.

Very recently, Goodarzi et al. *(87)* analyzed the relationship between insulin resistance, β-cell function, obesity, and androgen levels in patients with PCOS, using as controls a reference population derived from NHANES III. Multiple regression analyses demonstrated that insulin resistance and bioavailable testosterone were independent predictors of β-cell function, β-cell function and obesity were independent predictors of insulin resistance, and β-cell function was an independent predictor of bioavailable testosterone. Comparison with normal women from NHANES revealed a significantly stronger relationship between β-cell function and insulin resistance in PCOS, raising the possibility that an intrinsic defect in β-cell function, whereby increasing insulin resistance, leads to a higher than normal insulin response in PCOS. The authors conclude by underlining the importance of β-cell dysfunction as a central pathogenetic defect in patients with PCOS, leading to consider, in terms of therapy, more appropriate drugs modulating insulin secretion than those modulating insulin action commonly used today.

Gennarelli et al., in a very recent study *(88)* in normal-weight Mediterranean women with PCOS with no family history of type 2 diabetes mellitus, did not find evidence of abnormal insulin sensitivity and secretion, confirming previous results obtained in Scandinavian women with PCOS. A decreased activity of glucose *per se* on its own uptake was observed in this study, and the authors speculated that among various factors, the reduced glucose effectiveness could be considered an additional metabolic feature in at least some women with PCOS, although more data should be acquired concerning the role of glucose effectiveness in the abnormalities of glucose metabolism in PCOS.

CONCLUSIONS

Women with PCOS are considered to have an increased risk for the development of insulin resistance, the metabolic syndrome, glucose intolerance, and type 2 diabetes analogously to other diabetes-prone populations, such as nondiabetic first-degree relatives of type 2 diabetics. Obese patients have a higher risk with respect to lean ones.

Glucose intolerance is more frequent in the PCOS population than in age- and weight-matched women without PCOS, with small differences with regards to ethnicity or dietary composition. The conversion rate from normal to altered glucose tolerance and type 2 diabetes is accelerated in patients with PCOS, at least if left untreated. Glucose intolerance in PCOS appears earlier than expected in life. Obesity, strictly correlated with insulin resistance, represents the major predictor for the conversion from normal to altered glucose tolerance in almost all available studies. Other predictors may be represented by low birth weight and precocious menarche. β-cell dysfunction is an essential step for the development of glucose intolerance and type 2 diabetes, but it is still unclear if this is a consequence or not of increased insulin secretion, directly correlated to insulin resistance.

Several evidences suggest that insulin resistance/hyperinsulinemia cause hyperandrogenemia, but an opposite relationship is also likely to occur.

FUTURE AVENUES OF INVESTIGATION

Longitudinal studies, carried out over prolonged periods, may give more information about the role of insulin resistance/hyperinsulinemia and hyperandrogenemia as a primary cause of PCOS, leading to select, within the heterogeneous population of subjects with the syndrome, subgroups with different clinical and biochemical characteristics and, possibly, different evolution as far as it concerns the metabolic disorders and the cardiovascular risk. Moreover, microarray experiments or proteomic studies in the next 10 years will probably give precise answers to the open problems, evidentiating the genes responsible for the different clinical aspects of PCOS, probably allowing us to distinguish different subsets of patients within the heterogeneous group of women with PCOS.

REFERENCES

1. Revised 2003 consensus on diagnostic criteria and long-term health risks related to polycystic ovary syndrome (PCOS). Hum Reprod 2004;19:41–47.
2. Adams J, Polson DW, Franks S. Prevalence of polycystic ovaries in women with anovulation and idiopathic hirsutism. Br Med J (Clin Res Ed) 1986;293:355–359.
3. Ehrmann DA, Barnes RB, Rosenfield RL, Cavaghan MK, Imperial J. Prevalence of impaired glucose tolerance and diabetes in women with polycystic ovary syndrome. Diabetes Care 1999;22: 141–146.
4. Franks S. Adult polycystic ovary syndrome begins in childhood. Best Pract Res Clin Endocrinol Metab 2002;16:263–272.
5. Ibanez L, Valls C, Potau N, Marcos MV, de Zegher F. Polycystic ovary syndrome after precocious pubarche: ontogeny of the low birthweight effect. Clin Endocrinol (Oxf) 2001;55:667–672.
6. Eisner JR, Dumesic DA, Kemnitz JW, Abbott DH. Timing of prenatal androgen excess determines differential impairment in insulin secretion and action in adult female rhesus monkeys. J Clin Endocrinol Metab 2000;85:1206–1210.
7. Eisner JR, Dumesic DA, Kemnitz JW, Colman RJ, Abbott DH. Increased adiposity in female rhesus monkeys exposed to androgen excess during early gestation. Obes Res 2003;11:279–286.
8. Eisner JR, Barnett MA, Dumesic DA, Abbott DH. Ovarian hyperandrogenism in adult female rhesus monkeys exposed to prenatal androgen excess. Fertil Steril 2002;77:167–172.
9. Abbott DH, Dumesic DA, Franks S. Developmental origin of polycystic ovary syndrome—a hypothesis. J Endocrinol 2002;174:1–5.
10. Meas T, Chevenne D, Thibaud E, et al. Endocrine consequences of premature pubarche in post-pubertal Caucasian girls Clinical Endocrinology 2002;57:101–106.
11. Glueck CJ, Papanna R, Wang P, Goldenberg N, Sieve-Smith L. Incidence and treatment of metabolic syndrome in newly referred women with confirmed polycystic ovarian syndrome. Metabolism 2003;52:908–915.
12. National Cholesterol Education Program (NCEP) Expert Panel on Detection, Evaluation, and Treatment of High Blood Cholesterol in Adults (Adult Treatment Panel III). Third Report of the National Cholesterol Education Program (NCEP) Expert Panel on Detection, Evaluation, and Treatment of High Blood Cholesterol in Adults (Adult Treatment Panel III): final report. Circulation 2002;106:3143–3421.
13. Einhorn D, Reaven GM, Cobin RH, et al. American College of Endocrinology position statement on the insulin resistance syndrome. Endocr Pract 2003;9:237–252.
14. Legro RS, Kunselman AR, Dodson WC, Dunaif A. Prevalence and predictors of risk for type 2 diabetes mellitus and impaired glucose tolerance in polycystic ovary syndrome: a prospective, controlled study in 254 affected women. J Clin Endocrinol Metab 1999;84:165–169.
15. Krosnick A. The diabetes and obesity epidemic among the Pima Indians. N J Med 2000;97:31–37.
16. Norman RJ, Masters L, Milner CR, Wang JX, Davies MJ. Relative risk of conversion from normogly-caemia to impaired glucose tolerance or non-insulin dependent diabetes mellitus in polycystic ovarian syndrome. Hum Reprod 2001;16:1995–1998.
17. Dunaif A, Segal KR, Futterweit W, Dobrjansky A. Profound peripheral insulin resistance, independent of obesity, in polycystic ovary syndrome. Diabetes 1989;38:1165–1174.
18. Dunaif A. Insulin resistance and the polycystic ovary syndrome: mechanism and implications for pathogenesis. Endocr Rev 1997;18:774–800.

19. Dunaif A, Wu X, Lee A, Diamanti-Kandarakis E. Defects in insulin receptor signaling in vivo in the polycystic ovary syndrome (PCOS). Am J Physiol Endocrinol Metab 2001;281:E392–E399.

20. Kahn SE, Prigeon RL, McCulloch DK, et al. Quantification of the relationship between insulin sensitivity and B-cell function in human subjects: evidence for a hyperbolic function. Diabetes 1993;42: 1663–1672.

21. Polonsky KS, Sturis J, Bell GI. Noninsulin- dependent diabetes mellitus—a genetically programmed failure of the beta cell to compensate for insulin resistance. N Engl J Med 1996;334:777–783.

22. Ehrmann DA, Sturis J, Byrne MM, Karrison T, Rosenfield RL, Polonsky KS. Insulin secretory defects in polycystic ovary syndrome: relationship to insulin sensitivity and family history of non-insulin-dependent diabetes mellitus. J Clin Invest 1995;96:520–527.

23. O'Meara NM, Blackman JD, Ehrmann DA, et al. Defects in beta-cell function in functional ovarian hyperandrogenism. J Clin Endocrinol Metab 1993;76:1241–1247.

24. Ehrmann DA, Breda E, Cavaghan MK, et al. Insulin secretory responses to rising and falling glucose concentrations are delayed in subjects with impaired glucose tolerance. Diabetologia 2002;45: 509–517.

25. Ehrmann DA, Breda E, Corcoran MC, et al. Impaired beta-cell compensation to dexamethasone-induced hyperglycemia in women with polycystic ovary syndrome. Am J Physiol Endocrinol Metab 2004;287:E241–E246.

26. Dunaif A, Finegood DT. β-cell dysfunction independent of obesity and glucose intolerance in the polycystic ovary syndrome. J Clin Endocrinol Metab 1996;81:942–947.

27. Kousta E, Cela E, Lawrence N, et al. The prevalence of polycystic ovaries in women with a history of gestational diabetes. Clin Endocrinol (Oxf) 2000;53:501–507.

28. Ehrmann DA. Genetic contributions to glucose intolerance in polycystic ovary syndrome. Reprod Biomed Online 2004;9:28–34.

29. Yildiz BO, Yarali H, Oguz H, Bayraktar M. Glucose intolerance, insulin resistance, and hyperandrogenemia in first degree relatives of women with polycystic ovary syndrome. J Clin Endocrinol Metab 2003;88:2031–2036.

30. Norman RJ, Masters S, Hague W. Hyperinsulinemia is common in family members of women with polycystic ovary syndrome. Fertil Steril 1996;66:942–947.

31. Weyer C, Tataranni PA, Bogardus C, Pratley RE. Insulin resistance and insulin secretory dysfunction are independent predictors of worsening of glucose tolerance during each stage of type 2 diabetes development. Diabetes Care 2001;24:89–94.

32. Haffner SM, Miettinen H, Gaskill SP, Stern MP. Decreased insulin secretion and increased insulin resistance are independently related to the 7-year risk of NIDDM in Mexican-Americans. Diabetes 1995;44:1386–1391.

33. Ehrmann DA, Kasza K, Azziz R, Legro RS, Ghazzi MN, for the PCOS/Troglitazone Study Group. Effects of race and family history of type 2 diabetes on metabolic status of women with polycystic ovary syndrome. J Clin Endocrinol Metab 2005;90:66–71.

34. Colilla S, Cox N, Ehrmann D. Heritability of insulin secretion and insulin action in women with polycystic ovary syndrome and their first-degree relatives. J Clin Endocrinol Metab 2001;86: 2027–2031.

35. Legro RS, Bentley-Lewis R, Driscoll D, Wang SC, Dunaif A. Insulin resistance in the sisters of women with polycystic ovary syndrome: association with hyperandrogenemia rather than menstrual irregularity. J Clin Endocrinol Metab 2002;87:2128–2133.

36. Wagenknecht LE, Langefeld CD, Scherzinger AL, et al. Insulin sensitivity, insulin secretion, and abdominal fat: the Insulin Resistance Atherosclerosis Study (IRAS) Family Study. Diabetes 2003;52:2490–2496.

37. Burks DJ, White MF. IRS proteins and β-cell function. 2001;50:S140–S145.

38. El Mkadem SA, Lautier C, Macari F, et al. Role of allelic variants Gly972Arg of IRS-1 and Gly1057Asp of IRS-2 in moderate-to-severe insulin resistance of women with polycystic ovary syndrome. Diabetes 2001;50:2164–2168.

39. Hart LM, Stolk RP, Dekker JM, et al. Prevalence of variants in candidate genes for type 2 diabetes mellitus in The Netherlands: the Rotterdam study and the Hoorn study. J Clin Endocrinol Metab 1999;84:1002–1006.

40. Clausen JO, Hansen T, Bjorbaek C, et al. Insulin resistance: interactions between obesity and a common variant of insulin receptor substrate-1. Lancet 1995;346:397–402.

41. Porzio O, Federici M, Hribal ML, et al. The Gly972—>Arg amino acid polymorphism in IRS-1 impairs insulin secretion in pancreatic beta cells. J Clin Invest 1999;104:357–364.
42. Almind K, Bjorbaek C, Vestergaard H, Hansen T, Echwald S, Pedersen O. Aminoacid polymorphisms of insulin receptor substrate-1 in non-insulin-dependent diabetes mellitus. Lancet 1993;42:828–832.
43. Almind K, Inoue G, Pedersen O, Kahn CR. A common amino acid polymorphism in insulin receptor substrate-1 causes impaired insulin signaling. Evidence from transfection studies. J Clin Invest 1996;97:2569–2575.
44. Sir-Petermann T, Perez-Bravo F, Angel B, Maliqueo M, Calvillan M, Palomino A. G972R polymorphism of IRS-1 in women with polycystic ovary syndrome. Diabetologia 2001;44:1200–1201.
45. Florez JC, Sjogren M, Burtt N, et al. Association testing in 9,000 people fails to confirm the association of the insulin receptor substrate-1 G972R polymorphism with type 2 diabetes. Diabetes 2004;53:3313–3318.
46. Wu X, Sallinen K, Anttila L, et al. Expression of insulin-receptor substrate-1 and -2 in ovaries from women with insulin resistance and from controls. Fertil Steril 2000;74:564–572.
47. Hu FB, Manson JE, Stampfer MJ, et al. Diet, lifestyle, and the risk of type 2 diabetes mellitus in women. N Engl J Med 2001;345:790–797.
48. O'Dea K. Marked improvement in carbohydrate and lipid metabolism in diabetic Australian aborigines after temporary reversion to traditional lifestyle. Diabetes 1984;33:596–603.
49. Weiss R, Dziura J, Burgert TS, et al. Obesity and the metabolic syndrome in children and adolescents. N Engl J Med 2004;350:2362–2374.
50. Knowler WC, Barrett-Connor E, Fowler SE, et al. Diabetes Prevention Program Research Group. Reduction in the incidence of type 2 diabetes with lifestyle intervention or metformin. N Engl J Med 2002;346:393–403.
51. Pan XR, Li GW, Hu YH, et al. Effects of diet and exercise in preventing NIDDM in people with impaired glucose tolerance. The Da Qing IGT and Diabetes Study. Diabetes Care 1997; 20:537–544.
52. Tuomilehto J, Lindstrom J, Eriksson JG, et al. Finnish Diabetes Prevention Study Group. Prevention of type 2 diabetes mellitus by changes in lifestyle among subjects with impaired glucose tolerance. N Engl J Med 2001;344:1343–1350.
53. Rizkalla SW, Taghrid L, Laromiguiere M, et al. Improved plasma glucose control, whole-body glucose utilization, and lipid profile on a low-glycemic index diet in type 2 diabetes. Diabetes Care 2004;27:1866–1872.
54. Knowler WC, Barrett-Connor E, Fowler SE, et al. Reduction in the incidence of type 2 diabetes with lifestyle intervention or metformin. N Engl J Med 2002;346:393–403.
55. Norman RJ, Davies MJ, Lord J, Moran LJ. The role of lifestyle modification in polycystic ovary syndrome. Trends Endocrinol Metab 2002;13:251–257.
56. Tang T, Glanville J, Hayden CJ, White D, Barth JH, Balen AH. Combined lifestyle modification and metformin in obese patients with polycystic ovary syndrome. A randomized, placebo-controlled, double-blind multicentre study. Hum Reprod 2006;21:80–89.
57. Hoeger KM, Kochman L, Wixom N, Craig K, Miller RK, Guzick DS. A randomized, 48-week, placebo-controlled trial of intensive lifestyle modification and/or metformin therapy in overweight women with polycystic ovary syndrome: a pilot study. Fertil Steril 2004;82:421–429.
58. Kiddy DS, Hamilton-Fairley D, Bush A, et al. Improvement in endocrine and ovarian function during dietary treatment of obese women with polycystic ovary syndrome. Clin Endocrinol (Oxf) 1992;36:105–111.
59. Escobar-Morreale HF, Botella-Carretero JI, Alvarez-Blasco F, Sancho J, San Millan JL. The polycystic ovary syndrome associated with morbid obesity may resolve after weight loss induced by bariatric surgery. J Clin Endocrinol Metab 2005;90:6364–6369.
60. Weerakiet S, Srisombut C, Bunnag P, Sangtong S, Chuangsoongnoen N, Rojanasakul A. Prevalence of type 2 diabetes mellitus and impaired glucose tolerance in Asian women with polycystic ovary syndrome. Int J Gynaecol Obstet 2001;75:177–184.
61. Gambineri A, Pelusi C, Manicardi E, et al. Glucose intolerance in a large cohort of mediterranean women with polycystic ovary syndrome: phenotype and associated factors. Diabetes 2004;53:2353–2358.
62. Conn JJ, Jacobs HS, Conway GS. The prevalence of polycystic ovaries in women with type 2 diabetes mellitus. Clin Endocrinol (Oxf) 2000;52:81–86.

63. Holte J, Gennarelli G, Wide L, Lithell H, Berne C. High prevalence of polycystic ovaries and associated clinical, endocrine, and metabolic features in women with previous gestational diabetes mellitus. J Clin Endocrinol Metab 1998;83:1143–1150.

64. Harris MI, Hadden WC, Knowler WC, Bennett PH. Prevalence of diabetes and impaired glucose tolerance and plasma glucose levels in U.S. population aged 20–74 yr. Diabetes 1987;36:523–534.

65. Kjos SL, Peters RK, Xiang A, Henry OA, Montro M, Buchanan TA. Predicting future diabetes in Latino women with gestational diabetes. Utility of early postpartum glucose tolerance testing. Diabetes 1995;44:586–591.

66. Harris MI, Flegal KM, Cowie CC, et al. Prevalence of diabetes, impaired fasting glucose, and impaired glucose tolerance in U.S. adults. Diabetes Care 1998;21:518–524.

67. Legro RS, Gnatuk CL, Kunselman AR, Dunaif A. Changes in glucose tolerance over time in women with polycystic ovary syndrome: a controlled study. J Clin Endocrinol Metab 2005;90:3236–3242.

68. Phillips DI, Barker DJ, Hales CN, Hirst S, Osmond C. Thinness at birth and insulin resistance in adult life. Diabetologia 1994;37:150–154.

69. Ibanez L, Potau N, Francois I, de Zegher F. Precocious pubarche, hyperinsulinism, and ovarian hyperandrogenism in girls: relation to reduced fetal growth. J Clin Endocrinol Metab 1998;83:3558–3562.

70. Holte J. Polycystic ovary syndrome and insulin resistance: thrifty genes struggling withover-feeding and sedentary life style? J Endocrinol Invest 1998;21:589–601.

71. Martin BC, Warram JH, Krolewski AS, Bergman RN, Soeldner JS, Kahn CR. Role of glucose and insulin resistance in development of type 2 diabetes mellitus: results of a 25-year follow-up study. Lancet 1992;340:925–929.

72. Weyer C, Bogardus C, Mott DM, Pratley RE. The natural history of insulin secretory dysfunction and insulin resistance in the pathogenesis of type 2 diabetes mellitus. J Clin Invest 1999;104:787–794.

73. Gastaldelli A, Ferrannini E, Miyazaki Y, Matsuda M, DeFronzo RA, San Antonio metabolism study. Beta-cell dysfunction and glucose intolerance: results from the San Antonio metabolism (SAM) study. Diabetologia 2004;47:31–39.

74. Fukushima M, Usami M, Ikeda M, et al. Insulin secretion and insulin sensitivity at different stages of glucose tolerance: a crosssectional study of Japanese type 2 diabetes. Metabolism 2004;53:831–835.

75. Osei K, Rhinesmith S, Gaillard T, Schuster D. Impaired insulin sensitivity, insulin secretion, and glucose effectiveness, predict future development of impaired glucose tolerance and type 2 diabetes in pre-diabetic African Americans. Diabetes Care 2004;27:1439–1446.

76. Ovesen P, Moller J, Ingerslev HJ, et al. Normal basal and insulin-stimulated fuel metabolism in lean women with the polycystic ovary syndrome. J Clin Endocrinol Metab 1993;77:1636–1640.

77. Holte J, Bergh T, Berne C, Wide L, Lithell H. Restored insulin sensitivity but persistently increased early insulin secretion after weight loss in obese women with polycystic ovary syndrome. J Clin Endocrinol Metab 1995;80:2586–2593.

78. Dunaif A, Graf M, Mandeli J, Laumas V, Dobrjansky A. Characterization of groups of hyperandrogenic women with acanthosis nigricans, impaired glucose tolerance and/or hyperinsulinemia. J Clin Endocrinol Metab 1987;65:499–507.

79. Robinson S, Kiddy D, Gelding SV, et al. The relationship of insulin insensitivity to menstrual pattern in women with hyperandrogenism and polycystic ovaries. Clin Endocrinol (Oxf) 1993;39:351–355.

80. Sampson M, Kong C, Patel A, Unwin R, Jacobs HS. Ambulatory blood pressure profiles and plasminogen activator inhibitor (PAI-1) activity in lean women with and without the polycystic ovary syndrome. Clin Endocrinol (Oxf) 1996;45:623–629.

81. Bergman RN, Phillips LS, Cobelli C. Physiologic evaluation of factors controlling glucose tolerance in man: measurement of insulin sensitivity and beta-cell glucose sensitivity from the response to intravenous glucose. J Clin Invest 1981;68:1456–1467.

82. Bergman RN. Toward physiological understanding of glucose tolerance. Minimal model approach. Diabetes 1989;38:1512–1527.

83. O'Meara NM, Blackman JD, Ehrmann DA, et al. Defects in b-cell function in functional ovarian hyperandrogenism. J Clin Endocrinol Metab 1993;76:1241–1247.

84. Ehrmann DA, Sturis J, Byrne MM, Karrison T, Rosenfield RL, Polonksy KS. Insulin secretory defects in polycystic ovary syndrome. Relationship to insulin sensitivity and family history of non-insulin-dependent diabetes mellitus. J Clin Invest 1995;96:520–527.

85. Ryan EA, Imes S, Liu D, et al. Defects in insulin secretion and action in women with a history of gestational diabetes. Diabetes 1995;44:506–512.

86. Ehrmann DA, Breda E, Corcoran MC, et al. Impaired β-cell compensation to dexamethasone-induced hyperglycemia in women with polycystic ovary syndrome. Am J Physiol Endocrinol Metab 2004;287:E241–E246.

87. Goodarzi MO, Erickson S, Port SC, Jennrich RI, Korenman SG. β-Cell function: a key pathological determinant in polycystic ovary syndrome. J Clin Endocrinol Metab 2005;90:310–315.

88. Gennarelli G, Rovei V, Novi RF, et al. Preserved insulin sensitivity and β-cell activity, but decreased glucose effectiveness in normal-weight women with the polycystic ovary syndrome. J Clin Endocrinol Metab 2005;90:3381–3386.

15 "Secondary" Polycystic Ovary Syndrome

Gregory Kaltsas, MD, FRCP and George Chrousos, MD, FACP

Summary

Hyperandrogenism and menstrual irregularities are the most common endocrine symptoms in premenopausal women. The vast majority of these women suffer from the polycystic ovary syndrome (PCOS), which is defined as a state of "gonadotropin-dependent functional hyperandrogenism and oligo-anovulation" in which no distinct autonomous source of androgen secretion is identified. PCOS is a chronic disorder characterized by specific clinical, endocrine, and ultrasonographic features, and is commonly associated with insulin resistance. However, a number of women with PCOS have other underlying diagnoses, such as adrenal and ovarian androgen-secreting tumors, adrenal and/or ovarian steroidogenic deficiencies, other medical or endocrine disorders, and/or receive certain medications. These disorders may exhibit similar clinical, endocrine, and/or ultrasonographic features to PCOS, and their early identification may be based on the presence of distinct features and a high index of suspicion. In contrast to PCOS, some of these conditions can be life-threatening and require prompt diagnosis and treatment. In this chapter, we consider disorders

From: *Contemporary Endocrinology: Insulin Resistance and Polycystic Ovarian Syndrome: Pathogenesis, Evaluation, and Treatment*
Edited by: E. Diamanti-Kandarakis, J. E. Nestler, D. Panidis, and R. Pasquali © Humana Press Inc., Totowa, NJ

that can present as PCOS, discuss their pathogenesis and diagnosis and define the features that may help distinguish them from PCOS.

Key Words: Hyperandrogenism; anovulation; hyperinsulinemia; polycystic ovaries.

INTRODUCTION

Symptoms and signs of hyperandrogenism, menstrual irregularities, and chronic oligo-anovulation are among the most common endocrine abnormalities of premenopausal women *(1–3)*. The great majority of such women *(1–4)* suffer from the polycystic ovary syndrome (PCOS), a chronic disorder usually of peripubertal onset, that is characterized by distinct endocrine abnormalities and the presence of polycystic ovaries (PCO) on ovarian ultrasonography *(1,3–6)*. Of note, although PCO is found in approx 21–23% of premenopausal women, only about one-third to one-half of them develop the full clinical and endocrine manifestations of PCOS *(1,6–8)*. This suggests the presence of additional factors that may operate in the development of the syndrome, the most probable being hyperinsulinemia and insulin resistance *(1,6–8)*. Because the definition of PCOS has been a matter of debate for a long time, a recent International Consensus Group proposed that PCOS could be diagnosed when at least two of the following were present: oligo- or anovulation (usually reflected by oligo- or amenorrhea), clinical (hirsutism) and/or biochemical (elevated circulating androgen levels) features of hyperandrogenism, and PCO as defined by ultrasonography *(9)*. In addition, the same group incorporated into the diagnostic criteria the exclusion of other medical conditions, that could be associated with similar clinical, endocrine and ultrasonographic manifestations *(9,10)*.

The clinical and endocrine features of PCOS are heterogeneous and nonspecific, and there is still considerable debate as to whether PCOS represents a single syndrome, or whether it reflects a variety of disorders which may originate in different organs and/or be triggered by different as yet poorly understood mechanisms *(1,5,6)*. Current understanding of the pathogenesis of the syndrome suggests that it is a complex, multifactorial, and polygenic disorder *(10)*. Candidate genes that regulate the hypothalamic–pituitary–ovarian (HPO) and/or –adrenal axis (HPA), as well as those responsible for the development of insulin resistance have been studied and a number of them appear to be related to the development of PCOS *(11–13)*. Similarly, several disorders leading to either excessive androgen production from the steroidogenic organs, namely the adrenals and ovaries, or affecting steroid biosynthesis, secretion, metabolism, and/or action, may present with the clinical, endocrine, and/or ultrasonographic hallmarks of PCOS *(3)* (Table 1).

Insulin plays a key role in the pathogenesis of hyperandrogenemia and/or PCOS *(1,3,8,10)*. This hormone, along with luteinizing hormone (LH), enhances androgen production from the theca cells of the ovary and inhibits hepatic synthesis of sex hormone-binding globulin (SHBG) causing a decrease of its circulating concentration, and, hence, an increase of the biologically active free fraction of this hormone *(1,3,10)*. Hyperinsulinemia and insulin resistance is more evident in women with PCOS and menstrual irregularities irrespective of the presence of obesity and/or hyperandrogenism *(1,10,14)*. The severity of hyperinsulinemia correlates with the degree of clinical expression of the syndrome, with the ovaries being appropriately responsive to the elevated levels of the hormone. Insulin resistance and hence the effect of insulin on the ovaries is further exacerbated by obesity

Table 1
Disorders Associated With the PCOS Phenotype

Adrenal hyperandrogenism
CAH (both classic and nonclassic)
21-hydroxylase deficiency
11-hydroxylase deficiency
3β-hydroxysteroid dehydrogenase deficiency
Adrenal androgen-producing tumors (adenomas, carcinomas)
Abnormal cortisol action and/or metabolism
Glucocorticoid resistance
11-ketosteroid reductase type 1 deficiency

Ovarian hyperandrogenism
Ovarian steroidogenic defects
Side chain cleavage enzyme
17α-hydroxylase deficiency
3β-hydroxysteroid dehydrogenase deficiency
Ovarian androgen-producing tumors
Hyperthecosis, luteoma
Ectopic LH secretion

Endocrinopathies
Cushing's syndrome
Acromegaly
Hyperprolactinemia
Insulinoma
Ectopic LH secretion
Precocious puberty
Thyroid disorders (?)

Syndromes of hyperinsulinemia and insulin resistance states
Lipoatrophic diabetes, Leprechaunism, Rabson-Mendenhall
    syndrome, Kahn types A, and B insulin resistance
T2DM, GDM, obesity

Other nonendocrine disorders
Epilepsy (?), intracranial hypertension
Female to male transectualism

Drugs
Valproic acid
GH (?)
All atypical major anti-psychotics
Testosterone and other androgens

(1,15). It is, therefore, possible that insulin resistance may underlie the pathophysiology of several disorders with PCOS phenotype *(3)*. Although the role of hyperinsulinemia in the pathogenesis and treatment of PCOS and its implications to general health has been addressed extensively, there is not much information on its role in diseases with a PCOS-phenotype in which there is a known cause of hyperandrogenism. This is particularly important because hyperinsulinemia and insulin resistance are related to the metabolic syndrome and are associated with increased cardiovascular morbidity and mortality *(16)*.

The extent to which patients presenting with hyperandrogenism and chronic oligo-anovulation should be investigated to exclude such diseases is still not clear *(1,17,18)*. Findings from several series, including some recent ones, have revealed a relatively small prevalence (less than 7%) of disorders other than the classic PCOS in women presenting with the typical phenotype *(4,19,20)*. Some of these disorders may have subtle symptoms and run a chronic course, whereas others can develop a rapid course and be life-threatening *(3,21)*. It is, therefore, important for the practicing clinician to appropriately diagnose and manage these disorders.

DISORDERS ASSOCIATED WITH A PCOS PHENOTYPE

Disorders Associated With Altered Androgen Secretion, Metabolism, and/or Action

ADRENAL AND OVARIAN ANDROGEN-PRODUCING TUMORS

Androgen-producing tumors, adrenal carcinomas, and less commonly adenomas, and a wide variety of ovarian tumors can present with virilization (clitoromegaly, deepening of the voice, frontal balding, and muscle hypertrophy), hyperandrogenism and chronic oligo-anovulation *(17,22,23)*. Although virilization has been reported in women with PCOS, it is extremely rare *(24)*. Adrenal carcinomas are large tumors that secrete large quantities of testosterone or its precursors with or without concomitant cortisol hypersecretion *(7)*. Ovarian neoplasms can be of variable size secreting mainly testosterone although rarely can also cosecrete various androgen precursors *(25)*. Occasionally, ovarian neoplasms of epithelial origin may produce factors stimulating steroidogenesis in a paracrine fashion *(21)*. Sertoli-Leydig cell tumor, is the most common virilizing ovarian tumor that occurs during the second to fourth decade of life and may be gonadotrophin-responsive *(7,25)*. Other tumors that simulate the PCOS, are hilus cell tumors, benign cystic teratomas, and adrenal rest tumors; these tumors occur more frequently in postmenopausal women *(21)*.

Ovarian hyperthecosis (nests of luteinizing cells distributed throughout the ovarian stroma) can present as PCOS but is usually associated with severe insulin resistance *(21,26)*. The ovaries are enlarged and of an extremely firm texture as a result of extensive and dense fibroblast growth; the absence of follicle formation provides a clear morphologic distinction from the classic PCOS ovary *(21)*. Rapidly progressing symptoms of androgen excess should always suggest the presence of an androgen-secreting tumor. This rapid progression is typical of both ovarian and adrenal androgen producing tumors, although cases of slowly evolving tumors associated with endocrine and ultrasonographic features of PCOS have also been described *(17)*.

In general, patients with virilizing tumors usually present after puberty with rapidly progressing male-pattern alopecia, deepening of the voice, increased libido and a male body habitus. However, particular attention should be paid to cases of slowly evolving tumors, which can be clinically indistinguishable from PCOS *(3,7,17)*. Patients with tumors invariably have elevated androgen levels; however, only testosterone values greater than 200 ng/dL (7 nmol/L) are highly suggestive of autonomous production from an androgen-secreting tumor *(3,4,7,17)*. Elevated dehydroepiandrosterone-sulfate (DHEAS) may reflect autonomous androgen secretion by an adrenal androgen-secreting tumor, however, a number of patients with adrenal carcinomas do not have substantially raised DHEAS levels *(17,22)*. Prompt diagnosis and management of these tumors are important, particularly in cases of adrenal carcinoma, as patients with localized disease exhibit a much more favorable survival *(27)*.

Cushing's Syndrome

The great majority of women with Cushing's syndrome (CS) develop hirsutism, and between 70 to 80% of them menstrual irregularities *(28,29)*. These findings together with truncal obesity and acne may suggest the diagnosis of PCOS but the presence of specific Cushing stigmata, such as easy bruising, thinning of the skin, and proximal myopathy, are indicative of glucocorticoid excess and point to the correct diagnosis *(30)*. The presence of menstrual irregularities associated with high serum cortisol rather than androgen or estradiol levels, suggests that menstrual irregularities are directly related to the degree of hypercortisolemia *(28,29)*. A recent prospective study demonstrated attenuation of pulsatile LH secretion indicating gonadotrophin deficiency in the majority of women with CS; this suggests the presence of different mechanisms that alter LH pulsatile secretion between women with CS and PCOS *(31)*. PCO were also found in 46% of patients with CS, whereas all patients had low SHBG levels, presumably as a consequence of hypercortisolism-induced insulin resistance and hyper-insulinemia *(3,28)*. This could account for the development of hirsutism in patients with CS, even in the presence of normal androgen levels, owing to an increase in the free androgen index *(3,28)*.

It has been suggested that when cortisol levels are moderately elevated, gonadotrophin secretion is still preserved, maintaining ovarian steroid output and leading to menstrual irregularities and the development of a PCOS-phenotype while preserving an estradiol-sufficient state *(28)*. However, when cortisol concentration is higher than a critical level, a hypogonadotrophic hypogonadism state develops leading to estrogen deficiency *(31)*. In this situation, persistence of PCO morphology and/or PCOS phenotype could be attributed to the severe hyperinsulinemia and its effect on ovarian function and steroid output *(28)*.

Besides the presence of a characteristic phenotype, another feature that could distinguish women with CS from those with PCOS, particularly in subtle forms of CS, is the decrease of bone mineral density, which is usually decreased in women with CS as a result of the hypercortisolemia *(32,33)*. Although circulating cortisol levels can be elevated in patients with CS leading to increased urinary free cortisol (UFC) excretion, the hallmark of the diagnosis is abnormal cortisol secretion characterized by loss of circadian rhythm and failure to be suppressed by dexamethasone administration *(30)*.

Adrenal-Ovarian Steroidogenic Deficiencies

The disorder of adrenal steroidogenesis are comprised by several enzymatic defects, the most common of which is 21-hydroxylase (21-OH). Compared with classic congenital adrenal hyperplasia (CAH), which is recognized at birth or in childhood, the nonclassic, or late-onset or adult-onset, CAH (NCAH) form can fully simulate PCOS *(3,21)*. Late-onset 21-OH deficiency occurs in 1–5% of hyperandrogenic women depending on their ethnicity *(2)*. Both classic and late-onset CAH, secondary to 21-OH, 11-hydroxylase, or 3-β-hydroxysteroid dehydrogenase (3-β-OH-D) deficiency, are

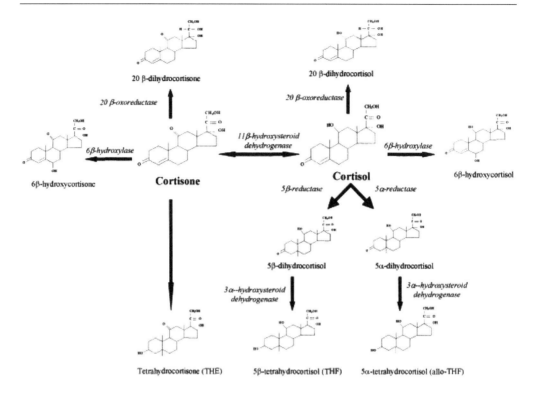

Fig. 1. Pathway of cortisol metabolism. 11β-hydroxysteroid (11β-HSD) isoenzymes convert cortisone and cortisol and reverse. 5α/β-reductase induces ring reduction.

associated with increased adrenocorticotrophin (ACTH) secretion and, respectively, 17-hydroxyprogesterone, 11-deoxycortisol, and 17-hydroxypregnenolone *(34–36)*. The diagnosis of late-onset CAH is made by measuring the accumulation of the appropriate steroid precursor after ACTH and/or cortisol releasing hormone (CRH) administration *(34,35)*. Interestingly, the 17-hydroxyprogesterone responses to the gonadotropin-releasing hormone agonist leuprolide in patients with classic CAH were similar to those of patients with PCOS, suggesting the presence of a common inherent steroidogenic defect at the level of the 17,20 lyase enzyme *(37)*; 83% of adult and 76% of postmenarchal patients with CAH have PCO *(38)*. Patients with CAH also have elevated insulin levels and are insulin-resistant *(34,39)*, further enhancing adrenal and ovarian androgen production and probably contributing to the development of PCO, PCOS and the metabolic syndrome (hyperinsulinemia, hyperlipidemia and reduced HDL levels, impaired glucose tolerance), and its complications *(34)*.

Adrenal and ovarian 3-β-(OHD) deficiency are extremely rare, and only a few cases of ovarian 17-ketosteroid reductase and aromatase deficiency have been described *(7)*. Similarly, girls with premature adrenarche (onset of pubic hair before the age of 8 years with no evidence of true puberty or adrenal dysfunction) have elevated adrenal androgen levels secondary to ACTH stimulation, and an increased risk of developing PCO and/or PCOS later in life *(40,41)*. Furthermore, girls with untreated central precocious puberty (initiation of puberty before the age of eight) have large volume ovaries and a greater than expected prevalence of PCO, which persists even after standard treatment with gonadotropin-releasing hormone analogues and growth hormone (GH) *(3,41)*.

Glucocorticoid-Resistance-States (Fig. 1)

Glucocorticoid resistance results from the partial inability of glucocorticoids to exert their effects on their target tissues. As a result, there is a compensatory increase in circulating pituitary ACTH, leading to excessive secretion of adrenal androgens *(42)*. In women, hyperandrogenism can result in acne, hirsutism, menstrual irregularity, oligo-anovulation, and infertility, therefore, mimicking the PCOS-phenotype *(42,43)*. The exact prevalence of glucocorticoid resistance-related PCO and/or PCOS has never been assessed, but it is probably very rare because of the rarity of the glucocorticoid resistance syndrome per se *(17)*. The hallmark for this diagnosis is elevated cortisol and ACTH levels in the absence of any Cushing features; although there is failure of cortisol suppression following dexamethasone administration, the normal circadian rhythm of cortisol secretion and the response of the HPA axis to stress are maintained albeit at higher levels of secretion *(42)*.

States of Altered Glucocorticoid Metabolism (Fig. 1)

Alterations of enzymatic pathways involved in cortisol metabolism are associated with increased ACTH secretion; this is associated with increased androgen secretion, mainly from the adrenals, although ACTH might also stimulate ovarian steroidogenesis *(44,45)*. Rare enzymatic defects, such as deficiency of 11-oxo-reductase, which converts inactive cortisone (E) to cortisol (F), are associated with enhanced cortisol metabolism, compensatory ACTH hypersecretion and hyperandrogenism leading to hirsutism and amenorrhea *(45,46)*. Overactivity of 5α-reductase, which is involved in both cortisol and testosterone metabolism, increases cortisol breakdown and causes subsequent ACTH hypersecretion and hyperandrogenism; in addition, it converts testosterone to more active metabolites, such as dehydrotestosterone, leading to hirsutism *(44)*. Both of these conditions are considered to be very rare causes of PCOS *(17)*.

DISORDERS ASSOCIATED WITH HYPERINSULINEMIA AND INSULIN RESISTANCE

Syndromes of Severe Hyperinsulinemia and Insulin Resistance

The HAIR-AN syndrome stands for hyperandrogenism (HA), insulin resistance (IR), and acanthosis nigricans (AN); the primary pathophysiologic derangements are insulin resistance and hyperandrogenism; the acanthosis nigricans being an epiphenomenon of IR *(8,47)*. In patients with the HAIR-AN syndrome, the degree of severity of insulin resistance is positively correlated with the severity of the hyperandrogenism *(47,48)*. It is thought that hyperinsulinemia stimulates ovarian androgen production directly and hyperandrogenism itself produces insulin resistance *(8)*. The relation between insulin resistance and hyperandrogenism might explain the hyperandrogenemia seen in lipoatrophic diabetes, leprechaunism and Kahn types A and B insulin resistance, and the development of PCO even before puberty in women with hepatic glycogen storage diseases *(8,47,48)*.

Diabetes-Mellitus Type 2

Between 68 and 82% of women of reproductive age and type 2 diabetes mellitus (T2DM) have PCO, and more than half have evidence of hyperandrogenism and menstrual irregularities *(15,49)*. Several correlations exist between indices of the metabolic and reproductive features, suggesting an overall stimulatory effect of insulin to the ovary; however, although it has been suggested that patients with T2DM and PCOS are more insulin-resistant than those without PCOS, this has not been reproduced in all studies *(15,50)*. It seems that the mechanism of insulin resistance in patients with PCOS might be different to that found in patients with T2DM *(8)*. However, as not all women with hyperinsulinemia associated with T2DM develop PCO and/or PCOS, it is probable that hyperinsulinemia alone is insufficient for the development of this ovarian morphology *(3,15)*.

Gestational-Diabetes-Mellitus

Women with gestational-diabetes-mellitus (GDM) have a higher incidence of PCO, (approx 30–50%) *(51–53)* and higher adrenal androgen secretion *(53)*. Women with GDM and PCO morphology also have increased frequency of menstrual irregularities and increased ovarian androgen production *(51,53)*. The lower prevalence of PCO in GDM compared with T2DM it probably relates to the fact that only women with proven fertility, and, hence, less severe PCOS, develop GDM *(51–53)*. In all of these studies, PCO on ultrasound was used as the main criterion to identify patients with a PCOS-like phenotype *(51–53)*. As women with GDM and PCOS demonstrate abnormalities in insulin action and secretion and are at increased risk for developing T2DM, the ultrasonographic appearance of PCO may be a predictive factor of altered glucose tolerance during and after pregnancy *(54)*.

Obesity

Obesity modifies insulin sensitivity and gonadotrophin secretory dynamics, and can be associated with hyperandrogenemia and oligo-amenorrhea, thereby mimicking PCOS *(55)*. Testosterone formation from androstenedione (Δ_4) is increased and, because of the hyperinsulinemia-induced reduction of SHBG levels, the free androgen index is increased *(3)*. A negative correlation between free testosterone and SHBG has been found particularly in upper body obesity, and this is associated with a high prevalence of PCOS symptoms in adulthood *(3)*.

ENDOCRINE DISORDERS ASSOCIATED WITH INCREASED ANDROGEN SECRETION, BIOAVAILABILITY, AND/OR INSULIN RESISTANCE

Acromegaly

Hirsutism and menstrual irregularities are found in approx 40–80% of patients with acromegaly *(56)*. Although the majority of patients have large tumors with complete or partial gonadotropin deficiency with or without concomitant hyperprolactinemia, there is a predilection for the development of PCOS *(56,57)*. Such patients may be estrogen-deficient but also severely insulin resistant and hyperinsulinemic, with insulin exerting a stimulatory effect on the ovary *(3,56)*. The low serum SHBG concentration found in these patients and the inverse association of SHBG with GH, even in estrogen-deficient patients, could explain the development of hirsutism in the presence of normal androgen levels as a result of an increase in the free androgen index *(56)*. In contrast, patients with small size tumors maintain their gonadotropin secretion and remain estrogen-sufficient, exhibiting an endocrinologic profile similar to that of PCOS *(56)*. Although ovarian ultrasonography has not been systematically performed in such patients, it has been suggested that either GH or insulin growth factor-I excess or the associated insulin resistance can affect steroid production, SHBG levels and ovarian function, ultimately leading to the development of PCOS *(56)*.

Hyperprolactinemia

Hyperprolactinemia mainly presents with menstrual irregularities with or without galactorrhea; hirsutism, seborrhea, increased androgen levels, particularly serum DHEAS; PCO have also been described in such patients *(2)*. Some retrospective studies have demonstrated a high prevalence of hirsutism and PCO (56 and 50–67%, respectively), in women with hyperprolactinemia *(58)*. In addition, hyperprolactinemia was shown to perpetuate insulin resistance contributing further to the development of PCOS *(59)*. A direct effect of elevated prolactin levels on adrenal steroidogenesis was suggested further by the demonstration of high expression of prolactin receptors in the adrenal gland *(60)*. However, currently there are no well-conducted prospective studies that have investigated the prevalence of PCO and/or PCOS in women with different causes of hyperprolactinemia.

Thyroid Dysfunction

Decreased SHBG and increased free testosterone levels and altered estradiol metabolism have been described in hypothyroid patients, whereas PCO has been detected in 36.5% of hypothyroid patients *(61)*. Precocious puberty and severe PCO have also been described in women with long-standing acquired hypothyroidism *(62)*. However, there are no large-scale studies examining the impact of thyroid dysfunction on ovarian function and morphology and the development of PCOS. Hypothyroidism might enhance the PCOS-phenotype and there may be a relation between insulin secretion and thyroid and ovarian function in patients with PCOS *(3)*. Hyperthyroidism has also been associated with increased SHBG and subnormal cortisol, free testosterone, and DHEA levels *(61)*.

Less Common Endocrine Disorders Associated With PCOS

A few cases of ectopic LH secretion from pancreatic endocrine tumors presenting with menstrual irregularities and PCOS were recently described *(63,64)*. Androgen levels were related to LH bioactivity and patients exhibited a PCOS-like phenotype *(63,64)*. However, no increased incidence of PCO or PCOS has been described in female carriers of activating mutations of the LH receptor or the Gs protein (familial male sexual precocity and McCune–Albright syndromes, respectively). Hyperandrogenism, menstrual irregularity, and PCOS were also described in patients with insulin-secreting tumors that resolved after the removal of the insulinoma *(65,66)*. It was hypothesized that insulin directly affected androgen secretion either acting as a co-gonadotrophin to coexistent PCO or inducing PCOS per se as previously described *(7,8,65)*. However, this has not been the case in patients with nesidioblastosis *(66)*.

OTHER DISORDERS ASSOCIATED WITH PCOS

It has been reported that women with epilepsy have a high prevalence of menstrual irregularities, hyperandrogenism, and PCO or PCOS *(67,68)*. Although this association was originally attributed to the effects of treatment with valproic acid, subsequent studies revealed that it was not related to any specific anti-epileptic drugs, as it was also observed in drug-free patients *(69)*. An association of idiopathic intracranial hypertension with PCOS was also described recently *(70)*.

DRUGS ASSOCIATED WITH PCOS

Initial studies suggested that patients treated with valproic acid are at increased risk of developing PCO and/or PCOS compared to patients receiving other antiepileptic treatment but not in drug-free epileptic women *(71,72)*. However, subsequent studies did not confirm these findings that await to be confirmed in large sample studies *(3)*. Treatment with GH increases the prevalence of PCO in children with precocious puberty *(41)*. Drugs such as diazoxide, phenytoin, cyclosporin, and minoxidil have been associated with hirsutism but there is no firm evidence that they can induce either PCO or PCOS *(3)*. Although exogenous androgen administration is associated with a hirsutism and other signs of androgen excess it is not entirely clear whether they can initiate PCO *(3)*. In addition, psychiatric conditions and psychiatric medications may mimic PCOS through abnormalities of insulin secretion and/or action.

CLINICAL, BIOCHEMICAL, AND RADIOLOGICAL
CONFIRMATION OF SECONDARY CAUSES OF PCOS (TABLE 2, FIG. 2)

In most cases the diagnosis of a disorder other than PCOS can be made clinically and substantiated with biochemical and, when necessary, imaging confirmation *(3,21)*. Clinical history of virilization, particularly if it is of a later onset and not from the time of puberty, is highly suggestive of an androgen-producing tumor *(3,7,17)*. Particular attention should be paid to exclude cases of slowly evolving tumors *(3,17)*, which can be clinically indistinguishable from PCOS *(17)*. It has been suggested that testosterone and DHEAS levels in excess of 200 ng/dL (7 nmol/L) and 7000 ng/mL (19 µmol/L), respectively, suffice to distinguish such patients *(4,17,21)*. However, cases of androgen secreting tumors with androgen levels below these cut-off numbers have been described *(3)*. To identify patients harboring such tumors, which may also develop in the context of coexisting PCOS, the testosterone response during a 48-hour low-dose (2 mg) dexamethasone-suppression test (LDDST) can be used *(7,17,22)*. Of 17 patients with androgen-secreting tumors, none showed either a greater than 40% reduction or normalization of the previously elevated testosterone levels, whereas 88% of patients with PCOS showed such a response (100% sensitivity and 73% specificity in distinguishing virilizing tumors from PCOS) *(17)*. Measurement of androstenedione and DHEAS might also be necessary to identify patients whose tumors preferentially secrete these androgens rather than testosterone, although this is rare *(4,7,17)*.

Table 2

Clinical, Biochemical, and Ultrasonographic Features in Secondary Causes of PCOS[a,b,c]

Disease or other state	Hirsutism	Anovulation	17OHPG	E_2	Testosterone	Δ_4	DHEAS	LH	FSH	SHBG	IR	PCO
CAH	+	+	↑↑	→↓	→↑	→↑	→↑	→↑	→↓	→↓	→↓	82%
Virilizing adrenal tumors	+	+	→↑	→↑	↑↑	→↑	↑↑	→↑	→↓	→↓↑	→↑	25%
Virilizing ovarian tumors	++	+	→↑	↑↑	↑↑	↑↑	→↑	→↓	→↓	↓	↑	>80%
CS	+	+	→↑	→↓	→↑	→↑	→↓↑	→↓↑	→↓	→↓	→↑	46%
Acromegaly	+	+	→↑	→↓	→↑	→↑	→↑	→↓↑	→↓	→↑	→↑	NK
Hyperprolactinemia	+	+	→↑	→↓	→↑	→↑	→↑	→↓↑	→↓	→↑	→↑	50–67%
Glucocorticoid resistance	+	+	→↑	→↑	→↑	→↑	→↑	→↓↑	→↓	→↑	→↓	NK
Altered cortisol metabolism	+	+	→↑	→↑	→↑	→↑	→↑	→↑	→↓	→↑	→↓	NK
Severe forms of IR	++	++	→↑	→↑	→↑	→↑	→↑	→↑	↑	→↓	↑↑	80–100%
T2DM	+	+	→↑	↑←	→↑	→↑	↑	→↑	↑	→↑	→↑	68–82%
Gestational DM	–	–	→	↑↑	→↑	→↑	→↑	→↓	→	↑↑	→↑	30–50%
Exogenous androgen administration (Testosterone)	++	+/–	→	→↑	↑↑	→	→	→↓	→↓	→	→↑	NK

[a]Modified from ref. 3.

[b](+), present; (++), present in severe form; (–), absent; (→), normal; (↑), elevated; (↓), decreased.

[c]CAH, congenital adrenal hyperplasia; IR, insulin resistance (lipoatrophic diabetes, leprechaunism, Rabson-Mendenhall, Kahn types A and B insulin resistance); T2DM, diabetes mellitus type 2; CS, Cushing's syndrome; PCO, polycystic ovaries; NK, not known; 17OHPG, 17-hydroxy-progesterone; E2, estradiol; Δ_4, androstenedione; DHEAS, dehydroepiandrosterone sulfate; LH, luteinizing hormone; FSH, follicle stimulating hormone; SHBG, sex hormone-binding globulin.

207

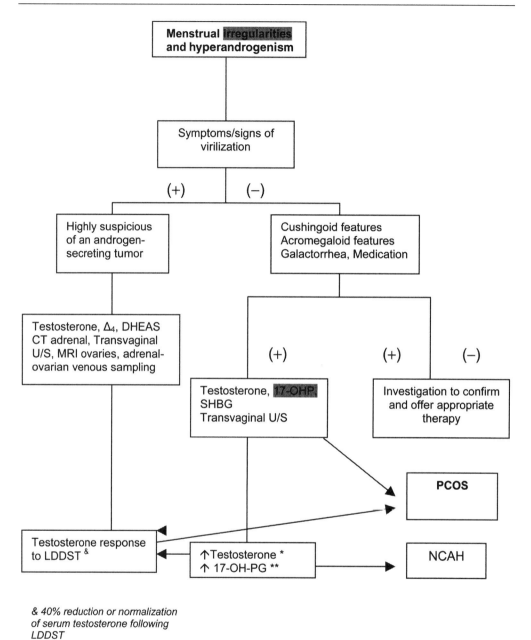

Fig. 2. Proposed investigational algorithm for the exclusion of secondary causes of PCOS. * Testosterone levels (200 ng/dL) (7 nmol/L). ** 17-OH-PG levels (3 ng/mL). LDDST: low-dose dexamethasone suppression test (0.5 mg every 6 hours for 48 hours). NCAH: Non classic congenital adrenal hyperplasia.

In cases of high clinical and biochemical suspicion of an androgen-producing tumor, computerized tomography imaging of the adrenals identifies adrenal tumors and transvaginal ultrasonography or magnetic resonance imaging ovarian tumors (7,17,21). In the very unusual cases, where imaging studies are negative, venous catheterization and sampling to demonstrate a testosterone or other androgen gradient can be of value, although this requires particular experience and expertise *(25)*.

Late-onset CAH is clinically indistinguishable from PCOS and the diagnosis is based on either basal morning or stimulated early follicular 17-OH-PG measurements *(7,17)*. A circulating level of 17-OH-PG greater than 3 ng/mL obtained during the follicular phase warrants further evaluation by an ACTH stimulation test *(7,17,21)*. Because there is a wide variation in the prevalence of this disorder among different ethnicities, this should always be considered when patients from a high-risk population are evaluated. In cases of inconclusive results, genetic analysis for particular mutations may provide important diagnostic information.

Patients with CS can be distinguished from patients with PCOS from their distinct clinical picture *(30)*. In cases with subtle disease without the typical clinical features of CS, measurement of urinary free cortisol (UFC) only may not suffice to distinguish them from patients with PCOS, who may also have mildly raised UFC *(73)*. In such cases, the degree of cortisol suppression following the administration of 1 mg of dexamethasone offers high sensitivity and specificity in identifying patients with CS, as they fail to obtain adequate cortisol suppression *(73)*. Biochemical evidence of hypercortisolism and hyperandrogenism without the clinical features of CS suggests the presence of glucocorticoid resistance and/or alterations of glucocorticoid metabolism *(17,42)*. Although patients with glucocorticoid resistance fail to achieve adequate cortisol suppression to dexamethasone administration they do retain normal cortisol circadian rhythm and may have a relevant family history. However, the final diagnosis may have to rely on genetic screening *(42)*.

Clinical signs of acromegaly and hyperprolactinemia should be looked for, particularly when low SHBG but relatively normal androgen levels are found *(3)*. Prolactin and insulin growth factor-I levels should be measured, and a GH suppression test performed, when indicated *(3)* (Table 2). Pituitary magnetic resonance imaging with gadolinium enhancement usually demonstrates the presence of a pituitary tumor in the majority of patients. Stigmata of insulin resistance and dyslipidemia (acanthosis nigricans and xanthomata) indicate the presence of severe insulin resistance, whereas an oral glucose tolerance test may confirm the diagnosis of T2DM or GDM in the relevant clinical setting. A detailed history can also reveal other underlying abnormalities or the intake of medications related to the development of PCOS.

CONCLUSIONS

The great majority of women with hyperandrogenism and chronic anovulation have PCOS. However, the clinical, endocrinologic and ultrasonographic features are not specific to PCOS, and can be found in a number of other disorders, particularly when associated with insulin resistance and hyperinsulinemia. Although the majority of these disorders exhibit distinct clinical history and phenotype a high index of clinical suspicion is required in the relevant clinical setting to identify such cases and distinguish them from PCOS. This is particularly important in cases of androgen-secreting tumors and/or systemic disorders such as CS and acromegaly, which need to be diagnosed promptly to choose the most effective treatment and minimize short and long-term morbidity.

FUTURE AVENUES

PCOS is a complex and heterogenous disorder exhibiting a wide spectrum of non-specific clinical, biochemical and radiological features shared by a number of other disorders. Further research is required to delineate the exact underlying pathophysiologic mechanisms and develop sensitive and specific markers that suggest the diagnosis and the severity of the disorder.

KEY POINTS

PCOS is the most common endocrine disorder of women within the reproductive age range that runs a chronic course. However, before making the diagnosis a number of disorders with similar clinical, biochemical, and radiological features need to be considered as a number of them may be life threatening and require urgent management.

REFERENCES

1. Franks S. Polycystic ovary syndrome. N Engl J Med 1995;333:853–861.
2. Balen AH, Conway GS, Kaltsas G, et al. Polycystic ovary syndrome: the spectrum of the disorder in 1741 patients. Hum Reprod 1995;10:2107–2111.
3. Kaltsas GA, Isidori AM, Besser GM, Grossman AB. Secondary forms of polycystic ovary syndrome. Trends Endocrinol Metab 2004;15:204–210.
4. O'Driscoll JB, Mamtora H, Higginson J, Pollock A, Kane J, Anderson DC. A prospective study of the prevalence of clear-cut endocrine disorders and polycystic ovaries in 350 patients presenting with hirsutism or androgenic alopecia. Clin Endocrinol (Oxf) 1994;41:231–236.
5. Carmina E, Lobo RA. Polycystic ovaries in Hirsute women with normal menses. Am J Med 2001; 111:602–606.
6. Lobo RA, Carmina E. The importance of diagnosing the polycystic ovary syndrome. Ann Intern Med 2000;132:989–993.
7. Barnes RB. Diagnosis and therapy of hyperandrogenism. Baillieres Clin Obstet Gynaecol 1997;11: 369–396.
8. Dunaif A. Insulin resistance and the polycystic ovary syndrome: mechanism and implications for pathogenesis. Endocr Rev 1997;18:774–800.
9. Revised 2003 consensus on diagnostic criteria and long-term health risks related to polycystic ovary syndrome (PCOS). Hum Reprod 2004;19:41–47.
10. Ehrmann DA. Polycystic ovary syndrome. N Engl J Med 2005;352:1223–1236.
11. Wood JR, Nelson VL, Ho C, et al. The molecular phenotype of polycystic ovary syndrome (PCOS) theca cells and new candidate PCOS genes defined by microarray analysis. J Biol Chem 2003;278: 26,380–26,390.
12. Roldan B, San Millan JL, Escobar-Morreale HF. Genetic basis of metabolic abnormalities in polycystic ovary syndrome: implications for therapy. Am J Pharmacogenomics 2004;4:93–107.
13. Carmina E. Genetic and environmental aspect of polycystic ovary syndrome. J Endocrinol Invest 2003; 26:1151–1159.
14. Adams JM, Taylor AE, Crowley WF Jr., Hall JE. Polycystic ovarian morphology with regular ovulatory cycles: insights into the pathophysiology of polycystic ovarian syndrome. J Clin Endocrinol Metab 2004; 89:4343–4350.
15. Conn JJ, Jacobs HS, Conway GS. The prevalence of polycystic ovaries in women with type 2 diabetes mellitus. Clin Endocrinol (Oxf) 2000;52:81–86.
16. Apridonidze T, Essah PA, Iuorno MJ, Nestler JE. Prevalence and characteristics of the metabolic syndrome in women with polycystic ovary syndrome. J Clin Endocrinol Metab 2005;90:1929–1935.
17. Kaltsas GA, Isidori AM, Kola BP, et al. The value of the low-dose dexamethasone suppression test in the differential diagnosis of hyperandrogenism in women. J Clin Endocrinol Metab 2003;88: 2634–2643.

18. Murray RD, Davison RM, Russell RC, Conway GS. Clinical presentation of PCOS following development of an insulinoma: case report. Hum Reprod 2000;15:86–88.

19. Glinthorg D, Henriksen JE, Andersen M, et al. Prevalence of endocrine diseases and abnormal glucose tolerance tests in 340 Caucasian premenopausal women with hirsutism as the referral diagnosis. Fertil Steril 2004;82:1570–1579.

20. Azziz R, Sanchez LA, Knochenhauer ES, et al. Androgen excess in women: experience with over 1000 consecutive patients. J Clin Endocrinol Metab 2004;89:453–462.

21. Chang RJ. A practical approach to the diagnosis of polycystic ovary syndrome. Am J Obstet Gynecol 2004;191:713–717.

22. Derksen J, Nagesser SK, Meinders AE, Haak HR, van de Velde CJ. Identification of virilizing adrenal tumors in hirsute women. N Engl J Med 1994;331:968–973.

23. Miller WL. The molecular basis of premature adrenarche: an hypothesis. Acta Paediatr Suppl 1999; 88:60–66.

24. Cela E, Robertson C, Rush K, et al. Prevalence of polycystic ovaries in women with androgenic alopecia. Eur J Endocrinol 2003;149:439–442.

25. Kaltsas GA, Mukherjee JJ, Kola B, et al. Is ovarian and adrenal venous catheterization and sampling helpful in the investigation of hyperandrogenic women? Clin Endocrinol (Oxf) 2003;59:34–43.

26. Rittmaster RS. Polycystic ovary syndrome, hyperthecosis and the menopause. Clin Endocrinol (Oxf) 1997;46:129–130.

27. Icard P, Goudet P, Charpenay C, et al. Adrenocortical carcinomas: surgical trends and results of a 253-patient series from the French Association of Endocrine Surgeons study group. World J Surg 2001; 25:891–897.

28. Kaltsas GA, Korbonits M, Isidori AM, et al. How common are polycystic ovaries and the polycystic ovarian syndrome in women with Cushing's syndrome? Clin Endocrinol (Oxf) 2000;53: 493–500.

29. Lado-Abeal J, Rodriguez-Arnao J, Newell-Price JD, et al. Menstrual abnormalities in women with Cushing's disease are correlated with hypercortisolemia rather than raised circulating androgen levels. J Clin Endocrinol Metab 1998;83:3083–3088.

30. Newell-Price J, Trainer P, Besser M, Grossman A. The diagnosis and differential diagnosis of Cushing's syndrome and pseudo-Cushing's states. Endocr Rev 1998;19:647–672.

31. Penezic Z, Zarkovic M, Vujovic S, et al. Gonadotropin pulsatility in Cushing's syndrome compared with polycystic ovary syndrome. Gynecol Endocrinol 2005;20:150–154.

32. Leong GM, Mercado-Asis LB, Reynolds JC, Hill SC, Oldfield EH, Chrousos GP. The effect of Cushing's disease on bone mineral density, body composition, growth, and puberty: a report of an identical adolescent twin pair. J Clin Endocrinol Metab 1996;81:1905–1911.

33. Good C, Tulchinsky M, Mauger D, Demers LM, Legro RS. Bone mineral density and body composition in lean women with polycystic ovary syndrome. Fertil Steril 1999;72:21–25.

34. Charmandari E, Weise M, Bornstein SR, et al. Children with classic congenital adrenal hyperplasia have elevated serum leptin concentrations and insulin resistance: potential clinical implications. J Clin Endocrinol Metab 2002;87:2114–2120.

35. Chrousos GP, Loriaux DL, Mann DL, Cutler GB, Jr. Late-onset 21-hydroxylase deficiency mimicking idiopathic hirsutism or polycystic ovarian disease. Ann Intern Med 1982;96:143–148.

36. Kelestimur F, Sahin Y, Ayata D, Tutus A. The prevalence of non-classic adrenal hyperplasia due to 11 beta-hydroxylase deficiency among hirsute women in a Turkish population. Clin Endocrinol (Oxf) 1996;45:381–384.

37. Ghizzoni L, Virdis R, Vottero A, et al. Pituitary-ovarian responses to leuprolide acetate testing in patients with congenital adrenal hyperplasia due to 21-hydroxylase deficiency. J Clin Endocrinol Metab 1996;81:601–606.

38. Hague WM, Adams J, Rodda C, et al. The prevalence of polycystic ovaries in patients with congenital adrenal hyperplasia and their close relatives. Clin Endocrinol (Oxf) 1990;33:501–510.

39. Speiser PW, Serrat J, New MI, Gertner JM. Insulin insensitivity in adrenal hyperplasia due to non-classical steroid 21-hydroxylase deficiency. J Clin Endocrinol Metab 1992;75:1421–1424.

40. Silfen ME, Manibo AM, Ferin M, McMahon DJ, Levine LS, Oberfield SE. Elevated free IGF-I levels in prepubertal Hispanic girls with premature adrenarche: relationship with hyperandrogenism and insulin sensitivity. J Clin Endocrinol Metab 2002;87:398–403.

41. Bridges NA, Cooke A, Healy MJ, Hindmarsh PC, Brook CG. Ovaries in sexual precocity. Clin Endocrinol (Oxf) 1995;42:135–140.

42. Chrousos GP, Detera-Wadleigh SD, Karl M. Syndromes of glucocorticoid resistance. Ann Intern Med 1993;119:1113–1124.

43. Lamberts SW, Poldermans D, Zweens M, de Jong FH. Familial cortisol resistance: differential diagnostic and therapeutic aspects. J Clin Endocrinol Metab 1986;63:1328–1333.

44. Stewart PM, Shackleton CH, Beastall GH, Edwards CR. 5 alpha-reductase activity in polycystic ovary syndrome. Lancet 1990;335:431–433.

45. Walker EA, Stewart PM. 11beta-hydroxysteroid dehydrogenase: unexpected connections. Trends Endocrinol Metab 2003;14:334–339.

46. Rodin A, Thakkar H, Taylor N, Clayton R. Hyperandrogenism in polycystic ovary syndrome. Evidence of dysregulation of 11 beta-hydroxysteroid dehydrogenase. N Engl J Med 1994;330:460–465.

47. Pfeifer SL, Wilson RM, Gawkrodger DJ. Clearance of acanthosis nigricans associated with the HAIR-AN syndrome after partial pancreatectomy: an 11-year follow-up. Postgrad Med J 1999;75:421–422.

48. Barbieri RL, Ryan KJ. Hyperandrogenism, insulin resistance, and acanthosis nigricans syndrome: a common endocrinopathy with distinct pathophysiologic features. Am J Obstet Gynecol 1983;147:90–101.

49. Stamataki KE, Spina J, Rangou DB, Chlouverakis CS, Piaditis GP. Ovarian function in women with non-insulin dependent diabetes mellitus. Clin Endocrinol (Oxf) 1996;45:615–621.

50. Peppard HR, Marfori J, Iuorno MJ, Nestler JE. Prevalence of polycystic ovary syndrome among premenopausal women with type 2 diabetes. Diabetes Care 2001;24:1050–1052.

51. Holte J, Gennarelli G, Wide L, Lithell H, Berne C. High prevalence of polycystic ovaries and associated clinical, endocrine, and metabolic features in women with previous gestational diabetes mellitus. J Clin Endocrinol Metab 1998;83:1143–1150.

52. Kousta E, Cela E, Lawrence N, et al. The prevalence of polycystic ovaries in women with a history of gestational diabetes. Clin Endocrinol (Oxf) 2000;53:501–507.

53. Koivunen RM, Juutinen J, Vauhkonen I, Morin-Papunen LC, Ruokonen A, Tapanainen JS. Metabolic and steroidogenic alterations related to increased frequency of polycystic ovaries in women with a history of gestational diabetes. J Clin Endocrinol Metab 2001;86:2591–2599.

54. Kousta E, Efstathiadou Z, Lawrence NJ, et al. The impact of ethnicity on glucose regulation and the metabolic syndrome following gestational diabetes. Diabetologia 2005;49:1–5.

55. Galtier-Dereure F, Pujol P, Dewailly D, Bringer J. Choice of stimulation in polycystic ovarian syndrome: the influence of obesity. Hum Reprod 1997;12:88–96.

56. Kaltsas GA, Mukherjee JJ, Jenkins PJ, et al. Menstrual irregularity in women with acromegaly. J Clin Endocrinol Metab 1999;84:2731–2735.

57. Unal A, Sahin Y, Kelestimur F. Acromegaly with polycystic ovaries, hyperandrogenism, hirsutism, insulin resistance and acanthosis nigricans: a case report. Endocr J 1993;40:207–211.

58. Isik AZ, Gulekli B, Zorlu CG, Ergin T, Gokmen O. Endocrinological and clinical analysis of hyperprolactinemic patients with and without ultrasonically diagnosed polycystic ovarian changes. Gynecol Obstet Invest 1997;43:183–185.

59. Bahceci M, Tuzcu A, Bahceci S, Tuzcu S. Is hyperprolactinemia associated with insulin resistance in non-obese patients with polycystic ovary syndrome? J Endocrinol Invest 2003;26:655–659.

60. Glasow A, Breidert M, Haidan A, Anderegg U, Kelly PA, Bornstein SR. Functional aspects of the effect of prolactin (PRL) on adrenal steroidogenesis and distribution of the PRL receptor in the human adrenal gland. J Clin Endocrinol Metab 1996;81:3103–3111.

61. Tagawa N, Tamanaka J, Fujinami A, et al. Serum dehydroepiandrosterone, dehydroepiandrosterone sulfate, and pregnenolone sulfate concentrations in patients with hyperthyroidism and hypothyroidism. Clin Chem 2000;46:523–528.

62. Chattopadhyay A, Kumar V, Marulaiah M. Polycystic ovaries, precocious puberty and acquired hypothyroidism: The Van Wyk and Grumbach syndrome. J Pediatr Surg 2003;38:1390–1392.

63. Piaditis G, Angellou A, Kontogeorgos G, et al. Ectopic bioactive luteinizing hormone secretion by a pancreatic endocrine tumor, manifested as luteinized granulosa-thecal cell tumor of the ovaries. J Clin Endocrinol Metab 2005;90:2097–2103.

64. Hirshberg B, Conn PM, Uwaifo GI, Blauer KL, Clark BD, Nieman LK. Ectopic luteinizing hormone secretion and anovulation. N Engl J Med 2003;348:312–317.

65. Stanciu IN, Pitale S, Prinz RA, et al. Insulinoma presenting with hyperandrogenism: a case report and a literature review. J Intern Med 2003;253:484–489.

66. Witteles RM, Straus II FH, Sugg SL, Koka MR, Costa EA, Kaplan EL. Adult-onset nesidioblastosis causing hypoglycemia: an important clinical entity and continuing treatment dilemma. Arch Surg 2001;136:656–663.
67. Luef G, Abraham I, Haslinger M, et al. Polycystic ovaries, obesity and insulin resistance in women with epilepsy. A comparative study of carbamazepine and valproic acid in 105 women. J Neurol 2002;249:835–841.
68. Duncan S. Polycystic ovarian syndrome in women with epilepsy: a review. Epilepsia 2001;42:60–65.
69. Meo R, Bilo L. Polycystic ovary syndrome and epilepsy: a review of the evidence. Drugs 2003;63: 1185–1227.
70. Glueck CJ, Iyengar S, Goldenberg N, Smith LS, Wang P. Idiopathic intracranial hypertension: associations with coagulation disorders and polycystic-ovary syndrome. J Lab Clin Med 2003;142:35–45.
71. Isojarvi JI, Laatikainen TJ, Pakarinen AJ, Juntunen KT, Myllyla VV. Polycystic ovaries and hyperandrogenism in women taking valproate for epilepsy. N Engl J Med 1993;329:1383–1388.
72. Isojarvi JI, Rattya J, Myllyla VV, et al. Valproate, lamotrigine, and insulin-mediated risks in women with epilepsy. Ann Neurol 1998;43:446–451.
73. Putignano P, Bertolini M, Losa M, Cavagnini F. Screening for Cushing's syndrome in obese women with and without polycystic ovary syndrome. J Endocrinol Invest 2003;26:539–544.

16 Lipid Abnormalities in Polycystic Ovary Syndrome

Djuro Macut, MD, PhD

CONTENTS

Summary

Polycystic ovary syndrome (PCOS) is a complex reproductive disorder with the consequent clinical and metabolic derangements. In the natural disease course, an increased cardiovascular risk has to be anticipated in a metabolically unstable condition.

Among risk factors, dyslipidemia is certainly the most persistent with high prevalence. Consequently, it is reasonable to conclude that women with PCOS may indeed be at significantly increased risk for developing coronary heart disease. The effect of aging on the pattern of dyslipidemia in PCOS, with increase of total cholesterol and low-density lipoprotein (LDL)-cholesterol, is causing almost stable cardiovascular risk over a lifetime. Predominant observation of the most studies in women with PCOS was an elevation of LDL-cholesterol in both lean and obese patients. Decreased concentrations of total high-density lipoprotein (HDL) was found in obese patients with PCOS from the third decade of life onward, whereas triglycerides start to rise from the second decade of life in both younger and older subgroups. Prevalence of metabolic syndrome was 43–46% in women with PCOS, with lipid abnormalities as the most frequent component of the syndrome.

Women with PCOS have 7.4-fold relative risk for myocardial infarction. Different surrogate tools could be of clinical importance in evaluation of the cardiovascular derangement. Therapeutic interventions, including dietary regiments and exercise, led to amelioration of dyslipidemia, whereas some therapeutic agents, such as metformin, troglitazone, and antiobesity drugs as adjuvant therapy, did not succeed in improvement of the lipid profile. Novel intervention modalities with confirmation in longitudinal studies are needed in prospect for more specific and efficacious amelioration of lipid profile in women with PCOS.

Key Words: PCOS; lipids; metabolic syndrome; atherosclerosis; cardiovascular risk.

From: *Contemporary Endocrinology: Insulin Resistance and Polycystic Ovarian Syndrome: Pathogenesis, Evaluation, and Treatment*
Edited by: E. Diamanti-Kandarakis, J. E. Nestler, D. Panidis, and R. Pasquali © Humana Press Inc., Totowa, NJ

INTRODUCTION

Polycystic ovary syndrome (PCOS) is today acknowledged by many investigators to be the most common endocrine disorder among women of reproductive age and the major cause of anovulatory infertility *(1)*. Reproductive consequences of PCOS have been recognized for several decades, although in the last two decades, an increasing number of studies demonstrated an association between the syndrome and a characteristic metabolic disorder. That, in turn, has led to concern about the effect of PCOS on long-term health, particularly with regard to diabetes and coronary heart disease.

The central features of the metabolic disturbance are peripheral insulin resistance and hyperinsulinemia, with the evidence of causative abnormalities in both insulin action and pancreatic β-cell function *(2)*. These metabolic features, together with centripetal fat distribution, constitute a cluster of risk factors for cardiovascular disease and have been a major concern in considering the long-term management of patients with PCOS. The finding of disturbances in lipid and lipoprotein metabolism is fairly common in women with PCOS. However, interpreting the relevance of these abnormalities in terms of cardiovascular risk is not easy. First, there are inconsistencies among studies in the features of the dyslipidemia. Second, it is not yet clear how the combined risk factors translate into a real risk of developing cardiovascular disease *(3)*.

Therefore, it is necessary to address both physiological issues of the metabolism of lipoproteins and their specificities between the sexes at the onset of reproductive period and in further life, and the specific pattern of the lipid metabolism in PCOS, as the most common disorder of the female reproductive period. As previously mentioned, the role of lipids in the possible early atherosclerosis in PCOS is still controversial issue.

METABOLISM OF LIPOPROTEINS

Lipoproteins are macromolecular aggregates of lipids and apolipoproteins. Lipids can be divided into two main groups: simple and complex. The two most important simple lipids are cholesterol and fatty acids. Lipids become complex lipids when fatty acids undergo esterification to produce esters *(4,5)*.

Simple Lipids

Cholesterol is a soft waxy substance present in all cells of the body. Cholesterol is synthesized primarily in the liver and small intestine. Fatty acids are the simplest form of lipid found in the body and are an important energy source. They are present as saturated, monounsaturated, and polyunsaturated forms. Fatty acids exist freely in the plasma mostly bound to albumin, and could be stored in adipose tissue as triglycerides *(4)*.

Complex Lipids

Triglycerides are mainly stored in adipose tissue and are the main lipid currency of the body. Phospholipids are glycerol esters being an important component of the cell membrane *(4)*.

Apolipoproteins

In order for the water-insoluble lipids to be transported around the body in the aqueous medium (blood), they are aggregated with apolipoproteins to form lipoproteins. These multimolecular packages consist of a hydrophobic core containing cholesteryl esters and triglyceride, surrounded by a hydrophilic surface layer of phospholipids, proteins, and some free cholesterol. Although structurally similar, lipoproteins vary in their proportions of component molecules and the type of proteins present *(4)*.

TYPES OF LIPOPROTEINS

There are four types of lipoprotein particles. Chylomicrons and very low-density lipoproteins (VLDL) are the two triglyceride-rich lipoproteins, whereas low-density lipoprotein (LDL) and high-density lipoprotein (HDL) are the two cholesterol-rich lipoproteins.

Chylomicrons are the largest in size, lowest in density, and are not associated with atherosclerosis. They transport dietary triglyceride from the intestine to the sites of use and storage, and are cleared rapidly from the bloodstream *(4)*. Each chylomicron also contains many different apolipoproteins, including one molecule of Apo-B45 and others, such as Apo-E and Apo-CII.

VLDL particles are similar in structure to chylomicrons but are smaller. They are produced in the liver and are the main carriers of endogenous triglycerides and cholesterol to sites for use or storage. As the triglycerides are removed, the VLDL remnants continue to circulate as LDL particles. Thus, VLDL are implicated in atherosclerosis development *(4)*.

LDL particles are the principal lipoproteins involved in atherosclerosis. Oxidized LDL (OxLDL) is the most atherogenic form of LDL. They are the main carriers of cholesterol—as cholesteryl ester or free cholesterol—accounting for 60–70% of plasma cholesterol. Thus, the concentration of LDL-cholesterol provides a good estimate of the total concentration of serum cholesterol. LDL particles are remnants of VLDL particles, but they contain only a single apolipoprotein, Apo-B100 *(4,5)*.

LDL-cholesterol has been shown to be strongly associated with the development of atherosclerosis and the risk of coronary heart disease (CHD) events in patients with established CHD (history of angina pectoris, myocardial infarction, and so on) and in those without CHD. This applies to women as well as men, but in women, the general level of CHD risk is lower *(6)*. A 10% increase in LDL-cholesterol is associated with an approx 20% increase in risk for CHD *(4)*.

Most of the cholesterol present in plasma is found in LDL particles. LDL particles vary in size depending of the amount of cholesterol they contain. The smaller particles contain fewer lipids per particle and, hence, are denser than the larger particles. Smaller, denser LDL are more atherogenic than larger, buoyant particles *(4,5)*.

HDL particles are the smallest but most abundant of the lipoproteins, and contain almost one-quarter of serum cholesterol. They do not cause atherosclerosis, but actually protect against its development. This is because they return about 20–30% of cholesterol in the blood to the liver from peripheral tissue for excretion (reverse cholesterol transport). They also inhibit the oxidation of LDL and they decrease the attraction of macrophages to the artery wall. HDL particles also contain apolipoproteins, including apolipoprotein (Apo)-AI *(7)*.

There is a strong inverse association between plasma HDL-cholesterol and the risk of CHD. This has been shown in both patients with CHD and asymptomatic subjects, in men and women, and is independent of LDL-cholesterol and other risk factors.

The lower the HDL-cholesterol level, the higher the risk for CHD; a low level (<40 mg/dL, 1.0 mmol/L) increases risk and a higher level (≥60 mg/dL, 1.6 mmol/L) considered a decreased risk *(5)*. Concentrations of HDL-cholesterol tend to be low when triglycerides are high. It is thought that the HDL-cholesterol goal should be higher for women than that for men. Apo-AI is the major apolipoprotein in HDL and an elevated Apo-AI is linked to reduced risk for cardiovascular disease (CVD) *(7)*.

Controversy exists whether hypertriglyceridaemia is associated with increased risk of CVD events. However, the association is not as strong as that of LDL-cholesterol, and becomes much weaker when other risk factors are taken into account. The link between triglycerides and increased CVD risk is complex. It may reflect the athero-genic effects of the triglyceride-rich lipoproteins themselves, particularly the smaller particles. It may also mark the presence of other atherogenic risks, such as low levels of HDL, the presence of small dense LDL particles, and the presence of the metabolic syndrome (MS) *(5,7)*. In fasting plasma, triglycerides are transported in VLDL synthe-sised in the liver, and after meals are also found in chylomicrons. Catabolism of these triglyceride-rich lipoproteins produces remnant lipoproteins that have atherogenic potential.

APOLIPOPROTEINS

Apolipoproteins are the protein constituents of lipoproteins. There are eight broad groups of apolipoproteins that have currently been identified. These are designated Apo-A to F, Apo-H, and Apo-J.

Each VLDL and LDL particle contains one molecule of apolipoprotein-B100 (Apo-B), whereas each chylomicron particle contains one molecule of Apo-B40. Because there is one Apo-B molecule per particle, the level of Apo-B gives a good estimate of LDL particle number and is an important marker for atherosclerosis. Apo-AI is the major apolipoprotein in HDL and is linked to reduced CVD risk *(4,7)*.

LIPID CHANGES DURING LIFE

Determinants of Dyslipidemia in the Young

Clinical and epidemiological studies, such as the Framingham Study *(8)*, demon-strated 40 years ago that the probability of a person developing coronary artery disease (CAD), stroke, or peripheral arterial disease could be predicted years in advance by measuring a few individual characteristics that became known as risk factors. Among few conditions associated with higher risk of disease, high total serum cholesterol concentration, high LDL-cholesterol level, and low HDL-cholesterol level are undoubtedly forming the core of CVD risk *(9)*. It is known that the existence of the familial hypercholesterolemia characterized by elevated levels of total cholesterol and LDL-cholesterol from birth onward is caused by mutations in LDL receptor genes *(10)*. LDL-cholesterol levels vary between children with familial hypercholes-terolemia, partly as a result polymorphisms in the Apo ε gene. In particular, the ε4 allele is associated with higher, and the ε2 with lower, total cholesterol and LDL-cholesterol levels *(11)*. This early association strongly predisposes the early initiation of athero-genesis and premature CVD. Therefore, together with regulation of hypertension, reduction of LDL-cholesterol levels became a part of the major strategy for prevention of CAD, decreasing the probability of clinical disease manifestations in middle age and later *(12)*.

From the 1970s onward, a number of epidemiological surveys of children showed that, although the average plasma cholesterol and blood pressure levels were lower in children than in adults, a wide range of these indices existed *(13)*, influencing the attempts to control these risk factors. At that time, it was not known whether these variables were associated with the progression of atherosclerosis early in life *(14)*.

In recent years, attempts were made to answer the questions of the possible influence of gender, age, ethnic, or geographical distribution on various lipids and their possible causative development of CVD. Meta-analysis of the worldwide investigations on lipids and lipoproteins distribution in young age confirmed variations in different observed indices *(15)*.

The overall curve of cholesterol during life indicates a type of curvilinear pattern: a preadolescent peak and then a slightly inverse change are observed for both boys and girls from 3 to 12 years old being almost coincident absolute values. Beyond age 12, values for boys continue to slightly decrease to age 16, whereas for girls, they tend to increase through this age range. The curve in the late teens (16–18 years) tends to reach preteen levels for both sexes, although girls have consistently higher absolute values than boys. This pattern might reflect differences in growth and physical maturation by sex *(15)*.

Ethnic comparisons show higher mean values of total cholesterol in Caucasians and North American blacks than in Asians, North American Indians, and African blacks. It is interesting, however, how Asians and North American Indians reach similar values to black and white Americans at the end of childhood. This fact might reflect an adaptation of these adolescents to a universal lifestyle, even if they come from populations with different cultures *(15)*.

Geographical distribution suggests consistent differences between Northern European and Mediterranean countries, except for Greece, where total cholesterol levels are clearly higher than the ones observed in Spain, Italy, or Portugal. Results obtained for total cholesterol in children in the Athens study were explained in the light of recent dietary habits and overall "Westernization." These undoubted changes in lifestyle, and their consequences over time, might have an impact on the steady increase of the incidence of CVD in the Greek population over the last decades *(16)*.

DEVELOPMENT OF EARLY STAGES OF ATHEROSCLEROSIS

It was previously shown that atherosclerosis begins in childhood, with deposits of cholesterol and its esters in macrophages of the intima of large muscular and elastic arteries forming early lesions called fatty streaks that are, themselves, innocuous. In metabolically susceptible persons, lipids continue to accumulate, becoming extracellular, and together with changes in macrophages, smooth muscle, and connective tissue, proliferate toward forming a fibrous plaque or raised lesion further leading to the occlusion of the arterial vessel *(17)*.

High serum VLDL associated with high LDL-cholesterol, low HDL-cholesterol, hypertension, and hyperglycemia are associated with more rapid progression of atherosclerosis from fatty streaks to raised lesion. This transformation begins in high-risk persons in their early 20s, and the process accelerates at about 25 years of age, leading to the well-established raised lesions in their 30s. The extent of raised lesions increases with age in both men and women. Women lag behind men by about 5 years, and by age 30–34 years, have about half the extent of raised lesions. This sex difference cannot be accounted for by differences in serum lipoproteins, elevated HbA1c, hypertension, or smoking *(17)*.

Lipid Changes in Adulthood

Whereas measurement of total cholesterol, LDL-cholesterol, and HDL-cholesterol are recommended in most current cardiovascular screening algorithms in the general population *(18)*, several investigations have suggested that superior risk prediction might be achieved by alternatively measuring Apo-B and Apo-AI *(19)*. At the same time, recent guidelines have emphasized the importance of non-HDL-cholesterol as a predictor of cardiovascular risk *(18)*, whereas others have strongly advocated use of specific lipid ratios, such as total cholesterol to HDL-cholesterol, LDL-cholesterol to HDL-cholesterol, Apo-B to Apo-AI, and Apo-B to HDL-cholesterol *(20)*. A recently published prospective study on more than 15,000 initially healthy women in the United States older than 45 years analyzed hazard ratios for first-ever major cardiovascular events according to baseline levels of each lipid marker. It was shown that hazard ratios for future cardiovascular events for those in the extreme quintiles were 1.62 for LDL-cholesterol, 1.75 for Apo-AI, 2.08 for total cholesterol, 2.32 for HDL-cholesterol, 2.50 for Apo-B, and 2.51 for non-HDL-cholesterol, whereas hazard ratios for the lipid ratios were 3.01 for Apo-B to Apo-AI, 3.18 for LDL-cholesterol to HDL-cholesterol, and 3.81 for total cholesterol to HDL-cholesterol ratio. Overall, it was suggested that the magnitude of the association was greater for Apo-B than for either total cholesterol or LDL-cholesterol *(21)*.

Another follow-up of initially healthy middle aged subjects indicated strong CHD prediction based on LDL-cholesterol, HDL-cholesterol, triglycerides, and Lp(a), with relative risks of 4.9 in men and 13.5 in women when non-lipid risk factors are included. The same study showed that lipid concentrations were associated with greater relative risk for CHD in women (4.7) than men (2.1). Association of triglycerides and CHD in women persisted in analyses that included LDL-cholesterol, HDL-cholesterol and Lp(a). Overall conclusion was that LDL-cholesterol, HDL-cholesterol, triglycerides, and Lp(a), without additional apolipoproteins or lipid subfractions, provide substantial CHD prediction with much higher relative risk in women than men. This study also indicated that CHD risk is elevated for approx 40% for every millimole per liter increment in LDL-cholesterol, and that optimal LDL values are those of less than 100 mg/dL in both women and men *(22)*.

An important proatherogeneric relation exists between triglycerides and LDL-cholesterol particle size. It was confirmed both in children and adult populations that triglyceride concentration was the strongest independent predictor of LDL particle size and accounted for approx 33% of the variance in LDL particle size *(23)*. In fact, small, dense LDL has been detected even in early childhood and has been shown to be associated with obesity and/or hypertriglyceridemia *(24)*. Gender differences in LDL particle size, as reported in adults (diameters in females greater than those in males) may develop with age, possibly because of the increasing influence of sex hormones after puberty *(25)*. Another important proatherogenic factor seems to be the lipid ratio of

Apo-B to Apo-AI. Besides the known predictive power of Apo-AI and Apo-B when considered alone in prediction of CHD, their ratio is strongly associated with incident cardiovascular events independent of the non-lipid covariates typically used in global risk prediction scores *(21)*.

Surrogate Indices of Cardiovascular Disease

Endothelial dysfunction and increased intima-media thickness (IMT) have both been validated as predictive for future CVD *(26)*. Familial-hypercholesterolemic children had a fivefold more rapid increase of carotid arterial wall IMT during childhood years than their affected siblings. This increase led to a significant deviation in terms of IMT values from the age of 12 years onward. LDL-cholesterol proved a strong and independent predictor of carotid artery IMT, highlighting the pivotal role of this lipoprotein for the development of atherosclerosis in this condition, already at a young age *(27)*.

Arterial calcium can be detected with simple radiographic techniques, but newer, more sophisticated techniques may be more useful in detecting and quantifying coronary calcium. The electronbeam computed tomography calcium score has been shown to correlate strongly with the number of segments showing 20% or greater stenosis by angiography and with total plaque burden in autopsy *(28)*.

Cardiac magnetic resonance (CMR) imaging of the carotid arteries is a relatively new in vivo technique that has the ability to characterize carotid plaque. CMR imaging also may be used to identify qualitative changes in plaque and monitor the impact of lipid-lowering therapy on plaque size and regression *(29)*.

Left ventricular hypertrophy may be determined by echocardiography and may predict cardiovascular events independent of age, diabetes, smoking, or lipid profile. It was shown that the relative risk of CVD for every increase of 50 g/m in left ventricular mass is higher in women (1.57) than in men (1.49) *(30)*.

Ankle–brachial index (ABI) is measured as the ratio of the systolic blood pressure in the ankle (posterior tibial and dorsalis pedis arteries) over the systolic blood pressure in the arm (brachial artery). Studies in patients with diabetes found that ABI cannot be reliably used for the diagnosing peripheral artery disease or monitor the response to lipid-lowering therapy. Because patients with diabetes often have increased stiffness of the arterial wall, impaired blood flow may be present even when the ABI is normal *(31)*.

Brachial artery reactivity testing represents a technique that could estimate release of nitric oxide from activated endothelial cells in response to shear stress. This vasodilatory reaction is among the earliest physiological impairments during the development of atherosclerosis and the time leading up to anatomic obstruction. This test may be useful in detecting early changes in the endothelium before more obvious atherosclerotic changes happen in younger people who are at risk of developing glucose impairment or the MS *(32)*.

LIPID CHANGES IN WOMEN WITH PCOS

Prevalence of Dyslipidemia in PCOS

Dyslipidemia may be the most common metabolic abnormality in PCOS, although the type and extent of the findings have been variable. Borderline or high prevalence of an abnormal lipid level in PCOS approaches 70% according to the National Cholesterol

Education Program (NCEP) guidelines *(33)*. Thus, a substantial portion of women with PCOS may have a completely normal circulating lipid profile. In large published studies of lipid levels in women with PCOS, mean levels of total cholesterol, LDL-cholesterol, HDL-cholesterol, and triglycerides—for the most part—fall within normal limits as determined by NCEP cutoffs *(33,34–38)*.

Influence of Aging and Body Mass Index

The effect of aging on the pattern of dyslipidemia in PCOS was well analyzed in the studies by Talbott et al. *(36,39)*. In the first study, they included patients mostly in their fourth decade of life *(36)*. This study was extended with repeat lipid phenotyping in the cohort, and changes over time have been reported in the second study *(39)*. This subsequent report showed persistent lipid abnormalities in the PCOS population. Important observation was that the slope of increasing total cholesterol and LDL-cholesterol with age is almost flat for the patients with PCOS, while it was increasing in controls. These data were interpreted as an increased cardiovascular risk over a lifetime, given the prolonged exposure of women with PCOS from an early age to abnormal circulating lipid values. Another alternative interpretation is that the stability of the risk profile into and through menopause in women with PCOS may offer them a favorable risk profile compared with the worsening levels of the control population *(40)*. Recently, a study on postmenopausal women in their sixth decade of life pointed out that of those who had PCOS earlier in life, 85% had characteristic dyslipidemia of the MS (i.e., high triglycerides and/or low HDL-cholesterol) *(41)*.

Even younger studied populations of women with PCOS showed aggravation in assessed cardiovascular risk factors with ageing *(42)*, therefore confirming previous observation. A significant increase in lipids and a positive correlation with age was found for total cholesterol, LDL-cholesterol, triglycerides, and Apo-B at the transition from the second to third decade of life in obese women with PCOS. Therefore, it seems that the youngest obese population with PCOS represents a cohort with potential cardiovascular disease in adulthood *(42)*.

Obesity is common among women with PCOS and is affected by a variety of factors, including genetics, physical activity, and diet. It has been estimated to affect more than 50% of women with PCOS *(43)*. Body fat distribution, especially an android or centripetal fat distribution, has been independently associated with cardiovascular mortality, being a stronger predictor than obesity alone *(44)*. This could be a case in women with PCOS because of the frequently present android habitus *(33,36)*. The most consistently reported alterations in obese compared to non-obese PCOS subgroups included elevated triglycerides and lower HDL-cholesterol *(45–47)*. Therefore, controlling for the confounder of obesity has become the standard for analysis of lipids in women with PCOS who have parallel analyses in both obese and non-obese groups, with more abnormal levels usually found in the obese groups *(38,45,46,48)*.

Total Cholesterol and LDL-Cholesterol Subfractions in PCOS

Although concentrations of total cholesterol in plasma were inconsistently higher, the predominant observation of the most studies in women with PCOS was an elevation of LDL-cholesterol in both lean and obese patients *(33,39)*. However, a simple quantitative measurement of LDL concentration may be misleading because LDL do not exist as homogenous particles. Rather, LDL comprises several subpopulations of particles differing in lipid composition, density, size, and atherogenic potential. LDL particles that are small and dense (LDL-III) are considered to be more atherogenic than larger buoyant LDL species (LDL-I and LDL-II) and their presence in circulation, even in the presence of normal LDL-cholesterol concentration, is associated with a higher incidence of CAD *(49)*. Study in women with PCOS found an existence of higher concentrations and proportion of the more atherogenic LDL-III subfraction. This difference in LDL subfractions occurs despite similar and normal total LDL-cholesterol concentrations, indicating that in women with PCOS measurement of total LDL-cholesterol may not reflect true magnitude of vascular risk *(50)*.

Accordingly, measurement of the LDL particle size showed that women with PCOS had smaller diameter LDL particles. Obtained correlation of LDL particle size and decreased sex hormone-binding globulin as a marker of androgen excess, could lead to the conclusion that androgen excess may have an early modifying effect on LDL size in women with PCOS *(51)*.

Besides density and particle size of LDL-cholesterol, metabolic change of LDL-cholesterol by increased oxidation could also indicate a higher atherogenic potential of such modified particles. An elevated level of OxLDL have been detected in patients with CAD *(52,53)* establishing the role of OxLDL in the initiation and progression of atherosclerosis. Among others, clinical predictor of elevated OxLDL levels was shown to be female sex *(52)*.

HDL-Cholesterol Composition in PCOS

A number of studies have demonstrated that women with PCOS had significantly lower levels of HDL-cholesterol particles that were thought to be the strongest metabolic predictor of CHD *(39,45,54)*. In contrast, others described HDL-cholesterol levels that were higher than normal, although this difference was not significant after adjusting for other variables, such as body mass index (BMI) and fasting insulin *(33)*.

Variations in HDL-cholesterol concentration have to be evaluated in the light of age and BMI of patients, and the compositional derangements of HDL. Age distribution showed a decreased level of total HDL to be started from the third decade of life onward. The same tendency was found for HDL2 from the fourth decade of life *(39)*. This led to the conclusion that changes in HDL concentration, as with all lipid parameters, are time-dependent and, at the same time, accumulating during time. When BMI was taken into consideration, only obese women with PCOS showed decreased HDL concentrations in comparison with obese controls *(48)*. It was suggested that PCOS selectively reduced HDL. Hepatic lipase and phospholipids transfer protein remove lipid from HDL, and are induced by obesity and consequent insulin resistance *(37)*. Therefore, obesity represents the common soil for various metabolic derangements, including unfavorable lipid depletion of HDL. The absence of dyslipidemia in the lean subjects with PCOS further supports the conclusion of the majority of other studies on the importance of obesity *(34,46)*.

Relation to Triglycerides

As previously mentioned, elevated triglycerides represent common and fairly consistent lipid disturbance in women with PCOS *(39,42,45,50,55)*. Elevated triglycerides in women with PCOS compared with controls were consistently found with ageing, starting from the second decade of life. Triglycerides were predicted in both younger and older groups with PCOS when the multiple linear regression analyses were performed *(39)*. Relation of triglycerides to obesity, insulin resistance, and MS in PCOS is addressed in the next paragraph.

There is considerable evidence suggesting that postprandial triglyceride response has a significant role in the development of CAD. The only study that analyzed this issue found a significant postprandial triglyceride and insulin response in patients with the higher waist-to-hip ratio and BMI. Interestingly, the non-obese subgroup of patients with PCOS had a higher postprandial triglyceride response than did non-obese controls, suggesting that even in absence of obesity, intrinsic lipid abnormality could be present in this condition *(56)*. It was shown that extended postprandial lipemia may increase the uptake of triglyceride-rich remnants by arterial cells, and thus increasing atherogenic intracellular accumulation of cholesterol esters *(57)*. The demonstration of an amplified postprandial triglyceride response in overweight and normal-weight women with PCOS completes the list of metabolic abnormalities in this condition, contributing to increase the risk for CAD *(56)*.

Prevalence of the MS in PCOS

The major components of the MS include atherogenic dyslipidemia, increased blood pressure, elevated glucose, and a prothrombotic state. Atherogenic dyslipidemia generally manifests as elevated serum triglycerides, increased LDL particles, and decreased HDL-cholesterol levels. There is growing evidence that each of the components of the MS is independently atherogenic. At the same time, each of these risk factors suggests the presence of other components of MS. It was supposed that insulin resistance at the cellular level appears to play a pathogenic role in MS *(58)*.

The NCEP ATP III guidelines recently confirmed by American Diabetes Association/European Association for the Study of Diabetes Statement *(59,60)* define the MS as a condition with three or more of the following abnormalities: waist circumference in females greater than 88 cm, fasting serum glucose greater than 6.1 mmol/L (>5.6 mmol/L may be applicable), fasting serum triglycerides greater than 1.7 mmol/L, serum HDL-cholesterol less than 1.3 mmol/L in women, and blood pressure higher than 130/85 mmHg. Data from NHANES III survey gave the prevalence of the MS among women in age groups 20–29 and 30–39 years of 6 and 15%, respectively *(59)*.

Recently published studies found a prevalence of 43–46% of MS in women with PCOS *(61,62)*. Obtained prevalence of MS among examined women with PCOS under age 40 was comparable to the 44% rate reported for women aged 60–69 years in the general population. Such high prevalence of the MS in young women with PCOS is in relation to the verified manifest increased atherosclerosis *(63)*, and a sevenfold increased risk of myocardial infarction *(64)* in these patients.

Further analyses of the data showed that majority (91%) of women with PCOS had at least one abnormality of the MS present, 69% had two or more of the abnormalities, whereas only 9% did not have any abnormality. Lipid abnormalities are the most frequent abnormalities within the components of the MS, namely with the prevalence of low HDL-cholesterol in 42% and elevated triglycerides in 32% of the patients with PCOS having MS *(62)*.

What is the important outcome of the study of Apridonidze et al. is that higher prevalence of the MS in women with PCOS compared with the respective US female population persisted even when stratified by both age and BMI. It could be concluded that obesity itself interferes with the age-related differences in the prevalence of the MS between women with PCOS and general population. It was suggested that the presence of PCOS by itself confers increased risk of the MS, perhaps secondary to the intrinsic insulin resistance of PCOS. The specific type of insulin resistance in PCOS was explained by altered visceral lipolysis, different from that observed in visceral fat cells in the insulin resistance syndrome, and that occurs at the level of adrenergic receptors *(65)*.

Cardiovascular Risk in PCOS

It is known that major modifiable CVD risk factors in women with PCOS are hypertension, dyslipidemia, obesity, diabetes, smoking, and physical inactivity. On the other hand, non-modifiable CVD risk factors include age, gender, and family history of premature CVD *(40)*.

The study of Wild et al. *(66)* gave the prevalence of CHD and CHD risk factors in women with history of PCOS. In spite of insignificant prevalence for overall CHD (4.7 vs 4.0%), patients with PCOS in comparison to controls had significantly higher prevalence of high cholesterol (30 vs 17%), obesity (26 vs 18%), diabetes (6.9 vs 3.0%), cerebrovascular disease (3.1 vs 1.2%), and family history of CHD (47 vs 40%). On the other hand, it was shown that women with PCOS have 7.4-fold relative risk for myocardial infarction *(64)*.

Among cardiovascular risk factors, hypertension was occasionally noted in women with PCOS *(67)*, and large clinical studies of women with PCOS have reported normal mean baseline blood pressures *(33,39)*. Increases in blood pressure, when noted, are usually mild and of questionable clinical significance. This may be because hypertension is a late-developing sequelae of insulin resistance and is not found in reproductive-age women with PCOS *(67)*.

Dyslipidemia seems to be the most common metabolic abnormality in PCOS with the variable extent of the findings, as it was analyzed before. As it was mentioned previously, LDL subclasses are among important predictors of CVD *(49)*. Small, dense LDL particles have been associated with an increased relative risk of CAD that ranges from three- to sevenfold *(68)*. It was shown in women with PCOS the existence of small-diameter LDL particles that could itself promote atherosclerosis, and contribute to the higher risk of CVD reported in this syndrome *(51)*.

Obesity is common among women with PCOS and is estimated to affect more than 50% of the patients, but it is suggested that this is a possible underestimation, at least for the US population *(43)*. Android or centripetal fat distribution has been independently associated with cardiovascular mortality and was stronger predictor than obesity alone in women with PCOS *(44)*.

Impaired glucose tolerance or type 2 diabetes appears to be common among women with PCOS. It was reported a prevalence of around 10% in women with PCOS of the reproductive age, with a further 30% with impaired glucose tolerance. A strong family history of type 2 diabetes was found in families of women with PCOS affecting about one-third of the first-degree relatives *(69)*.

SURROGATE TOOLS IN DIAGNOSIS

Functional and morphological cardiovascular changes in women with PCOS were demonstrated using different surrogate tools.

Vascular lesions on coronary arteries had been diagnosed by coronary angiography. It was shown that coronary calcification was more prevalent in PCOS with odds ratio 2.52. When electron beam computed tomography was used, the prevalence of coronary artery calcification in premenopausal women with PCOS is significantly greater than community-dwelling women (odds ratio 5.9), and is similar to that of men of comparable age *(70)*. Lesions on the carotid artery assessed by ultrasound measurement of IMT showed that women with PCOS had greater IMT, leading to the increased risk of subclinical atherosclerosis in their 40s *(71)*. Talbott and collaborators in further studies found that among patients with PCOS, 7.2% had a plaque index of three or greater compared with 0.7% in controls *(72)*. Among women 45 years of age or older, PCOS cases had significantly greater mean IMT compared with controls (0.78 vs 0.7 mm), suggesting that lifelong exposure to an adverse cardiovascular risk profile in women with PCOS may lead to premature atherosclerosis, and that PCOS–IMT association could be explained in part by weight and fat distribution *(72)*. These results should be considered because carotid change could be a potential surrogate marker for potential CAD, and arteriosclerotic changes do not necessarily lead to more events.

Dysfunctional endothelium represents an early step in the process of atherosclerosis. Data on the functional assessment of the endothelium are partly controversial. Examining vascular function of the brachial artery in women with PCOS, some authors did not find more frequent endothelial dysfunction in the brachial artery in women with PCOS compared with healthy controls *(73)*. However, others found on the same vascular model that a functional defect exists in women with PCOS who have insulin resistance and elevated serum endothelin-1 levels *(74)* in subjects that were non-hypertensive and without overt cardiovascular disease.

Left ventricular hypertrophy have been shown to be independently associated with an increased cardiovascular risk. Recently, it was suggested that young women with PCOS have increased left ventricular mass and diastolic dysfunction, neither of which is weight dependent *(55)*. These data are in concert with the previous functional studies, demonstrating that women with PCOS are candidates for early cardiovascular disease.

Implications for Preventive Regiments and Therapeutic Modalities

It was previously explained the relation of age and the formation of fibrous plaque leading to further development of cardiovascular disease. The relation of the risk factors to the increasing extent of plaque formation at about age 25 suggests that risk factor modification should be initiated by about age 15–20 years *(17)*. When talking about hyperlipidemia as the most prevalent risk factor for CVD, the age at which HMG-CoA (3-hydroxy-3-methylglutaryl coenzyme A) reductase inhibitors (statin) therapy should be initiated it is still unclear. The age of the youngest patients with familial hypercholesterolemia in the studies assessing trials with statins varied from 4 to 10 years, which indicates that patients can be treated safely from an age of 10 years onward *(75)*.

Reduction of unfavorable lipid profile in women with PCOS was analyzed through various preventive and therapeutic trials. In adult women with PCOS, even modest weight loss of less than 10% of initial body weight has been shown to reduce hyperlipidemia among other followed clinical and biochemical parameters *(76)*. However, apart from the assessment of the efficacy of dietary or exercise regiments in women with PCOS with lipid derangements, there are no literature data concerning therapeutic or preventive use of any antilipemic drugs for the treatment of dyslipidemic states in this potential CVD risk group.

Metformin, an insulin-senzitizing agent, is one of the most investigated drugs in women with PCOS with the aim to examine possible effectiveness in improving clinical and biochemical features of the syndrome. Recent meta-analysis on the overall benefits of metformin in PCOS found the positive effect on reduction of fasting insulin, ovulation, and pregnancy rates. When the effect on lipids was assessed, total cholesterol showed no evidence of a significant decrease on therapy with metformin, but LDL cholesterol was significantly reduced in the metformin group, with a weighted mean difference of –0.44. No evidence was found of an effect on HDL cholesterol or on triglyceride concentrations from metformin *(77)*.

Another insulin-senzitizer, troglitazone, showed a significant dose–response improvement in ovulation and circulating hyperandrogenemia or hirsutism *(78)*, resembling on the same effects obtained with widely used metformin. On the other hand, there was a favorable, but non-significant, increase of HDL-cholesterol, decrease of LDL-cholesterol, and a trend toward decreased circulating triglycerides, only in patients treated with a high dose of troglitazone. It was concluded that treatment with troglitazone in women with PCOS may have minimal impact on lipids as a cardiovascular risk factor. Therefore, it should not be assumed that this treatment alone is sufficient to treat dyslipidemia in women with PCOS *(79)*.

In the recent years, treatment of obesity by various means gave another possibility for the reduction of cardiovascular risk factors. Orlistat is a potent and irreversible inhibitor of gastric and pancreatic carboxylester lipase, inhibiting the digestion of dietary triglycerides and decreasing the absorption of lipids. Despite previous results on the favorable effect of orlistat on improvement in lipid parameters associated with weight loss *(22–25)*, a similar effect on lipids in women with PCOS was not obtained *(80)*. Sibutramine, an inhibitor of norepinephrine and serotonin reuptake, is another anti-obesity drug that results in enhancing satiety and weight reduction. As with orlistat, sibutramine was investigated for possible metabolic intervention in PCOS. It was shown that treatment with sibutramine alone led to the decrease of plasma triglycerides giving this novel agent a possible influence on the reduction of cardiovascular risk in PCOS *(81)*.

A study by Ciampelli et al. showed the potential influence of acipimox, an anti-lipolytic nicotinic acid analog that decreases plasma free fatty acids, on the lipid levels in women with PCOS *(82)*. The results of this pilot study showed that, in spite of its influence on glucose and insulin metabolism, administration of acipimox did not influence insulin sensitivity in women with PCOS but led to decrease of cholesterol, LDL-cholesterol, and triglycerides in obese subjects. Therefore, this agent appeared as a potential additional therapeutic agent to ameliorate atherogenic lipid profile in PCOS.

CONCLUSION

PCOS is a complex reproductive disorder that cause with the affected women numerous clinical as well as metabolic derangements. From the metabolic point of view, PCOS is an insulin-resistant state closely related to the MS having decreased HDL-cholesterol and increased triglyceride levels, as a pattern of dyslipidemia that is frequently found in PCOS. In the natural disease course, a cardiovascular disease risk has to be anticipated in a metabolically unstable condition. From the previously mentioned facts in favor to cardiovascular disease risk, certainly there is substantial evidence that known risk factors for CHD (obesity, type 2 diabetes, dyslipidemia, hypertension) are generally more prevalent in women with PCOS than respective controls. Among there risk factors, dyslipidemia is certainly the most persistent with high prevalence. Consequently, it is reasonable to conclude that women with PCOS may indeed be at significantly increased risk for developing CHD. Most of the therapeutic interventions, to ameliorate dyslipidemia and decrease cardiovascular risk, were based on dietary regiments and improvement of physical activity. In the past decade, some therapeutic agents like metformin, troglitazone, and antiobesity drugs as adjuvant therapy, did not succeed in attaining satisfactory decrease of unfavorable lipids. Therefore, novel intervention modalities with confirmation in longitudinal studies are needed in prospect for more specific and efficacious amelioration of lipid profile in women with PCOS.

FUTURE AVENUES OF INVESTIGATION

Cardiovascular endocrinology represents an exciting field for the analyzes of molecular basis for the development of atherosclerosis and CVD. Dyslipidemia in PCOS, much like PCOS, is a heterogeneous disorder. Together with other traditional and non-traditional CHD risk factors, PCOS represents a multifactorial condition that significantly increases risk for developing CHD. There is still an unsolved investigation field, as well as a concomitant therapeutic intervention possibility in investigation of possible pathophysiological mechanisms of influence of deranged lipid milieu on the initiation of process of atherosclerosis. Therefore, the years to come will bring us further exploration of the interrelation between various cytokines and lipid particles or their structural derangements in the process of plaque formation. Novel technologies would possibly enable us to follow this process by the novel diagnostic surrogate tools or to examine surrogate endpoints for CHD, not only by examining the endothelial function-ality but also endothelial structure during the process of incorporation of various lipids metabolic intermediaries on predilection sites. The next period will possibly bring the PCOS closer to the MS with subpopulation specificities. Therefore, analyses of lipids as the most prevalent risk factor for CHD, also present in the core of MS, should be one of the essential tools in the further larger epidemiological studies.

In the therapeutic modalities, longitudinal studies are needed in PCOS population, presumably on the potential role of statins and other novel antilipemic drugs in the treatment of the subclinical or premature CVD in women over 40 years of age, and even in youngest subpopulation of subjects with the potential to develop CVD. Genetic therapeutic intervention, although in early development, could be a possible therapeutic tool at least for patients with the familial forms of hypercholesterolemia.

KEY POINTS

• Apart from the known reproductive consequences, PCOS has been characterized as a metabolic disorder. That has led to concern about the long-term health consequences, particularly with regard to diabetes and coronary heart disease.

- Dyslipidemia seems be the most common metabolic abnormality in PCOS. Borderline or high prevalence of an abnormal lipid concentrations in PCOS approaches 70% according to the NCEP guidelines. In addition, of those postmenopausal women who had PCOS earlier in life, 85% had characteristic dyslipidemia of the metabolic syndrome, high triglycerides, and/or low HDL-cholesterol.
- The effect of aging on the pattern of dyslipidemia in PCOS, with increasing of total cholesterol and LDL-cholesterol, is causing almost stable cardiovascular risk over a lifetime.
- The most consistently reported alterations in obese compared to non-obese PCOS subgroups included elevated triglycerides and lower HDL-cholesterol.
- The predominant observation of most studies in women with PCOS was an elevation of LDL-cholesterol in both lean and obese patients. In the structure, an existence of higher concentrations and proportion of the more atherogenic LDL-III subfraction was confirmed together with smaller diameter of LDL particles.
- Decreased concentrations of total HDL was found from the third decade of life onward. Only obese women with PCOS showed decreased HDL concentrations.
- Elevated triglycerides concentration is common lipid disturbance in women with PCOS being consistently found with ageing, starting from the second decade of life, but found in both younger and older subgroups.
- Prevalence of the metabolic syndrome (MS) was 43–46% in women with PCOS. This prevalence of MS among patients with PCOS under the age 40 was comparable to the 44% rate reported for women aged 60–69 in the general population. Lipid abnormalities are the most frequent within the components of the MS, namely with the prevalence of low HDL-cholesterol in 42% and elevated triglycerides in 32% of the patients with PCOS who have MS.
- Analyzing cardiovascular risk, PCOS in comparison with controls had significantly higher prevalence of high cholesterol, obesity, diabetes, cerebrovascular disease, and family history of CHD. Women with PCOS have 7.4-fold relative risk for myocardial infarction.
- Different surrogate tools, i.e., coronary angiography assessing coronary calcification, ultrasound measurement of intima-media thickness, brachial artery flow for assessment of vascular endothel dysfunction, or left ventricular mass and diastolic function evaluation could be of clinical importance in evaluation of the cardiovascular derangement.
- Therapeutic interventions, including dietary regiments and exercise, led to amelioration of dyslipidemia, whereas some therapeutic agents such as metformin, troglitazone, and anti-obesity drugs as adjuvant therapy, did not succeed in improvement of lipid profile.

REFERENCES

1. Franks S. Medical progress article: polycystic ovary syndrome. N Engl J Med 1995;333:853–861.
2. Dunaif A. Insulin resistance and the polycystic ovary syndrome: mechanism of action and implications for pathogenesis. Endocr Rev 1996;18:774–800.
3. Franks S. Are women with polycystic ovary syndrome at increased risk of cardiovascular disease? Too early to be sure, but not too early to act! Am J Med 2001;111:665–666.
4. Stamler J, Daviglus ML, Garside DB, Dyer AR, Greenland P, Neaton JD. Relationship of baseline serum cholesterol levels in 3 large cohorts of younger men to long-term coronary, cardiovascular, and all-cause mortality and to longevity. JAMA 2000;284:311–318.
5. Expert panel on detection, evaluation, and treatment of high blood cholesterol in adults. JAMA 2001;285:2486–2497.
6. Wood D, De Backer G, Faergeman O, Graham I, Mancia G, Pyorala K. Prevention of coronary heart disease in clinical practice: recommendations of the Second Joint Task Force of European and other Societies on Coronary Prevention. Atherosclerosis 1998;140:199–270.

7. Assmann G, Gotto AM Jr. HDL cholesterol and protective factors in atherosclerosis. Circulation 2004;109(23 Suppl 1):III8–III14.

8. Dawber TR, Moore FE, Mann GV. Coronary heart disease in the Framingham Study. Am J Public Health 1957;47:4–23.

9. Pooling Project Research Group. Relationship of blood pressure, serum cholesterol, smoking habit, relative weight and ECG abnormalities to incidence of major coronary events: final report of the Pooling Project. J Chronic Dis 1978;31:201–306.

10. Goldstein JL, Hobbs HH, Brown HS. Familial hypercholesterolemia. In: Scriver CR, Beaudet AL, Sly WS, Valle D, eds. The Metabolic Basis of Inherited Disease. 8th ed. New York: McGraw-Hill, 2001, pp. 2863–2913.

11. Davignon J, Gregg RE, Sing CF. Apolipoprotein E polymorphism and atherosclerosis. Arteriosclerosis 1988;8:1–21.

12. Forrester JS, Merx NB, Bush TL, et al. Task Force 4. Efficacy of risk factor management. J Am Coll Cardiol 1996;27:964–1047.

13. Berenson GS, Srinivasan SR, Nicklas TA, Webber LS. Cardiovascular risk factors in children and early prevention of heart disease. Clin Chem 1988;34:B115–B122.

14. Donahue RP, Jacobs DR Jr, Sidney S, Wagenknecht LE, Albers JJ, Hulley SB. Distribution of lipoproteins and apolipoproteins in young adults. The Cardia Study. Artzzeriosclerosis 1989;9:656–664.

15. Brotons C, Ribera A, Perich RM, et al. Worldwide distribution of blood lipids and lipoproteins in childhood and adolescence: a review study. Atherosclerosis 1998;139:1–9.

16. Adamopoulos PN, Papamechael C, Frida H, et al. Precursors of atherosclerosis in a random sample from a Hellenic population: the Athens Study. J Cardiovasc Risk 1995;2:525–531.

17. McGill HC Jr, McMahan CA. Determinants of atherosclerosis in the young. Pathobiological Determinants of Atherosclerosis in Youth (PDAY) Research Group. Am J Cardiol 1998;82(10B): 30T–36T.

18. Executive Summary of The Third Report of The National Cholesterol Education Program (NCEP) Expert Panel on Detection, Evaluation, And Treatment of High Blood Cholesterol In Adults (Adult Treatment Panel III). JAMA 2001;285:2486–2497.

19. Lamarche B, Moorjani S, Lupien PJ, et al. Apolipoprotein A-I and B levels and the risk of ischemic heart disease during a five-year follow-up of men in the Quebec Cardiovascular Study. Circulation 1996;94:273–278.

20. Kinosian B, Glick H, Garland G. Cholesterol and coronary heart disease: predicting risks by levels and ratios. Ann Intern Med 1994;121:641–647.

21. Ridker PM, Rifai N, Cook NR, Bradwin G, Buring JE. Non-HDL cholesterol, apolipoproteins A-I and B100, standard lipid measures, lipid ratios, and CRP as risk factors for cardiovascular disease in women. JAMA 2005;294:326–333.

22. Sharrett AR, Ballantyne CM, Coady SA, et al. Coronary heart disease prediction from lipoprotein cholesterol levels, triglycerides, lipoprotein(a), apolipoproteins A-I and B, and HDL density subfractions: the Atherosclerosis Risk in Communities (ARIC) Study. Circulation 2001;104:1108–1113.

23. Kojima M, Kanno Y, Yamazaki Y, Koyama S, Kanazawa S, Arisaka O. Association of low-density lipoprotein particle size distribution and cardiovascular risk factors in children. Acta Paediatrica 2005;94:281–286.

24. Freedman DS, Bowman BA, Otvos JD, Srinivasan SR, Berenson GS. Levels and correlates of LDL and VLDL particle size among children: Bogalusa Heart Study. Atherosclerosis 2000;152:441–449.

25. Freedman DS, Bowman BA, Srinivasan SR, Berenson GS, Otvos JD. Distribution and correlates of high density lipoprotein subclasses among children and adolescents. Metabolism 2001;50:370–376.

26. Schachinger V, Britten MB, Zeiher AM. Prognostic impact of coronary vasodilator dysfunction on adverse long- term outcome of coronary heart disease. Circulation 2000;101:1899–1906.

27. Wiegman A, Groot E, Hutten BA, et al. Arterial intima-media thickness in children heterozygous for familial hypercholesterolemia. Lancet 2004;363:369–370.

28. Schmermund A, Denktas AE, Rumberger JA, et al. Independent and incremental value of coronary artery calcium for predicting the extent of angiographic coronary artery disease: comparison with cardiac risk factors and radionuclide perfusion imaging. J Am Coll Cardiol 1999;34:777–786.

29. Corti R, Fuster V, Fayad ZA, et al. Lipid lowering by simvastatin induces regression of human atherosclerotic lesions: two years' follow-up by high-resolution noninvasive magnetic resonance imaging. Circulation 2002;106:2884–2887.

30. Levy D, Garrison RJ, Savage DD, Kannel WB, Castelli WP. Prognostic implications of echocardio-graphically determined left ventricular mass in the Framingham Heart Study. N Engl J Med 1990;322:1561–1566.

31. Suzuki E, Egawa K, Nishio Y, et al. Prevalence and major risk factors of reduced flow volume in lower extremities with normal ankle-brachial index in Japanese patients with type 2 diabetes. Diabetes Care 2003;26:1764–1769.

32. Rajaram V, Pandhya S, Patel S, et al. Role of surrogate markers in assessing patients with diabetes mellitus and the metabolic syndrome and in evaluating lipid-lowering therapy. Am J Cardiol 2004;93(11A):32C–48C.

33. Legro RS, Kunselman AR, Dunaif A. Prevalence and predictors of dyslipidemia in women with poly-cystic ovary syndrome. Am J Med 2001;111:607–613.

34. Wild RA, Painter PC, Coulson PB, Carruth KB, Ranney GB. Lipoprotein lipid concentrations and cardiovascular risk in women with polycystic ovary syndrome. J Clin Endocrinol Metab 1985;61:946–951.

35. Norman RJ, Hague WM, Masters SC, Wang XJ. Subjects with polycystic ovaries without hyperandro-genaemia exhibit similar disturbances in insulin and lipid profiles as those with polycystic ovary syndrome. Hum Reprod 1995;10:2258–2261.

36. Talbott E, Guzick D, Clerici A, et al. Coronary heart disease risk factors in women with polycystic ovary syndrome. Arterioscler Thromb Vasc Biol 1995;15:821–826.

37. Robinson S, Henderson AD, Gelding SV, et al. Dyslipidaemia is associated with insulin resistance in women with polycystic ovaries. Clin Endocrinol (Oxf) 1996;44:277–284.

38. Mather KJ, Kwan F, Corenblum B. Hyperinsulinemia in polycystic ovary syndrome correlates with increased cardiovascular risk independent of obesity. Fertil Steril 2000;73:150–156.

39. Talbott E, Clerici A, Berga SL, et al. Adverse lipid and coronary heart disease risk profiles in young women with polycystic ovary syndrome: results of a case-control study. J Clin Epidemiol 1998;51:415–422.

40. Legro RS. Polycystic ovary syndrome and cardiovascular disease: a premature association? Endocr Rev 2003;24:302–312.

41. Margolin E, Zhornitzki T, Kopernik G, Kogan S, Schattner A, Knobler H. Polycystic ovary syndrome in post-menopausal women—marker of the metabolic syndrome. Maturitas 2005;50:331–336.

42. Macut D, Mićić D, Cvijović G, et al. Cardiovascular risk in adolescent and young adult obese females with polycystic ovary syndrome (PCOS). J Pediatr Endoccrinol Metab 2001;14(Suppl. 5):1353–1359.

43. Legro RS, Finegood D, Dunaif A. A fasting glucose to insulin ratio is a useful measure of insulin sen-sitivity in women with polycystic ovary syndrome. J Clin Endocrinol Metab 1998;83:2694–2698.

44. Folsom AR, Kaye SA, Sellers TA, Hong CP, Cerhan JR, Potter JD. Body fat distribution and 5-year risk of death in older women. JAMA 1993;269:483–487.

45. Conway GS, Agrawal R, Betteridge DJ, Jacobs HS. Risk factors for coronary artery disease in lean and obese women with the polycystic ovary syndrome. Clin Endocrinol (Oxf) 1992;37:119–125.

46. Holte J, Bergh T, Berne C, Lithell H. Serum lipoprotein lipid profile in women with the polycystic ovary syndrome: relation to anthropometric, endocrine and metabolic variables. Clin Endocrinol (Oxf) 1994;41:463–471.

47. Silfen ME, Denburg MR, Manibo AM, et al. Early endocrine, metabolic, and sonographic character-istics of polycystic ovary syndrome (PCOS): comparison between nonobese and obese adolescents. J Clin Endocrinol Metab 2003;88:4682–4688.

48. Rajkhowa M, Neary RH, Kumpatla P, et al. Altered composition of high density lipoproteins in women with the polycystic ovary syndrome. J Clin Endocrinol Metab 1997;82:3389–3394.

49. Crouse JR, Parks JS, Schey HM, Kahl FR. Studies of low density lipoprotein molecular weight in human beings with coronary artery disease. J Lipid Res 1985;26:566–574.

50. Pirwany IR, Fleming R, Greer IA, Packard CJ, Sattar N. Lipids and lipoprotein subfractions in women with PCOS: relationship to metabolic and endocrine parameters. Clin Endocrinol (Oxf) 2001;54:447–453.

51. Dejager S, Pichard C, Giral P, et al. Smaller LDL particle size in women with polycystic ovary syn-drome compared to controls. Clin Endocrinol (Oxf) 2001;54:455–462.

52. Mosca L, Rubenfire M, Tarshis T, Tsai A, Pearson T. Clinical predictors of oxidized low-density lipoprotein in patients with coronary artery disease. Am J Cardiol 1997;80:825–830.

53. Holvoet P, Mertens A, Verhamme P, et al. Circulating oxidized LDL is a useful marker for identifying patients with coronary artery disease. Arterioscler Thromb Vasc Biol 2001;21:844–848.

54. Legro RS, Blanche P, Krauss RM, Lobo RA. Alterations in low-density lipoprotein and high-density lipoprotein subclasses among Hispanic women with polycystic ovary syndrome: influence of insulin and genetic factors. Fertil Steril 1999;72:990–995.

55. Orio F Jr., Palomba S, Spinelli L, et al. The cardiovascular risk of young women with polycystic ovary syndrome: an observational, analytical, prospective case-control study. J Clin Endocrinol Metab 2004;89:3696–3701.

56. Velázquez E, Bellabarba GA, Mendoza S, Sánchez L. Postprandial triglyceride response in patients with polycystic ovary syndrome: relationship with waist-to-hip ratio and insulin. Fertil Steril 2000;74:1159–1163.

57. Nestel PJ, Billinton T, Bazelmans J. Metabolism of human triacylglycerol-rich lipoproteins in rodent macrophages: capacity for interaction at beta-VLDL receptor. Biochim Biophys Acta 1985;837:314–324.

58. Grundy SM. Hypertriglyceridemia, insulin resistance, and the metabolic syndrome. Am J Cardiol 1999;83:25F–29F.

59. Third Report of the National Cholesterol Education Program (NCEP). Expert panel on detection, evaluation, and treatment of high blood cholesterol in adults (Adult Treatment Panel III) final report. Circulation 2002;106:3143–3421.

60. Kahn R, Buse J, Ferrannini E, Stern M. The metabolic syndrome: time for a critical appraisal. Diabetologia 2005;48:1684–1699.

61. Glueck CJ, Papanna R, Wang P, Goldenberg N, Sieve-Smith L. Incidence and treatment of metabolic syndrome in newly referred women with confirmed polycystic ovarian syndrome. Metabolism 2003;52:908–915.

62. Apridonidze T, Essah PA, Iuorno MJ, Nestler JE. Prevalence and characteristics of the metabolic syndrome in women with polycystic ovary syndrome. J Clin Endocrinol Metabol 2005;90:1929–1935.

63. Reaven GM. Insulin resistance, hyperinsulinemia, hypertriglyceridemia, and hypertension. Parallels between human disease and rodent models. Diabetes Care 1991;14:195–202.

64. Dahlgren E, Janson PO, Johansson S, Lapidus L, Oden A. Polycystic ovary syndrome and risk for myocardial infarction. Evaluated from a risk factor model based on a prospective population study of women. Acta Obstet Gynecol Scand 1992;71:599–604.

65. Ek I, Arner P, Rydén M, et al. A unique deffect in the regulation of visceral fat cell lipolysis in the polycystic ovary syndrome as an early link to insulin resistance. Diabetes 2002;51:484–492.

66. Wild S, Pierpoint T, McKeigue P, Jacobs H. Cardiovascular disease in women with polycystic ovary syndrome at long-term follow-up: a retrospective cohort study. Clin Endocrinol (Oxf) 2000;52:595–600.

67. Sampson M, Kong C, Patel A, Unwin R, Jacobs HS. Ambulatory blood pressure profiles and plasminogen activator inhibitor (PAI-1) activity in lean women with and without the polycystic ovary syndrome. Clin Endocrinol (Oxf) 1996;45:623–629.

68. Austin MA, Breslow JL, Hennekens CH, Buring JE, Willett WC, Krauss RM. Low-density lipoprotein subclass patterns and risk of myocardial infarction. JAMA 1988;260:1917–1921.

69. Legro RS, Kunselman AR, Dodson WC, Dunaif A. Prevalence and predictors of risk for type 2 diabetes mellitus and impaired glucose tolerance in polycystic ovary syndrome: a prospective, controlled study in 254 affected women. J Clin Endocrinol Metab 1999;84:165–169.

70. Christian RC, Dumesic DA, Behrenbeck T, Oberg AL, Sheedy PF 2nd, Fitzpatrick LA. Prevalence and predictors of coronary artery calcification in women with polycystic ovary syndrome. J Clin Endocrinol Metab 2003;88:2562–2568.

71. Guzick DS, Talbott EO, Sutton-Tyrrell K, Herzog HC, Kuller LH, Wolfson SK Jr. Carotid atherosclerosis in women with polycystic ovary syndrome: initial results from a case–control study. Am J Obstet Gynecol 1996;174:1224–1229.

72. Talbott EO, Guzick DS, Sutton-Tyrrell K, et al. Evidence for association between polycystic ovary syndrome and premature carotid atherosclerosis in middle-aged women. Arterioscler Thromb Vasc Biol 2000;20:2414–2421.

73. Mather KJ, Verma S, Corenblum B, Anderson TJ. Normal endothelial function despite insulin resistance in healthy women with the polycystic ovary syndrome. J Clin Endocrinol Metab 2000;85:1851–1856.

74. Orio F Jr., Palomba S, Cascella T, et al. Early impairment of endothelial structure and function in young normal-weight women with polycystic ovary syndrome. J Clin Endocrinol Metab 2004;89:4588–4593.

75. Rodenburg J, Vissers MN, Wiegman A, Trip MD, Bakker HD, Kastelein JJP. Familial hypercholesterolemia in children. Curr Opin Lipidol 2004;15:405–411.

76. Moran LJ, Noakes M, Clifton PM, Tomlinson L, Galletly C, Norman RJ. Dietary composition in restoring reproductive and metabolic physiology in overweight women with polycystic ovary syndrome. J Clin Endocrinol Mctab 2003;88:812 819.
77. Lord JM, Flight IHK, Norman RJ. Metformin in polycystic ovary syndrome: systematic review and meta-analysis. BMJ 2003;327:951–915.
78. Azziz R, Ehrmann D, Legro RS, et al. Troglitazone improves ovulation and hirsutism in the polycystic ovary syndrome: a multicenter, double blind, placebo-controlled trial. J Clin Endocrinol Metab 2001;86:1626–1632.
79. Legro RS, Azziz R, Ehrmann D, Gmerek Fereshetian A, O'Keefe M, Ghazzi MN, for the PCOS/Troglitazone Study Group. Minimal response of circulating lipids in women with polycystic ovary syndrome to improvement in insulin sensitivity with troglitazone. J Clin Endocrinol Metab 2003;88:5137–5144.
80. Jayagopal V, Kilpatrick ES, Holding S, Jennings PE, Atkin SL. Orlistat is as beneficial as metformin in the treatment of polycystic ovarian syndrome. J Clin Endocrinol Metab 2005;90:729–733.
81. Sabuncu T, Harma M, Harma M, Nazligul Y, Kilic F. Sibutramine has a positive effect on clinical and metabolic parameters in obese patients with polycystic ovary syndrome Fertil Steril 2003;80: 1199–1204.
82. Ciampelli M, Leoni F, Lattanzi F, Guido M, Apa R, Lanzone A. A pilot study of the long-term effects of acipimox in polycystic ovarian syndrome. Human Reprod 2002;17:647–653.

17 Fat Distribution and Adipose Products in Polycystic Ovary Syndrome

Enrico Carmina, MD

CONTENTS

Summary

Because adipose tissue is a complex endocrine organ that secretes many substances with profound effects on metabolism and the cardiovascular (CV) system, most obese subjects have an increased CV risk. However, 20% of obese subjects are metabolically healthy, and many studies suggest that fat distribution, in particular abdominal fat excess, is the most important factor that determines a secretion of adipose products that may increase CV risk.

Women with polycystic ovary syndrome (PCOS) present abdominal fat excess that is related to their androgen and/or insulin excess and that is present not only in the obese, but also in overweight and normal weight patients. Altered fat distribution plays an important role in the increased metabolic and CV risk observed in PCOS.

Key Words: PCOS; hyperandrogenism; visceral fat; subcutaneous fat; cardiovascular risk.

INTRODUCTION

Increased body weight is a classic characteristic of polycystic ovary syndrome (PCOS) *(1)*. Although the prevalence of obesity in women with PCOS may vary in different countries *(2)*, even in countries with relatively low prevalence of obesity, as in Southern Italy, patients with PCOS have a much higher body weight than the normal population

From: *Contemporary Endocrinology: Insulin Resistance and Polycystic Ovarian Syndrome:*
Pathogenesis, Evaluation, and Treatment
Edited by: E. Diamanti-Kandarakis, J. E. Nestler, D. Panidis, and R. Pasquali © Humana Press Inc., Totowa, NJ

of similar age, and patients with normal body weight represent only about 30% of all patients with PCOS, the others being overweight or obese *(3,4)*.

However, for many years there was little understanding of the possible role of increased body weight on metabolic risk of patients with PCOS. In fact, initial studies focused on the role of adipose tissue in regulating sex hormone balance *(5,6)*, whereas only recently the effects of increased body fat on metabolic and cardiovascular (CV) risk of PCOS have received attention *(3)*. On the other hand, it has been known for several years that PCOS is characterized by an accumulation of fat in some particular districts, the so-called "visceral obesity" *(7)*. This finding in the general population has been associated with an increased risk for type 2 diabetes and CV disease *(8,9)*, and it has raised the possibility that visceral obesity may play the main role in determining insulin resistance and metabolic risk in women with PCOS *(10)*.

This chapter discusses the evidence that adipose tissue is an endocrine organ, but that fat distribution is very important in modifying the hormonal activity of fat. In particular, this chapter focuses on hormones and products that may have a role in CV morbidity induced by obesity. Finally, the role of fat distribution on CV risk of PCOS is discussed.

ENDOCRINE FUNCTION OF ADIPOSE TISSUE

It is now clear that adipose tissue is a complex endocrine organ that secretes hormones, cytokines, free fatty acids, and various proteins that have profound effects on metabolism and CV system *(11)*.

The first adipose hormone discovered was leptin *(12)*, a 146-amino acid protein that acts mostly as a signaling factor from adipose tissue to the central nervous system, serving as a metabolic indicator of energy sufficiency *(13)*. Leptin has many other, not well-understood, functions including regulation of timing of puberty *(14)* and inhibition of bone development *(15)*. It has been suggested that leptin increases blood pressure *(16)* and promotes the inflammatory response, which is involved in the development of atherosclerosis *(17)*, but no conclusive data regarding these effects of leptin in humans have been presented.

The adipose tissue also produces adiponectin *(18)*, a large protein with 244 amino acids that plays a major role in preventing or counteracting the development of diet-induced insulin resistance *(19)*. Moreover, adiponectin seems to have an important function in protecting endothelial cells from injury *(18)*. In humans, adiponectin has been shown to enhance endothelium-dependent and -independent vasodilatation, reduce levels of tumor necrosis factor (TNF)-α, and suppress the inflammatory effects of TNF-α on endothelial cells *(18,19)*. Surprisingly, adiponectin is decreased in obesity *(20)*—probably because of negative feedback driven by hyperinsulinemia—and its reduction may contribute to the effects of obesity on insulin resistance and endothelial disease. A further adipocyte factor, resistin, which, at least in animals, has been linked to insulin resistance *(21)*, may influence blood pressure and increase vascular endothelial inflammation *(22)*. However, resistin values are not increased in obesity *(23,24)* and the role of this adipose hormone in humans is still unclear.

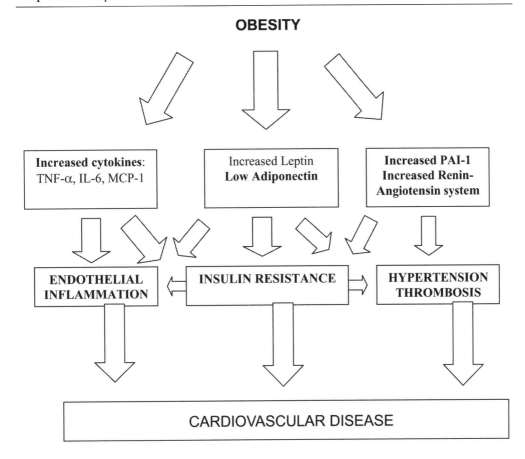

Fig. 1. Effect of adipose products on cardiovascular risk.

Adipose tissue is also a very important producer of different cytokines, including TNF-α, interleukin (IL)-6, and monocyte chemoattractant protein (MCP)-1 *(11)*, and in obese subjects the circulating levels of these products are elevated. Increased production of cytokines from adipose tissue probably plays an important role in determining endothelial inflammation and atherosclerosis. TNF-α also seems to be important in inducing insulin resistance by impairing insulin signaling both directly (by activation of serine kinases) and indirectly (by increasing mobilization of free fatty acids [FFA]) *(25,26)*.

Adipose tissue is an important source of plasminogen activator inhibitor (PAI)-1 *(27)*, a factor correlated to insulin resistance and that may be important in thrombogenesis because it is the main inhibitor of fibrinolysis.

Finally, adipocytes also produce components of the renin–angiotensin system, in particular angiotensinogen and angiotensin-converting enzyme *(28)*, and may raise aldosterone levels and favor the appearance of hypertension.

In summary, the combined effect of an increase of adipose products may determine insulin resistance, vascular inflammation, hypertension, and thrombogenesis and, therefore, it is not surprising that obesity is associated with increased CV morbidity and mortality. In Fig. 1, a scheme of main adipose tissue products and their effects on CV system is presented.

DIFFERENTIAL HORMONAL ACTIVITY OF SUBCUTANEOUS AND VISCERAL FAT

Although obesity is associated with increased insulin resistance and CV risk, a subgroup of obese individuals does not display these characteristics *(29)*. At least 20% of obese individuals have normal or high insulin sensitivity and favorable CV risk profiles *(30)*. These findings have reemphasized the old notion that abdominal or male-type obesity is more often associated with metabolic and CV diseases than the gluteo-femoral or female-type fat distribution *(31)*. In fact, waist circumference has proven useful in predicting metabolic and CV risk of obese subjects and has been included in most diagnostic definitions of metabolic syndrome *(32)*. However, the finding of abdominal obesity does not distinguish between accumulation of visceral (omentum and mesentery) and subcutaneous abdominal fat. Using imaging techniques such as computed tomography, it has been demonstrated that the accumulation of visceral fat is strongly associated with insulin resistance and CV morbidity *(31,33)*. Even excessive subcutaneous abdominal fat is associated to insulin resistance *(31)*, whereas gluteo-femoral subcutaneous fat has little metabolic activity and may be protective *(34)*. Therefore, it is clear that obese subjects who have a preferential increase of visceral fat have a greater metabolic and CV risk *(31)*.

Because of the different metabolic consequences of visceral and subcutaneous (at least gluteo-femoral) fat, several studies have tried to understand the differences in metabolic and hormonal activity of the different adipose tissues *(35)*. Many studies have been presented, and it is actually difficult to understand what the real relevance of the different proposed mechanisms is. Most likely, a main role is played by increased production of FFA by visceral fat. It has been shown that excessive influx of FFA into the muscle and the liver leads to insulin resistance *(32)*. In fact, visceral fat has a higher lipolytic activity compared with the subcutaneous adipose tissue because of a higher sensitivity to catecholamines and a lower sensitivity to the antilipolytic effect of insulin *(31)*. Therefore, the contribution of visceral fat to the circulating levels of FFA is much higher than that expected on the basis of its mass. Moreover, only FFA coming from visceral fat tissue are directly drained by the portal venous system to the liver.

Other mechanisms may be equally important. In fact, many differences in production of hormones and cytokines between subcutaneous and visceral fat have been shown. In particular, visceral fat produces more resistin, IL-6, TNF-α, and PAI-1, whereas subcutaneous fat produces more leptin, and adiponectin *(1,34–36)*. Differences also exist between abdominal and gluteo-femoral subcutaneous fat. Because of this, abdominal obesity is characterized by lower levels of adiponectin and by higher levels of some cytokines; this profile may increase insulin resistance and determine endothelial inflammation and CV morbidity. In Table 1, a summary of the differential production of adipose factors in abdominal and gluteofemoral obesity is presented.

FAT DISTRIBUTION AND ADIPOSE PRODUCTS IN OBESE WOMEN WITH PCOS

For many years, it has been known that abdominal-type obesity is largely prevalent in obese women with PCOS *(7,37)*. Because of this, it is not surprising that the same

Table 1
Differences in Adipose Products Between Gluteo-Femoral
and Abdominal Obesity

	Gluteo-femoral obesity	Abdominal obesity
FFA	+	+++
Leptin	+++	+++
Adiponectin	+++	+
Resistin	+	+
TNF-α	+	+++
IL-6	+	+++
PAI-1	++	+++

alterations of abdominal obesity have been found in obese patients with PCOS. In fact, compared with normal-weight controls, obese women with PCOS present lower levels of adiponectin *(38)*, increased levels of PAI-1 *(39)*, increased activity of the angiotensin–renin system *(40,41)*, and increased cytokines and inflammatory markers *(42)*. However, obese patients with PCOS present two important differences in comparison with non-PCOS women with abdominal obesity: more severe insulin resistance and higher androgen levels. Because both of these factors may affect adipocyte function, it is important to understand whether there are differences in production of adipose factors between obese women with PCOS and non-PCOS women with abdominal obesity. However, only in a few studies, obese women with PCOS have been matched against obese women with similar fat distribution. In most studies, obese controls have been matched only according to age and body mass index (BMI) and because of this, it still unclear what differences there are, if any, between obese patients with PCOS and non-PCOS women with abdominal obesity. The available data indicate the following:

1. Adipose hormones. There are no differences in levels of leptin, resistin, and adiponectin between obese women with PCOS and obese controls *(43)*. Therefore, it is unlikely that the hormonal activity of obese patients with PCOS is different from obese patients with similar fat distribution.
2. Cytokines. There are no differences in levels of TNF-α, IL-6, and markers of inflammation between obese women with PCOS and obese controls *(42,44)*. Therefore, it is unlikely that the cytokine production of obese patients with PCOS is different from obese patients with similar fat distribution.
3. PAI-1. A significant increase in PAI-1 levels between obese women with PCOS and obese controls has been reported by some authors *(45)*, but not by others *(46)*.
4. Angiotensin–renin system. Very few data are available.

Most likely, when frank obesity is present, most obese subjects present some degree of abdominal or visceral obesity. It has been reported that in women, an abdominal visceral fat area higher than 100 cm^2 is sufficient to determine significant alterations of CV risk profile *(47)*. Therefore, when using sufficiently large control groups, it is probably acceptable to compare obese patients with PCOS with obese controls.

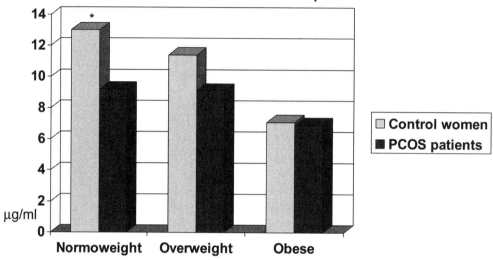

Adiponectin serum levels in control women and PCOS patients

* p<0.05 versus normoweight women with PCOS

Fig. 2. Adiponectin serum levels in normal controls and patients with polycystic ovary syndrome matched by body mass index. (Modified from ref. *43*.)

FAT DISTRIBUTION AND ADIPOSE PRODUCTS IN NORMOWEIGHT PCOS

The situation is different in normal-weight patients with PCOS. In fact, comparing these patients with controls of similar BMI, the following pattern of adipose products has been found:

1. Adipose hormones. There are no differences in serum leptin and resistin, but adiponectin is significantly lower in normoweight women with PCOS than in controls matched for BMI but not for fat distribution *(43)* (Fig. 2).
2. Cytokines. Normoweight patients with PCOS have higher serum levels of TNF-α than normoweight women *(42)*.
3. PAI-1. Normoweight women with PCOS have higher serum levels of PAI-1 than normoweight women *(48,49)*.
4. Angiotensin–renin system. Normoweight women with PCOS have higher levels of renin and components of the system than normoweight controls *(40)*.

All these data suggest that normoweight women with PCOS have an increased production of adipose factors that is similar to that found in abdominal obesity. At the moment, no sure explanation of this phenomenon can be given. Several hypotheses may be considered. Because these patients present a mild hyperinsulinemia and insulin resistance *(50)*, it is possible that it is sufficient to alter the adipocyte function. Consistent with this hypothesis, serum PAI-1 correlates with serum insulin in normoweight women with PCOS *(48,49)*. However, in the same group of patients, no correlation was found between serum adiponectin *(43)* or serum TNF-α *(42)* and serum insulin levels or indices of insulin resistance. Even in overweight patients with PCOS, no correlation between serum adiponectin and serum insulin or indices of insulin resistance was found *(43)*.

Hyperisulinemia alone is likely not sufficient to explain adipocyte dysfunction of normoweight women with PCOS. A partially different possibility is that normoweight and overweight women with PCOS have some degree of visceral (or, in general, abdominal) obesity that is not sufficient to determine an increase of body weight so to be defined "obesity," but that may be sufficient to determine increased production of some adipose products *(43)*. On the other hand, visceral obesity and hyperinsulinemia are generally strictly related, and it is always difficult to separate the two phenomena.

Data on fat distribution in normoweight patients with PCOS are very few. Recently, it has been shown that normoweight patients with PCOS have higher fat accumulation in visceral deposit *(51)* and lower subcutaneous fat in gluteo-femoral area *(52)*. Although greater experiences and studies on the correlation between fat distribution and adipose products in normoweight and overweight women with PCOS are needed, the available data suggest that in these patients, increased abdominal fat participates in the increased CVD risk. Of course, insulin resistance is linked to the increase of visceral fat, and it may contribute to the adipocyte dysfunction of normoweight women with PCOS.

CONCLUSIONS

Abdominal obesity determines an excessive adipose production of hormones, cytokines, and other products that are associated with an increased risk for CV disease. Patients with PCOS present excessive fat accumulation in abdominal and visceral deposits, and it plays an important role in their increased risk for CV disease. This altered fat distribution is present not only in the obese, but also in overweight and in normoweight patients with PCOS.

FUTURE AVENUES

Although it is clear that excessive abdominal fat has an important role in increased CVD and metabolic risk of PCOS, it remains to be determined what is the cause of this kind of fat distribution. Is it the consequence of insulin resistance or of androgen excess or of both? Is it genetically determined or is a consequence of environmental factors? What is the relationship between the number or the size of fat cells and their function? What is the relationship between adipose function and insulin resistance? Many questions remain unanswered, and the resolution of these questions will be very important in understanding the pathogenesis of PCOS.

KEY POINTS

1. Fat distribution is very important in determining metabolic and CVD risk.
2. Visceral fat is linked to increased CVD risk; however, excessive subcutaneous abdominal fat may alter the risk factors.
3. Excessive abdominal and visceral fat is present not only in obese patients with PCOS but also, although to lesser degree, in overweight and normoweight patients with PCOS.

4. Altered fat distribution may, at least in part, explain the increased risk of overweight and normoweight PCOS.

5. Abdominal obesity of women with PCOS may be linked to hyperinsulinemia and/or androgen excess.

REFERENCES

1. Stein IF, Leventhal ML. Amenorrhea associated with bilateral polycystic ovaries. Am J Obstet Gynecol 1935;29:181–186.

2. Carmina E, Legro R, Stamets K, Lowell J, Lobo RA. Differences in body weight between American and Italian women with the polycystic ovary syndrome: influence of the diet. Hum Reprod 2003; 11:2289–2293.

3. Carmina E, Longo RA, Rini GB, Lobo RA. Phenotypic variation in hyperandrogenic women influences the finding of abnormal metabolic and cardiovascular risk parameters. J Clin Endocrinol Metab 2005;90:2545–2549.

4. Carmina E. Relative prevalence of different androgen excess disorders in 950 women referred because clinical hyperandrogenism. J Clin Endocrinol Metab 2006;91:2–6.

5. Siiteri PK. Adipose tissue as a source of hormones. Am J Clin Nutr 1987;45:227–282.

6. Pasquali R, Casimirri F. The impact of obesity on hyperandrogenism and polycystic ovary in premenopausal women. Clin Endocrinol (Oxf) 1993;39:1–16.

7. Bringer J, Lefebrve P, Boulet F, et al. Body composition and regional fat patterning in polycystic ovarian syndrome: relationship to hormonal and metabolic profiles. Ann NY Acad Sci 1993; 687:115–123.

8. Peiris A, Sothmann M, Hoffman R, et al. Adiposity, fat distribution and cardiovascular risk. Ann Intern Med 1989;110:867–872.

9. Williams MJ, Hunter GR, Kekes-Szabo T, Snyder S, Treuth MS. Regional fat distribution in women and risk for cardiovascular disease. Am J Clin Nutr 1997;65:855–860.

10. Lord J, Wilkin T. Polycystic ovary syndrome and fat distribution: the central issue? Hum Fertil (Camb) 2002;5:67–71.

11. Kershaw EE, Flier JS. Adipose tissue as an endocrine organ. J Clin Endocrinol Metab 2004; 89:2548–2556.

12. Zhang Y, Proenca R, Maffei M, Barone M, Leopold L, Friedman JM. Positional cloning of the mouse obese gene and its human homologue. Nature 1994;372:425–432.

13. Friedman JM, Halaas JL. Leptin and the regulation of body weight in mammals. Nature 1998; 395:763–770.

14. Hileman SM, Pierroz DD, Flier JS. Leptin, nutrition and reproduction: timing is everything. J Clin Endocrinol Metab 2000;85:804–807.

15. Cock TA, Auwers J. Leptin: cutting the fat of the bone. Lancet 2003;362:1572–1574.

16. Matsumura K, Tsuchihashi T, Fujii K, Iida M. Neural regulation of blood pressure by leptin and the related peptides. Regul Pep 2003;114:79–86.

17. Fantuzzi G, Faggioni R. Leptin in the regulation of immunity, inflammation and hematopoiesis. J Leuk Biol 2003;68:437–446.

18. Goldstein BJ, Scalia R. Adiponectin: a novel adipokine linking adipocytes and vascular function. J Clin Endocrinol Metab 2004;89:2563–2568.

19. Fernandez-Real JM, Lopez-Bermejo A, Casamitjana R, Ricart W. Novel interactions of adiponectin with the endocrine system and inflammatory parameters. J Clin Endocrinol Metab 2003;88: 2714–2718.

20. Ryan AS, Berman DM, Nicklas BJ, et al. Plasma adiponectin and leptin levels, body composition and glucose utilization in adult women with wide ranges of age and obesity. Diabetes Care 2003;26:2283–2288.

21. Steppan CM, Bailey ST, Bhat S, et al. The hormone resistin links obesity to diabetes. Nature 2001; 409:307–312.

22. Kawanami D, Maemura K, Takeda N, et al. Direct reciprocal effects of resistin and adiponectin on vascular endothelial cells: a new insight into adipocytokine-endothelial interactions. Biochem Biophys Res Comm 2004;314:415–419.

23. Lee JH, Chan L, Yiannakouris N, et al. Circulating resistin levels are not associated with obesity or insulin resistance in humans and are not regulated by fasting leptin administration: cross-sectional

and interventional study in normal, insulin-resistant and diabetic subjects. J Clin Endocrinol Metab 2003;88:4848–4856.

24. Silha JV, Krsek M, Skrha JV, Sucharda P, Nyomba BL, Murphy LJ. Plasma resistin, adiponectin and leptin levels in lean and obese subjects: correlations with insulin resistance. Eur J Endocrinol 2003; 149:331–335.

25. Ruan H, Lodish HT. Insulin resistance in adipose tissue: direct and indirect effects of tumor necrosis factor-α. Cytokine Growth Factor Rev 2003;14:447–455.

26. Hotamisligil GS. Inflammatory pathways and insulin action. Int J Obes Relat Metab Disord 2003;27 (Suppl 3):S53–S55.

27. Mertens I, Van Gaal LF. Obesity, homeostasis and the fibrinolytic system. Obes Rev 2002;3:85–101.

28. Engeli S, Schling P, Gorzelniak K, et al. The adipose tissue renin-angiotensin-aldosterone system: role in the metabolic syndrome. Int J Biochem Cell Biol 2003;35:807–825.

29. Karelis AD, St-Pierre DH, Conus F, Rabasa-Lhoret R, Poehlman ET. Metabolic and body composition factors in subgroups of obesity: what do we know? J Clin Endocrinol Metab 2004;89:2569–2575.

30. Brochu M, Tchernof A, Dionne IJ, et al. What are the physical characteristics associated with normal metabolic profile despite a high level of obesity in postmenopausal women? J Clin Endocrinol Metab 2001;86:1020–1025.

31. Wajchenberg BL. Subcutaneous and visceral adipose tissue: their relation to metabolic syndrome. Endocr Rev 2000;21:697–738.

32. Grundy SM. Obesity, metabolic syndrome and cardiovascular disease. J Clin Endocrinol Metab 2004; 89:2595–2600.

33. Bosello O, Zamboni M. Visceral obesity and metabolic syndrome. Obes Rev 2000;1:47–56.

34. Van Pelt RE, Jankowski CM, Gozansky WS, Schwartz RS, Kohrt WM. Lower-body adiposity and metabolic protection in postmenopausal women. J Clin Endocrinol Metab 2005;90:4573–4578.

35. Fain JN, Madan AK, Hiler ML, Cheema P, Bahouth SW. Comparison of the release of adipokines by adipose tissue, adipose tissue matrix, and adipocytes from visceral and subcutaneous abdominal adipose tissues of obese humans. Endocrinology 2004;145:2273–2282.

36. Tsigos C, Kyrou I, Chala E, et al. Circulating tumor necrosis factor alpha concentrations are higher in abdominal versus peripheral obesity. Metabolism 1999;48:1332–1335.

37. Futterweit W. Clinical features of polycystic ovarian disease. In: Futterweit W, ed, Polycystic Ovarian Disease. Berlin: Springer-Verlag, 1984, pp. 83–95.

38. Panidis D, Kourtis A, Farmakiotis D, Mouslech T, Rousso D, Koliakos G. Serum adiponectin levels in women with polycystic ovary syndrome. Hum Reprod 2003;18:1790–1796.

39. Kelly CJ, Lyall H, Petrie JR, et al. A specific elevation in tissue plasminogen antigen in women with polycystic ovary syndrome. J Clin Endocrinol Metab 2002;87:3287–3290.

40. Jaatinen TA, Matinlauri I, Anttila L, Koskinen P, Erkkola R, Irjala K. Serum total renin is elevated in women with polycystic ovarian syndrome. Fertil Steril 1995;63:1000–1004.

41. Morris RS, Wong IL, Hatch IE, Gentzschein E, Paulson RJ, Lobo RA. Prorenin is elevated in polycystic ovary syndrome and may reflect hyperandrogenism. Fertil Steril 1995;64:1099–1103.

42. Gonzalez F, Thusu K, Abdel-Rahman E, Prabhala A, Tomani M, Dandona P. Elevated serum levels of tumor necrosis alpha in normal-weight women with polycystic ovary syndrome. Metabolism 1999; 48:437–441.

43. Carmina E, Orio F, Palomba S, et al. Evidence for altered adipocyte function in polycystic ovary syndrome. Eur J Endocrinol 2005;152:389–394.

44. Escobar-Morreale HF, Villuendas G, Botella-Carretero JI, Sancho J, San Millan JL. Obesity, and not insulin resistance, is the major determinant of serum inflammatory cardiovascular risk markers in premenopausal women. Diabetologia 2003;46:625–633.

45. Orio F, Palomba S, Cascella T, et al. Is plasminogen activator inhibitor-1 a cardiovascular risk in young women with polycystic ovary syndrome? Reprod Biomed Online 2004;9:505–510.

46. Atiomo WU, Fox R, Condon JE, et al. Raised plasminogen activator inhibitor-1 (PAI-1) is not an independent risk factor in the polycystic ovary syndrome. Clin Endocrinol (Oxf) 2000; 52: 487–492.

47. Lamarche B. Abdominal obesity and its metabolic complications: implications for the risk of ischemic heart disease. Coronary Artery Dis 1988;9:473–481.

48. Sampson M, Kong C, Patel A, Unwin R, Jacobs HS. Ambulatory blood pressure profiles and plasminogen activator inhibitor (PAI-1) activity in lean women with and without the polycystic ovary syndrome. Clin Endocrinol (Oxf) 1996;45:623–629.

49. Sills ES, Dreaws CD, Perloe M, Tucker MJ, Kaplan CR, Palermo GD. Absence of profound hyper-insulinism in polycystic ovary syndrome is not associated with subtle elevations in the plasminogen activator inhibitor system. Gynecol Endocrinol 2003;17:231–237.
50. Dunaif A. Insulin resistance and the polycystic ovary syndrome: mechanisms and implications for pathogenesis. Endocr Rev 1997;18:774–800.
51. Kirchengast S, Huber J. Body composition characteristics and body fat distribution in lean women with polycystic ovary syndrome. Hum Reprod 2001;16:1255–1260.
52. Horejsi R, Moller R, Rackl S, et al. Android subcutaneous adipose topography in lean and obese suffering from PCOS: comparison with type II diabetic women. Am J Phys Anthropol 2004;124: 275–281.

18 Long-Term Sequelae of Polycystic Ovary Syndrome

Association With Insulin Resistance and the Metabolic Syndrome

Richard S. Legro, MD

CONTENTS

INTRODUCTION
THE METABOLIC SYNDROME AND PCOS:
    SEPARATE AND NOT EQUAL
PREVALENCE OF GLUCOSE INTOLERANCE AND TYPE 2 DIABETES
    IN PCOS
PCOS AND CVD
ENDOMETRIAL CANCER AND INSULIN RESISTANCE
FUTURE AVENUES
KEY POINTS
REFERENCES

Summary

Insulin resistance is associated with reproductive abnormalities in women with polycystic ovary syndrome (PCOS) including hyperandrogenemia, anovulation, and polycystic ovaries, as well as long-term risk for developing diabetes and most likely also for cardiovascular disease (CVD) and endometrial cancer. There is emerging evidence of increased subclinical CVD in women with PCOS. But it may not be apparent until the perimenopause. Currently there are scant data that markers of insulin resistance predict response to treatment. Therefore, the role of these markers in selecting and following response to specific treatments is uncertain.

Further research that examines the long-term effects of improving insulin resistance on such important clinical endpoints as the development of diabetes, overt CVD, and endometrial cancer are needed.

Key Words: PCOS; insulin resistance; metabolic syndrome; cardiovascular disease; endometrial carcinoma.

From: *Contemporary Endocrinology: Insulin Resistance and Polycystic Ovarian Syndrome: Pathogenesis, Evaluation, and Treatment*
Edited by: E. Diamanti-Kandarakis, J. E. Nestler, D. Panidis, and R. Pasquali © Humana Press Inc., Totowa, NJ

Table 1
Criteria for the Metabolic Syndrome in Women With PCOS[a]

Risk factor	Cutoff
1. Abdominal obesity women	>88 cm (>35 in.)
2. Triglycerides	≥150 mg/dL
3. HDL-C women	<50 mg/dL
4. Blood pressure	≥130/≥85
5. Fasting and 2-hour glucose from OGTT	110–126 mg/dL and/or 2h glucose 140–199 mg/dL

[a]Three of five qualify for the syndrome (2).

INTRODUCTION

Establishing the long term sequelae of polycystic ovary syndrome (PCOS) and their relationship to the underlying insulin resistance that characterizes the disorder should be a fundamental priority of research in the 21st century. Unfortunately much of the hype surrounding long term sequelae of PCOS has focused on risk factors and risk factor modeling. As an example of this, one of the most frequently cited (perhaps miscited is the proper term) publication notes a sevenfold increased risk of myocardial infarction in women with PCOS (1), and this has gone on to be written in stone and is used to guide patient counseling and care, though this conclusion was not based on events but risk factor modeling. One must occasionally stand back from the strong convictions that suffuse the long term risks of PCOS and ask where are the event data? Without these, we remain in the realm of speculation. This chapter will examine a variety of sequelae in women with PCOS linked to insulin resistance in women with PCOS including diabetes, heart disease, and endometrial cancer.

THE METABOLIC SYNDROME AND PCOS: SEPARATE AND NOT EQUAL

The current literature has so wedded the concepts of PCOS and the insulin resistance syndrome that the two have become almost interchangeable. In such an environment there is substantial encouragement to publish data supporting this connection. The metabolic syndrome (Table 1), as defined by the National Cholesterol Education Program (2), has been promoted as a method for identifying high-risk individuals for type 2 diabetes and cardiovascular disease (CVD), though there is controversy about its utility (3). But it is important to note that about 20% of the population meet criteria for the metabolic syndrome (2), a substantial lower proportion of the female population (well under 10%) meet diagnostic criteria for PCOS (4). Although metabolic syndrome is very common in women with PCOS, it is not ubiquitous (5). One large series from a multicenter trial in women with PCOS examined 394 women (6). Three or more of these individual criteria were present in 123 (33.4%) subjects overall. The prevalence of the metabolic syndrome did not differ significantly between racial/ethnic groups. Increasing body weight was critical to the development of the syndrome, none of the 52 women with a body mass index (BMI) <27.0 kg/m^2 had the metabolic syndrome; those in the top BMI quartile were 13.7 times more likely (95% CI 5.7–33.0) to have the metabolic syndrome compared with those in the lowest quartile.

Similarly reproductive age women with the metabolic syndrome do not invariantly have PCOS. When these women are studied for reproductive stigmata of PCOS, they are no more likely to have PCO than other segments of the population, only about half have a history of oligomenorrhea (though oligomenorrhea was twice as common in the affected population than the controls) *(7)*. Higher rates of obesity in the United States and corresponding increases in waist circumference and other related components of the metabolic syndrome will markedly increase the prevalence.

PREVALENCE OF GLUCOSE INTOLERANCE AND TYPE 2 DIABETES IN PCOS

Women with PCOS have multiple factors that contribute to increased diabetes risk including: insulin resistance, β-cell dysfunction, obesity and especially centripetal obesity, a family history of type 2 diabetes, a personal history of gestational diabetes. Additionally there is some evidence to suggest polycystic ovaries and chronic anovulation are risk factors. Studies of large cohorts of women with PCOS in the United States have demonstrated that the prevalence rates of glucose intolerance are as high as 40% in PCOS women when the less stringent WHO criteria are used (Fig. 1) *(8–10)*, These studies are of interest because they have shown nearly identical rates of impaired glucose tolerance and type 2 diabetes among a diverse cohort, both ethnically and geographically as well as from different investigational groups.

Undiagnosed diabetes based on 2-hour glucose challenged glucose levels approaches 10% in these cohorts. The majority of affected women are in their third and fourth decade of life, but we have encountered PCOS adolescents with impaired glucose tolerance or type 2 diabetes, and also lean individuals with glucose intolerance. Based on the prevalence of glucose intolerance in women in the US population (7.8% impaired glucose tolerance and 1.0% undiagnosed diabetes by WHO criteria in women ages 20–44 years old) *(11)*, the prevalence of glucose intolerance in PCOS (40%) and on population-based study of the prevalence of PCOS (~5%) *(12)*, it can be extrapolated that PCOS contributes to approx 20% of impaired glucose tolerance and 40% of type 2 diabetes in reproductive-aged women. It is important to note that these series report fasting normoglycemia in the majority of women, and that although elevated fasting levels tend to predict elevated 2-hour glucose challenged levels, even women with glucose intolerance tend to have fasting glucose levels less than 100 mg/dL (Fig. 2).

This would suggest that these abnormalities may represent a universal characteristic of women with PCOS, at least those diagnosed on the basis of hyperandrogenic chronic anovulation. Less stringent, more inclusive criteria are more likely to include a group of metabolically normal women with lower prevalence rates of glucose intolerance. The inclusion of both ovulatory and anovulatory women may explain the failure of a previous large study of glucose tolerance in hyperandrogenic women to detect glucose intolerance using the more stringent National Diabetes Data Group (NDDG) criteria (Falsetti and Eleftheriou, 1996). Also rates of glucose intolerance and diabetes in a thinner European population with PCOS are lower *(13)*.

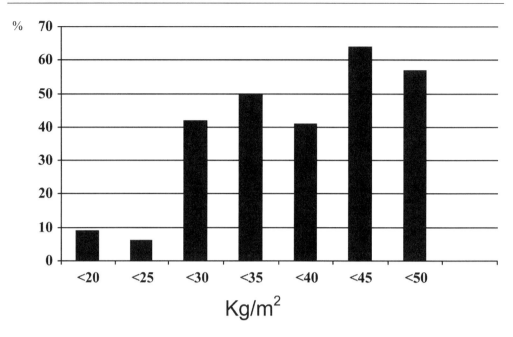

Fig. 1. Increasing prevalence of glucose intolerance by increasing body mass index among 254 women with PCOS. (Adapted from ref. 9.)

Prospective Studies of Conversion to Diabetes in PCOS

Natural history supportive of significant worsening of glucose tolerance would support more aggressive identification and treatment of this disorder in PCOS women. To date there have been several small published studies of conversion rates to diabetes over time, and rates, although clinically meaningful, do not approach the magnitude found in other high-risk populations such as women with gestational diabetes *(14)*. Ehrmann reported in a follow-up study of 25 PCOS women a significant increase in the mean 2-hour glucose value over a 3-year average period of follow-up to 161 ± 9 mg/dL compared to the baseline 2-hour value of 139 ± 6 mg/dL *(8)*. Recently Norman et al. have also noted a trend toward worsening glucose tolerance in a study of 67 women who were followed up after an average time of 6.2 years *(15)*. All women followed prospectively had normal glucose tolerance ($n = 54$) or IGT ($n = 13$) at the start of the study. Conversion rate was high with 5/54 (9%) of normoglycemic women at baseline developing IGT and a further 4/54 (8%) moving directly from normoglycaemic to type 2 diabetes. For women with IGT at baseline, 7/13 (54%) had type 2 diabetes at follow-up. BMI at baseline was an independent significant predictor of conversion risk.

Another follow up study of women with PCOS ($n = 71$) also included a group of control women ($n = 23$) with regular menstrual cycles and baseline normal glucose tolerance *(16)*. Mean follow-up was between 2 and 3 years for both groups (PCOS: 2.5 $\pm$ 1.7 years; controls: 2.9 $\pm$ 2.1 years). Based on WHO glucose tolerance categories there was no significant difference in the prevalence of glucose intolerance at follow-up in the PCOS group. At the follow-up visit the mean glycohemoglobin level was 6.1 $\pm$ 0.9% in women with PCOS vs 5.3 $\pm$ 0.7% in the control women ($p < 0.001$). Women with PCOS and baseline IGT had a low conversion risk of 6% to type 2 diabetes over

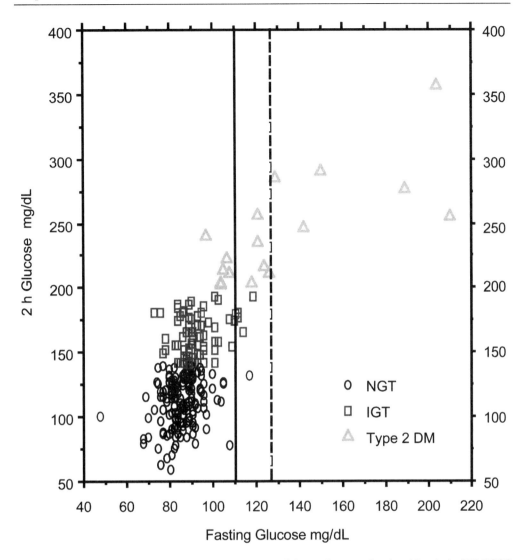

Fig. 2. Scattergram of fasting blood glucose levels vs 2-hour glucose stimulated levels in 254 PCOS women. Points on the graph are coded to reflect the WHO status based on OGTT. The solid vertical line is the threshold for impaired fasting glucose (110 mg/dL) by the 1997 ADA Criteria and the dashed vertical line (126 mg/dL) is the threshold for type 2 diabetes by the same criteria. Most PCOS women, regardless of WHO OGTT status have normal fasting glucose levels. (Adapted from ref. 9).

approx 3 years, or 2% per year. The effect of PCOS, given normal glucose tolerance (NGT) at baseline, is more pronounced with 16% conversion to IGT per year. These data do however, support a worsening of glucose intolerance over time and the need for periodic screening.

PCOS AND CVD

When approached by the more stringent requirement of cardiovascular events, i.e., increased mortality from CVD, premature mortality from CVD, or an increased incidence of cardiovascular events (stroke and/or myocardial infarction), there is little published evidence to support that PCOS women are unduly affected. The increased cardiovascular risk ascribed to women with PCOS is almost entirely inferential, based on risk factors *(17)*, including such surrogate markers as inflammatory markers *(18,19)*. There are multiple potential reasons for the lack of published data confirming increased cardiovascular events in this group. Varying or age specific diagnostic criteria have limited both clinical trials and long-term follow-up of women with PCOS. This heterogeneity of diagnostic criteria is both confounding and confusing, when assessing CVD in women with PCOS. The lack of any measure of hyperinsulinemia and/or insulin resistance in any of the current diagnostic criteria diminishes recognition of the most plausible link between PCOS and CVD.

The study of women with PCOS has been characterized by small sample sizes, usually in a premenopausal reproductive age population with limited follow-up. There have been few large-scale epidemiological trials of this younger female population that could document relatively rare events such as stroke and myocardial infarction. The lack of a menopausal PCOS phenotype, or more importantly the fading of the reproductive phenotype with age *(20,21)*, inhibits the linking of past, seemingly irrelevant, reproductive problems with current CVD in older populations.

There is the additional confounding effect of treatment on future complications of PCOS. Long-term benefits may have resulted from ovarian wedge resection or other forms of ovarian surgery. The current widespread use of insulin sensitizing agents for women of all ages with PCOS may contend ongoing or future studies of CVD, by ameliorating risk. Finally, the alternate hypothesis must always be entertained, i.e., PCOS is not associated with an increased CVD risk (or an earlier presentation).

PCOS and CVD Events

A large-scale epidemiologic case control study from the University of Pittsburgh, initiated in 1992 has identified cases with PCOS, primarily based on hyperandrogenic chronic anovulation ($n > 200$), and concurrently recruited community based controls ($n > 200$) *(22)*. The investigators have now followed this cohort for a decade. In preliminary data reported from the follow-up, there was an increased trend toward events/disease in the PCOS group compared to the control group. Among 126 Caucasian PCOS cases, there were two myocardial infarctions, four cases of angina pectoris, and two cases of surgical cardiac intervention (an angioplasty and a coronary bypass surgery). Among 142 controls of similar age there were no events. The odds ratio of a CV event in a PCOS woman compared to a control was 5.91 (95% CI, 0.7–135.6) *(23)*. One criticism of this study, that is not addressed in this preliminary data, but which has consistently been controlled for in published analyses, is the greater BMI in the PCOS group compared to controls. Nonetheless, the abnormal cardiovascular risk profile has persisted in women with PCOS, even after adjustment for differences in BMI, lipids, fat distribution, and compared to the reference population.

Another study from the Czech Republic with a much smaller case group ($n = 28$) noted a higher prevalence of self-reported coronary heart disease symptoms when compared with age-matched controls ($n = 752$) (21% of PCOS vs 5.2% of controls, $p = 0.001$) *(24)*. This group used diagnostic criteria of both hyperandrogenic chronic anovulation and past histopathologic evidence of PCO to identify cases, but only 28 of 61 cases identified responded to the questionnaire. Within the University of Pittsburgh study, the presence or absence of PCO had little effect on their cardiovascular risk (25), and the presence of PCO was primarily associated with increased incidence of reproductive abnormalities.

Utilizing a prospective cohort design from the Nurse's Health Study 82,439 female nurses provided information in 1982 on prior menstrual regularity (at ages 20–35 years) and were followed through 1996 for cardiovascular events (26). Incident reports of nonfatal myocardial infarction, fatal coronary heart disease (CHD), and nonfatal and fatal stroke were made and confirmed by review of medical records.

Compared with women reporting a history of very regular menstrual cycles, women reporting usually irregular or very irregular cycles had an increased risk for nonfatal or fatal CHD (Table 2) (26). This increasing risk with increasing menstrual irregularity suggests a dose–response effect. Increased risks for CHD associated with prior cycle irregularity remained significant after adjustment for BMI and other several potential confounders, including family history of myocardial infarction and personal exercise history. There was a nonsignificant increase in overall stroke risk as well as in ischemic stroke risk associated with very irregular cycles. There was unfortunately no further characterization of the etiology of the oligomenorrhea, for instance, quantifying the amount of clinical or biochemical androgen excess among the study cohort, to make a diagnosis of the etiology of the anovulation.

In a retrospective cohort study from the United Kingdom, ~800 women diagnosed with PCO, primarily by histopathology at the time of an ovarian wedge resection, were followed up after an average interval of 30 years after the procedure (27). Observed death rates were compared to expected death rates using standardized mortality ratios. There was no increased death from cardiovascular related causes, although there was an increased number of deaths as a result of complications of diabetes in the PCO group. In a follow up study by the same investigative group of 345 of these women with PCO and 1060 age-matched control women there was no increased long-term coronary heart disease mortality in the PCO group, although there was evidence of increased stroke related mortality even after adjustment for BMI (28).

PCOS and Increased Subclinical CVD

Several surrogate markers for atherosclerotic disease, including carotid wall thickness as determined by B-mode ultrasonography and coronary/aortic calcification as determined by electron beam computed tomography (EBCT) have been studied in women with PCOS. The University of Pittsburgh performed ultrasonography of the carotid arteries on 125 women with PCOS and 142 control women from their original cohort, and found a significantly higher prevalence of abnormal carotid plaque index in women with PCOS (7.2 vs 0.7% in controls) (29). Thus, the vast majority of predominantly premenopausal women with PCOS (93%) had no evidence for subclinical carotid atherosclerosis. No difference was noted in the intima-media thickness between PCOS and controls until the age group 45–49, a difference which persisted and increased in the age group in the menopausal range (≥50 years). These data would suggest that an increased risk for subclinical atherosclerotic disease is not

Table 2

Relative Risks (RRs With 95% Confidence Intervals) for Coronary Heart Disease as a Function of Menstrual Cycle Regularity at Ages 20–35 Years Data From the Nurse's Health Study[a]

Menstrual cycle regularity ages 20–35 years	Regular	Usually regular	Usually irregular	Very irregular	P trend
Total CHD					
No. of cases	810	327	184	96	
Person-year	715,293	264,924	126,406	49,292	
Age-adjusted RR (95% CI)	1.0	1.02 (0.90–1.16)	1.25 (1.07–1.47)	1.67 (1.35–2.06)	<0.001
Multivariate1 RR (95% CI)	1.0	1.02 (0.89–1.16)	1.22 (1.04–1.44)	1.53 (1.24–1.90)	<0.001
Nonfatal CHD					
No. of cases	562	210	132	60	
Age-adjusted RR (95% CI)	1.0	0.95 (0.81–1.11)	1.30 (1.07–1.60)	1.50 (1.15–1.96)	0.001
Multivariate1 RR (95% CI)	1.0	0.96 (0.82–1.12)	1.27 (1.05–1.54)	1.38 (1.06–1.80)	0.005
Fatal CHD					
No. of cases	248	117	52	36	
Age-adjusted RR (95% CI)	1.0	1.17 (0.94–1.46)	1.16 (0.86–1.56)	2.04 (1.44–2.89)	0.001
Multivariate1 RR (95% CI)	1.0	1.12 (0.90–1.40)	1.11 (0.82–1.50)	1.88 (1.32–2.67)	0.005

Adjusting for age, body mass index, cigarette smoking, menopausal status/postmenopausal hormone use, parental history of MI before age 60 years, parity, alcohol intake, aspirin use, multivitamin use, vitamin E supplement use, physical activity level, and history of oral contraceptive use.

[a]Adapted from ref 26.

apparent until the perimenopause in women with PCOS. A recent study from Greece studied intima media thickness and other CVD-associated parameters in 75 young women with PCOS and 55 healthy, age- and BMI-matched women. The PCOS women in this series also had significantly increased carotid IMT (0.58 vs 0.47 mm, $p < 0.001$) (30).

Coronary artery calcification correlates with the degree of histopathologic atherosclerosis and has been found to predict actual events (23). More recently, the University of Pittsburgh group has performed a pilot study of coronary and aortic calcification in a group of 32 women with PCOS and 30 controls. There was a significantly higher rate of detectable coronary artery calcification among PCOS women compared to controls (54 vs 24%, $p < 0.05$), with no difference noted in the abdominal aorta. Another investigative group recently reported a higher prevalence of coronary artery calcification in women with PCOS (31). Healthy, community-dwelling, ovulatory controls ($n = 71$) were matched by age and BMI to PCOS women ($n = 36$). Women with diabetes or known coronary heart disease were excluded. Coronary artery calcification was more prevalent in PCOS women (39%) than in matched controls (21%; odds ratio, 2.4; $p = 0.05$) or community-dwelling women (9.9%; odds ratio, 5.9; $p < 0.001$).

ENDOMETRIAL CANCER AND INSULIN RESISTANCE

Although endometrial cancer is viewed as the classic example of a hormone dependent neoplasias (increased risk with unopposed estrogen), more recently insulin resistance and hyperinsulinemia have been implicated as contributory agents to this cancer. Smaller studies of women with endometrial cancer have shown increased fasting and glucose stimulated insulin levels compared to controls *(32,33)*. Another study found a similar result among women with endometrial cancers both in relation to controls and women with other hormone dependent neoplasias such as breast cancer *(34)*. Insulin is a powerful mitogenic influence on a variety of tissues including endometrium and breast epithelial tissues and this proliferative effect may contribute to the appearance of oncogenes and transformation of benign tissue. In vitro studies of cancer cell lines has shown that insulin is mitogenic and most cell cultures of tumor cells require the presence of insulin to survive *(35)*. Studies of endometrial cancer lines have shown that the insulin receptor is expressed in a variety of cell lines, and that there is increased expression in poorly differentiated cell lines, specifically estrogen receptor negative cell lines HEC-1-A and HEC-1-B *(36)*. This suggested that insulin may play a role in the development of estrogen receptor negative endometrial cancers, cancers that usually are more aggressive and have a poorer prognosis. Insulin may also stimulate steroidogenesis in these tissues, through such mechanisms as increased expression of key enzymes such as aromatase, increased the bioavailability of sex steroids through suppression of binding proteins such as sex hormone-binding globulin, and increased biopotency of potent growth factors, such as IGF-1 through a similar mechanism of suppression of binding proteins *(35)*.

Endometrial Cancer and PCOS

Cancer of the endometrium is the most common cancer of the lower genital tract and is the fourth most common cancer diagnosed in women *(38)*. However only 4% of cases occur in women less than 40 years of age. Women with PCOS have often been noted to have an especially high risk for developing endometrial cancer and often at an early age *(39)*. However the majority of these studies are only case series or case reports or inferential based on stigmata of PCOS such as hirsutism, obesity, and anovulation (Table 3) *(39)*.

Chronic anovulation is associated with endometrial cancer *(40)*. In case series, women with PCOS have been over-represented in developing endometrial cancer and often at an early age. The fact that it is not noted in reference to a postmenopausal PCOS population reflects our difficulty in making the diagnosis after ovarian failure and cessation of menses. A Scandinavian study which looked at a group of both pre-menopausal and postmenopausal women with endometrial carcinoma, found hirsutism and obesity in both affected groups more often compared to controls *(41)*. In the younger group, they additionally noted a recent history of anovulation and infertility, two of the most common presenting complaints of women with PCOS (in addition to hirsutism and obesity).

Endometrial hyperplasia has also often been noted in association with anovulation and infertility *(42)*. In a large case/control study increased endometrial cancer risk was noted in women with lower levels of sex hormone-binding globulin and elevated insulin

Table 3
Summary of Publications Linking Women With PCOS to Endometrial Cancer[a]

Authors	Study design	Subjects	Findings	Comments
Speert 1949 (46)	Case series	14 women under 40 years with endometrial carcinoma	8 with cystic and 1 with sclerotic ovaries	No controls
Dockerty 1951 (47)	Case series	36 women under 40 years with endometrial carcinoma	14 with cystic ovaries (no histology in 8)	No controls
Jackson 1957 (48)	1. Case series	1. "Many thousands" of endometrial cancer cases	1. 16 women with PCOS.	No evidence of association
	2. Cross sectional	2. 27 women with PCO on biopsy	2. None had endometrial carcinoma	
Ramzy 1978 (49)	Case control	15 ovaries from cases of endo-metrial cancer, 25 from women with PCOS, 21 from controls	Ovaries from endometrial carcinoma cases more similar to the normal than to PCO	No evidence of association
Coulam 1983 (40)	Retrospective cohort	1270 women with chronic anovulation	SMR for endometrial carcinoma 3.1	No data for women with PCOS
Gallup 1984 (50)	Case series	111 cases of endometrial cancer	PCO in 31.2% of women under 40; 2.3% over 40	No controls
Escobedo 1991 (51)	Case control	399 cases of endometrial carcinoma; 3040 controls	Odds ratio for endo-metrial carcinoma 4.2 for "ovarian factor" infertility	No data for women with PCOS
Dahlgren 1991 (41)	Case control	147 cases of endo-metrial cancer; 409 controls	↑ hirsuitism in cases with endometrial cancer	No data for PCOS
Ho 1997 (42)	Retrospective cohort	116 patients with endometrial hyperplasia	Prevalence of endo-metrial carcinoma not ↑in cases with PCO	No evidence of association
Pierpoint 1998 (52)	Retrospective cohort	786 women with PCOS	Mortality from "miscellaneous cancers" not ↑	No data for endometrial cancer
Wild 2000 (28)	Retrospective cohort	345 surviving women from Pierpoint cohort	Odds ratio for endo-metrial cancer 5.3	Obesity a possible confounder

[a]The majority are small cases series, usually uncontrolled. Adapted from ref. 37.

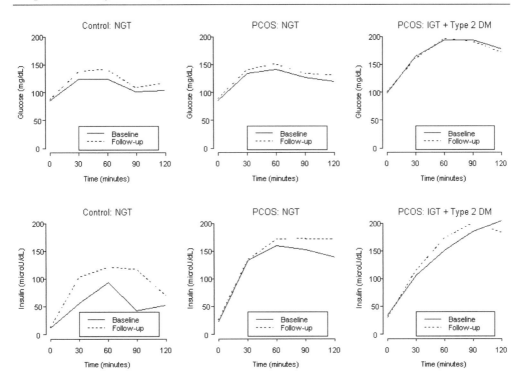

Fig. 3. Glucose and insulin levels during a 2-hour OGTT in control women and women with PCOS at baseline and follow-up 2–3 years later. There are no significant changes. (Adapted from ref. *16*).

levels *(43)*, both biochemical stigmata noted in women with PCOS. There are no systematic prospective studies of the prevalence of endometrial hyperplasia/neoplasia in a population with PCOS, or conversion rates over time. The true risk of endometrial cancer in women with PCOS, thus, is difficult to ascertain.

FUTURE AVENUES

1. Large-scale epidemiologic studies that focus on cardiovascular events in prospective cohorts are needed. The identification of a postmenopausal PCOS phenotype would allow utilization of existing cohorts.
2. Further research that examines the long-term effects of improving insulin resistance on such important clinical endpoints as the development of diabetes, overt CVD, and endometrial cancer are needed.

KEY POINTS

- Insulin resistance is associated with reproductive abnormalities in women with PCOS including hyperandrogenemia, anovulation, and polycystic ovaries, as well as long-term risk for developing diabetes and most likely also for CVD and endometrial cancer.
- There is emerging evidence of increased subclinical CVD in women with PCOS. But it may not be apparent until the perimenopause.
- Currently there are scant data that markers of insulin resistance predict response to treatment *(42,43)*. Therefore, the role of these markers in selecting and following response to specific treatments is uncertain.

REFERENCES

1. Dahlgren E, Janson PO, Johansson S, Lapidus L, Oden A. Polycystic ovary syndrome and risk for myocardial infarction. Evaluated from a risk factor model based on a prospective population study of women. Acta Obstetricia et Gynecologica Scandinavica 1992;71:599–604.
2. Ford ES, Giles WH, Dietz WH. Prevalence of the metabolic syndrome among US adults: findings from the third National Health and Nutrition Examination Survey. JAMA 2002;287:356–359.
3. Kahn R, Buse J, Ferrannini E, Stern M. The metabolic syndrome: time for a critical appraisal: joint statement from the American Diabetes Association and the European Association for the Study of Diabetes. Diabetes Care 2005;28:2289–2304.
4. Diamanti-Kandarakis E, Kouli CR, Bergiele AT, et al. A survey of the polycystic ovary syndrome in the Greek island of Lesbos: hormonal and metabolic profile. J Clin Endocrinol Metab 1999;84: 4006–4011.
5. Apridonidze T, Essah PA, Iuorno MJ, Nestler JE. Prevalence and characteristics of the metabolic syndrome in women with polycystic ovary syndrome. J Clin Endocrinol Metab 2005;90:1929–1935.
6. Ehrmann DA, Liljenquist DR, Kasza K, Azziz R, Legro RS, Ghazzi MN. Prevalence and predictors of the metabolic syndrome in women with polycystic ovary syndrome (PCOS). J Clin Endocrinol Metab 2006;91:48–53.
7. Korhonen S, Hippelainen M, Niskanen L, Vanhala M, Saarikoski S. Relationship of the metabolic syndrome and obesity to polycystic ovary syndrome: a controlled, population-based study. Am J Obstet Gynecol 2001;184:289–296.
8. Ehrmann DA, Barnes RB, Rosenfield RL, Cavaghan MK, Imperial J. Prevalence of impaired glucose tolerance and diabetes in women with polycystic ovary syndrome. Diabetes Care 1999;22:141–146.
9. Legro RS, Kunselman AR, Dodson WC, Dunaif A. Prevalence and predictors of risk for type 2 diabetes mellitus and impaired glucose tolerance in polycystic ovary syndrome: a prospective, controlled study in 254 affected women. J Clin Endocrinol Metab 1999;84:165–169.
10. Ehrmann DA, Kasza K, Azziz R, Legro RS, Ghazzi MN. Effects of race and family history of type 2 diabetes on metabolic status of women with polycystic ovary syndrome. J Clin Endocrinol Metab 2005;90:66–71.
11. Harris MI, Hadden WC, Knowler WC, Bennett PH. Prevalence of diabetes and impaired glucose tolerance and plasma glucose levels in U.S. population aged 20–74 yr. Diabetes 1987;36:523–534.
12. Azziz R, Woods KS, Reyna R, Key TJ, Knochenhauer ES, Yildiz BO. The prevalence and features of the polycystic ovary syndrome in an unselected population. J Clin Endocrinol Metab 2004;89: 2745–2749.
13. Pasquali R, Pelusi C, Ragazzini C, Hasanaj R, Gambineri A. Glucose tolerance, insulin secretion and insulin sensitivity in polycystic ovary syndrome. JOP 2002;3:1–7.
14. Kjos SL, Peters RK, Xiang A, Henry OA, Montoro M, Buchanan TA. Predicting future diabetes in Latino women with gestational diabetes. Utility of early postpartum glucose tolerance testing. Diabetes 1995;44:586–591.
15. Norman RJ, Masters L, Milner CR, Wang JX, Davies MJ. Relative risk of conversion from normoglycaemia to impaired glucose tolerance or non-insulin dependent diabetes mellitus in polycystic ovarian syndrome. Hum Reprod 2001;16:1995–1998.
16. Legro RS, Gnatuk CL, Kunselman AR, Dunaif A. Changes in glucose tolerance over time in women with polycystic ovary syndrome: a controlled study. J Clin Endocrinol Metab 2005;90:3236–3242.
17. Legro RS. Polycystic ovary syndrome and cardioivascular disease: A premature association? Endocr Rev 2003;24:302–312.
18. Diamanti-Kandarakis E, Spina G, Kouli C, Migdalis I. Increased endothelin-1 levels in women with polycystic ovary syndrome and the beneficial effect of metformin therapy. J Clin Endocrinol Metab 2001;86:4666–4673.
19. Diamanti-Kandarakis E, Paterakis T, Alexandraki K, et al. Indices of low-grade chronic inflammation in polycystic ovary syndrome and the beneficial effect of metformin. Hum Reprod 2006;21:1426–1431.
20. Elting MW, Korsen TJ, Rekers-Mombarg LT, Schoemaker J. Women with polycystic ovary syndrome gain regular menstrual cycles when ageing. Hum Reprod 2000;15:24–28.
21. Winters SJ, Talbott E, Guzick DS, Zborowski J, McHugh KP. Serum testosterone levels decrease in middle age in women with the polycystic ovary syndrome. Fertil Steril 2000;73:724–729.
22. Talbott E, Guzick D, Clerici A, et al. Coronary heart disease risk factors in women with polycystic ovary syndrome. Arterioscler Thromb Vasc Biol 1995;15:821–826.

23. Talbott EO, Zborowski JV, Sutton-Tyrrell K, McHugh-Pemu KP, Guzick DS. Cardiovascular risk in women with polycystic ovary syndrome. Obstet Gynecol Clin North Am 2001;28:111–133.

24. Cibula D, Cifkova R, Fanta M, Poledne R, Zivny J, Skibova J. Increased risk of non-insulin dependent diabetes mellitus, arterial hypertension and coronary artery disease in perimenopausal women with a history of the polycystic ovary syndrome. Hum Reprod 2000;15:785–789.

25. Loucks TL, Talbott EO, McHugh KP, Keelan M, Berga SL, Guzick DS. Do polycystic-appearing ovaries affect the risk of cardiovascular disease among women with polycystic ovary syndrome? Fertil Steril 2000;74:547–552.

26. Solomon CG, Hu FB, Dunaif A, et al. Menstrual cycle irregularity and risk for future cardiovascular disease. J Clin Endocrinol Metab 2002;87:2013–2037.

27. Pierpoint T, McKeigue PM, Isaacs AJ, Wild SH, Jacobs HS. Mortality of women with polycystic ovary syndrome at long-term follow-up. J Clin Epidemiol 1998;51:581–586.

28. Wild S, Pierpoint T, Jacobs H, McKeigue P. Long-term consequences of polycystic ovary syndrome: results of a 31 year follow-up study. Hum Fertil (Camb) 2000;3:101–105.

29. Talbott EO, Guzick DS, Sutton-Tyrrell K, et al. Evidence for association between polycystic ovary syndrome and premature carotid atherosclerosis in middle-aged women. Arterioscler Thromb Vasc Biol 2000;20:2414–2421.

30. Vryonidou A, Papatheodorou A, Tavridou A, et al. Association of hyperandrogenemic and metabolic phenotype with carotid intima-media thickness in young women with polycystic ovary syndrome. J Clin Endocrinol Metab 2005;90:2740–2746.

31. Christian RC, Dumesic DA, Behrenbeck T, Oberg AL, Sheedy PF, Fitzpatrick LA. Prevalence and predictors of coronary artery calcification in women with polycystic ovary syndrome. J Clin Endocrinol Metab 2003;88:2562–2568.

32. Nagamani M, Hannigan EV, Dinh TV, Stuart CA. Hyperinsulinemia and stromal luteinization of the ovaries in postmenopausal women with endometrial cancer. J Clin Endocrinol Metab 1988;67: 144–148.

33. Rutanen EM, Nyman T, Lehtovirta P, Ammala M, Pekonen F. Suppressed expression of insulin-like growth factor binding protein-1 mrna in the endometrium: a molecular mechanism associating endometrial cancer with its risk factors. Int J Cancer 1994;59:307–312.

34. Gamayunova VB, Bobrov YuF, Tsyrlina EV, Evtushenko TP, Berstein LM. Comparative study of blood insulin levels in breast and endometrial cancer patients. Neoplasma 1997;44:123–126.

35. Straus DS. Growth-stimulatory actions of insulin in vitro and in vivo. Endocr Rev 1984;5:356–369.

36. Nagamani M, Stuart CA. Specific binding and growth-promoting activity of insulin in endometrial cancer cells in culture. Am J Obstet Gynecol 1998;179:6–12.

37. Kaaks R, Lukanova A, Kurzer MS. Obesity, endogenous hormones, and endometrial cancer risk: a synthetic review. Cancer Epidemiol Biomarkers Prev 2002;11:1531–1543.

38. Landis SH, Murray T, Bolden S, Wingo PA. Cancer statistics, 1998. CA Cancer J Clin 1998;48: 6–29.

39. Hardiman P, Pillay OS, Atiomo W. Polycystic ovary syndrome and endometrial carcinoma. Lancet 2003;361:1810–1812.

40. Coulam CB, Annegers JF, Kranz JS. Chronic anovulation syndrome and associated neoplasia. Obstet Gynecol 1983;61:403–407.

41. Dahlgren E, Friberg LG, Johansson S, Lindstrom B, Oden A, Samsioe G. Endometrial carcinoma; ovarian dysfunction—a risk factor in young women. Eur J Obstet Gynecol Reprod Biol 1991;41: 143–150.

42. Ho SP, Tan KT, Pang MW, Ho TH. Endometrial hyperplasia and the risk of endometrial carcinoma. Singapore Med J 1997;38:11–15.

43. Potischman N, Hoover RN, Brinton LA, et al. Case-control study of endogenous steroid hormones and endometrial cancer. J Natl Cancer Inst 1996;88:1127–1135.

44. Moghetti P, Castello R, Negri C, et al. Metformin effects on clinical features, endocrine and metabolic profiles, and insulin sensitivity in polycystic ovary syndrome: a randomized, double-blind, placebo-controlled 6-month trial, followed by open, long-term clinical evaluation. J Clin Endocrinol Metab 2000;85:139–146.

45. Azziz R, Ehrmann D, Legro RS, et al. Troglitazone improves ovulation and hirsutism in the polycystic ovary syndrome: a multicenter, double blind, placebo-controlled trial. J Clin Endocrinol Metab 2001;86:1626–1632.

46. Speert, H. Carcinoma of the endometrium in young women. Surg Gynecol Obstet 1949;88:332–336.

47. Dockerty MB, Lovelady SB, Faust GT. Carcinoma of the corpus uteri in young women. Am J Obstet Gynecol 1951;61:966–981.
48. Jackson RL, Dockerty MB. The Stein-Leventhal syndrome. Analysis of 43 cases with special reference to endometrial cancer. Am J Obstet Gynecol 1957;73:161–173.
49. Ramzy I, Nisker JA. Histologic study of ovaries from young women with endometrial adenocarcinoma. Am J Clin Pathol 1979;71:253–256.
50. Gallup DG, Stock RJ. Adenocarcinoma of the endometrium in women 40 years of age or younger. Obstet Gynecol 1984;64:417–420.
51. Escobedo LG, Lee NC, Peterson HB, Wingo PA. Infertility-associated endometrial cancer risk may be limited to specific subgroups of infertile women. Obstet Gynecol 1991;77:124–128.
52. Pierpoint T, McKeigue PM, Isaacs AJ, Wild SH, Jacobs HS. Mortality of women with polycystic ovary syndrome at long-term follow-up. J Clin Epidemiol 1998;51:581–586.

19 Cardiovascular Disease and Inflammation

Francesco Orio, Jr., MD, PhD,
Evanthia Diamanti-Kandarakis, MD, PhD,
and Stefano Palomba, MD

CONTENTS

Summary

Polycystic ovary syndrome (PCOS) is not only a reproductive disorder, but also a complex, multifaceted, endocrine disease with several associated health complications. In fact, multiple lines suggest an increased cardiovascular risk and cardiovascular disease characterized by an impairment of cardiac structure and function, endothelial dysfunction, lipid abnormalities, and low-grade chronic inflammation. The increased prevalence of low-grade chronic inflammation in women with PCOS represents an emerging novel mechanism for cardiovascular disease in these women. All these features are likely linked to the insulin-resistance often present in women with PCOS. Cardiovascular disease and inflammation represent important long-term sequelae of PCOS that warrant further in-depth investigation.

Key Words: Cardiovascular disease (CVD); cardiovascular risk (CVR); inflammation; leukocytes; endothelial dysfunction; heart; inflammation.

INTRODUCTION

Polycystic ovary syndrome (PCOS) is one of the most common endocrine disorders in women, affecting 6–7% of women of reproductive age *(1)*. PCOS is not only one of the main causes of infertility in women, but is also considered a plurimetabolic syndrome *(2–4)*. Obesity *(5)*, insulin-resistance (IR) *(6)*, dyslipidemia *(7)*, and an altered fibrinolytic system *(8)* are metabolic comorbidities often evident in the syndrome. Moreover, PCOS

From: *Contemporary Endocrinology: Insulin Resistance and Polycystic Ovarian Syndrome:*
Pathogenesis, Evaluation, and Treatment
Edited by: E. Diamanti-Kandarakis, J. E. Nestler, D. Panidis, and R. Pasquali © Humana Press Inc., Totowa, NJ

is associated with long-term health risks, including type 2 diabetes mellitus *(9)* and cardiovascular disease (CVD) *(10–14)*. In particular, IR, hyperandrogenism, and dyslipidemia are likely the major risk factors for the occurrence of CVD in PCOS. These cardiovascular risk (CVR) factors are often evident at an early age, suggesting that women with PCOS represent a large group of women at increased risk for developing early-onset CVD, even if this has not yet been confirmed in long-term studies *(15)*.

The risk of coronary artery disease and myocardial infarction has been reported to be increased in patients with PCOS compared with regularly cycling women *(10)*; however, to date, no prospective study of cardiovascular mortality in PCOS has been performed *(16)*. Several studies *(8,17–20)* report alterations in intermediate end points for CVR in this population. In fact, endothelial *(21)* and diastolic *(22)* dysfunction have been demonstrated in PCOS and have been associated with both elevated androgen levels and IR. Recently, together with classical CVR factors, such as elevated total cholesterol (TC) levels and low high-density lipoprotein cholesterol (HDL-C) levels, obesity, elevated homocysteine, and left ventricular hypertrophy (LVH) have been shown to be independently associated with an increased CVR *(23)*. The scientific interest *vis-a-vis* CVR in PCOS is increasing in recent years; in particular, biochemical, morphological, and functional markers of early CVD have been evaluated to correctly identify the CV morbidity of this syndrome. Several studies *(17–20,24)* have reported alterations in intermediate end points for CVR in women with PCOS, and have attempted to demonstrate an association between PCOS and CVR factors and CVD (Table 1). Furthermore, it is possible that genetic factors associated with PCOS could cause an increased CVR profile. One such factor is IR, which is considered the main factor leading to the development of the increased low-grade chronic inflammation and CVD in PCOS (Fig. 1).

CARDIOVASCULAR DISEASE

At the moment, there is no single, universally accepted definition for PCOS. This may be a contributing reason as to why published studies on PCOS have not yet provided a conclusive answer on the incidence of CVD in PCOS.

Women with PCOS represent an intriguing biological model of the effects of hormonal abnormalities on CVR. Several findings indicate a relationship between heart disease and PCOS, i.e., dyslipidemia *(25)*, insulin resistance *(6)*, increased left ventricular mass (LVM) *(17)*, and diastolic dysfunction *(14,22)*.

CVR factors and precocious cardiovascular abnormalities are often evident at an early age in PCOS, suggesting that the chronically abnormal hormonal and metabolic milieu found in women with PCOS, starting from adolescence, may predispose these women to premature atherosclerosis and making them candidates for early CVD.

Visceral obesity is present in about 50% of women with PCOS *(1)* and is a recognized risk factor for IR/hyperinsulinemia, dyslipidemia, type 2 diabetes, hypertension, coagulation abnormalities, and premature CVD. It can worsen all these metabolic and CV features present in PCOS, but it does not represent the only or the first etiopathogenetic factor for the increase of CVR in PCOS. As mentioned previously, IR is a determinant of overall CVR independent of obesity. In fact, increased CVR is related to the degree of IR among women with PCOS *(26)*.

Table 1
Evidence for Association Between PCOS and CVD

Known CVR factors	○ Atherosclerosis
	○ Coronary artery disease
	○ Myocardial infarction
	○ Atherogenic lipid profile: $\uparrow$Col tot, $\uparrow$LDL, $\uparrow$Tg, $\downarrow$HDL
Emerging/new CVR factors	○ $\uparrow$CRP
	○ $\uparrow$WBC (lymphocytes and monocytes)
	○ $\uparrow$TNF-α
	○ $\uparrow$IL-6 and IL-18
Subclinical CVD	○ LVH
	○ Diastolic dysfunction
	○ $\uparrow$IMT
	○ Endothelial dysfunction: $\downarrow$FMD, $\uparrow$ET-1
	○ Impaired fibrinolysis ($\uparrow$PAI-1)
Clinical CVD	○ No increased mortality for CVD in PCOS
	○ Insulin resistance as the first cause of an increased CVR and CVD

CVR, cardiovascular risk; CVD, cardiovascular disease; Col tot, total cholesterol; LDL, low-density lipoprotein; TG, triglycerides; HDL, high-density lipoprotein; CRP, C-reactive protein; WBC, white blood cell; TNF, tumor necrosis factor; IL, interleukin; LVH, left ventricular hypertrophy; IMT, intima media thickness; FMD, flow-mediated dilation; ET, endothelin.

However, different confounding factors may co-exist in patients with PCOS, such as obesity, arterial hypertension, impaired glucose tolerance and/or type 2 diabetes, hyperinsulinemia, dyslipidemia, and coagulation disorders that could increase, *per se*, the risk for CVD in these subjects.

Scientific interest in the CVR of PCOS has increased in recent years because of the crucial consequences for the overall health of women with PCOS. In particular, biochemical, morphological, and functional markers of early CVD have been evaluated to correctly identify CV morbidity in this syndrome. Recently, together with classical CVR factors, such as elevated TC, low HDL-C levels and obesity, homocysteine, LVH, and low-grade chronic inflammation have also been shown to be independently associated with an increased CVR *(23)*.

An uncalculated but significantly increased risk of atherosclerosis *(13)* and a sevenfold increased risk of CVD *(10)* have been reported in subjects with PCOS. As a consequence of IR, patients with PCOS often have an abnormal lipid profile and increased incidence of CVR factors *(28)*. In fact, IR has been associated with elevated triglyceride levels, increased levels of low-density lipoprotein (LDL), and decreased levels of HDL *(25)*. These CVR factors are often evident at an early age, suggesting that women with PCOS represent a large group of women at increased risk for developing early-onset CVD.

One of the early signs of CVD is endothelial injury. Precocious anatomical and functional arterial changes have been reported in women with PCOS. Even in this case, IR is likely the major risk factor for the occurrence of CVD in PCOS, and could play a key role in the development of endothelial damage, which is an early sign of atherosclerosis.

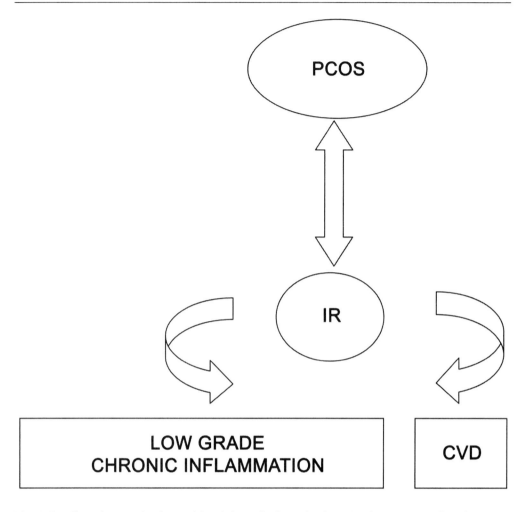

Fig. 1. Insulin resistance that is considered the main factor leads to the development of the increased low-grade chronic inflammation and cardiovascular disease in polycystic ovary syndrome.

Data on endothelial dysfunction in patients with PCOS are poor and conflicting *(18,21,28–33)*. An association between PCOS and early carotid atherosclerosis was demonstrated in several studies *(13,18,34)*. Some authors *(18)* reported no difference in flow-mediated dilation, which is a measure of reactive vascular hyperemia, between patients with PCOS and controls. Conversely, others *(21)* showed markedly diminished endothelium-dependent and insulin-mediated flow responses in the femoral artery of women with PCOS. Furthermore, endothelin (ET)-1, a marker of vasculopathy and of endothelial dysfunction, has been reported to be increased in women with PCOS *(18,34)*. Hyperandrogenism in women with PCOS may result in a male pattern of lipoproteins, resulting in an increased atherogenic potential in patients with PCOS *(25)*. In addition, some authors *(32)* have reported impaired carotid viscoelastic properties in women with PCOS, providing additional evidence of vascular dysfunction in women with this syndrome.

An interesting study *(29)* reported increased vascular stiffness and a functional defect in the vascular action of insulin in patients with PCOS. In young, normal-weight women with

PCOS who had normal lipids and blood pressure, endothelial function was altered and intimal media thickness (IMT) was increased, suggesting early functional and structural preatherosclerotic vascular impairment *(18,33)*. Furthermore, some studies have recently shown that a 6-month course of metformin improves endothelial structure and function in these young, normal-weight women with PCOS *(35,36)*, supporting a role for IR in the pathogenesis of these abnormalities. In contrast, some authors have hypothesized a cardioprotective effect of androgens on the vascular wall in women with PCOS *(30,37)*.

As noted earlier, in addition to classical CVR factors, even elevated homocysteine, LVH, and oxidative stress appear to be independently associated with an increased CVR *(23)*. Although data on homocysteine levels in subjects with PCOS are inconclusive and conflicting *(38,39)*, an early and IR-related impairment of endothelial structure and function *(12)*, specifically diastolic dysfunction and LVH *(11)*, have been demonstrated in young, normal-weight women with PCOS. LVH is an important predictor of CV mortality and morbidity *(40)*, and is one of several metabolic and CVR factors associated with IR and/or visceral obesity.

Impaired fibrinolysis, one of the more important co-factors in the development of fatal ischemic heart disease in women *(41)*, has also been demonstrated in PCOS. Specifically, a significant increase in serum plasminogen activator inhibitor (PAI)-1 activity *(42,43)* has been reported. This increase was again positively related to IR, but independent of obesity *(42)*.

Hyperinsulinemia, with or without diabetes, likely plays a pivotal role in the acceleration of macrovascular disease in women with PCOS *(28)*, and is a predictor of coronary artery disease; furthermore, IR has been proposed as the key factor linking hypertension, glucose intolerance, obesity, lipid abnormalities, and coronary heart disease in the association called "metabolic syndrome X" *(44)*. Moreover, as noted earlier, 50–60% of women with PCOS are obese *(1)* and obesity itself could further worsen the metabolic pattern and CVR of this group of patients. However, results of two important studies suggest that the apparent increase in CVD in women with PCOS does not increase CV mortality *(16,45)*.

It seems that PCOS may accelerate the development of an adverse CVR profile or even of sub-clinical atherosclerosis. IR is frequently cited as the cause of an increased risk for CVD among women with PCOS, even if no measure of insulin sensitivity is included in the current diagnostic criteria for PCOS *(36)*. Finally, phenotypic variation in hyperandrogenic women was reported to influence the findings of abnormal metabolic and CVR parameters *(45)*. In fact, the prevalence of metabolic and CV abnormalities was higher in classic PCOS (i.e., oligo- or anovulation with androgen excess), followed by normal ovulatory-PCOS, and then women with idiopathic hyperandrogenism *(46)*. This is a critical point because it demonstrates the importance of a homogeneous PCOS group in the effort to define the true CVR and putative CVD. In the future, all studies of CVR in PCOS should be conducted using not only the new diagnostic criteria for PCOS, but also subsetting subjects according to the different phenotypes of this complex disorder.

At the moment, large clinical trials evaluating the morbidity and mortality for CVD in women with PCOS are lacking. No long-term data of well-characterized women with PCOS and primary CV events, such as stroke or myocardial infarction, exist in the literature.

INFLAMMATION

Recently, original and interesting data have demonstrated a correlative and causative relationship between IR and inflammation *(47)*. Subclinical inflammation and IR are important predictors of CVD *(48)*.

Furthermore, in light of the role of IR in PCOS and of the increased CVR of affected women, a relationship between inflammation and hormonal–metabolic features of women with PCOS was also demonstrated *(49)*. It has been reported that women with PCOS have significantly increased C-reactive protein (CRP) concentrations *(50)*, suggesting CRP, a marker of low-grade chronic inflammation, as a predictor of coronary heart disease and CV events in PCOS that is also independently related to IR. The leukocyte count was found to be significantly higher in women with PCOS compared with healthy women, although no case of leukocytosis was found in either group *(49)*. Regarding the leukocyte differential, significant increases in lymphocytes and monocytes were observed in women with PCOS compared with controls *(49)*, which might have been expected considering that they play a key role in the pathophysiological mechanism of atherosclerosis. Inflammation has been recognized to play a central role in both initiation and progression of the atherosclerotic process *(51)*; therefore, an elevated leukocyte count should be directly associated with increased incidence of coronary heart disease, ischemic stroke, and mortality from CVD. Although this finding appears clear and interesting, further studies need to confirm this novel data.

In patients with PCOS, circulating levels of tumor necrosis factor (TNF)-α, interleukin (IL)-6, highly sensitive serum CRP (hs-CRP), as well as white blood cell count (WBC) and neutrophil count have been found to be elevated compared with age- and/or body mass index (BMI)-matched controls *(50,52–56)*. In contrast, recent reports found that obesity, and not PCOS status *per se*, was a major determinant of the circulating inflammatory markers TNF-α, soluble type 2 TNF receptor, IL-6, and hs-CRP *(57,58)*. Recently, Puder *(59)* demonstrated that the increase in both low-grade chronic inflammation and IR in women with PCOS is associated with increased central fat excess rather than PCOS status *(59)*. Conversely, it remains controversial whether the elevated CRP levels observed in women with PCOS are a function of obesity.

Furthermore, TNF-α is overexpressed in adipose tissue *(60)* and induces IR through acute and chronic effects on insulin-sensitive tissues. The source of excess circulating TNF-α in PCOS is likely to be adipose tissue in the obese, but remains unknown in lean women with the disorder. Increased visceral adiposity could be a source of excess TNF-α in lean women with PCOS.

Another proinflammatory cytokine is IL-18, which was reported to be increased in PCOS by Escobar-Morreale *(61)*. Furthermore, IL-18 induces the production of TNF-α, which promotes the synthesis of IL-6 *(62)*, which is also considered a strong risk marker for CVD *(63)*.

Collectively, the above findings indicate that low-grade chronic inflammation could be a novel mechanism contributing to increased risk of coronary heart disease in PCOS.

CONCLUSIONS

Although consistent and well-characterized phenotypes of reproductive and metabolic abnormalities have been demonstrated in PCOS, suggesting an increased risk for inflammation and CVD in women with PCOS, prospective studies and clinical trials with large sample sizes and long-term follow-up are lacking.

Several factors considered important to the development of CVD, such as lipoprotein abnormalities, hypertension, left ventricular mass index, endothelial dysfunction, and low-grade chronic inflammation have been described in women with PCOS, even at an early age, but these studies were limited by their small samples sizes.

Preliminary studies suggested a slight increase in CV events in women with PCOS. Overall, the small size and number of these epidemiological studies have been inadequate for conditions as common as PCOS and CVD in women. Therefore, larger prospective trials with long-term follow-up are needed to better define the incidence of CVR and subsequent CVD in PCOS.

FUTURE AVENUES

An early diagnosis of PCOS could provide an important opportunity to begin primary prevention of CVD.

There are multiple and several surrogate variables in PCOS, including anthropometrical and biochemical parameters. Their poor validity in relation to primary clinical end points represents major problems and needs to be considered in the design of future trials in women with PCOS.

CVD is among several clinical end points in PCOS studies, and until now, it has not been suitable as the primary outcome of clinical studies. Future multicenter studies in women with PCOS should focus on CVD as the primary clinical end point.

Emerging and future biomarkers of chronic low-grade inflammation should be assessed in PCOS.

Therapeutic effects of lifestyle modification (i.e., diet and physical exercise), oral contraceptives, and insulin-sensitizing drugs (metformin, thiazolidinediones, and so on) should be carefully investigated in well-designed studies investigating CVR and CVD in women with PCOS.

KEY POINTS

- PCOS could be associated to an increased cardiovascular risk and cardiovascular disease.
- There is a relationship between heart disease and PCOS, i.e., dyslipidemia, insulin resistance, increased LVM, and diastolic dysfunction; endothelial dysfunction and PCOS, i.e., flow-mediated dilation, endothelin-1; inflammation and PCOS, i.e., PCR, white blood cells, TNF-α, IL-6, and IL-18.
- Prospective studies and clinical trials from large sample sizes and from long-term follow-up are needed.

REFERENCES

1. Ehrmann DA. Polycystic ovary syndrome. N Engl J Med 2005;352:1223–1236.
2. Scarpitta AM, Sinagra D. Polycystic ovary syndrome: an endocrine and metabolic disease. Gynecol Endocrinol 2000;14:392–395.
3. Lobo RA, Carmina E. The importance of diagnosing the polycystic ovary syndrome. Ann Intern Med 2000;132:989–993.

4. Franks S. Are women with polycystic ovary syndrome at increased risk of cardiovascular disease? Too early to be sure, but not too early to act! Am J Med 2001;111:665–666.

5. Elting MW, Korsen TJM, Shoemaker J. Obesity rather than menstrual cycle pattern or follicle cohort size, determines hyperinsulinemia, dyslipidemia and hypertension in ageing women with polycystic ovary syndrome. Clin Endocrinol 2001;55:767–776.

6. Dunaif A. Insulin resistance and the polycystic ovary syndrome: mechanism and implications for pathogenesis. Endocr Rev 1997;18:774–800.

7. Legro RS, Kunselman AR, Dunaif A. Prevalence and predictors of dyslipidemia in women with polycystic ovary syndrome. Am J Med 2001;111:607–613.

8. Yildiz BO, Haznedaroglu IC, Kirazli S, Bayraktar M. Global fibrinolytic capacity is decreased in polycystic ovary syndrome, suggesting a prothrombotic state. J Clin Endocrinol Metab 2002;87:3871–3875.

9. Ovalle F, Azziz R. Insulin resistance, polycystic ovary syndrome, and type 2 diabetes mellitus. Fertil Steril 2002;77:1095–1105.

10. Dahlgren E, Janson PO, Johansson S, Lapidus L, Oden A. Polycystic ovary syndrome and risk for myocardial infarction. Evaluated from a risk factor model based on a prospective population study of women. Acta Obstet Gynecol Scand 1992;71:599–604.

11. Talbott E, Guzick D, Clerici A, et al. Coronary heart disease risk factors in women with polycystic ovary syndrome. Arter Thromb Vascul Biol 1995;15:821–826.

12. Conway GS, Agrawal R, Better, Guzi DJ, Jacobs HS. Risk factors for coronary heart disease in lean and obese women with the polycystic ovary syndrome. Clin Endocrinol (Oxf) 1992;37:119–125.

13. Talbott E, Guzick DS, Sutton-Tyrrell K, et al. Evidence for association between polycystic ovary syndrome and premature carotid atherosclerosis in middle-aged women. Arterioscler Thromb Vasc Biol 2000;20:2414–2421.

14. Tiras MB, Yalcin R, Noyan V, Maral I, Yildirim M, Dortlemez O, Daya S. Alterations in cardiac flow parameters in patients with polycystic ovarian syndrome. Hum Reprod 1999;14:1949–1952.

15. Legro RS. Polycystic ovary syndrome and cardiovascular disease: a premature association? Endocr Rev 2003;24:302–312.

16. Pierpoint T, McKeigue PM, Isaacs AJ, Wild SH, Jacobs HS. Mortality of women with polycystic ovary syndrome at long-term follow-up. J Clin Epidemiol 1998;51:581–586.

17. Orio F Jr., Palomba S, Spinelli L, et al. The cardiovascular risk of young women with polycystic ovary syndrome: an observational, analytical, prospective case-control study. J Clin Endocrinol Metab 2004;89:3696–3701.

18. Orio F Jr., Palomba S, Cascella T, et al. Early impairment of endothelial structure and function in young normal-weight women with polycystic ovary syndrome. J Clin Endocrinol Metab 2004;89:4588–4593.

19. Cibula D, Cifkova R, Fanta M, Poledne R, Zivny J, Skibova J. Increased risk of non-insulin dependent diabetes mellitus, arterial hypertension and coronary artery disease in perimenopausal women with a history of the polycystic ovary syndrome. Hum Reprod 2000;15:785–789.

20. Taponen S, Martikainen H, Jarvelin MR, et al. Metabolic cardiovascular disease risk factors in women with self-reported symptoms of oligomenorrhea and/or hirsutism: Northern Finland Birth Cohort 1966 Study. J Clin Endocrinol Metab 2004;89:2114–2118.

21. Paradisi G, Steinberg HO, Hempfling A, et al. Polycystic ovary syndrome is associated with endothelial dysfunction. Circulation 2001;103:1410–1415.

22. Yarali H, Yildirir A, Aybar F, et al. Diastolic dysfunction and increased serum homocysteine concentrations may contribute to increased cardiovascular risk in patients with polycystic ovary syndrome. Fertil Steril 2001;76:511–516.

23. Harjai KJ. Potential new cardiovascular risk factors: left ventricular hypertrophy, homocysteine, lipoprotein(a), triglycerides, oxidative stress, and fibrinogen. Ann Intern Med 1999;131:376–386.

24. Yildiz BO, Haznedaroglu IC, Kirazli S, Bayraktar M. Global Fibrinolytic capacity is decreased in polycystic ovary syndrome, suggesting a prothrombotic state. J Clin Endocrinol Metab 2002;87:3871–3875.

25. Wild RA, Painter PC, Coulson PB, Carruth KB, Ranney GB. Lipoprotein lipid concentrations and cardiovascular risk in women with polycystic ovary syndrome. J Clin Endocrinol Metab 1985;61:946–951.

26. Mather KJ, Kwan F, Corenblum B. Hyperinsulinemia in polycystic ovary syndrome correlates with increased cardiovascular risk independent of obesity. Fertil Steril 2000;73:150–156.

27. Amowitz LL, Sobel BE. Cardiovascular consequences of polycystic ovary syndrome. Endocrinol Metab Clin North Am 1999;28:439–458.
28. Mather KJ, Verma S, Corenblum B, Anderson T. Normal endothelial function despite insulin resistance in healthy women with the polycystic ovary syndrome. J Clin Endocrinol Metab 2000;85: 1851–1856.
29. Kelly CJG, Speirs A, Gould GW, Petrie JR, Lyall H, Connell JMC. Altered vascular function in young women with polycystic ovary syndrome. J Clin Endocrinol Metab 2002;87:742–746.
30. Meyer C, McGrath BP, Cameron J, Kotsopoulos D, Teede HJ. Vascular dysfunction and metabolic parameters in polycystic ovary syndrome. J Clin Endocrinol Metab 2005;90(8):4630–4635.
31. Tarkun I, Arslan BC, Canturk Z, Turemen E, Sahin T, Duman C. Endothelial dysfunction in young women with polycystic ovary syndrome: relationship with insulin resistance and low-grade chronic inflammation. J Clin Endocrinol Metab 2004;89:5592–5596
32. Lakhani K, Seifalian AM, Hardiman P. Impaired carotid viscoelastic properties in women with polycystic ovaries. Circulation 2002;106:81–85.
33. Kravariti M, Naka KK, Kalantaridou SN, et al. Predictors of endothelial dysfunction in young women with polycystic ovary syndrome. J Clin Endocrinol Metab 2005;90(9):5088–5095.
34. Diamanti-Kandarakis E, Spina G, Kouli C, Migdalis I. Increased endothelin-1 levels in women with polycystic ovary syndrome and the beneficial effect of metformin therapy. J Clin Endocrinol Metab 2001;86:4666–4673.
35. Vryonidou A, Papatheodorou A, Tavridou A, et al. Association of hyperandrogenemic and metabolic phenotype with carotid intima-media thickness in young women with polycystic ovary syndrome. J Clin Endocrinol Metab 2005;90(5):2740–2746.
36. Orio F Jr., Palomba S, Cascella T, et al. Improvement in endothelial structure and function after metformin treatment in young normal-weight women with polycystic ovary syndrome: results of a six-month study. J Clin Endocrinol Metab 2005;90(11):6072–6076.
37. Diamanti-Kandarakis E, Alexandraki K, Protogerou A, et al. Metformin administration improves endothelial function in women with polycystic ovary syndrome. Eur J Endocrinol 2005;152(5): 749–756.
38. Orio F Jr., Palomba S, Di Biase S, et al. Homocysteine levels and C677T polymorphism of methylenetetrahydrofolate reductase in women with polycystic ovary syndrome. J Clin Endocrinol Metab 2003;88:673–679.
39. Yilmaz M, Biri A, Bukan N, et al. Levels of lipoprotein and homocysteine in non-obese and obese patients with polycystic ovary syndrome. Gynecol Endocrinol 2005;20:258–263.
40. Levy D, Garrison RH, Savage DD, Kannell WB, Castelli WP. Prognostic implication of echocardiographically determined left ventricular mass in the Framingham Heart Study. New Engl J Med 1991;322:1561–1566.
41. Meade TW, Cooper JA, Chakrabarti R, Miller GJ, Stirling Y, Howarth DJ. Fibrinolytic activity and clotting factor in ischaemic heart disease in women. Br Med J 1996;312:1581.
42. Orio F Jr., Palomba S, Cascella T, et al. Is plasminogen activator inhibitor-1 (PAI-1) a cardiovascular risk factor in young women with polycystic ovary syndrome? RBM Online 2004;9:505–510.
43. Diamanti-Kandarakis E, Palioniko G, Alexandraki K, Bergiele A, Koutsouba T, Bartzis M. The prevalence of 4G5G polymorphism of plasminogen activator inhibitor-1 (PAI-1) gene in polycystic ovarian syndrome and its association with plasma PAI-1 levels. Eur J Endocrinol 2004;150:793–798.
44. Reaven GM. Banting lecture 1988. Role of insulin resistance in human disease. Diabetes 1988;37: 1595–1607.
45. Wild S, Pierpoint T, McKeigue P, Jacobs H. Cardiovascular disease in women with polycystic ovary syndrome at long-term follow-up: a retrospective cohort study. Clin Endocrinol 2000;52:595–600.
46. Carmina E, Longo RA, Rini GB, Lobo RA. Phenotypic variation in hyperandrogenic women influences the findings of abnormal metabolic and cardiovascular risk parameters. J Clin Endocrinol Metab 2005;90:2545–2549.
47. Bloomgarden ZT. Inflammation and insulin resistance. Diabetes Care 2003;26:1922–1926.
48. Frishman WH. Biologic markers as predictors of cardiovascular disease. Am J Med 1998;104: 18S–27S.
49. Orio F Jr., Palomba S, Cascella T, et al. The increase of leukocytes as a new putative marker of low-grade chronic inflammation and early cardiovascular risk in polycystic ovary syndrome. J Clin Endocrinol Metab 2005;90:2–5.
50. Kelly CC, Lyall H, Petrie JR, Gould GW, Connell JM, Sattar N. Low grade chronic inflammation in women with polycystic ovarian syndrome. J Clin Endocrinol Metab 2001;86:2453–2455.

51. Gonzalez F, Thusu K, Abdel-Rahman E, Prabhala A, Tomani M, Dandona P. Elevated serum levels of tumor necrosis factor alpha in normal-weight women with polycystic ovary syndrome. Metabolism 1999;48:437–441.

52. Alexander RW. Inflammation and coronary artery disease. N Engl J Med 1994;331:468–469.

53. Sayin NC, Gucer F, Balkanli-Kaplan P, et al. Elevated serum TNF-alpha levels in normal-weight women with polycystic ovaries or the polycystic ovary syndrome. J Reprod Med 2003;48:165–170.

54. Amato G, Conte M, Mazziotti G, et al. Serum and follicular fluid cytokines in polycystic ovary syndrome during stimulated cycles. Obstet Gynecol 2003;101:1177–1182.

55. Fenkci V, Fenkci S, Yilmazer M, Serteser M. Decreased total antioxidant status and increased oxidative stress in women with polycystic ovary syndrome may contribute to the risk of cardiovascular disease. Fertil Steril 2003;80:123–127.

56. Ibanez L, Jaramillo AM, Ferrer A, de Zegher F. High neutrophil count in girls and women with hyper-insulinaemic hyperandrogenism: normalization with metformin and flutamide overcomes the aggravation by oral contraception. Hum Reprod 2005;20:2457–2462.

57. Escobar-Morreale HF, Villuendas G, Botella-Carretero JI, Sancho J, San Millan JL. Obesity, and not insulin resistance, is the major determinant of serum inflammatory cardiovascular risk markers in pre-menopausal women. Diabetologia 2003;46:625–633.

58. Mohlig M, Spranger J, Osterhoff M, et al. The polycystic ovary syndrome per se is not associated with increased chronic inflammation. Eur J Endocrinol 2004;150:525–532.

59. Puder J, Vargas S, Kraenzlin M, De Geyter C, Keller U, Muller B. Central fat excess in polycystic ovary syndrome: relation to low-grade inflammation and insulin resistance. J Clin Endocrinol Metab 2005 16;[Epub ahead of print].

60. Hotamisligal GS, Shargill NS, Spiegelman BM. Adipose expression of tumor necrosis factor α: direct role in obesity linked insulin resistance. Science 1993;259:87–91.

61. Escobar-Morreale HF, Botella-Carretero JI, Villuendas G, Sancho J, San Millan JL. Serum interleukin-18 concentrations are increased in the polycystic ovary syndrome: relationship to insulin resistance and to obesity. J Clin Endocrinol Metab 2004;89:806–811.

62. Stephens JM, Butts MD, Pekala PH. Regulation of transcription factor mRNA accumulation during 3T3–L1 preadipocyte differentiation by tumour necrosis factor-α. J Mol Endocrinol 1992;9:61–72.

63. Blankenberg S, Tiret L, Bickel C, et al. Interleukin-18 is a strong predictor of cardiovascular death in stable and unstable angina. Circulation 2002;106:24–30.

20 Nonalcoholic Fatty Liver Disease in Polycystic Ovary Syndrome

Walter Futterweit, MD, FACP

CONTENTS

Summary

Nonalcoholic fatty liver disease (NAFLD) is the most common form of liver pathology. It is frequently associated with insulin resistance and obesity. Because no previous study has been described of its prevalence in polycystic ovary syndrome (PCOS), it was hypothesized that NAFLD may be more frequent in PCOS. A retrospective study of 88 consecutive women with PCOS, using the classic 1990 National Institutes of Health criteria, was studied, with ultrasonography of the liver. Its severity was graded as absent, mild, moderate, or severe by radiological criteria. The overall incidence of NAFLD in the group was 55%. An increased rate of steatosis was associated with a higher median body mass index (BMI) and homeostasis model assessment insulin resistance. Only 15% of women in the PCOS group had abnormal liver chemistries. Nonobese women with PCOS also demonstrated a significant prevalence of NAFLD when compared with control subjects. In conclusion, NAFLD is very common in women with PCOS, even in nonobese women with the syndrome, and appears to be associated with higher BMI and insulin resistance.

Key Words: Polycystic ovary syndrome; nonalcoholic fatty liver disease; steatosis; insulin resistance.

INTRODUCTION

Nonalcoholic fatty liver disease (NAFLD) is probably the most common liver disease in the general population. Hyperinsulinemia and insulin resistance may play a role in the pathogenesis of NAFLD *(1)*. NAFLD is associated with the metabolic

From: *Contemporary Endocrinology: Insulin Resistance and Polycystic Ovarian Syndrome: Pathogenesis, Evaluation, and Treatment*
Edited by: E. Diamanti-Kandarakis, J. E. Nestler, D. Panidis, and R. Pasquali © Humana Press Inc., Totowa, NJ

syndrome, with a significant increased presence of insulin resistance (1–6). Frequently, the presence of steatosis alone in NAFLD is associated with a good prognosis. If there is further hepatic inflammation and fibrosis, there may be progression to nonalcoholic steatohepatitis (NASH) leading to fibrosis and cirrhosis in 30% of subjects with NASH (7). There is concern that the increased incidence of obesity, type 2 diabetes mellitus, and their association with fatty liver disease (1,8) make them risk factors for the development of hepatocellular carcinoma (HCC) (9–11).

Insulin resistance and hyperinsulinemia are frequently found in obese subjects with NAFLD but are also noted in lean subjects who have fatty liver disease with normal glucose tolerance (12). An association between hepatic histology and the severity of the metabolic syndrome (insulin-resistance syndrome) (13) was noted in 46 patients with biopsy-proven NAFLD (7). An increased number of features of the insulin-resistance syndrome was associated with increased degrees of hepatic fibrosis and NASH in 78% of the patients, 48% of whom had type 2 diabetes mellitus (7).

Another entity associated with metabolic syndrome and insulin resistance is poly-cystic ovary syndrome (PCOS). Insulin resistance, the hallmark of the metabolic syndrome, is present in the majority of women with PCOS (14–19). Lean women with PCOS also have appreciable insulin resistance, but less so than their obese counterparts because of the presence of the unique form of the postreceptor defect present in women with PCOS (14). The most common endocrinopathy in reproductive-aged women, PCOS is prevalent in 5–9% of premenopausal women (20–23), and was shown to be as common in black as well as white women of the southeastern United States (20). Approximately 50–55% of patients with PCOS are obese, particularly in the United States when compared with European countries (24). Metabolic abnormalities are often seen in PCOS, which primarily is reflected as insulin resistance leading to compensatory hyperinsulinemia. The latter contributes to hyperandrogenism by stimulation of androgen biosynthesis in the ovarian theca cell (25) and by suppression of sex hormone-binding globulin (SHBG) production by the liver. Alternatively, reducing the degree of insulin resistance and hyperinsulinemia leads to a decrease of hyper-androgenemia in women with PCOS (26).

The literature on NAFLD and NASH in PCOS is sparse. To the best of our knowledge there has been no previous reported study of this association. In view of the high preva-lence of insulin resistance in PCOS and potential adverse consequences of NAFLD, a study of the prevalence of NAFLD in PCOS was initiated. The aim of this study was to estimate the prevalence of NAFLD in women with PCOS by ultrasound criteria and to note the presence and severity in both obese and nonobese women with PCOS. Our second goal was to identify associated factors for NAFLD in women with PCOS. Given the high prevalence of insulin resistance in PCOS and the potential adverse con-sequences of NAFLD, it is of interest to assess the impact of various metabolic factors that may be present and associated with NAFLD in PCOS.

METHODS

Medical records of 88 premenopausal women seen consecutively between April and November 2004, in a single endocrinology practice in New York City with expert-ise in the evaluation and management of PCOS, were retrospectively reviewed. Women

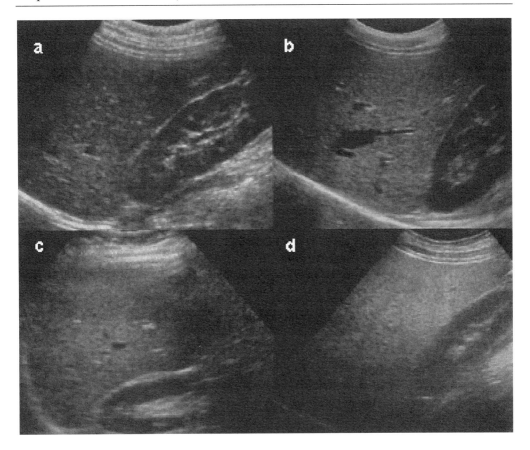

Fig. 1. Ultrasonographic criteria for severity of hepatic steatosis. (a) Absent: the echogenicity of the liver parenchyma is slightly greater or equal to that of the renal cortex; *clear visualization of diaphragm and intrahepatic vessels.* (b) Mild: slight diffuse increase in echoes liver parenchyma with *normal visualization of diaphragm and intrahepatic vessel borders.* (c) Moderate: moderate diffuse increase in fine echoes in liver parenchyma with *slightly impaired visualization of intrahepatic vessels and diaphragm.* (d) Severe: marked increase in fine echoes with *poor visualization of intrahepatic vessel borders and diaphragm.*

were included in the study population if they were 18 years of age or older at the time of the initial evaluation and met the following consensus criteria obtained by majority opinion for PCOS from the 1990 National Institutes of Health conference in Bethesda, MD *(27)*:

1. Menstrual dysfunction.
2. Hyperandrogenism.
3. The exclusion of other causes.

Subjects were excluded if they had a history of heavy alcohol use—defined as more than two drinks or 20 g of alcohol per day—or known liver disease. Data were collected from the medical records of the subjects' office encounters, including clinical history, height, weight, and laboratory values. Fasting measurements of untreated and premetformin levels of glucose and insulin, lipid profile, and liver chemistries were recorded.

The lipid profile, including serum high-density lipoprotein (HDL)-cholesterol and triglyceride levels, may have been variably affected by women who were already on oral contraceptives at the time of the study.

All women underwent abdominal ultrasonography, and the severity of hepatic steatosis was graded as absent, mild, moderate, or severe (Fig. 1) based on the echogenicity of the liver parenchyma and the visualization of intrahepatic vessels, the diaphragm, and renal cortex as described previously (28). Ultrasonography was performed with commercially available scanners (Advanced Technology Laboratories, Bothell, WA). Curved array transducers with wide-based frequency 4-2 or 5.1 MHz were used for routine abdominal scanning. In obese women or in women where there was difficulty in penetrating with sound beam, wide-band frequency 4-1, 4-2, or 3-2 MHz phase array transducer was used for scanning. The scans were performed in sagittal, coronal, and oblique subcostal planes on supine and left posterior decubitus positions. Ultrasound images were graded by an experienced radiologist who was blinded to the clinical characteristics of the patient, except for the diagnosis of PCOS.

All but 1 of the 88 subjects underwent pelvic ultrasonography, and the presence or absence of polycystic ovary morphology was noted as previously described (29).

Subjects were grouped into the following three categories according to their body mass index (BMI):

1. "Lean" with a BMI >25 kg/m^2.
2. "Overweight" with a BMI <25, but >30 kg/m^2.
3. "Obese" with a BMI <30 kg/m^2.

Insulin resistance was assessed by homeostasis model assessment insulin resistance (HOMA-IR) as calculated from fasting glucose and insulin values measured prior to the onset of those who were later treated with metformin (HOMA-IR = fasting insulin [mIU/L] × fasting glucose [mg/dL]/405) (30).

Data were analyzed and significance was determined for continuous variables using the Mann-Whitney U test and for proportions using the χ-square test with $\alpha - 0.05$.

The study was approved by the hospital IRB (Institutional Review Board) ethics committee and conforms to the ethical guidelines of the 1975 Declaration of Helsinki.

RESULTS

Eighty-eight women were identified who fit our inclusion criteria. Demographic and clinical data of the study population are reported in Table 1. Forty-three percent of the study population was found to be lean, 15% were overweight, and 42% were obese by BMI criteria. The overall prevalence of hepatic steatosis (mild, moderate, or severe) as assessed by abdominal ultrasonography was 55% (48/88 subjects). The presence of steatosis was associated with a greater median BMI than those without steatosis (31.1 vs 24.3 kg/m^2, $p = 0.009$) (Table 1). The prevalence of hepatic steatosis in the lean, overweight, and obese groups was 39, 54, ($p = 0.366$ vs lean), and 70% ($p = 0.007$ vs lean, $p = 0.282$ vs overweight), respectively (Fig. 2). Population estimates were significantly less other than in obese subjects with PCOS (Fig. 3). The prevalence and severity of steatosis in relation to BMI and population data are also shown in Fig. 2. Determinations of HDL: cholesterol levels were significantly lower in the women with PCOS who had steatosis when compared with the non-steatosis group (Table 1).

Table 1
Clinical and Laboratory Characteristics

Variable	All subjects (n = 88)	Steatosis absent (n = 40)	Steatosis present (n = 48)	p-value
Age	31.3 (27.3, 32.0)	29.0 (24.6, 32.0)	32.0 (27.3, 36.1)	0.280
BMI, kg/m^2	26.9 (24.4, 30.9)	24.3 (22.4, 26.8)	31.1 (26.8, 36.4)	**0.009**
Glucose, mg/dL	86 (84, 88)	86 (80, 88)	86 (84, 89)	0.150
Insulin, mIU/L	9.7 (6.9, 12.6)	7.0 (5.5, 11.0)	12.6 (9.1, 18.1)	0.059
HOMA-IR, mmol mIU/L^2	2.04 (1.53, 3.10)	1.50 (1.06, 2.29)	3.53 (1.79, 3.86)	**0.033**
Total cholesterol, mg/dL	193 (185, 196)	195 (184, 205)	187 (181, 198)	0.443
HDL cholesterol, mg/dL	60 (56, 64)	64 (59, 74)	54 (44, 63)	**0.003**
LDL cholesterol, mg/dL	105 (98, 113)	105 (97, 126)	105 (95, 118)	0.792
Triglycerides, mg/dL	97 (84, 111)	92 (63, 110)	107 (82, 134)	0.155
Presence of splenomegaly	6 (6.8%)	1 (2.5%)	5 (10.4%)	0.142
Presence of hepatomegaly	4 (4.5%)	0 (0%)	4 (8.3%)	0.062
Presence of PCO	64 (72.7%)	28 (70.0%)	36 (75.0%)	0.487
Abnormal ALT or GGT	9 (10.2%)	2 (5.0%)	7 (14.6%)	0.139

All data are medians with associated 95% confidence intervals or counts with proportions of the column using fasting laboratory specimens. p-values reflect results of Mann–Whitney U-tests or χ-square tests, as appropriate. Boldface indicates a significant p-value.

BMI, body mass index; HOMA-IR, homeostasis model assessment insulin resistance; HDL, high-denisty lipoprotein; LDL, low-density lipoprotein; PCO, polycystic ovaries; ALT, alanine aminotransferase; GGT, γ-glutamyl transferrase.

Patients in the higher HOMA-IR quartiles had significantly higher prevalence and higher severity of steatosis (Table 1, Fig. 4). Trends were noted toward greater premetformin fasting insulin and greater triglycerides, and increased prevalence of splenomegaly, hepatomegaly, and abnormal liver chemistries were present in those with steatosis. These differences, however, did not reach statistical significance, with α = 0.05. In addition, there were no significant differences in median age, premetformin fasting glucose, total cholesterol, or low-density lipoprotein cholesterol when compared with the women who had normal liver ultrasound imaging.

The presence of the PCO morphology on ultrasonography was 76.6 and 70.0% in the study subjects with steatosis or without steatosis, respectively ($p = 0.487$).

Addendum

Preliminary results comparing the prevalence and grade of steatosis was studied in 38 lean and 13 overweight women with PCOS from the previously listed study and compared with 22 controls also stratified into the lean and overweight category. Median age and BMI values in the control group were 38.3 years and 25.4 kg/m^2, respectively.

Prevalence of Non-alcoholic Fatty Liver Disease (NAFLD) by Body Mass Index (BMI)

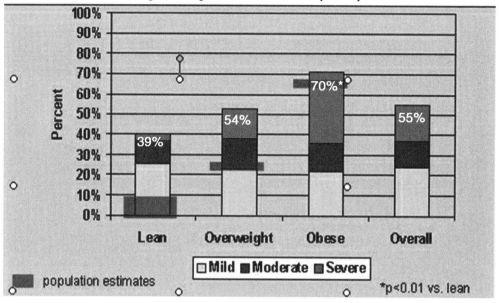

Fig. 2. Prevalence of nonalcoholic fatty liver disease (NAFLD) by body mass index (BMI).

The overall prevalence of hepatic steatosis in PCOS (mild and moderate) assessed by abdominal ultrasonography was 43.1% (22/51 subjects), whereas that of mild and moderately obese controls was 18.2% (4/22 subjects). A significant increased incidence of steatosis was noted in both the lean and overweight women with PCOS when compared with similarly categorized controls (39 and 54% vs 20 and 17% in the lean and overweight controls; $p = 0.03$). The severity of steatosis was associated with a greater BMI in both categories of PCOS compared with that of controls ($p = 0.02$). The prevalence and severity of steatosis in relation to BMI are presented in Table 2. HOMA-IR values in 47 of the lean and overweight women with PCOS were compared with 18 controls. The median HOMA-IR score was 1.4 mmol mIU/L (range 0.35 to 9.50) in the former and 1.3 (range 0.62 to 2.30) in the latter. No statistical difference was noted between the two groups of subjects ($p = 0.40$ by Wilcoxon rank sum test). (The data are preliminary and further controls are currently being studied.)

DISCUSSION

The high, almost global, prevalence of obesity has made fatty liver disease and its complications a leading public health issue. This asymptomatic entity, as well as the absence of specific surrogate markers, has made it difficult to diagnose and estimate its true prevalence in the population. However, some may have the capacity to develop later hepatic complications, particularly those with significant obesity and/or associated type 2 diabetes mellitus.

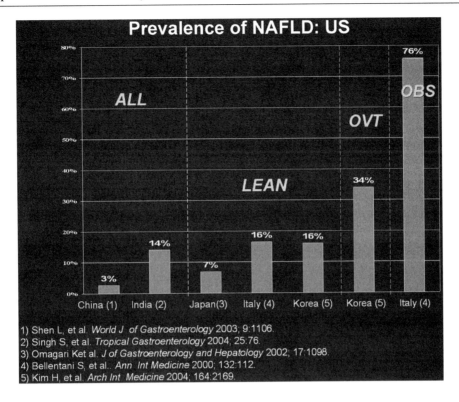

Fig. 3. Prevalence of nonalcoholic fatty liver disease (NAFLD) as observed by ultrasound.

NAFLD is associated with features of the metabolic syndrome *(1)* and the present study noted an increased prevalence in subjects with PCOS. The exclusion of overweight and obese subjects does not change the results. Insulin resistance and hyperinsulinemia may thus be found even in lean subjects with NAFLD who have normal glucose tolerance. There appears to be an association between liver histology and to the severity of the metabolic syndrome when liver biopsies are performed in patients with NAFLD *(7)*. An increase in the number of features of the metabolic syndrome was associated with increased degrees of hepatic fibrosis in 46 subjects with NAFLD *(7)*.

Data from the Third National Health and Nutrition Examination Survey (NHANES III) revealed that 30% of the US population is obese and almost three-quarters have fatty liver disease and NASH, which may progress in some to later hepatic complications *(31,32)*. The risk for HCC is increased two- to threefold in patients with diabetes mellitus in a population-based study of more than 2061 patients with liver cancer over the age of 65 years compared with more than 6000 noncancer controls *(11)*. This suggests that diabetes mellitus is an independent risk factor for HCC.

NAFLD is probably the most common cause of cryptogenic cirrhosis *(33)*. Skelly et al. *(34)* demonstrated histological evidence of steatosis or steatohepatitis (NASH) in approx 70% of asymptomatic patients with mild, cryptogenic liver enzyme elevations in the United Kingdom. A strong association between increased BMI and cryptogenic aminotransferase elevations was demonstrated in a large study of 18,825 adult subjects in the United States, with 1% having abnormal enzyme activity in the lean group, 3.3%

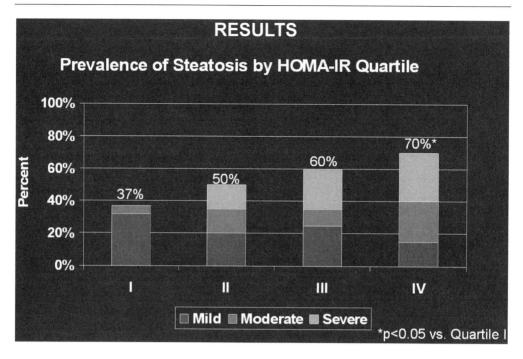

Fig. 4. Results of the prevalence of steatosis by homeostasis model assessment insulin resistance (HOMA-IR) quartile.

in the overweight, 5.5% in class I obesity, and 6.6% in class II/III obesity *(35)*. Other studies noted an incidence of cryptic elevated alanine aminotransferase values in 7.9% in the United States *(36)*, and 5–6% of moderate to severely obese women *(37)*.

Ultrasonographic grading of fatty infiltration of the liver has been described by Scatarige et al. *(28)*. They reported grades 0 (normal), grade 1 (mild to slight diffuse increase in fine echoes in the hepatic parenchyma), grade 2 (moderate to diffuse increase in echoes with slightly impaired visualization of intrahepatic vessels and diaphragm), and grade 3 (severe to marked increased echoes with poor visualization of intrahepatic vessel borders and diaphragm). In their study, they found a good correlation between the sonographic findings and unenhanced computed tomography of the liver.

A review of 73 consecutive infertile women, most of whom had been nulliparous, with PCOS demonstrated that where serum ALT was recorded, 30% had elevation of ALT *(38)*. Serum aspartate aminotransferase (AST) levels were elevated in 12%. In the present study, the history excluded those women with excessive alcohol intake, prior hepatitis, and use of hepatotoxic medications. Studies were performed to exclude hepatitis B and C, and hemochromatosis. Total and direct bilirubin levels were normal in our subjects. A significant association was found in those with elevated ALT levels and higher BMI, waist circumference, serum triglycerides, total cholesterol/HDL ratio, hirsutism, and insulin resistance as defined, to some extent, by the elevated serum insulin levels and the quantitative insulin sensitivity check index.

It appears that insulin resistance and the association of the metabolic syndrome explains the elevated ALT levels in overweight women with PCOS who have an approximately fivefold increase of this liver function test as compared with a non-PCOS

Table 2
Comparing Steatosis in PCOS Patients With That in Controls All Patients
and Controls are Lean or Overweight (Obese Patients are Excluded)

Number	Steatosis	Present N (%)
BMI < 25	PCOS patients 38	15 (39%)
	Controls 10	2 (20%)
BMI 25–30	PCOS patients 13	7 (54%)
	Controls 12	2 (17%)

The proportion of patients with steatosis differs significantly between PCOS patients and controls, $p = 0.03$ by Mantel-Haenszel test, stratifying on BMI category.

Number	Steatosis	Ultrasound steatosis grade (No. [%])			
		0	1	2	3
BMI < 25	PCOS pts 38	23 (61%)	10 (26%)	4 (11%)	1 (3%)
Controls	10	8 (80%)	2 (20%)	0	0
BMI 25–30	PCOS pts 13	6 (46%)	3 (23%)	2 (15%)	2 (15%)
Controls	12	10 (83%)	1 (8%)	1 (8%)	0

The grade of steatosis differs significantly between PCOS patients and controls, p = 0.02 by Mantel-Haenszel test ordered outcomes, stratifying on BMI category.

population. It should be noted, however, that radiological methods including ultrasonography are unable to differentiate NAFLD from NASH (39). Only a liver biopsy can distinguish the two entities (39,40).

In this study's cohort of premenopausal women having PCOS, we found a high prevalence of NAFLD in both lean and obese subjects. Prior studies from India, China, Italy, Japan, Korea, and the United States noted a 3–16% prevalence of NAFLD by ultrasound criteria in lean or general populations and up to 70% of obese men and women in a Northern Italian study (41–44), with evidence of steatosis in 16% of lean, nonheavily drinking participants (44) (Fig. 3). Our study demonstrated, however, a significant 40% prevalence of steatosis in lean (BMI >25 kg/m^2) women with PCOS and a 70% incidence of steatosis in the obese women with PCOS, similar to the obese Northern Italian population. On the other hand, this study is consistent with previous work in the field, in which insulin resistance and obesity appear to be important associated factors with NAFLD. The HOMA-IR score was significantly greater and HDL was significantly lower in subjects with steatosis than in those without steatosis. Both reflect greater insulin resistance in the subjects with steatosis. Most importantly, there was a substantial prevalence of NAFLD in lean women with PCOS. This may reflect the impact of insulin resistance in PCOS, whereas greater prevalence of NAFLD in the obese women with PCOS as compared with the lean women may reflect the additive effect of obesity in augmenting insulin resistance.

We found a relatively low prevalence of liver enzyme abnormalities in subjects who demonstrated hepatic steatosis by ultrasound (7 of the 48 subjects, 15%). Because advanced liver disease, including cirrhosis, may be present in the absence of abnormal liver chemistries, the presence of NAFLD by ultrasound and normal liver chemistries in a large group of these young women is of concern. Currently, there are no noninvasive tests to diagnose and stage NAFLD. Liver biopsy remains the most sensitive diagnostic test but cannot distinguish NAFLD from other causes of fatty liver disease, such as alcohol abuse. Elevated serum aminotransferase levels can suggest a diagnosis of NAFLD; however, these liver function tests are both insensitive and nonspecific indicators of NAFLD-related liver damage. For instance, the degree of liver enzyme elevation does not correlate with the level of damage on histological analysis; thus, these tests cannot reliably distinguish steatosis from steatohepatitis or cirrhosis. Serum aminotransferase levels may indeed be normal or only slightly elevated, although liver disease is advanced. Sorrentino et al. *(45)* demonstrated that more than 70% of patients with metabolic syndrome and normal liver enzymes may have varying degrees of nonalcoholic steatohepatitis, with 33% having evidence of fibrosis and 10% of cirrhosis.

To our knowledge, this is the first study to estimate the prevalence of NAFLD in premenopausal women with PCOS. Our study has shown that NAFLD is common in PCOS regardless of BMI. As expected, however, obesity and insulin resistance are associated with even higher prevalence rates. Despite varying degrees of hepatic steatosis, elevated liver chemistries are not common in PCOS. Because NASH is a risk factor for the development of cirrhosis, and occasionally HCC, the high prevalence of hepatic steatosis in young lean and obese women having PCOS and mostly in the absence of abnormal liver chemistries is of concern. It appears prudent to perform liver ultrasonography in patients with PCOS, regardless of their BMI and whether liver chemistry tests are abnormal. In view of data demonstrating that the frequently measured HOMA-IR and other indices of insulin resistance in all weight groups of PCOS tend to underestimate its prevalence compared with the euglycemic clamp technique *(46)*, the treatment of NAFLD should be targeted accordingly. An unsatisfactory response to the above may possibly necessitate the use of liver biopsy to make a diagnosis and define the stage of liver disease. A case report of a young woman with PCOS and NASH proven by liver biopsy revealed a very significant improvement in liver histopathology and liver chemistries 1 year after instituting a significant weight-loss program *(47)*.

Although weight reduction is the cornerstone for patients with obesity in PCOS as well as NAFLD, it is not feasible to achieve adequate clinical results in many with a normal body weight. Metformin has been amply shown to affect significant changes in insulin resistance in PCOS, and is often used in many women with the syndrome *(16,48)*. Because insulin sensitizers such as metformin and other drugs such as the thiozolidinediones are part of the armamentarium to treat PCOS as well as NAFLD *(49–55)*, their use in conjunction with a change in lifestyle is of great import in patients with PCOS who have hepatic steatosis.

In summary, there is a high incidence of NAFLD as determined by ultrasonography of the liver in obese and non-obese women with PCOS. Obesity and insulin resistance are important associated factors with NAFLD in PCOS as in other population studies. Of clinical relevance is the fact that the majority of subjects with NAFLD do not demonstrate elevated liver chemistries, and those that demonstrate abnormalities are usually in the obese category. Because NASH is a potential risk factor for the development of later hepatic complications, its high prevalence in young women with PCOS in association with mostly normal liver function tests should be addressed. Further studies of treatment modalities to modify NAFLD in subjects with PCOS would be of interest and importance.

FUTURE AVENUES OF INVESTIGATION

The relationship between NALFD and the cluster of features comprising the metabolic syndrome in PCOS remain to be determined. The high frequency of insulin resistance in nonobese women with NAFLD and PCOS suggests that imaging of the liver may be a marker of the presence and/or likelihood of a cluster of features of the metabolic syndrome. Further studies are indicated to assess this hypothesis and the role of lifestyle modification and pharmacological treatment, such as insulin sensitizers. A proactive approach may not only delay or prevent the progression of NAFLD to NASH, but possibly address some of the risk factors associated with the metabolic syndrome.

KEY POINTS

- NAFLD is present in 40–54% of lean and overweight women with PCOS, respectively. This is a threefold increased prevalence over that of global population studies. Its presence in obese women with PCOS is 70%.
- Insulin resistance appears to be a significant association of NAFLD in PCOS.
- Ultrasonography of the liver is a useful noninvasive tool in assessing its presence.
- A majority of women with NAFLD have normal liver enzymes, and does not indicate its presence.

ACKNOWLEDGMENT

My sincerest thanks for the technical assistance of Richard Weiss and the help of my office staff—Luba Dronova and Roni Malinbaum. I also wish to thank Dr. Carol Bodian for her expert statistical analysis.

REFERENCES

1. Marchesini G, Brizi M, Morselli-Labate AM, et al. Association of nonalcoholic fatty liver disease with insulin resistance. Am J Med 1999;107:450–455.
2. Friis-Liby I, Aldenborg F, Jerlstad P, Rundsröm K, Björnsson E. High prevalence of metabolic complications in patients with non-alcoholic fatty liver disease. Scand J Gastroenterol 2004;39:868–869.
3. Marchesini G, Brizi M, Bianchi G, et al. Nonalcoholic fatty liver disease: a feature of the metabolic syndrome. Diabetes 2001;50:1844–1850.
4. Angelico F, Del Ben M, Conti R, et al. Insulin resistance, the metabolic syndrome, and nonalcoholic fatty liver disease. J Clin Endocrinol Metab 2005;90:1578–1582.
5. Knobler H, Schattner A, Zhornicki T, et al. Fatty liver—an additional and treatable feature of the insulin resistance syndrome. QJM 1999;92:73–79.
6. Marceau P, Biron S, Hould FS, et al. Liver pathology and the metabolic syndrome X in severe obesity. J Clin Endocrinol Metab 1999;84:1513–1517.
7. Ryan MC, Best JD, Wilson AM, Jenkins AJ, Slavin J, Desmond PV. Associations between liver histology and severity of the metabolic syndrome in subjects with nonalcoholic fatty liver disease. Diabetes Care 2005;28:1222–1224.
8. Andersen T, Gluud C. Liver morphology in morbid obesity: a literature study. Int J Obes 1984;8:97–106.
9. Caldwell SH, Crespo DM, Kang HS, Al-Osaimi AM. Obesity and hepatocellular carcinoma. Gastroenterology 2004;127:S97–S103.
10. El-Serag HB. Hepatocellular carcinoma: recent trends in the United States. Gastroenterology 2004; 127:S27–S34.
11. Davila JA, Morgan RO, Shaib Y, McGlynn KA, El-Serag HB. Diabetes increases the risk of hepatocellular carcinoma in the United States: a population based case control study. Gut 2005; 54:533–539.

12. Kim HJ, Kim HJ, Kwang EL, et al. Metabolic significance of nonalcoholic fatty liver disease in nonobese, nondiabetic adults. Arch Intern Med 2004;164:2169–2175.

13. Valantine H, Rickenbacker P, Kemna M, et al. Metabolic abnormalities characteristic of dysmetabolic syndrome predict the development of transplant coronary artery disease: a prospective study. Circulation 2001;103:2144–2152.

14. Dunaif A, Segal KR, Futterweit W, Dobrjansky A. Profound insulin resistance independent of obesity in polycystic ovary syndrome. Diabetes 1989;38:1165–1174.

15. Dunaif A. Insulin resistance and the polycystic ovary syndrome: mechanism of action and implications for pathogenesis. Endocr Rev 1996;18:774–800.

16. Apridonidze T, Essah PA, Iuorno MJ, Nestler JE. Prevalence and characteristics of the metabolic syndrome in women with polycystic ovary syndrome. J Clin Endocrinol Metab. 2005;90:1929–1935.

17. DeUgarte CM, Bartolucci AA, Azziz R. Prevalence of insulin resistance in the polycystic ovary syndrome using the homeostasis model assessment. Fertil Steril 2005;83:1454–1460.

18. Azziz R. Polycystic ovary syndrome, insulin resistance, and molecular defects of insulin signaling. J Clin Endocrinol Metab 2002;89:4085–4087.

19. PCO Writing Committee: Cobin RH, Futterweit W, Nestler JE, et al. AACE Position Statement on metabolic and cardiovascular consequences of polycystic ovary syndrome. Endocr Pract 2005;11: 125–134.

20. Knochenhauer ES, Key TJ, Kahsar-Miller M, Waggoner W, Boots LR, Azziz R. Prevalence of the polycystic ovary syndrome in unselected black and white women of the southeastern United States: a prospective study. J Clin Endocrinol Metab 1998;83:3078–3082

21. Diamanti-Kandarakis E, Kouli CR, Bergiele AT, et al. A survey of the polycystic ovary syndrome in the Greek island of Lesbos: hormonal and metabolic profile. J Clin Endocrinol Metab 1999;84: 4006–4011.

22. Asuncion M, Calvo RM, San Millan JL, Sancho J, Avila S, Escobar-Morreale HF. A prospective study of the prevalence of polycystic ovary syndrome from Spain. J Clin Endocrinol Metab 2000;85: 2434–2438.

23. Azziz R, Yildiz B, Woods KS, et al. The prevalence of polycystic ovary syndrome among unselected consecutive premenopausal women. J Clin Endocrinol Metab 2004;89:2745–2749.

24. Carmina E, Legro RS, Stamets K, Lowell J, Lobo RA. Difference in body weight between American and Italian women with polycystic ovary syndrome. Hum Reprod 2003;11:2289–2293.

25. Nestler JE, Jakubowicz DJ, de Vargas AF, Brik C, Quintero N, Medina F. Insulin stimulates testosterone biosynthesis by human theca cells from women with polycystic ovary syndrome by activating its own receptor and using inositolglycan mediators as the signal transduction system. J Clin Endocrinol Metab 1998;83:2001–2005.

26. Nestler JE, Jakubowicz DJ. Lean women with polycystic ovary syndrome respond to insulin reduction with decreases in P450c alpha activity and serum androgens. J Clin Endocrinol Metab 1997;82: 4075–4079.

27. Zawadsky JK, Dunaif A. Diagnostic criteria for polycystic ovary syndrome: towards a rational approach. In: Dunaif A, Givens JR, Haseltine FP, Merriam GR, eds. Polycystic Ovary Syndrome, Boston, MA: Blackwell Scientific Publications; 1992, pp. 377–384.

28. Scatarige JC, Scott WW, Donovan PJ, Siegelman SS, Sanders RC. Fatty infiltration of the liver: ultrasonographic and computed tomographic correlation. J Ultrasound Med 1984;3:9–14.

29. Yeh HC, Futterweit W, Thornton JC. Polycystic ovarian disease: US features in 104 patients. Radiology 1987;163:111–116.

30. Matthews DR, Hosker JP, Rudenski AS, Naylor BA, Treacher DF, Turner RC. Homeostasis model assessment: insulin resistance and beta-cell function from fasting plasma glucose and insulin concentrations in man. Diabetologia 1985;28:412–419.

31. Flegal KM, Carroll MD, Ogden CL, Johnson CL. Prevalence and trends in obesity among US adults, 1999–2000. JAMA 2002;288:1723–1727.

32. Wanless IR, Lentz JS. Fatty liver hepatitis (steatohepatitis) and obesity: an autopsy study with analysis of risk factors. Hepatology 1990;12:1106–1110.

33. Caldwell SH, Oelsner DH, Iezzoni JC, Hespenheide EE, Battle EH, Driscoll CJ. Cryptogenic cirrhosis: clinical characterization and risk factors for underlying disease. Hepatology 1999;29:664–669.

34. Skelly MM, James PD, Ryder SD. Findings on liver biopsy to investigate abnormal liver function tests in the absence of diagnostic serology. J Hepatol 2001;35:195–199.

35. Erbey JR, Silberman C, Lydick E. Prevalence of abnormal serum alinine aminotransferase levels in obese patients and patients with type 2 diabetes. Am J Med 2000;109:588–590.

36. Clark JM, Brancati FL, Diehl AM. The prevalence and etiology of elevated aminotransferase levels in the United States. Am J Gastroenterol 2003;98:960–967.

37. Ruhl C, Everhart J. Determinations of the association of overweight with elevated serum alanine aminotransferase activity in the United States. Gastroenterology 2003;124:71–79.

38. Schwimmer JB, Khorram O, Chiu V, Schwimmer WB. Abnormal aminotransferase activity in women with polycystic ovary syndrome. Fert Steril 2005;83:494–497.

39. Saadeh S, Younossi ZM, Remer EM, et al. The utility of radiological imaging in nonalcoholic fatty liver disease. Gastroenterology 2002;123:745–750.

40. Sanyal AJ. AGA technical review on nonalcoholic fatty liver disease. Gastroenterology 2002;123: 1705–1725.

41. Shen L, Fan J-G, Shao Y, et al. Prevalence of nonalcoholic fatty liver among administrative officers in Shanghai: an epidemiologic survey. World J Gastroenterol 2003;9:1106–1110.

42. Singh SP, Nayak S, Swain M, et al. Prevalence of nonalcoholic fatty liver disease in coastal eastern India: a preliminary ultrasonographic survey. Trop Gastroenterol 2004;25:76–79.

43. Omagari K, Kadokawa Y, Masuda J-I, et al. Fatty liver in non-alcoholic non-overweight Japanese adults: incidence and clinical characteristics. J Gastroenterol Hepatol 2002;17:1098–1105.

44. Bellentani S, Saccoccio G, Masutti F, et al. Prevalence of and risk factors for hepatic steatosis in northern Italy. Ann Int Med 2000;132:112–117.

45. Sorrentino P, Tarantino G, Conca P, et al. Silent non-alcoholic fatty liver disease—a clinical–histological study. J Hepatol 2004;41:751–757.

46. Diamanti-Kandarakis E, Kouli C, Alexandraki K, Spina G. Failure of mathematical indices to accurately assess insulin resistance in lean, overweight, or obese women with polycystic ovary syndrome. J Clin Endocrinol Metab 2004;89:1273–1276.

47. Brown AJ, Tendice DA, McMurray RG, Setji TL. Polycystic ovary syndrome and severe nonalcoholic steatohepatitis: beneficial effect of modest weight loss and exercise on liver biopsy findings. Endocr Pract 2005;11:319–324.

48. Nestler JE. Should patients with polycystic ovarian syndrome be treated with metformin? An enthusiastic endorsement. Hum Reprod 2002;17:1950–1953.

49. Neuschwander-Tetri BA, Brunt EM, Wehmeier KR, Oliver D, Bacon BR. Improved nonalcoholic steatohepatitis after 48 weeks of treatment with the PPAR-gamma ligand rosiglitazone. Hepatology 2003;38:1008–1013.

50. Shadid S, Jensen MD. Effect of pioglitazone on biochemical indices of non-alcoholic fatty liver disease in upper body obesity. Clin Gastroenterol Hepatol 2003;1:384–387.

51. Promrat K, Lutchman G, Uwaifo GI, et al. A pilot study of pioglitazone treatment for nonalcoholic steatohepatitis. Hepatology 2004;39:188–196.

52. Bugianesi E, Gentilcore E, Manini R, et al. A randomized controlled trial of metformin versus vitamin E or prescriptive diet in nonalcoholic fatty liver disease. Am J Gastroenterol 2005;100:1082–1090.

53. Marchesini G, Brizi M, Bianchi G, Tomassetti S, Zoli M, Melchionda N. Metformin in nonalcoholic steatohepatitis. Lancet 2001;358:893–894.

54. Urso R, Visco-Comandini U. Metformin in non-alcoholic steatohepatitis. Lancet 2002;359:893–894.

55. Schwimmer JB, Middleton MS, Deutsch R, Lavine JE. A phase 2 clinical trial of metformin as a treatment for non-diabetic paediatric non-alcoholic steatohepatitis. Aliment Pharmacol Ther 2005;21:871–879.

21 Endometrial Carcinoma in Polycystic Ovary Syndrome

Emmanuel Diakomanolis, MD

CONTENTS

Summary

Endometrial carcinoma is the most common malignancy of the female genital tract, accounting for 6% of all cancers among women, and exceeded in overall frequency only by breast, lung, and colorectal cancers.

Retrospective studies from the 1970s revealed that unopposed estrogen, both exogenous and endogenous, was a leading factor in the development of endometrial cancer. Although the average age of women developing endometrial cancer secondary to unopposed estrogen is 63 years, 25% of all endometrial cancers occur in premenopausal women. The main explanation for the development of endometrial cancer in young women is unopposed estrogen secondary to anovulation. Polycystic ovary syndrome (PCOS) is thought to explain a majority of those cases.

The true risk of endometrial cancer in women with PCOS, however, is difficult to ascertain. A substantial proportion of endometrial cancer could be avoided with the maintenance of a normal weight throughout life. There is no effective way of screening for endometrial cancer. Abnormal uterine bleeding is the most frequent symptom, and surgery is the cornerstone of treatment. During the last decade, efforts have focused on attempting to identify cytocinetic or molecular events that correlate with the malignant potential of endometrial cancer.

We are going to discuss our approach to screening, cancer risk assessment, and the therapeutic intervention in patients with endometrial cancer.

From: *Contemporary Endocrinology: Insulin Resistance and Polycystic Ovarian Syndrome:*
Pathogenesis, Evaluation, and Treatment
Edited by: E. Diamanti-Kandarakis, J. E. Nestler, D. Panidis, and R. Pasquali © Humana Press Inc., Totowa, NJ

Key Words: Endometrial cancer; polycystic ovary syndrome (PCOS); risk factors; prognostic factors; treatment options; surgical staging; oncogene expression.

INTRODUCTION

All malignancies have increased in incidence this century and disease patterns have changed. The incidence of endometrial cancer is rising as life expectancy increases. Age-adjusted incidence is increasing, even when corrected for hysterectomy. The rise has been associated with an epidemic of obesity and physical inactivity *(1,2)*.

Worldwide, endometrial cancer is the seventh most common malignant disorder, but incidence varies among regions. In less-developed countries, risk factors are less common and endometrial cancer is rare, although specific mortality is higher. The incidence is 10 times higher in North America and Europe than in less developed countries.

In North America, endometrial cancer is the eighth most common cause of cancer-related death in the female population. It is estimated that 36,100 new cases of endometrial cancer will be diagnosed in the United States during 2000 and that 6500 women will die *(3)*. Each year in Europe, an estimated 9000 women die of endometrial cancer. Substantial decreases in the incidence and mortality are unlikely in the next few years because early detection and treatment modalities have not had a major influence on mortality.

Although the incidence of endometrial carcinoma has remained relatively stable during the past decade, the number of deaths from this disease has more than doubled since 1987 (from 2900 to 6400 deaths). Presumably, the explanations for these statistics are multifactorial, but we are obligated to reassess more objectively and critically the processes that guide the overall management of this neoplasm.

PATHOGENESIS

Any factor that increases exposure to unopposed estrogen (e.g., hormone replacement therapy, obesity, anovulatory cycles, estrogen secreting tumors) increases the risk of endometrial cancer, whereas factors that decrease exposure to estrogens or increase progesterone levels (e.g., oral contraceptives or smoking) tend to be protective.

The importance of understanding pathogenesis is that it affects how we treat young women with endometrial cancers. If an elevated estrogen state is thought to cause the malignancy, a reduction in the estrogen stimulation, and even a reversal of the estrogen-induced lesion by progesterone, has been advocated. There are data to show that progesterone can reverse premalignant endometrial lesions. However, if the reason for the development of cancer is secondary to a defect in mismatch repair genes or other tumor suppressor genes, there are no data to suggest that progesterone will treat the cancer.

The mechanism that is generally assumed to be responsible for any increased risk of endometrial carcinoma in women with polycystic ovary syndrome (PCOS) relates to prolonged anovulation with consequent secretion of estrogen unopposed by progesterone. However, hypersecretion of luteinizing hormone, a feature of PCOS, has also been implicated in the development of endometrial cancer in women with PCOS. Receptors for luteinizing hormone and human chorionic gonadotropin are overexpressed at both the mRNA and protein levels in endometrial adenocarcinomas *(4)*. It seems that over-expression of receptors for luteinizing hormone and human chorionic gonadotropin is a feature of endometrial hyperplasia and endometrial carcinoma, developing in younger anovulating women, including those with PCOS *(5)*.

Long-lasting unopposed estrogen exposure leads to endometrial hyperplasia, which increases the chance of development of atypical hyperplasia and, eventually, type 1 endometrial cancer. The molecular basis of this process is still not known because the involvement of only a minority of factors is reproducible. The classic teaching has been that endometrial hyperplasia represents a continuum of morphological severity; the most severe form, termed *atypical hyperplasia*, was considered the immediate precursor of endometrial carcinoma.

Molecular research supports the view of a dualistic model of endometrial carcinogenesis. Phosphatase and tensin homolog deleted on chromosome ten (PTEN) is a tumor-suppressor gene that is expressed most highly in an estrogen-rich environment; progestagens affect PTEN expression and promote involution of PTEN-mutated endometrial cells in various histopathological settings *(6)*. These observations are consistent with the well-documented clinical effect of progestagen-mediated suppression of human endometrial precancer, and even ablation of some cancers. Apart from *PTEN* mutations typically seen in type 1 endometrial cancers, there are other gene alterations that are specific for cancers of types 1 and 2, which support a dualistic model of endometrial carcinogenesis *(7)*. Type 1 carcinomas are associated with mutations in the *KRAS2* oncogene, PTEN tumor-suppressor gene, and near-diploid karyotype. By contrast, type 2 carcinomas are associated with mutations in *TP53* and *ERBB-2* (HER-2/neu) expression and more are non-diploid *(8)*.

We have come to the point of changing from descriptive pathology to a functional or genetic description of the disease. In other words, we are changing to molecular oncology. In this way, we may base our therapeutic decisions on the genetic profiles of tumors for the better management of our patients.

Most endometrioid carcinomas are well to moderately differentiated and arise on a background of endometrial hyperplasia. These tumors, also known as type 1 (low-grade) endometrial carcinomas, have a favorable prognosis *(9)*. They are associated with long-duration unopposed estrogenic stimulation and are histologically of the endometrioid type in 80% of cases. About 10% of endometrial cancers are type 2 (high-grade) lesions. Women with such tumors are at high risk of relapse and metastatic disease. These tumors are not estrogen-driven, and most are associated with endometrial atrophy; surgery is commonly followed by adjuvant therapy.

Serous carcinoma is the most aggressive type of nonendometrioid endometrial carcinoma *(10)*. Myometrial invasion is prominent in most cases, and vascular invasion is common. Clear-cell carcinoma is another type of nonendometrioid endometrial carcinoma (up to 40% of nonendometrioid endometrial cancers are mixed with an endometrioid component). World Health Organization histological classification of endometrial carcinoma is shown in Table 1. Histological grading applies only to endometrioid carcinomas; serous and clear-cell carcinomas are classed as high-grade by definition.

PCOS AND ENDOMETRIAL CARCINOMA

Data from many previous studies suggest that infertility is a risk factor for endometrial cancer. Case series of epidemiological studies have identified an association between infertility and endometrial cancer *(11)*. However, it is uncertain whether this association varies according to the cause of infertility.

Table 1
WHO Histological Classification of Endometrial Carcinoma

Endometrioid adenocarcinoma
Variants: with squamous differentiation
                 villoglandular, secretory
                 with ciliated cells
Other adenocarcinomas:
Mucinous carcinoma
Serous carcinoma
Clear-cell carcinoma
Mixed carcinoma
Squamous-cell carcinoma
Transitional-cell carcinoma
Small-cell carcinoma
Undifferentiated carcinoma

PCOS is the most common endocrinopathy in women, affecting 5–10% of women of reproductive age. Consequently, it is the most common cause of anovulatory infertility, oligomenorrhea, amenorrhea, and hirsutim. PCOS is also associated with type 1 and 2 gestational diabetes, as well as many risk factors for coronary heart disease and cancer.

The association between PCOS and endometrial adenocarcinoma has been reported for many years *(12)*, but a search of current literature provides surprisingly little evidence to support this association. Many of the published studies have no controls and their interpretation is further complicated by the variety of diagnostic criteria used to define the syndrome.

There is considerable heterogeneity of symptoms and signs among women with PCOS, and for an individual these may change overtime. Furthermore, polycystic ovaries can exist without clinical signs of the syndrome, which may then become expressed over time.

There is still lack of consensus as to the definition of PCOS. Criteria for making the diagnosis have been the basis of several "consensus conferences" on PCOS. As a result of the lack of clearly defined and universally accepted criteria, research studies have been based on a variety of signs, symptoms, and laboratory results in the patient populations enrolled. It has long been recognized that the presence of enlarged ovaries with multiple small cysts (2–8 mm) and a hypervascularized androgen-secreting stroma are associated with signs of androgen excess, hirsutism, acne, and menstrual irregularities (oligomenorrhea or amenorrhea).

Approximately 20% of women of reproductive age will have polycystic ovaries on ultrasound scan, whereas up to 10% will have symptoms consistent with the diagnosis of PCOS *(13)*. In North America, clinicians tend to use the "NIH definition" *(14)* of hyperandrogenism, chronic anovulation, and exclusion of other known disorders, such as congenital adrenal hyperplasia, Cushing's Syndrome, and androgen-producing tumors.

The European definition of the syndrome tends to be based on ultrasound appearances of the ovaries and one of several clinical symptoms, including hirsutism, oligomenorrhea, or amenorrhea and infertility. A recent practice bulletin from the American College of Obstetricians and Gynecologists (15) discusses the diagnosis and clinical management of PCOS. It is noted that chronic anovulation, obesity, hyperinsulinemia, and decreased concentrations of sex-hormone binding globulin are associated with endometrial cancer.

The true risk of endometrial carcinoma in women with PCOS, however, is difficult to ascertain. Studies to date have been limited by the relatively small number of cases of endometrial carcinoma identified specifically in women with PCOS.

An early study published in 1957 by Jackson and Dockerty (12) showed a 37% prevalence of endometrial carcinoma in women with polycystic ovaries. This study and many other studies that continue to be cited today unfortunately have differences in diagnostic criteria and absence of suitable controls. For these reasons it is not possible to do a meta-analysis to calculate an estimate of the relative risk of endometrial carcinoma in women with PCOS.

In a more recent study (16) of women with endometrial carcinoma, obese subjects were found to have a 2.6- to 3-fold increased risk of endometrial carcinoma compared with nonobese patients. This finding suggests that anovulation may not be an independent risk factor for endometrial carcinoma and that the apparent association between PCOS and endometrial carcinoma could be caused by specific endocrine or metabolic abnormalities occurring as a result of the syndrome.

Women with type 1 endometrial cancer are likely to have been exposed to unopposed estrogens (Table 2). Excessive fat consumption and overweight (defined as body mass index [BMI] of at least 25 kg/m^2) are important risk factors present in almost 50% of women with endometrial cancer (17).

A BMI higher than 25 kg/m^2 doubles a woman's risk of endometrial cancer and a BMI higher than 30 kg/m^2 triples the risk (17). High BMI in young age and BMI gain are also associated with endometrial cancer (5).

Obesity seems to remain a risk factor for endometrial cancer even when circulating concentrations of estrogen are normal. It alters concentrations of insulin-like growth factor and its binding proteins. Physical inactivity, high-energy intake, blood pressure higher than 140/90 mmHg, and high serum glucose concentrations are BMI-independent risk factors, whereas the presence of polycystic ovaries depends on the BMI (3).

In premenopausal women, overweight causes insulin resistance, ovarian androgen excess, anovulation, and chronic progesterone deficiency. In postmenopausal women, it causes a higher circulating concentration of bioavailable estrogens from extraglandular conversion of androgens. This change stimulates endometrial cell proliferation, inhibits apoptosis, and promotes angiogenesis.

Diabetes mellitus is well recognized as a risk factor for endometrial cancer. The association may partly relate to obesity, but there is evidence for a specific effect of hyperinsulinemia, and increased concentrations of plasma insulin were found in patients with endometrial cancer (18).

Because insulin upregulates aromatase activity in endometrial glands and stroma, endogenous estrogen production is enhanced in women with high circulating insulin. By contrast, the argument linking hyperinsulinemia with endometrial cancer is not supported by other studies. On the basis of the available evidence, it is reasonable to conclude that the interaction between endocrine and metabolic factors and endometrial neoplasia in women with PCOS is more complex than originally believed.

Table 2
Risk Factors for Endometrial Cancer

Increasing age
Long-term exposure to unopposed estrogens
High concentrations of estrogens postmenopausally
Metabolic syndrome (obesity, diabetes)
Years of menstruation
Nulliparity
Hormone-replacement therapy with less than 12–14 days of progestagens

It seems likely that women with PCOS who have irregular periods or amenorrhea are at greatest risk because of the stimulatory effects of unopposed estrogen secretion. There is evidence that women with anovulatory infertility are at risk of developing endometrial hyperplasia, and in some cases, this will be atypical in type and, therefore, potentially premalignant. However, we cannot conclude that women with PCOS will necessarily have a high risk of developing endometrial cancer, despite the fact that PCOS is the most common cause of anovulation. It is more likely that the risk applies only to a subgroup of women, possibly those who are also obese.

PREVENTION AND SCREENING

A substantial proportion of endometrial cancers could be avoided with the maintenance of normal weight and physical activity throughout life, an inexpensive way to lower bioavailable estrogens (19). Pregnancy with intense placental production of progestagens protects against endometrial cancer. Nulliparity is a risk factor that is more important if infertility is also present; grand multiparity protects from endometrial cancer (20).

Contraceptive pills containing estrogens and progestogens lower the endometrial cancer risk (21). After menopause, for women taking hormone-replacement therapy, the addition of progestogens to estrogen (generally for 10–14 days per month or daily) counteracts the adverse effects of estrogens on the endometrium.

There is no effective way of screening for endometrial cancer. The ideal method for outpatient sampling of the endometrium has not yet been devised. Furthermore, minimally invasive modalities potentially suitable for mass screening, including transvaginal ultrasonography (TVU) and cytology from a Pap smear or endometrial brush, have limited accuracy for the diagnosis of endometrial cancer in an asymptomatic population, mass screening of the population not being practical. However, screening for endometrial carcinoma or its precursors is justified for certain high-risk people, including those with PCOS.

Only 50% of women with endometrial cancer have malignant cells on their Pap smear; therefore, cytology from a Pap smear has limited accuracy. However, the appearance of normal as well as abnormal-appearing endometrial cells in cervical smears taken in the second half of the menstrual cycle or in postmenopausal women should alert the clinician to the possibility of endometrial disease.

The unsatisfactory results with conventional Pap smears are caused by the indirect sampling of the endometrium, thus, several commercially available devices have been developed to allow direct sampling (e.g., Pipelle de Cornier® Cooper Surgical, vabra aspirator). Although the accuracy of endometrial sampling has not been definitely determined, it is probably in the order of 90%.

In the 1990s, TVU was investigated as a screening technique. There is strong association between the thickness of the endometrium and endometrial disease, with a normal endometrium being usually less than 5 mm thick. Finally, education about the importance of investigation if any vaginal bleeding occurs in postmenopausal women should be given to health care workers and women themselves.

SYMPTOMS AND DIAGNOSIS

Abnormal uterine bleeding is the most frequent symptom of endometrial cancer. Intermenstrual bleeding or heavy prolonged bleeding in perimenopausal or anovulatory premenopausal women should arouse suspicion. The diagnosis may be delayed unnecessarily in these women because the bleeding is usually ascribed to "hormonal imbalance." A high index of suspicion also is needed to make an early diagnosis in women younger than 40 years of age.

All postmenopausal women with vaginal bleeding and those with abnormal uterine bleeding associated with risk factors for endometrial cancer or hyperplasia (e.g., PCOS, obesity, hormone replacement therapy) should undergo further diagnostic endometrial assessment. The probability of endometrial cancer in women presenting with postmenopausal bleeding is 5–10%, but the chances increase with age and risk factors.

Endometrial cancer is usually diagnosed histologically from endometrial tissue obtained with curettage or miniature endometrial biopsy devices in the form of plastic disposable Pipelle. Endometrial cytology from an endometrial brush has a lower sensitivity to detect endometrial cancer than endometrial biopsy.

A Pipelle biopsy for the diagnosis of atypical hyperplasia or endometrial cancer has a calculated sensitivity of 81–99% *(22)*. Some people will consider TVU as the first step in any woman presenting with abnormal uterine bleeding. A thin and regular endometrial line is associated with a very low risk of endometrial cancer. Normality is defined as a thickness of less than 4–5 mm *(23)*. The value of TVU in symptomatic premenopausal women and those using hormone replacement therapy is lower because the normal endometrial thickness varies with circulating concentrations of female steroid hormones.

Hysteroscopy is used as an outpatient procedure to exclude intracavitary lesions such as submucous fibroids and endometrial polyps that might also contain endometrial cancers. With this method, there is a small risk of the spread of malignant cells to the peritoneal cavity *(24)*.

STAGING

In 1988, the Cancer Committee at FIGO introduced a surgical staging system for endometrial cancer because clinical staging is incorrect in more than 20% of cases *(25)*. The depth of myometrial invasion and extrauterine disease have all been incorporated into the FIGO staging scheme as shown in Table 3.

Useful preoperative assessment includes clinical examination, transvaginal sonography, and a computed tomography scan of the lungs, liver, and retroperitoneal lymph nodes.

Table 3
Surgical Staging of Carcinoma of the Uterus (1988)

Stage and grade	Features
Stage IA; grade 1, 2, or 3	Tumor limited to endometrium
Stage IB; grade 1, 2, or 3	Invasion of less than half of the myometrium
Stage IC; grade 1, 2, or 3	Invasion of more than half of the myometrium
Stage IIA; grade 1, 2, or 3	Endocervical glandular involvement only
Stage IIB; grade 1, 2, or 3	Cervical stromal invasion
Stage IIIA; grade 1, 2, or 3	Tumor invading serosa or adnexa, or malignant peritoneal cytology
Stage IIIB; grade 1, 2, or 3	Vaginal metastasis
Stage IIIC; grade 1, 2, or 3	Metastasis to pelvic or para-aortic lymph nodes
Stage IVA; grade 1, 2, or 3	Tumor invasion of the bladder or bowel mucosa
Stage IVB	Distant metastases including intraabdominal or inguinal nodes

TVU is simple, readily available, and has reasonable accuracy in predicting cervical and myometrial invasion from endometrial cancer. It is almost as accurate as magnetic resonance imaging and most other proposed methods for measuring depth of myometrial invasion, including computed tomography scan and frozen section of the hysterectomy specimen. Intraoperative visual estimation of the depth of myometrial invasion is accurate in 90% of cases *(26)*.

Although the histological assessment of the hysterectomy specimen remains the gold standard, the combination of a preoperatively known tumor grade and visual estimation of the depth of myometrial invasion will enable the surgeon to select candidates for lymphadenectomy.

Although more accurate information should be obtained if surgical staging was carried out on all patients, this is unlikely to happen for a number of reasons:

1. Many patients with endometrial carcinoma are treated in the community, where the necessary surgical skills to perform lymphadenectomy may not be available.
2. Many patients are obese and not suitable for extensive nodal resections.
3. Patients with early tumors do not justify a routine lymphadenectomy, but a few of these patients will have positive notes. In addition, the extent of the lymphadenectomy has not been defined.

Endometrial carcinoma spreads by direct extension to adjacent structures, by lymphatic and hematogenous dissemination, and by transtubal passage of exfoliated cells.

PROGNOSTIC VARIABLES AND SURVIVAL

Although stage of disease is the most significant prognostic variable, a number of factors have been shown to correlate with the outcome in patients with the same stage of disease. Some of the traditional and most important prognostic factors in endometrial cancer include histological type, histological grade, myometrial invasion, tumor size, and peritoneal cytology findings.

There is a strong correlation between histological grade, myometrial invasion, and prognosis. Increasing tumor grade and myometrial penetration are associated with an increasing risk of pelvic and para-aortic lymph node metastases, adnexal metastases, positive peritoneal cytology findings, local vault recurrence, and hematogenous spread. Positive peritoneal washings are most common in patients with grade 3 histological type, metastases to the adnexal, deep myometrial invasion, and positive pelvic or para-aortic nodes. The new FIGO grading system takes into account the nuclear grade of the tumor and "nuclear atypia" inappropriate for the architectural grade raises the grade by 1. However, there is grade variability in the literature regarding the criteria for nuclear grading and intra-observer reproducibility of nuclear grading is poor. Tumor size is reported to be an independent prognostic factor and the incidence of nodal metastases increases in relation to the tumor size and depth of invasion.

During the last decade efforts have focused on attempting to identify cytokinetic or molecular events that correlate with the malignant potential of endometrial cancers. Some centers have evaluated the expression of oncogenes and tumor suppressor genes, such as the *HER-2/neu* oncogene, *bcl-2 protein*, and *p53* tumor suppressor gene *(27)*. Furthermore, markers of cell proliferation, such as DNA ploidy, S-phase fraction, proliferation index, and proliferating cell nuclear antigen have been evaluated *(28)*.

The preoperative assessment of markers predictive of patients outcomes in pre-treatment endometrial curettage samples would assist the clinician in stratifying women into risk groups. The idea being that patients at risk for aggressive or advanced disease could be referred to clinicians with special expertise in managing advanced endometrial carcinoma, an approach that would permit the tailoring of treatment according to the estimated risk of recurrence of the disease.

Analysis of cytokinetic and molecular parameters in preoperative endometrial samples showed a significant correlation between advanced surgical stage and p53, histological subtype, ploidy, and S-phase fraction *(29)*. In the same paper, recurrence-free survival was significantly linked with *p53, MIB1, bcl-2*, and *HER-2/neu*, but the prognostic value derivable only from assessment in a curettage specimen is limited, and the subjective nature of the analysis prompts concern about the reproducibility. Furthermore, high-grade cases are missed in 10–26% of preoperative endometrial samples, and the aggressive histological subtypes may escape recognition in 36–54% of preoperative biopsy samples.

Nonendometrioid endometrial cancers, such as serous and clear-cell carcinomas, make up about 10% of endometrial cancers, but account for more than 50% of recurrences and deaths from endometrial cancer *(30)*.

Ideally, the identification of variables in a pretreatment endometrial specimen could predict extrauterive spread of disease and facilitate treatment selection.

Flow cytometic-determined ploidy and cytokinetic variables are well-recognized prognostic factors in endometrial cancer that can effectively predict advanced disease and patient outcome *(31)*.

The strong association of ploidy with extrauterine disease suggests a possible role for flow cytometry in the preoperative "molecular staging" of endometrial cancer. With only a few exceptions, the literature also recognizes the *p53* tumor suppressor gene as an important prognostic factor *(32)*. It seems that the role of *p53* in the pretreatment prognosis and molecular staging of endometrial cancer is of paramount importance.

It is suggested that the evaluation of ploidy MIB1 and *p53* in preoperative endometrial samples may enable the clinician to stratify endometrial cancer patients into low- and high-risk groups before the commencement of definite therapy.

The possibility that PCOS could influence the prognosis of women with endometrial cancer was investigated in the past *(33)*. In the paper by Jafari et al. it was suggested that the presence of PCOS was associated with favorable prognosis, but because of a small number of patients it is clearly impossible to draw any firm conclusions from this study.

TREATMENT OPTIONS

The cornerstone of treatment for endometrial cancer is surgery. The procedure includes total abdominal hysterectomy, bilateral salpingo-ophorectomy, and peritoneal fluid or washings for cytology. In selected cases, laparoscopic-assisted vaginal hysterectomy is feasible when operating for endometrial cancer, although the results of randomized trials are still lacking. In addition, many patients require some type of adjuvant radiation therapy to help prevent vaginal vault recurrence and to sterilize occult disease on lymph nodes.

With the increasing emphasis on surgicopathological staging, a more individualized approach to adjuvant radiation is now possible.

The initial approach for all medically fit patients should be total abdominal hysterectomy and bilateral salpingo-oophorectomy. The ovaries should be removed because they maybe the site of microscopic metastases. In addition, patients with endometrial carcinoma are at increased risk for ovarian cancer. Such tumors sometimes occur concurrently. Recent data suggest that concurrent ovarian malignancies are much more common than previously thought. Walsh et al.'s article highlights this problem in a recent publication where 25% of 102 women with endometrial cancer were found to have coexisting ovarian malignancies *(1)*. These patients had endometrioid (96%) or adenosquamous (4%) histology and many of them did not have a physical or histological profile of unopposed estrogen exposure.

Although early endometrial cancers are thought to be easily cured by the surgical removal of the uterus, ovarian cancer is deadly and rarely identified at an early stage. Because of this, the standard of care is to remove the ovaries and tubes in women who develop endometrial cancer.

Surgical staging should be performed in those patients with grade 2 and 3 lesions, tumors greater than 2 cm in diameter, with clear-cell or papillary serous carcinomas, with greater than 50% of myometrial invasion, and with cervical extension of the disease.

Surgical staging requirements have not been detailed by the Cancer Committee of FIGO. If accurate surgical staging is to be obtained, full pelvic lymphadenectomy should be performed and dissection should include any enlarged paraortic nodes.

Type 1 endometrial cancer has a primarily lymphatic spread in most cases limited to pelvic nodes. Isolated involvement of the para-aortic nodes is rare. Complete excision of the nodes located around the iliac vessels and above the obtuvator nerve allows identification of 90% of node-positive patients *(34)*.

The decision on whether to undertake lymphadenectomy should not be based on palpation of the nodal area because less than 10% of the patients with nodal metastases have grossly enlarged nodes. For example, patients with grade 1 endometrial cancer with deep myometrial invasion, grade 2 with any myometrial invasion, and grade 3 endometrioid cancer have at least a 5% risk of having positive pelvic lymph nodes *(35)*, and some physicians will propose routine lymphadenectomy for this group of patients.

Type 2 endometrial cancers have a different spread pattern, with a higher likelihood of extrauterine disease, and for these reasons, a thorough lymphatic dissection is recommended in women with such tumors. The transperitoneal spread of type 2 endometrial cancer resembles that of ovarian cancer and women with such lesions require similar surgical management *(36)*.

Whether lymphadenectomy is curative in endometrial cancer remains controversial. Recent findings suggest the therapeutic benefit of lymphadenectomy, but confirmation of this must await randomized studies.

The feasibility of using the results of lymphadenectomy to modify adjuvant radiation therapy has been addressed in several nonrandomized trials. All reports would suggest that if the lymph nodes are negative, it may be reasonable to omit external-beam therapy and rely on brachytherapy to prevent vault recurrence.

The goal of adjuvant radiotherapy is to treat the pelvic lymph node regions that might contain microscopic disease, as well as the central pelvic region, including the upper vagina.

Regarding patient with PCOS, some authors have reported conservative management of endometrial adenocarcinoma in women with PCOS. The rationale is that cancer of the endometrium often presents at an early stage, is well differentiated, and there is a low risk of metastasis and therefore is not perceived as being life-threatening.

Furthermore, these women are young and usually desirous of fertility. Some authors *(37)* used a combination of curettage and high-dose progestogens in a few young women with well-differentiated lesions, some of whom later bore children. Nevertheless, most of the patients who they reported required hysterectomy.

Few other authors have also advocated different conservative approaches but, in general, the literature on women with PCOS and endometrial hyperplasia or adenocarcinoma suggests that this group of patients have a poor prognosis for fertility.

This may be because of the factors that predispose to the endometrial pathology—chronic anovulation combined often with severe obesity—or secondary to the endometrial pathology disrupting potential embryonic implantation. Case studies and small series of patients treated successfully may be subjected to publication bias and may not represent widespread medical opinion. Thus, a more traditional and radical surgical approach is suggested as the safest way to prevent progression of the cancer.

In women with PCOS with symptoms of amenorrhea or oligomenorrhea, we recommend cyclical hormone therapy for the induction of artificial withdrawal bleeding to prevent endometrial hyperplasia.

Theoretically, metformin, a treatment that is now widely used to treat infertile women with PCOS, may have a role in preventing endometrial hyperstimulation by lowering insulin concentrations and restoring ovulation *(38)*. However, the long-term effects of this drug in women with PCOS are not known and more studies are required before suggesting its use for preventing endometrial cancer.

At present, therefore, there is little choice other than to advise oligomenorrhoic women with PCOS that they may be at increased risk of developing endometrial cancer and to suggest treatment in the form of combined oral contraceptive pills or cyclic progestagens.

CONCLUSIONS

The risk of developing endometrial cancer has been shown to be adversely influenced by a number of factors including obesity, long-term use of unopposed estrogens, multiparity, and infertility.

The evidence for increased risk of endometrial carcinoma in PCOS is incomplete and contradictory. PCOS is the most common cause of anovulation and there seems to be an association between PCOS and endometrial cancer.

Published data exist relating to a few cases that indicate that patients with well-differentiated adenocarcinoma of the endometrium may also be treated conservatively with progestogens and ovulation induction, although only a few pregnancies are reported, and the safest approach is probably still hysterectomy.

The cornerstone of treatment for endometrial cancer is surgery, which is not only important for staging purposes but also enables appropriate tailoring of adjuvant treatment modalities that benefit high-risk patients only.

There is a substantial prognostic difference between the histological types of endometrial cancers. The most common lesions (type 1) are typically hormone sensitive and low stage and have an excellent prognosis, whereas tumors of type 2 are high grade with a tendency to recur, even in early stage.

Traditional prognostic features in endometrial cancer are the surgical FIGO stage, myometrial invasion, histological type, and differentiation grade. Indications for radiotherapy are generally in the adjuvant setting.

FUTURE AVENUES OF INVESTIGATION

Issues that form areas of current research in endometrial cancer include the following:

1. Microarray analysis and evaluation of prognostic and predictive factors from molecular findings.
2. Cost–benefit analysis of screening tests and assessment of the role of three-dimensional ultrasonography in the diagnosis and management of endometrial cancer.
3. Conservative management with antiestrogens or local progestagens to conserve fertility in young women with well-differentiated lesions.
4. Definition of correct surgical staging in relation to lymphadenectomy and resolve the question of the therapeutic role of lymphadenectomy and its ability to modify adjuvant therapy.

KEY POINTS

- Adenocarcinoma of the endometrium is the most common malignancy of the female genital tract, accounting for 6% of all cancers among women. The incidence is rising as life expectancy increases, and this rise has been associated with an epidemic of obesity and physical inactivity.

- The PCOS is the most common endocrine disturbance affecting women. There seems to be an association between PCOS and endometrial cancer, but disagreements in diagnostic criteria make it difficult to compare epidemiological studies on long-term health risks such as cancer.
- During the last decade, efforts have focused on attempting to identify cytokinetic or molecular events that correlate with the malignant potential of endometrial cancers.
- The preoperative identification of high-risk endometrial cancer cases is currently suboptimal. High-grade cases are missed in 10–26% of preoperative endometrial samples.
- The use of preoperative analysis of endometrial cancer specimens is recommended with a panel of cytokinetic and molecular variables such as flow cytometry-determined ploidy and p53 overexpression.
- Endometrial cancer is a surgically staged cancer because clinical estimates and preoperative imaging of the extent of the disease are incorrect in more than 20% of cases.
- The most important therapy for endometrial cancer is surgery. The procedure includes total abdominal hysterectomy, bilateral salpingo-ophorectomy, and acquisition of peritoneal fluid or washings for cytology; in selected cases, retroperitoneal lymph node dissection is recommended.

REFERENCES

1. Walsh C, Holschneider C, Hoang Y, Tieu K, Karlan B, Cass I. Coexisting ovarian malignancy in young women with endometrial cancer. Obstet Gynecol 2005;106:693–699.
2. Farhi DC, Nosanchuk J, Silverberg SG. Endometrial adenocarcinoma in women under 25 years of age. Obstet Gynecol 1986;68:741–745.
3. Schouten LJ, Goldbohm RA, van den Brandt PA. Anthropometry, physical activity and endometrial cancer risk: results from the Netherlands Cohort Study. J Natl Cancer Inst 2004;96:1635–1638.
4. Lincoln SR, Lei ZM, Ackermann DM. The expression of human chorionic gonadotrophin/human luteinizing hormone receptors in human endometrial and myometrial blood vessels. J Clin Endocrinol Metab 2002;76:1140–1144.
5. Konishi I, Koshiyama M, Mandai M, et al. Increased expression of LH/hCG receptors in endometrial hyperplasia and carcinoma in anovulatory women. Gynecol Oncol 1997;65:273–280.
6. Zheng W, Baker HE, Mutter GL. Involution of PTEN-null endometrial glands with progestin therapy. Gynecol Oncol 2004;92:1008–1013.
7. Stefansson IM, Salvesen HB, Immervoll H, Akslen LA. Prognostic impact of histological grade and vascular invasion compared with tumor cell proliferation in endometrial carcinoma of endometrioid type. Histopathology 2004;44:472–479.
8. Santin AD. HER2/neu overexpression has the Achiles' heel of uterine serous papillary carcinoma been exposed. Gynecol Oncol 2003;88:263–295.
9. Bokhman JV. Two pathogenetic types of endometrial carcinoma. Gynecol Oncol 1983;15:10–17.
10. Darvishian F, Hummer AJ, Thaler HT, et al. Serous endometrial cancers that mimic endometrioid adenocarcinomas: a clinicopathologic and immunohistochemical study of a group of problematic cases. Am J Surg Pathol 2004;28:1568–1578.
11. Kelsey JL, LiVolsi VA, Holford TR, et al. A case-control study of cancer of the endometrium. Am J Epidemiol 1982;116:333–342.
12. Jackson RL, Dockerty MB. The Stein-Leventhal syndrome: analysis of 43 cases with special reference to association with endometrial carcinoma. Am J Obstet Gynecol 1957;73:161–173.
13. Polson DW, Adams J, Wadsworth J, Franks S. Polycystic ovaries-a common finding in normal women. Lancet 1988;1:870–872.
14. Chang RJ. Polycystic ovary syndrome: diagnostic criteria. In: Chang RJ, Heindel JJ, Dunaif A, eds. *Polycystic Ovary Syndrome*. New York: Marcel Dekker, 2002, pp. 361–365.
15. ACOG practice bulletin. Polycystic ovary syndrome. Obstet Gynecol 2002;100:1389–1402.
16. Furberg A, Thune I. Metabolic abnormalities (hypertension, hyperglycaemia and overweight), lifestyle (high energy intake and physical inactivity) and endometrial cancer risk in a Norwegian cohort. Int J Cancer 2003;104:669–676.

17. Calle EE, Rodriguez C, Walker-Thurmond K, Thun MJ. Overweight, obesity, and mortality from cancer in a prospectively studied cohort of U.S. adults. N Engl J Med 2003;348:1625–1638.

18. Bershtein LM, Gamaiunova VB, Kvachevskaia IuO, Tsyrlina EV, Kovalenko IG. The nature of hyper-insulinaemia (insulin resistance) in endometrial carcinoma: of plasma levels of insulin and c-peptide. Vopr Onkol 2000;46:191–195.

19. McTiernan A, Tworoger SS, Ulrich GM, et al. Effect of exercise on serum estrogen in postmenopausal women: a 12-month randomized clinical trial. Cancer Res 2004;64:2923–2928.

20. Hinkula M, Pukkala E, Kyyronen P, Kauppila A. Grand multiparity and incidence of endometrial cancer: a population-based study in Finland. Int J Cancer 2002;98:912–915.

21. Deligeoroglou E, Michailidis E, Creatsas G. Oral contraceptives and reproductive system cancer. Ann NY Acad Sci 2003;997:199–208.

22. Clark TJ, Mann CH, Shah N, et al. Accuracy of outpatient endometrial biopsy in the diagnosis of endometrial cancer: a systematic quantitative review. BJOG 2002;109:313–321.

23. Gupta JK, Chien PF, Voit D, Clark TJ, Khan KS. Ultrasonographic endometrial thickness for diagnosing endometrial pathology in women with postmenopausal bleeding: a meta-analysis. Acta Obstet Gynecol Scand 2002;81:799–816.

24. Revel A. Does hysteroscopy produce intraperitoneal spread of endometrial cancer cells? Obstet Gynecol Surv 2004;59:280–284.

25. Creasman WT. FIGO stage 1988 revision. Gynecol Oncol 1989;35:125–127.

26. Franchi M, Ghezzi F, Melpignano M, et al. Clinical value of entraoperative gross examination in endometrial cancer. Gynecol Oncol 2000;76:357–361.

27. Geisler JP, Geisler HE, Wiemann MC, Zhou Z, Miller GA, Crabtree W. Lack of bcl-2 persistence: an independent prognostic indicator of poor prognosis in endometrial carcinoma. Gynecol Oncol 1998;71:305–307.

28. Garzetti GG, Ciavattini A, Goteri G, De Nictolis M, Romanini C. Proliferating cell nuclear antigen in endometrial carcinoma: pre-treatment identification of high-risk patients. Gynecol Oncol 1996;61: 16–21.

29. Mariani A, Sebo TJ, Katzmann JA, et al. Pretreatment assessment of prognostic indicators in endometrial cancer. Am J Obstet Gynecol 2000;182:1535–1544.

30. Creasman WT, Kohler MF, Odicino F, Maisoneuve P, Boyle P. Prognosis of papillary serous, clear cell and grade 3 stage I carcinoma of the endometrium. Gynecol Oncol 2004;95:593–596.

31. Britton LC, Wilson TO, Gaffey TA, Cha SS, Wieand HS, Podratz KC. DNA ploidy in endometrial carcinoma: major objective prognostic factor. Mayo Clin Proc 1990;65:643–650.

32. Hamel NW, Sebo TJ, Wilson TO, et al. Prognostic value of p53 and proliferating cell nuclear antigen expression in endometrial carcinoma. Gynecol Oncol 1996;62:192–198.

33. Jafari K, Javaheri G, Ruiz G. Endometrial adenocarcinoma and the Stein-Leventhal syndrome. Obstet Gynecol 1978;51:97–100.

34. Benedetti-Panici P, Maneschi F, Cutillo G, et al. Anatomical and pathological study of retroperitoneal nodes in endometrial cancer. Int J Gynecol Cancer 1998;8:1837–1842.

35. Kilgore LC, Partridge EE, Alvarez RD, et al. Adenocarcinoma of the endometrium survival comparisons of patients with and without pelvic node sampling. Gynecol Oncol 1995;56:29–33.

36. Trimbos B, Vergote I, Bolis G, et al. Impact of adjuvant chemotherapy and surgical staging in early-stage ovarian carcinoma: European Organization for Research and Treatment of Cancer-Adjuvant Chemo Therapy in Ovarian Neoplasm Trial. J Natl Cancer Inst 2003;95:113–125.

37. Farhi DC, Nosanchuk J, Silverberg SG. Endometrial adenocarcinoma in women under 25 years of age. Obstet Gynecol 1986;68:741–745.

38. Nestler JE. Metformin and the polycystic ovary syndrome. J Clin Endocrinol Metab 2001;86:1430.

IV   INFERTILITY AND PCOS:
ROLE OF INSULIN RESISTANCE

22 Anovulation in Polycystic Ovary Syndrome

Stephen Franks, MD

Summary

Polycystic ovary syndrome (PCOS) is the most common cause of anovulatory infertility. Anovulation in PCOS is characterized by arrest of antral follicle growth in the final stages of maturation. There is evidence that the abnormal endocrine environment in PCOS (specifically elevation of serum levels of luteinizing hormone and/or insulin) plays an important role in arrest of antral follicles but, as a result of recent studies, abnormalities in early follicle development have also been shown to be present. This suggests that, in PCOS, the whole process of follicle development—from initiation of follicle growth to the late antral stage—is abnormal. These observations have important implications for understanding the pathogenesis of PCOS, and open the door to potential new methods of treatment for this very common endocrinopathy.

Key Words: Polycystic ovary syndrome; anovulation; luteinizing hormone; insulin; granulosa cells.

INTRODUCTION

Polycystic ovary syndrome (PCOS) is the most common cause of anovulatory infertility; however, the mechanism of anovulation remains uncertain (1). Antral follicles are typically arrested at around 5–10 mm, i.e., before final maturation prior to ovulation, and this appears to reflect the abnormal endocrine environment. However, there is also emerging evidence to suggest that there is an intrinsic abnormality of early follicle development that may have a profound impact on later follicle function. This chapter addresses these issues and highlights the clinical significance of these phenomena.

From: *Contemporary Endocrinology: Insulin Resistance and Polycystic Ovarian Syndrome:*
Pathogenesis, Evaluation, and Treatment
Edited by: E. Diamanti-Kandarakis, J. E. Nestler, D. Panidis, and R. Pasquali © Humana Press Inc., Totowa, NJ

ANORMALITIES OF ANTRAL FOLLICLE FUNCTION
IN POLYCYSTIC OVARIES

It appears that in PCOS the tight coordination that links growth and differentiation of granulosa cells during the final stages of preovulatory follicle maturation is disrupted. Granulosa cells of follicles from anovulatory women with PCOS appear to stop dividing but remain steroidogenically competent and, indeed, show evidence of both increased aromatase activity and progesterone production when compared with follicles of similar size from ovulatory women with either normal or polycystic ovaries (PCO) *(2–4)*. Estradiol production by medium-sized antral follicles is typically increased in anovulatory women with PCO (i.e., the "classic" syndrome of hyperandrogenism with anovulation), but not in subjects with PCO who have regular menses *(3,4)*.

Steroidogenesis by theca cells is, by contrast, abnormal in both anovulatory and ovulatory subjects with PCO. After measurement of steroids in theca-conditioned medium, we observed that concentrations of androstenedione (20-fold), 17α-hydroxy-progesterone (10-fold), and progesterone (5-fold) were significantly greater in cultures from PCO compared with control cultures, regardless of menstrual cycle history *(5)*. In summary, follicular cells from ovulatory subjects with PCO hypersecrete androgen but not estrogen, whereas cells from anovulatory women with PCO are characterized by excessive production of both androgen and estrogen. Because increased androgen production is common to both ovulatory and anovulatory women with PCO, it is unlikely that hyperandrogenism is the major cause of anovulation. It is possible, however, that excessive androgen production contributes to the etiology of anovulation by contributing to the accumulation of cyclic AMP (cAMP) in granulosa cells, as discussed next.

We suggest that the explanation for the apparent disparity between follicle growth between ovulatory and anovulatory women with PCO may be the abnormal endocrine environment. Anovulation in women with PCOS is characterized by hypersecretion of luteinzing hormone (LH), insulin, and androgens. The interaction of these three factors may influence development of the maturing follicle by each contributing to an inappropriately high concentration of cAMP in the granulosa cell of large antral follicles. In the normal primate menstrual cycle, granulosa cells in the dominant follicle acquire responsiveness to LH in the mid-follicular phase. LH stimulates steroidogenesis by granulosa cells, but also triggers terminal differentiation and arrest of follicle growth in the normal, mature, preovulatory follicle *(6)*. The switch from growth to terminal differentiation of granulosa cells in the preovulatory follicle is thought to be activated by exceeding a notional "ceiling" level of intracellular cAMP triggered by the onset of the mid-cycle LH surge *(6)*. PCOS is characterized by hypersecretion of LH, and it is possible that this alone may promote premature arrest of follicular growth. However, many patients have normal serum concentrations of LH *(7–9)*. In these subjects (as well as in those with elevated serum LH concentrations), the gonadotrophic action of insulin may be a crucial factor in the mechanism of disordered follicular function.

In human granulosa cells of both normal and PCO, insulin, in the absence of gonadotrophins, stimulates estradiol and progesterone secretion *(10)*. Significantly, it has also been shown to augment, synergistically, LH-induced steroidogenesis by isolated granulosa cells *(10)*. Thus, tonically elevated levels of LH and/or amplification of LH action on the follicle by hyperinsulinemia could account for the arrest of follicle

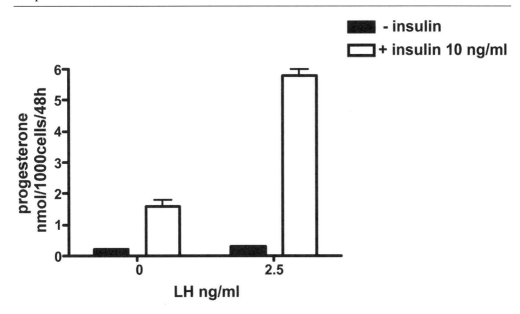

Fig. 1. Effect of insulin preincubation on luteinizing hormone (LH)-induced progesterone production by human granulosa cells in monolayer culture. Note synergistic interaction of insulin and LH. (Adapted from ref. *10*).

growth, but at the same time enhancement of estradiol and progesterone production *(1)* (Fig. 1). Although there is little evidence that insulin has any direct effect on cAMP production, it is likely that the mechanism whereby insulin amplifies LH action involves an increase in the number of LH receptors on the maturing granulosa cells *(11)*.

PCOS is also characterized by peripheral insulin resistance. It may therefore appear to be paradoxical that we are suggesting that the elevated levels of insulin have an impact on follicular growth and steroidogenesis in the ovary. Recent studies have, however, pointed to selective, signaling-pathway-specific differences in sensitivity to insulin action between normal and PCO *(12)*. Insulin action on glucose uptake and metabolism in granulosa–lutein cells from anovulatory women with PCOS is impaired, but steroidogenesis is unaffected *(13)*.

Androgens may also contribute to the disordered folliculogenesis of PCOS. In granulosa cell cultures, androgens augment gonadotrophin-induced cAMP production *(14)*, and it is therefore possible that the hypersecretion of ovarian androgens, which is typical of the polycystic ovary, can, by the same common intracellular mechanism, add to the effects of LH and insulin on follicle maturation.

There is evidence that antral follicles of anovulatory women with PCO respond inappropriately to LH. Normally, granulosa cells from the dominant follicle of normal ovaries (or of PCO from ovulatory women) secrete estradiol in response to LH when the follicle has reached about 10 mm in diameter. By contrast, in cells derived from anovulatory women with PCO, LH stimulates secretion of estradiol and progesterone in granulosa cells from follicles as small as 4 mm *(4)*. Furthermore, antral follicles approx 6–8 mm in diameter produce levels of estradiol and progesterone that are more akin to those found in the normal, preovulatory follicle. The mechanism of this "premature" response to LH remains to be determined. It could represent an effect of endogenous hyper-insulinemia (with or without the influence of hyperandrogenism), but may also reflect an intrinsic abnormality of the control of follicle development. Inappropriate steroidogenesis by prematurely advanced antral follicles may also help explain the slightly, but significantly, lower levels of serum follicle-stimulating hormone (FSH) in anovulatory women with PCOS. Using mathematical modeling, it can be predicted that enhanced estradiol production by a proportion of small antral follicles in a "cohort" would—by a negative feedback effect—tend to suppress FSH and prevent further development of "healthy" follicles within that cohort (15). This would also explain why low-dose FSH—presumably by promoting growth of those healthy follicles—can lead to normal development of a dominant follicle in women with PCOS.

PRE-ANTRAL FOLLICULAR DEVELOPMENT IN PCOS

It is clear that the population of antral follicles is increased in the PCO, but there is evidence that disordered folliculogenesis also involves the smaller, pre-antral follicles (16). The numbers of primary and secondary follicles in the PCO are about twice those observed in the normal ovary. Recently, work from the author's laboratory has shown increased density of small pre-antral follicles in ovarian cortical biopsies from anovulatory women with PCOS compared with normal ovarian tissue (17). Furthermore, we observed a reduced proportion of primordial (resting) follicles and a reciprocally increased proportion of early growing follicles in tissue from women with PCO regardless of their ovulatory status. Development of pre-antral follicles does not appear to be primarily under endocrine control, but it is not yet clear which of the many candidates among the paracrine and autocrine factors that have been identified in small follicles are most important for early follicular growth (18–21). Currently, no clear candidate has emerged to explain the abnormalities of early follicle development in PCOS, but recent data indicate that primordial and transitional follicles in ovarian sections obtained from anovulatory women with PCOS lack anti-Mullerian hormone, a growth factor of the transforming growth factor-β superfamily that appears to have an autocrine or paracrine role in inhibition of initiation of follicle growth (22).

In conclusion, anovulation in PCOS appears to involve both abnormalities of pre-antral folliculogenesis (stages that are gonadotropin-independent) and of antral follicle maturation (likely to be a manifestation of the abnormal endocrine environment). It is, of course, possible that the abnormalities of early follicle development predispose to follicle dysfunction in the later stages and that the mechanism of anovulation therefore has its origins at the very earliest phases of the life cycle of the follicle.

FUTURE AVENUES

The challenge to understand the altered dynamics of follicle development and maturation that lead to anovulation in PCOS is a considerable task. However, our increasing knowledge of the factors involved in early follicle development offers the hope of providing clearer insight into what this author considers to be the fundamental abnormality in PCOS. In particular, it will be important to establish the link between the abnormalities of the earliest stages of folliculogenesis (which are not obviously influenced by the endocrine environment) and, at the other end of the follicle's life cycle, the mechanism of antral follicle arrest, which is almost certainly affected by endocrine factors.

KEY POINTS

- PCOS is the most common cause of anovulatory infertility and menstrual irregularity.
- Arrested antral follicle growth in PCOS probably reflects the abnormal endocrine environment.
- Ovulation can be restored by raising endogenous FSH or by giving exogenous FSH.
- Recent studies point to an abnormality of early follicle development that cannot readily be explained by endocrine dysfunction.

REFERENCES

1. Franks S, Mason H, Willis D. Follicular dynamics in the polycystic ovary syndrome. Mol Cell Endocrinol 2000;163:49–52.
2. Erickson GF, Magoffin DA, Garzo VG, Cheung AP, Chang RJ. Granulosa cells of polycystic ovaries: are they normal or abnormal? Hum Reprod 1992;7:293–299.
3. Mason HD, Willis DS, Beard RW, Winston RM, Margara R, Franks S. Estradiol production by granulosa cells of normal and polycystic ovaries: relationship to menstrual cycle history and concentrations of gonadotropins and sex steroids in follicular fluid. J Clin Endocrinol Metab 1994;79:1355–1360.
4. Willis DS, Watson H, Mason HD, Galea R, Brincat M, Franks S. Premature response to luteinizing hormone of granulosa cells from anovulatory women with polycystic ovary syndrome: relevance to mechanism of anovulation. J Clin Endocrinol Metab 1998;83:3984–3991.
5. Gilling-Smith C, Willis DS, Beard RW, Franks S. Hypersecretion of androstenedione by isolated thecal cells from polycystic ovaries. J Clin Endocrinol Metab 1994;79:1158–1165.
6. Hillier SG. Current concepts of the roles of follicle stimulating hormone and luteinizing hormone in folliculogenesis. Hum Reprod 1994;9:188–191.
7. Franks S. Polycystic ovary syndrome: a changing perspective. Clin Endocrinol (Oxf) 1989;31:87–120.
8. Conway GS, Jacobs HS. Acanthosis nigricans in obese women with the polycystic ovary syndrome: disease spectrum not distinct entity. Postgrad Med J 1990;66:536–538.
9. White D, Leigh A, Wilson C, Donaldson A, Franks S. Gonadotrophin and gonadal steroid response to a single dose of a long-acting agonist of gonadotrophin-releasing hormone in ovulatory and anovulatory women with polycystic ovary syndrome. Clin Endocrinol (Oxf) 1995;42:475–481.
10. Willis D, Mason H, Gilling-Smith C, Franks S. Modulation by insulin of follicle-stimulating hormone and luteinizing hormone actions in human granulosa cells of normal and polycystic ovaries. J Clin Endocrinol Metab 1996;81:302–309.
11. Hattori M, Horiuchi R. Biphasic effects of exogenous ganglioside GM3 on follicle-stimulating hormone-dependent expression of luteinizing hormone receptor in cultured granulosa cells. Mol Cell Endocrinol 1992;88:47–54.
12. Willis D, Franks S. Insulin action in human granulosa cells from normal and polycystic ovaries is mediated by the insulin receptor and not the type-I insulin-like growth factor receptor. J Clin Endocrinol Metab 1995;80:3788–3790.
13. Rice S, Christoforidis N, Gadd C, et al. Impaired insulin-dependent glucose metabolism in granulosa-lutein cells from anovulatory women with polycystic ovaries. Hum Reprod 2005;20:373–381.
14. Harlow CR, Winston RM, Margara RA, Hillier SG. Gonadotrophic control of human granulosa cell glycolysis. Hum Reprod 1987;2:649–653.
15. Chavez-Ross A, Franks S, Mason HD, Hardy K, Stark J. Modelling the control of ovulation and polycystic ovary syndrome. J Math Biol 1997;36:95–118.
16. Hughesdon PE. Morphology and morphogenesis of the Stein-Leventhal ovary and of so-called "hyperthecosis." Obstet Gynecol Surv 1982;37:59–77.

17. Webber LJ, Stubbs S, Stark J, et al. Formation and early development of follicles in the polycystic ovary. Lancet 2003;362:1017–1021.
18. Elvin JA, Yan C, Wang P, Nishimori K, Matzuk MM. Molecular characterization of the follicle defects in the growth differentiation factor 9-deficient ovary. Mol Endocrinol 1999;13:1018–1034.
19. Gougeon A. Regulation of ovarian follicular development in primates: facts and hypotheses. Endocrine Rev 1996;17:121–154.
20. McNatty KP, Heath DA, Lundy T, et al. Control of early ovarian follicular development. J Reprod Fertil Suppl 1999;54:3–16.
21. Hasegawa T, Zhao L, Caron KM, et al. Developmental roles of the steroidogenic acute regulatory protein (StAR) as revealed by StAR knockout mice. Mol Endocrinol 2000;14:1462–1471.
22. Stubbs SA, Hardy K, Da Silva-Buttkus P, et al. Anti-mullerian hormone protein expression is reduced during the initial stages of follicle development in human polycystic ovaries. J Clin Endocrinol Metab 2005;90:5536–5543.

23 Insulin Resistance and Early Pregnancy Loss in Polycystic Ovary Syndrome

Daniela Jakubowicz, MD
and Susmeeta T. Sharma, MBBS

CONTENTS

Summary

Polycystic ovary syndrome (PCOS), a prevalent disorder in young women, is characterized by chronic anovulation and hyperandrogenism. One of the major concerns in women with PCOS has been infertility, a consequence of chronic oligo- or anovulation. However, even after ovulation is restored, either pharmacologically or via lifestyle interventions, women with PCOS exhibit a surprisingly high rate of spontaneous miscarriage. Several studies have shown that insulin resistance and hyperinsulinemia play an integral role in early pregnancy loss in PCOS. However, the exact underlying mechanism remains poorly understood. Several different mechanisms for the effect of hyperinsulinemia have been proposed, including its effect on oocyte maturation, glucose uptake and metabolism, implantation, and alteration of expression of *HOXA10* genes. One of the most compelling hypotheses is the effect of hyperinsulinemic insulin resistance on decreasing serum and endometrial glycodelin and insulin-like growth factor binding protein-1 concentrations, major endometrial secretory proteins that play an important role in implantation and maintenance of pregnancy. The accumulated evidence supports the use of insulin sensitizing drugs like metformin in the treatment of infertility in PCOS, and suggests that it may reduce miscarriages in the disorder. However, the duration of metformin treatment during pregnancy in women with PCOS is controversial. Although metformin appears to have a reassuring safety profile during pregnancy, future

From: *Contemporary Endocrinology: Insulin Resistance and Polycystic Ovarian Syndrome:
Pathogenesis, Evaluation, and Treatment*
Edited by: E. Diamanti-Kandarakis, J. E. Nestler, D. Panidis, and R. Pasquali © Humana Press Inc., Totowa, NJ

rigorous, randomized controlled trials are needed to confirm its efficacy and safety under these conditions.

Key Words: Polycystic ovary syndrome; early pregnancy loss; insulin resistance; hyperinsulinemia; glycodelin; IGFBP-1; insulin sensitizing drugs; metformin.

OVERVIEW

Polycystic ovary syndrome (PCOS) is one of the most common endocrine disorders in women of reproductive age *(1,2)*. It is characterized by chronic anovulation and hyperandrogenism—either in the form of biochemical androgen excess or clinically as hirsutism, acne, and/or male pattern alopecia *(3,4)*. One of the major concerns in women with PCOS is infertility, a consequence of chronic oligo- or anovulation. However, even after ovulation is restored, either pharmacologically or via lifestyle interventions, women with PCOS exhibit a surprisingly low reproductive potential with higher-than-expected rates of spontaneous miscarriage. Rates of early pregnancy loss (EPL), defined as miscarriage of a clinically recognized pregnancy during the first trimester, are reported to be 30–50% in women with polycystic ovaries *(5,6)* or PCOS *(7,8)*. This is threefold higher than the 10–15% rate reported in retrospective studies for normal women *(9,10)*. Conversely, 36–82% of women with recurrent or habitual EPL are reported to have PCOS or polycystic ovaries *(6,10,11)*.

In the past, studies have suggested that hypersecretion of luteinizing hormone (LH) leads to an increased risk of miscarriage in women with PCOS *(7,8)*. However, a recent study showed that, in women with elevated circulating LH levels and history of recurrent miscarriage, suppression of endogenous LH release before conception does not improve live birth rates *(12)*. Hence, investigators have turned to alternative hypotheses, and obesity *(13)* and elevated serum androgen concentrations *(14)* have now been reported as risk factors for EPL in PCOS.

An important advance in our understanding of PCOS has been recent evidence of the central role of insulin resistance and compensatory hyperinsulinemia in the pathogenesis of the syndrome. Numerous studies have documented the presence of insulin resistance in both obese and lean women with PCOS *(15,16)*. Lean women with PCOS appear to have a form of insulin resistance that is intrinsic to the syndrome and poorly understood *(16)*. Obese women with PCOS not only have this intrinsic form of insulin resistance, but also have the added burden of insulin resistance owing to excess adiposity *(17)*. Hyperinsulinemia is now known to increase circulating ovarian androgen concentrations and impede ovulation. It has also been implicated as an independent risk factor for EPL in PCOS *(13)*. Moreover, studies have shown that administration of various insulin-sensitizing drugs, such as metformin, leads to a decrease in serum androgens, an increase in the ovulation rate, and is associated with a decrease in EPL in affected women *(18)*. These findings collectively suggest that insulin resistance with compensatory hyperinsulinemia, resulting in hyperandrogenemia, might be the inciting event in EPL in women with PCOS.

Hyperinsulinemic insulin resistance in PCOS presents a fascinating paradox, as peripheral tissues such as skeletal muscle are resistant to insulin in terms of glucose metabolism whereas the ovaries remain sensitive to insulin with regard to stimulation of testosterone biosynthesis. This may be a consequence of tissue specific differences in insulin sensitivity. Although several advances have been made in the field, the exact underlying mechanism of insulin resistance in PCOS remains poorly characterized. Our aim here is to emphasize the role of insulin resistance and hyperinsulinemia in EPL in PCOS, and to discuss the various possible mechanisms for this phenomenon.

INSULIN RESISTANCE AND OOCYTE MATURATION

The developmental competence of the oocyte is one of the factors that affect early embryonic survival, establishment and maintenance of pregnancy, and fetal development. Quality, or developmental competence, is acquired during folliculogenesis, as the oocyte grows, and during the period of oocyte maturation. Assisted reproductive technologies commonly used in women with PCOS, including ovarian hyperstimulation or in vitro maturation of oocytes, perturb this process and result in oocytes with reduced quality *(19)*. A poor quality oocyte, in turn, can lead to delayed embryonic development, abnormal blastocyst formation, fetal growth retardation, and increased fetal loss.

The growth and maturation of the oocyte are dependent on the nurturing capacity of the granulosa and cumulus cells. The highly specialized cumulus cells have distinctive transzonal cytoplasm processes that penetrate through the zona pellucida and the oolemma. Intimate metabolic contact between the oocyte and the cumulus cells is thought to play a role in disseminating nutritional, metabolic, and hormonal factors in the cumulus oocyte complex, promoting the developmental competence of the oocyte *(20,21)*. Intercellular connections, including connexin-43, connexin-37, and transzonal cytoplasm processes are also responsible for transfer of metabolites such as glucose, amino acids, purines, and pyrimidines from the granulosa cells to the oocyte *(22–24)*.

Insulin, an important factor influencing oocyte growth, exerts its effects on the oocyte via its own receptor in the granulosa cells *(25)*. The earliest stage at which the insulin receptor appears is the preantral stage, increasing thereafter with follicular growth *(26)*. Insulin, acting in concert with insulin-like growth factor (IGF)-1 and -2, LH, follicle stimulating hormone, and other intraovarian growth factors, influences steroidogenesis, mitogenic activity, and glucose metabolism in the granulosa cells leading to follicular development and maturation *(27)*. Phosphorylation of insulin receptor substrate (IRS)-1, a postreceptor substrate, by insulin is a key step in insulin mediated metabolic effects in the granulosa cells, including glucose uptake, glycogen synthesis, synthesis of pyruvate and lactate—the preferred substrates for the oocyte—and *de novo* purine synthesis via the stimulation of the pentose phosphate pathway *(28–30)*. The mitogenic effects of insulin, including activation of the meiosis promoting factor in cumulus oocyte complex, activation of cell differentiation of the granulosa cells, and oocyte maturation, are mediated via stimulation of IRS-2, another postreceptor substrate *(28,31)*.

Several studies have reported the presence of impaired insulin-mediated lactate production in human granulosa cells in PCOS ovaries compared to normal *(32–34)*. Lin et al. conducted a study looking at the effect of insulin on lactate accumulation in granulosa-luteal cells in women with PCOS compared with those with normal ovarian function. They observed that stimulation by insulin led to a dose-dependent increase in accumulation of lactate in the granulosa cells of normal ovaries but no change in the lactate levels of cells from PCOS ovaries. Moreover, basal and hCG-stimulated lactate accumulations in the two groups were similar *(33)*. These results implicate the presence of insulin resistance with regard to glucose metabolism in the granulosa cells in PCOS. Another study, conducted by Rice et al., demonstrated that insulin-dependent lactate production was markedly impaired in granulosa-lutein cells from anovulatory poly-cystic ovaries (PCOs) compared with either normal ($p = 0.002$) or ovulatory PCOs ($p < 0.0001$). However, there was no difference in insulin-stimulated progesterone production in granulosa-lutein cells between the PCOS and normal ovaries *(34)*. This supports the probability of impairment of a specific postreceptor signaling pathway of insulin action in PCOS.

Recent studies have also shown the existence of a selective impairment of insulin-stimulated glucose uptake in ovarian granulosa cells of PCOS women *(35,36)*. Wu et al., in their initial study, showed that, compared with follicles at a similar stage of devel-opment in ovulatory ovaries, follicles in polycystic ovaries had decreased concentration of IRS-1 in granulosa cells but increased levels of IRS-2 in theca interna cells *(35)*. In a subsequent study published in 2003, they further demonstrated that there was a signifi-cant decrease in insulin-stimulated glucose incorporation into glycogen, a metabolic action of insulin, in ovarian cells from PCOS women. However, IGF-1 stimulation of thymidine incorporation, a mitogenic action of insulin and its mediators, was found to be greater in PCOS cells compared with normal ovarian cells. Moreover, troglitazone, an insulin sensitizing drug of the thiazolidinedione class, reversed the expression imbalance between IRS-1 and -2 in PCOS cells; treatment with troglitzone increased insulin-induced glycogen synthesis but decreased the IGF-1-augmented responses of DNA synthesis in PCOS cells *(36)*.

These defects in glucose metabolism because of selective insulin resistance at the level of ovaries could adversely affect the flow of glucose, lactate, pyruvate, purines, and cAMP to the oocyte leading to an alteration in meiosis *(37)* and oocyte maturation, thus contributing to the anovulatory disturbances and EPL seen in women with PCOS.

INSULIN RESISTANCE AND ITS ROLE IN APOPTOSIS OF THE BLASTOCYST

Insulin and IGF-1 are known to be important in the maintenance of pregnancy as they stimulate glucose uptake in the preimplantation blastocyst, thereby sustaining cell growth. These effects are mediated via the IGF-1 receptor, which mediates trans-location of GLUT 8, an insulin-regulated glucose transporter in the blastocyst, toward the cell membrane *(38)*.

It has recently been proposed that high insulin and/or IGF-1 levels surrounding the preimplantation blastocyst downregulate the IGF-1 receptor, leading to decreased glucose uptake and attenuated cell growth. Impaired glucose uptake may then result in an increase in apoptosis and programmed cell death *(39–41)*. It has also been reported that hyperinsulinemia and hyperglycemia, frequent findings in women with PCOS, induce the expression of "caspase," an enzyme that attacks the cells of the blastocyst and triggers the cascade of programmed cell death *(41,42)*.

Another important glucose transporter regulated by insulin is GLUT 4, which is expressed in endometrial epithelial cells, primarily in the proliferative phase. Insulin, by binding to its receptor, induces the translocation of GLUT 4 to the surface of endometrial cells, facilitating glucose uptake into the cells *(43)*. Studies have clearly shown that expression of GLUT 4 is significantly diminished in adipocytes from women with PCOS compared with those from normal women *(44)*. Recently, Mioni et al. assessed GLUT 4 expression in endometrial cells of normal and PCOS women. GLUT 4 content was significantly lower in endometrial cells of hyperinsulinemic and obese PCOS women compared with those from normoinsulinemic PCOS women or controls *(43)*. The lowest expression of GLUT 4 was found in obese, hyperinsulinemic PCOS women, and no difference was observed between lean, normoinsulinemic PCOS women, and controls. These results indicate that hyperinsulinemia and obesity not only influence GLUT 4 expression through independent mechanisms, but that they also exert an additional injury on the insulin resistant state in the endometrium of PCOS women *(43,45)*.

Collectively, these findings suggest that an embryonic insult caused by high levels of insulin, glucose, and IGF-1 in women with PCOS may be responsible for the high rates of EPL seen in this population. Therefore, therapies aimed at decreasing the levels of insulin and IGF-1 may help to improve fertility and decrease miscarriage rates in women with PCOS.

INSULIN RESISTANCE AND IMPLANTATION

A principal function of the endometrium is to prepare for and sustain a pregnancy. Endometrial receptivity toward embryo implantation is a complex process that involves the ovaries, endometrium, and embryo itself. Estrogen and progesterone together stimulate the expression of key molecules necessary for implantation of the embryo.

It is generally accepted that initial attachment of the embryo is mediated via certain cell adhesion molecules located on the luminal surface of the endometrium *(46)*. One of the well-characterized cell adhesion molecules is the $\alpha_v\beta_3$ integrin, which facilitates adhesion of the embryo to the apical surface of the endometrium prior to invasion *(46,47)*. Lessey et al. assessed uterine receptivity in nulliparous women with unexplained infertility as well as in fertile and infertile parous controls. Women with unexplained infertility frequently had abnormal expression of integrin in the endometrium. Specifically, they identified two distinct defects in integrin expression: "out-of-phase" defects with lack of beta 3 because of histologic lag (type I defects) and "in-phase" endometrium that still failed to express this integrin (type II defects) *(48)*. Subsequently, Apparao et al. showed that women with PCOS have significantly lower levels of $\alpha_v\beta_3$ integrins in the endometrium and that this was closely associated with an increase in the endometrial androgen receptors *(49)*.

In normal fertile women, the quantity of androgen and estrogen receptors in the endometrium diminish during implantation and the expression of androgen receptors (AR) is negligible in the luteal phase. Androgens and estrogens are known to upregulate the expression of ARs in the endometrium while progestins downregulate them *(50,51)*. It is well established that women with PCOS have significantly higher concentrations of androgens and estrogens, and chronically decreased levels of progestins *(52)*. This combination of hormonal abnormalities may be responsible for the increased AR and decreased $\alpha_v\beta_3$ integrin expression seen in women with PCOS.

As discussed earlier, hyperinsulinemia leads to elevated androgen concentrations in women with PCOS. It has thus been suggested that insulin resistance and hyperinsulinemia, by causing hyperandrogenemia, may be responsible for the decreased uterine receptivity for implantation that is characteristic of this population.

HOXA10 GENES AND IMPLANTATION

Another factor that plays an important role in implantation and maintenance of pregnancy is a set of genes called "home box genes" or *HOXA10* genes. Adequate expression of *HOXA10* helps maintain the endometrial plasticity necessary for its sequential differentiation during each menstrual cycle. Upregulation of these genes is also essential for sustaining uterine receptivity for embryo implantation *(53,54)*.

Sex steroids regulate the expression of *HOXA10* genes. Estrogen and progesterone induce the expression of these genes while testosterone inhibits it *(55)*. In a recent study, Cermik et al. looked at mid-secretory phase endometrial samples obtained from seven hyperandrogenemic PCOS women and five normal controls. They observed that the expression of *HOXA10* and its mRNA was significantly reduced in women with PCOS. They also found that testosterone blocked the estradiol- and progesterone-induced increase in *HOXA10* mRNA expression in Ishikawa cells (a well-differentiated human endometrial adenocarcinoma cell line that expresses androgen, estrogen, and progesterone receptors). However, treatment with insulin did not directly affect expression of these genes *(56)*. These results suggest that hyperinsulinemia may indirectly affect the endometrium by increasing serum androgen levels, thus contributing to the decreased uterine receptivity and the high rates of spontaneous miscarriage seen in women with PCOS.

ROLE OF GLYCODELIN AND IGF-BINDING PROTEIN-1

One of the most compelling pieces of evidence suggesting a role for insulin resistance in the EPL of PCOS is the effect of insulin to decrease circulating levels of glycodelin and IGF-binding protein (IGFBP)-1 *(57)*, major endometrial secretory proteins that play an important role in implantation and maintenance of pregnancy.

Glycodelin is a glycoprotein produced by decidualized endometrial glands during the luteal phase, and it facilitates implantation by inhibiting the immune response of the endometrial natural killer cells to the embryo. Deficient production of endometrial glycodelin can result in a locally hostile immunological environment for the embryo. It is thus important for protection of the embryo from the maternal immune response during the implantation period *(58–61)*. Glycodelin appears in the endometrium at the time when the embryo enters the uterine cavity. Progesterone stimulates the synthesis and the cyclical expression of glycodelin in the endometrium. The maximum increase in the level of glycodelin is observed on the 10th and 12th day after ovulation *(58,62)*. Studies have shown that women with unexplained infertility, recurrent EPL, and retarded endometrial maturation have significantly lower levels of endometrial glycodelin (in samples obtained via uterine flushing) during the luteal phase compared with normal fertile women *(63,64)*.

IGFBP-1, another important endometrial protein, facilitates the adhesion process at the feto–maternal interface, maintains adequate utero-placental blood flow, and thus plays a central role in the peri-implantation period *(65–69)*. It is produced primarily by the liver during the non-pregnant state and is negatively regulated by insulin *(70,71)*. During pregnancy, IGFBP-1 is a major secretory product of the decidual stroma *(72)*.

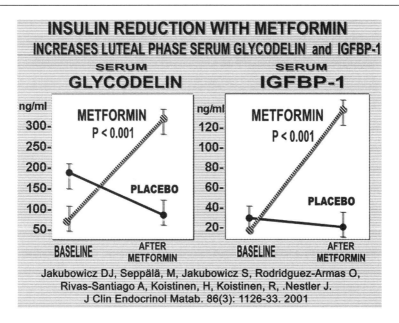

Fig. 1. Treatment with metformin was associated with a threefold increase in the luteal phase serum glycodelin concentrations (*p* < 0.001) and a significant increase in IGFBP-1 levels. No change was noted in these variables in the placebo group *(73)*.

It is thought to act locally by signaling through $\alpha_5\beta_1$ integrin, influencing endovascular trophoblastic invasion of the spiral arteries, primarily during the first trimester of pregnancy. This leads to a remodeling of the utero-placental arteries into dilated, low resistance, nonelastic tubes, with loss of maternal vasomotor control, which in turn increases the maternal blood flow and utero-placental perfusion necessary to meet the requirements of the fetus *(67–69)*.

Although the exact mechanism by which hyperinsulinemic insulin resistance contributes to EPL in PCOS is not known, it probably involves suppression of endometrial glycodelin and IGFBP-1 production, resulting in a hostile endometrial milieu. In support of this idea is a study conducted by Jakubowicz et al. that assessed 48 women with PCOS before and after 4 weeks of administration of 500 mg of metformin or placebo three times daily *(73)*. Serum glycodelin and IGFBP-1 levels were determined during the follicular and clomiphene-induced luteal phases of the menstrual cycle, and insulin sensitivity was determined by an oral glucose tolerance test. Treatment with metformin was associated with a 20-fold increase in the follicular phase and a 3-fold increase in the luteal phase serum glycodelin concentrations (*p* < 0.001). There was a significant increase in IGFBP-1 levels in the metformin group as well (Fig. 1). These changes in the metformin group were further accompanied by a substantial decrease in serum insulin and glucose concentrations, a 37% decrease in serum free testosterone levels, a significant increase in SHBG, and an increase in the uterine vasculature penetration as evident by a 20% decrease in the resistance index. No change was noted in these variables in the placebo group.

On the basis of the above findings, and to further confirm their hypothesis, Jakubowicz et al. subsequently conducted a study in 134 pregnant women—72 PCOS

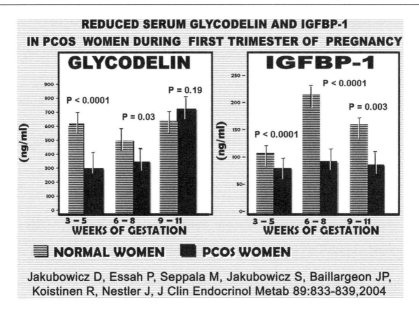

Fig. 2. Serum concentrations of both glycodelin and IGFBP-1 were markedly lower in women with PCOS (black bars) compared with normal women during 3–5, 6–8, and 9–11 weeks of pregnancy *(74)*.

women and 62 controls—during the first trimester assessing serum glycodelin and IGFBP-1 levels *(74)*. They found that serum concentrations of both glycodelin and IGFBP-1 were markedly lower in women with PCOS compared with controls. Specifically, in women with PCOS, serum glycodelin was 56% lower during weeks 3–5, 23% lower during weeks 6–8, but by weeks 9–11 the levels were similar between the two groups. Likewise, IGFBP-1 levels in women with PCOS were 60–70% lower during weeks 3–5 and 6–8, and 39% lower during weeks 9–11 (Fig. 2). Insulin sensitivity was markedly lower and serum total testosterone was significantly higher in women with PCOS throughout the first trimester. Moreover, women with PCOS had significantly more miscarriages compared with normal women (14 vs 3%, respectively) and within the PCOS group itself, serum glycodelin and IGFBP-1 levels were significantly lower in women with EPL.

Several other studies have documented decreased endometrial levels of IGFBP-1 and glycodelin during the first trimester of pregnancy in various insulin resistant and hyperinsulinemic states including PCOS *(18,69,75)*. Decreased secretion of IGFBP-1 from the secretory endometrium has been associated with retarded endometrial development, abnormal trophoblastic invasion, disturbed remodeling of spiral arteries, and recurrent miscarriage. Lower circulating concentrations of IGFBP-1 in the early half of pregnancy have also been associated with intrauterine growth restriction (IUGR) and preeclampsia *(67–69,76,77)*.

Given the consistency among these studies, it appears that insulin resistance, by decreasing the levels of these endometrial proteins, creates a hostile environment for implantation and fetal growth and, thus, plays an important role in EPL in women with PCOS.

INSULIN SENSITIZING DRUGS IN EPL IN PCOS

Numerous studies lend credence to the idea that insulin resistance contributes to endometrial dysfunction, infertility, and EPL in PCOS. Insulin sensitizing drugs may thus prove to be a novel therapeutic option to improve endometrial function and decrease the risk of miscarriage in this population.

Several studies have examined the effects of insulin-sensitizing drugs on the rate of miscarriage in PCOS. Glueck et al. *(78)* conducted a prospective cohort pilot study of women with PCOS, comparing those treated with metformin prior to conception who continued the drug throughout pregnancy to historical controls who did not receive metformin. Their results showed that the rate of first trimester pregnancy loss was 39% in the historical controls but only 11% in the metformin group. Ten women in the metformin group had had previous pregnancies while not receiving metformin. In this subcohort, the miscarriage rate decreased from 73 to 10% with the addition of metformin ($p < 0.002$). Overall, no evidence of teratogenicity was noted in the metformin group. Before metformin therapy, fasting serum insulin levels correlated positively with plasminogen activator inhibitor (PAI) activity ($r = 0.60$, $p = 0.004$). Over a median treatment period of 6 months (prior to conception), a reduction in fasting serum insulin was also positively correlated with a reduction in PAI activity ($r = 0.65$, $p = 0.04$), suggesting that hyperinsulinemia and PAI activity may be closely related; perhaps both can help explain the etiology of EPL in PCOS.

Glueck et al. *(79)* subsequently completed a larger but uncontrolled study that confirmed that EPL decreased from 62 to 26% ($p < 0.0001$) when women continued metformin throughout pregnancy. Again, no teratogenic adverse events occurred on metformin therapy.

These findings were later confirmed by Jakubowicz et al. in a larger, controlled, retrospective study of 96 pregnant PCOS women *(18)*. Among the 65 women who became pregnant on metformin and received metformin throughout pregnancy, there were a total of 68 pregnancies, of which 6 (8.8%) ended in EPL. In contrast, among the 31 control PCOS women who had not received metformin, there were 31 pregnancies, of which 13 (41.9%) ended in EPL (Fig. 3). The 41.9% rate of EPL in the control group is comparable with the 30–50% rate described in the literature for women with PCOS *(5–8)*. In contrast, the 8.8% rate of EPL in the women treated with metformin is similar to the 10–15% rate reported for clinically recognized pregnancies in normal women *(9,10)*, suggesting that metformin treatment removes any independent risk for EPL conferred by the disorder itself. Moreover, similarly to prior studies, metformin treatment resulted in a 57% decrease in free testosterone levels and an improvement in insulin sensitivity. These findings suggest that metformin treatment prior to conception and during pregnancy may dramatically decrease the rate of EPL in women with PCOS.

Of all the insulin-sensitizing drugs, metformin, which is designated a class B drug for use during pregnancy, is probably the safest therapeutic option given that thiazolidinediones are pregnancy class C drugs. However, the safety of metformin in pregnancy has come under question. Hellmuth et al. *(80)* performed a cohort study of pregnant diabetic women treated with metformin and compared them with women treated with a sulfonylurea or insulin. They reported an increased incidence of preeclampsia and perinatal mortality in the metformin group. However, the authors acknowledged that the reference group selected was not an ideal one, because the women in the metformin

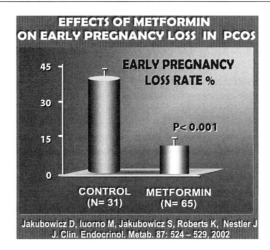

Fig. 3. Among the 65 women who became pregnant on metformin and received metformin through-out pregnancy, there were a total of 68 pregnancies, of which 6 (8.8%) ended in early pregnancy loss (control group). In contrast, among the 31 control PCOS women who had not received metformin, there were 31 pregnancies, of which 13 (41.9%) ended in early pregnancy loss *(18)*.

group had a significantly higher body mass index and worse diabetes control, both of which predispose to preeclampsia, than the women treated with sulfonylurea or insulin. In contrast, Glueck et al. *(81)* recently performed a prospective study to assess the growth and motor-social development in 126 live births to 109 women with PCOS, who conceived on and continued metformin throughout pregnancy. They found that metformin was not teratogenic and did not adversely affect birth length and weight, growth, or motor-social development in the first 18 months of life. Other studies have further substantiated this claim *(18,82)*. However, given the conflicting data, prospective randomized controlled trials are needed to more definitively assess metformin's safety profile and efficacy during pregnancy.

RESEARCH AGENDA AND CONCLUSIONS

PCOS, a prevalent disorder in young women, is characterized by chronic anovulation and hyperandrogenism. One of the major concerns in women with PCOS has been infertility, a consequence of chronic oligo- or anovulation. However, even after ovulation is restored, either pharmacologically or via lifestyle interventions, women with PCOS exhibit a surprisingly high rate of spontaneous miscarriage.

Several studies have shown that insulin resistance and hyperinsulinemia play an integral role in EPL in PCOS. However, the exact underlying mechanism remains poorly understood. Several different mechanisms for the effect of hyperinsulinemia have been proposed, including its effect on oocyte maturation, glucose uptake and metabolism, implantation, and alteration of expression of *HOXA10* genes. However, one of the most compelling hypotheses is the effect of hyperinsulinemic insulin resistance on decreasing serum and endometrial glycodelin and IGFBP-1 concentrations, major endometrial secretory proteins that play an important role in implantation and main-tenance of pregnancy. These findings raise the possibility that measurement of serum glycodelin and IGFBP-1 may be used to identify women at increased risk for spontaneous miscarriage. However, future prospective studies are required to further explore this concept.

Insulin sensitizing drugs, especially metformin, may prove to be a unique therapeutic option to decrease the rate of EPL in women with PCOS. The accumulated evidence supports the use of metformin in the treatment of infertility in PCOS, and suggests that it may reduce miscarriages in the disorder. However, the duration of metformin treatment during pregnancy in women with PCOS is controversial, and future long-term prospective studies are required for further evaluation. Studies are also needed to further elucidate and confirm the underlying mechanism of insulin resistance in PCOS. Although metformin appears to have a reassuring safety profile during pregnancy, future rigorous, randomized controlled trials are needed to confirm its efficacy and safety under these conditions.

Furthermore, the incidence of complications in the second and third trimester of pregnancy among PCOS patients has only been sparsely studied. PCOS has been associated with gestational diabetes mellitus, hypertensive disorders of pregnancy, preeclampsia, IUGR, and premature delivery, with hyperinsulinemic insulin resistance being an underlying factor for most of these complications (83–87). Metformin treatment during pregnancy has been shown to reduce severe pregnancy and postpartum complications (88). It is also increasingly evident that the foundations of lifelong health are built *in utero*, and that infants surviving IUGR are at increased risk for several long-term health problems including hypertension, dyslipidemia, obesity, diabetes, precocious adrenarche, and infertility (89–92). These observations suggest that interventions to reduce insulin resistance during pregnancy will not only reduce the risk for EPL, but may also exert beneficial effects by prevention of gestational diabetes, preeclampsia, and IUGR, and may ameliorate the risk of long-term health problems like coronary artery disease, dyslipidemia, hypertension, obesity, diabetes, and infertility during the adult life of infants born to PCOS women.

FUTURE AVENUES TO RESEARCH

Recent studies have clearly shown that insulin resistance and hyperinsulinemia play a central role in EPL in PCOS. However, the underlying pathophysiology is not clearly understood. Several different mechanisms for the effect of hyperinsulinemia have been proposed, including its effect on oocyte maturation, glucose uptake and metabolism, implantation, altered expression of *HOXA10* genes, and the effect of hyperinsulinemia on decreasing endometrial and serum glycodelin and IGFBP-1 concentrations.

Decreased serum and endometrial IGFBP-1 levels have been found to be correlated with abnormal endovascular trophoblastic invasion of the spiral arteries during the first trimester of pregnancy and also with inadequate establishment of the feto-maternal blood flow that is unable to meet the nutrition requirements of the fetus, leading to IUGR. Lower circulating concentrations of IGFBP-1 in the early half of pregnancy have also been associated with recurrent miscarriage and preeclampsia. These findings suggest that measurement of serum glycodelin and IGFBP-1 may be used to identify women at increased risk for spontaneous miscarriage. However, prospective studies are required to further explore this concept.

Current data suggests that insulin sensitizing drugs, especially metformin, if used prior to and during pregnancy, can reduce the incidence of EPL in women with PCOS. However, the duration of metformin treatment during pregnancy in women with PCOS remains controversial, and long-term prospective studies are required for further evaluation. Future rigorous, prospective, randomized controlled trials are also needed to confirm the beneficial effects of various interventions that reduce insulin resistance on the prevention of gestational diabetes, preeclampsia, IUGR, and possible amelioration of the risk of long-term health problems like coronary artery disease, dyslipidemia, hypertension, obesity, diabetes, and infertility during the adult life of infants born to PCOS women.

REFERENCES

1. Knochenhauer ES, Key TJ, Kahsar-Miller M, et al. Prevalence of the polycystic ovary syndrome in unselected black and white women of the Southeastern United States: a prospective study. J Clin Endocrinol Metab 1998;83:3078–3082.
2. Asuncion M, Calvo RM, San Millan JL, et al. A prospective study of the prevalence of the polycystic ovary syndrome in unselected Caucasian women from Spain. J Clin Endocrinol Metab 2000;85: 2434–2438.
3. Franks S. Polycystic ovary syndrome. N Engl J Med 1995;333:853–861.
4. Adams J, Polson DW, Franks S. Prevalence of polycystic ovaries in women with anovulation and idiopathic hirsutism. Br J Med (Clin Res Ed) 1986;293:355–359.
5. Balen AH, Tan SL, MacDougall J, Jacobs HS. Miscarriage rates following in vitro fertilization are increased in women with polycystic ovaries and reduced by pituitary desensitization with buserelin. Hum Reprod 1993;8:959–964.
6. Sagle M, Bishop K, Ridley N, et al. Recurrent early miscarriage and polycystic ovaries. Br J Med 1988;297:1027–1028.
7. Homburg R, Armar NA, Eshel A, et al. Influence of serum luteinising hormone concentrations on ovulation, conception, and early pregnancy loss in polycystic ovary syndrome. Br J Med 1988; 297:1024–1026.
8. Regan L, Owen EJ, Jacobs HS. Hypersecretion of luteinising hormone, infertility, and miscarriage. Lancet 1990;336:1141–1144.
9. Gray RH, Wu LY. Subfertility and risk of spontaneous abortion. Am J Public Health 2000;90: 1452–1454.
10. Regan L, Braude PR, Trembath PL. Influence of past reproductive performance on risk of spontaneous abortion. Br J Med 1989;299:541–545.
11. Liddle HS, Sowden K, Farquhar CM. Recurrent miscarriage: screening for polycystic ovaries and subsequent pregnancy outcome. Aust N Z J Obstet Gynaecol 1997;37:402–406.
12. Clifford K, Rai R, Watson H, et al. Does suppressing luteinising hormone secretion reduce the miscarriage rate? Results of a randomized controlled trial. Br J Med 1996;312:1508–1511.
13. Fedorcsak P, Storeng R, Dale PO, et al. Obesity is a risk factor for early pregnancy loss after IVF or ICSI. Acta Obstet Gynecol Scand 2000;79:43–48.
14. Okon MA, Laird SM, Tuckerman EM, Li TC. Serum androgen levels in women who have recurrent miscarriages and their correlation with markers of endometrial function. Fertil Steril 1998;69: 682–690.
15. Dunaif A, Segal KR, Futterweit W, et al. Profound peripheral resistance, independent of obesity, in polycystic ovary syndrome. Diabetes 1989;38:1165–1174.
16. Chang RJ, Nakamura RM, Judd HL, et al. Insulin resistance in nonobese patients with polycystic ovarian disease. J Clin Endocrinol Metab 1983;57:356–359.
17. Campbell PJ, Gerich JE. Impact of obesity on insulin action in volunteers with normal glucose tolerance: demonstration of a threshold for the adverse effect of obesity. J Clin Endocrinol Metab 1990;70: 1114–1118.
18. Jakubowicz DJ, Iuorno MJ, Jakubowicz S, Roberts KA, Nestler JE. Effects of metformin on early pregnancy loss in the polycystic ovary syndrome. J Clin Endocrinol Metab 2002;87:524–529.
19. Krisher RL. The effect of oocyte quality on development. J Anim Sci 2004;82:E14–E23.

20. Sutton ML, Gilchrist RB, Thompson JG. Effects of in-vivo and in-vitro environments on the metabolism of the cumulus-oocyte complex and its influence on oocyte developmental capacity. Hum Reprod Update 2003;9:35–48.

21. Colonna R, Mangia F. Mechanisms of amino acid uptake in cumulus-enclosed mouse oocytes. Biol Reprod 1983;28:797–803.

22. Simon AM, Goodenough DA, Li E, Paul DL. Female infertility in mice lacking connexin 37. Nature 1997;385:525–529.

23. Ackert CL, Gittens JE, O'Brien MJ, et al. Intercellular communication via connexin43 gap junctions is required for ovarian folliculogenesis in the mouse. Dev Biol 2001;233:258–270.

24. Epigg JJ, Downs SM. Chemical signals that regulate mammalian oocyte maturation. Biol Reprod 1984;30:1–11.

25. Willis D, Franks F. Insulin action in human granulosa cells from normal and polycystic ovaries is mediated by the insulin receptor and not the type-I insulin-like growth factor receptor. J Clin Endocrinol Metab 1995;80:3788–3790.

26. Samoto T, Maruo T, Ladines-Llave CA, et al. Insulin receptor expression in follicular and stromal compartments of the human ovary over the course of follicular growth, regression and atresia. Endocr J 1993;40:715–726.

27. Roy SK, Terada DM. Activities of glucose metabolic enzymes in human preantral follicles: in vitro modulation by follicle-stimulating hormone, luteinizing hormone, epidermal growth factor, insulin-like growth factor I, and transforming growth factor beta1. Biol Reprod 1999;60:763–768.

28. White MF, Yenush L. The IRS-signaling system: a network of docking proteins that mediate insulin and cytokine action. Curr Top Microbiol Immunol 1998;228:179–208.

29. Lawrence JC Jr., Roach PJ. New insights into the role and mechanism of glycogen synthase activation by insulin. Diabetes 1997;46:541–547.

30. Virkamaki A, Ueki K, Kahn CR. Protein-protein interaction in insulin signaling and the molecular mechanisms of insulin resistance. J Clin Invest 1999;103:931–943.

31. Saltiel AR. Diverse signaling pathways in the cellular actions of insulin. Am J Physiol 1996;270:E375–E385.

32. Fedorcsak P, Storeng R, Dale PO, et al. Impaired insulin action on granulosa-lutein cells in women with polycystic ovary syndrome and insulin resistance. Gynecol Endocrinol 2000;14:327–336.

33. Lin Y, Fridstrom M, Hillensjo T. Insulin stimulation of lactate accumulation in isolated human granulosa-luteal cells: a comparison between normal and polycystic ovaries. Hum Reprod 1997;12:2469–2472.

34. Rice S, Christoforidis N, Gadd C, et al. Impaired insulin-dependent glucose metabolism in granulosa-lutein cells from anovulatory women with polycystic ovaries. Hum Reprod 2005;20:373–381.

35. Wu X, Sallinen K, Anttila L, et al. Expression of insulin-receptor substrate-1 and -2 in ovaries from women with insulin resistance and from controls. Fertil Steril 2000;74:564–572.

36. Wu XK, Zhou SY, Liu JX, et al. Selective ovary resistance to insulin signaling in women with polycystic ovary syndrome. Fertil Steril 2003;80:954–965.

37. Colton SA, Pieper GM, Downs SM. Altered meiotic regulation in oocytes from diabetic mice. Biol Reprod 2002;67:220–231.

38. Crayannopoulos MO, Chi MM, Cui Y, et al. GLUT 8 is a glucose transporter responsible for insulin-stimulated glucose uptake in the blastocyst. Proc Natl Acad Sci USA 2000;97:7313–7318.

39. Chi MM, Schlein AL, Moley KH. High insulin-like growth factor 1 (IGF-1) and insulin concentrations trigger apoptosis in the mouse blastocyst via down-regulation of the IGF-1 receptor. Endocrinology 2000;141:4784–4792.

40. Chi MM, Pingsterhaus J, Crayannopoulos MO, et al. Decreased glucose transporter expression triggers BAX-dependent apoptosis in murine blastocyst. J Biol Chem 2000;275:40,252–40,257.

41. Pinto AB, Crayannopoulos MO, Hoehn A, et al. Glucose transporter 8 expression and translocation are critical for murine blastocyst survival. Biol Reprod 2002;66:1729–1733.

42. Hinck L, Thissen JP, De Hertogh R. Identification of caspase-6 in rat blastocysts and its implication in the induction of apoptosis by high glucose. Biol Reprod 2003;68:1808–1812.

43. Mioni R, Chiarelli S, Xamin N, et al. Evidence for the presence of glucose transporter 4 in the endometrium and its regulation in polycystic ovary syndrome patients. J Clin Endocrinol Metab 2004;89:4089–4096.

44. Rosenbaum D, Haber RS, Dunaif A. Insulin resistance in polycystic ovary syndrome: decreased expression of GLUT-4 glucose transporters in adipocytes. Am J Physiol 1993;264:E197–E202.

45. Mozzanega B, Mioni R, Granzotto M, et al. Obesity reduces the expression of GLUT4 in the endometrium of normoinsulinemic women affected by the polycystic ovary syndrome. Ann N Y Acad Sci 2004;1034:364–374.

46. Lessey BA. Adhesion molecules and implantation. J Reprod Immunol 2002;55:101–112.

47. Lessey BA, Damjanovich L, Coutifaris C, et al. Integrin adhesion molecules in the human endometrium. Correlation with the normal and abnormal menstrual cycle. J Clin Invest 1992;90: 188–195.

48. Lessey BA, Castelbaum AJ, Sawin SW, Sun J. Integrins as markers of uterine receptivity in women with primary unexplained infertility. Fertil Steril 1995;63:535–542.

49. Apparao KB, Lovely LP, Gui Y, et al. Elevated endometrial androgen receptor expression in women with polycystic ovarian syndrome. Biol Reprod 2002;66:297–304.

50. Fujimoto J, Nishigaki M, Hori M, et al. The effect of estrogen and androgen on androgen receptors and mRNA levels in uterine leiomyoma, myometrium and endometrium of human subjects. J Steroid Biochem Mol Biol 1994;50:137–143.

51. Lovely LP, Appa Rao KB, Gui Y, Lessey BA. Characterization of androgen receptors in a well-differentiated endometrial adenocarcinoma cell line (Ishikawa). J Steroid Biochem Mol Biol 2000;74: 235–241.

52. Apparao KB, Lovely LP, Gui Y, et al. Elevated endometrial androgen receptor expression in women with polycystic ovarian syndrome. Biol Reprod 2002;66:297–304.

53. Bagot CN, Troy PJ, Taylor HS. Alteration of maternal Hoxa10 expression by in vivo gene transfection affects implantation. Gene Ther 2000;7:1378–1384.

54. Bagot CN, Kliman HJ, Taylor HS. Maternal Hoxa10 is required for pinopod formation in the development of mouse uterine receptivity to embryo implantation. Dev Dyn 2001;222:538–544.

55. Cermik D, Karaca M, Taylor HS. HOXA10 expression is repressed by progesterone in the myometrium: differential tissue-specific regulation of HOX gene expression in the reproductive tract. J Clin Endocrinol Metab 2001;86:3387–3392.

56. Cermik D, Selam B, Taylor HS. Regulation of HOXA-10 expression by testosterone in vitro and in the endometrium of patients with polycystic ovary syndrome. J Clin Endocrinol Metab 2003;88: 238–243.

57. Jakubowicz DJ, Essah PA, Seppala M, et al. Reduced serum glycodelin and insulin-like growth factor-binding protein-1 in women with polycystic ovary syndrome during first trimester of pregnancy. J Clin Endocrinol Metab 2004;89:833–839.

58. Seppala M, Taylor RN, Koistinen H, et al. Glycodelin: a major lipocalin protein of the reproductive axis with diverse actions in cell recognition and differentiation. Endocr Rev 2002;23:401–430.

59. Bolton AE, Pockley AG, Clough KJ, et al. Identification of placental protein 14 as an immunosuppressive factor in human reproduction. Lancet 1987;1:593–595.

60. Kamarainen N, Leivo I, Koistinen R, et al. Normal human ovary and ovarian tumors express glycodelin, a glycoprotein with immunosuppressive and contraceptive properties. Am J Pathol 1996; 148:1435–1443.

61. Rachmilewitz J, Riely GJ, Tykocinski ML. Placental protein 14 functions as a direct T-cell inhibitor. Cell Immunol 1999;191:26–33.

62. Julkunen M, Koistinen R, Sjoberg J, et al. Secretory endometrium synthesizes placental protein 14. Endocrinology 1986;118:1782–1786.

63. Dalton CF, Laird SM, Serle E, et al. The measurement of CA 125 and placental protein 14 in uterine flushings in women with recurrent miscarriage; relation to endometrial morphology. Hum Reprod 1995;10:2680–2684.

64. Tulppala M, Julkunen M, Tiitinen A, et al. Habitual abortion is accompanied by low serum levels of placental protein 14 in the luteal phase of the fertile cycle. Fertil Steril 1995;63:792–795.

65. Guidice LC. Multifaceted roles for IGFBP-1 in human endometrium during implantation and pregnancy. Ann N Y Acad Sci 1997;828:146–156.

66. Jones JI, Doerr ME, Clemmons DR. Cell migration: interactions among integrins, IGFs and IGFBPs. Prog Growth Factor Res 1995;6:319–327.

67. Kaufmann P, Black S, Huppertz B. Endovascular trophoblast invasion: implications for the pathogenesis of intrauterine growth retardation and preeclampsia. Biol Reprod 2003;69:1–7.

68. Anim-Nyame N, Hills FA, Sooranna SR, Steer PJ, Johnson MR. A longitudinal study of maternal plasma insulin-like growth factor binding protein-1 concentrations during normal pregnancy and pregnancies complicated by pre-eclampsia. Hum Reprod 2000;15:2215–2219.

69. Gleeson LM, Chakraborty C, McKinnon T, Lala PK. Insulin-like growth factor binding protein 1 stimulates human trophoblast migration by signaling through alpha 5 beta 1 integrin via mitogen-activated protein kinase pathway. J Clin Endocrinol Metab 2001;86:2484–2493.

70. Suikkari AM, Angervo M, Koistinen R, et al. Insulin-like growth factor-binding protein-1 (IGFBP-1) in the human ovary. Ann N Y Acad Sci 1991;626:184–188.

71. Suikkari AM, Koivisto VA, Koistinen R, et al. Dose-response characterisitics for suppression of low molecular weight plasma insulin-like growth factor-binding protein by insulin. J Clin Endocrinol Metab 1989;68:135–140.

72. Rutanen EM, Seppala M. Insulin-like growth factor binding protein-1 in female reproductive functions. Int J Gynaecol Obstet 1992;39:3–9.

73. Jakubowicz DJ, Seppala M, Jakubowicz S, et al. Insulin reduction with metformin increases luteal phase serum glycodelin and insulin-like growth factor-binding protein 1 concentrations and enhances uterine vascularity and blood flow in the polycystic ovary syndrome. J Clin Endocrinol Metab 2001;86:1126–1133.

74. Jakubowicz DJ, Essah PA, Seppala M, et al. Reduced serum glycodelin and insulin-like growth factor-binding protein-1 in women with polycystic ovary syndrome during first trimester of pregnancy. J Clin Endocrinol Metab 2004;89:833–839.

75. Heitala R, Pohja-Nylander P, Rutanen EM, Laatikainen T. Serum IGFBP-1 at 16 weeks and subsequent preeclampsia. Obstet Gynecol 2000;95:185–189.

76. Crossey P, Pillai CC, Miell JP. Altered placental development and intrauterine growth restriction in IGF binding protein-1 transgenic mice. J Clin Invest 2002;110:411–418.

77. de Groot CJ, O'Brien TJ, Taylor RN. Biochemical evidence of impaired trophoblastic invasion of decidual stroma in women destined to have preeclampsia. Am J Obstet Gynecol 1996;175:24–29.

78. Glueck CJ, Phillips H, Cameron D, et al. Continuing metformin throughout pregnancy in women with polycystic ovary syndrome appears to safely reduce first-trimester spontaneous abortion: a pilot study. Fertil Steril 2001;75:46–52.

79. Glueck CJ, Wang P, Goldenberg N, Sieve-Smith L. Pregnancy outcomes among women with polycystic ovary syndrome treated with metformin. Hum Reprod 2002;17:2858–2864.

80. Hellmuth E, Damm P, Molsted-Pedersen L. Oral hypoglycaemic agents in 118 diabetic pregnancies. Diabet Med 2000;17:507–511.

81. Glueck CJ, Goldenberg N, Pranikoff J, et al. Height, weight, and motor-social development during the first 18 months of life in 126 infants born to 109 mothers with polycystic ovary syndrome who conceived on and continued metformin through pregnancy. Hum Reprod 2004;19:1323–1330.

82. Coetzee EJ, Jackson WP. The management of non-insulin-dependent-diabetes during pregnancy. Diabetes Res Clin Pract 1985;1:281–287.

83. Solomon CG, Seely EW. Hypertension in pregnancy. Endocrinol Metab Clin North Am 2006;35:157–171.

84. Gjonnaess H. The course and outcome of pregnancy after ovarian electrocautery in women with polycystic ovarian syndrome: the influence of body-weight. Br J Obstet Gynaecol 1989;96:714–719.

85. de Vries MJ, Dekker GA, Schoemaker J. Higher risk of preeclampsia in the polycystic ovary syndrome. A case control study. Eur J Obstet Gynecol Reprod Biol 1998;76:91–95.

86. Mikola M, Hiilesmaa V, Halttunen M, et al. Obstetric outcome in women with polycystic ovarian syndrome. Hum Reprod 2001;16:226–229.

87. Bjercke S, Dale PO, Tanbo T, et al. Impact of insulin resistance on pregnancy complications and outcome in women with polycystic ovary syndrome. Gynecol Obstet Invest 2002;54:94–98.

88. Vanky E, Salvesen KA, Heimstad R, et al. Metformin reduces pregnancy complications without affecting androgen levels in pregnant polycystic ovary syndrome women: results of a randomized study. Hum Reprod 2004;19:1734–1740.

89. Yiu V, Buka S, Zurakowski D, et al. Relationship between birthweight and blood pressure in childhood. Am J Kidney Dis 1999;33:253–260.

90. Barker DJ, Gluckman PD, Godfrey KM, et al. Fetal nutrition and cardiovascular disease in adult life. Lancet 1993;341:938–941.

91. Ibanez L, Potau N, de Zegher F. Recognition of a new association: reduced fetal growth, precocious pubarche, hyperinsulinism and ovarian dysfunction. Ann Endocrinol 2000;61:141–142.

92. Barker DJ, Osmond C, Forsen TJ, Kajantie E, Eriksson JG. Trajectories of growth among children who have coronary events as adults. N Engl J Med 2005;353:1802.

24 Late Pregnancy Complications in Polycystic Ovary Syndrome

Dimitrios Panidis, MD, PhD
and Neoklis A. Georgopoulos, MD

CONTENTS

Summary

Gestational diabetes mellitus and new-onset hypertension, which includes gestational hypertension and preeclampsia, are common complications of pregnancy. Many features of the insulin resistance syndrome have been associated with these conditions. These include glucose intolerance, hyperinsulinemia, hypertension, obesity, and lipid abnormalities. Other accompanying abnormalities may include elevated serum levels of leptin, tumor necrosis factor-α, plasminogen activator inhibitor-1, and testosterone. The establishment of these features before the onset of gestational diabetes mellitus and hypertension in pregnancy suggests that insulin resistance or associated abnormalities may play a role in these disorders. These observations suggest that therapeutic interventions to reduce insulin resistance may lower the risk of both gestational diabetes mellitus and hypertension in pregnancy.

Key Words: Pregnancy; insulin resistance; gestational diabetes mellitus; hypertension in pregnancy; preeclampsia.

INTRODUCTION

With a prevalence of 5–10%, polycystic ovary syndrome (PCOS) is probably the most common endocrine abnormality in women of reproductive age *(1–4)*. Aside from reproductive endocrine abnormalities, including amenorrhea or oligomenorrhea, hyperandrogenism, and chronic anovulation, a key feature of PCOS is insulin resistance

From: *Contemporary Endocrinology: Insulin Resistance and Polycystic Ovarian Syndrome:*
Pathogenesis, Evaluation, and Treatment
Edited by: E. Diamanti-Kandarakis, J. E. Nestler, D. Panidis, and R. Pasquali © Humana Press Inc., Totowa, NJ

(nearly 80% of obese and 30% of lean women with PCOS demonstrate insulin resistance), with compensatory hyperinsulinemia and β-cell dysfunction *(5,6)*.

The presence of insulin resistance in PCOS has important later consequences upon health. Insulin resistance is associated with an increased risk for several disorders, including type 2 diabetes, hypertension, dyslipidaemia, endothelial dysfunction, elevated endothelin-1, and cardiovascular disease. This group of abnormalities coupled with insulin resistance constitutes the so-called "metabolic syndrome" *(7)*. Many women with PCOS show a phenotype similar to Syndrome X. Therefore, PCOS may be considered a component of the metabolic syndrome *(8)*.

It has been demonstrated that women with PCOS present an increased risk for diabetes development and hypertension during pregnancy *(9–18)*. These complications might be attributed to the coexistence of insulin resistance and β-cell dysfunction in a significant percentage of women with PCOS before conception *(5,6)*.

INSULIN RESISTANCE OF NORMAL PREGNANCY

Pregnancy is a complex metabolic entity that involves major alterations in the hormonal status, as well as an increasing burden of fuel utilization by the conceptus. In normal pregnancy, insulin resistance and compensatory hyperinsulinemia occur in the second and maximize in the third trimester of pregnancy. The insulin resistance of normal pregnancy is advantageous. It is regulated by placental hormones and is a physiological adaptation that ensures adequate amounts of maternal glucose meet the increasing nutritional and growth demands of the developing fetus *(17,19–22)*.

The insulin resistance of normal pregnancy is probably mediated by several hormonal changes, including increases in serum levels of estradiol, progesterone, prolactin, cortisol, human chorionic gonadotropin, placental growth hormone (PGH), and human placental lactogen (hPL). hPL has been considered the main insulin-resistance hormone of pregnancy *(23)*. hPL presents its peak at 30 weeks of gestation and has been shown to have both insulin and anti-insulin effects. The major role of hPL may be the adaptive increase in insulin secretion necessary for pregnancy, rather than the induction of insulin resistance. Tumor necrosis factor (TNF)-α was recently demonstrated to have a strong correlation with the insulin resistance of pregnancy, but its role is not yet clear *(24)*.

Human PGH (hPGH) is probably the main factor to mediate the insulin resistance of pregnancy because it is known that chronically elevated levels of pituitary GH have diabetogenic effects. hPGH differs from pituitary growth hormone by 13 amino acids *(25)*. It is not regulated by growth hormone-releasing hormone (GH-RH) or inhibited by somatostatin analogs, but has the same affinity for the GH receptor as the pituitary GH. By 20 weeks of gestation, it replaces pituitary GH almost completely in the maternal circulation. hPGH does not cross the placenta and appears to regulate the maternal levels of insulin-like growth factor (IGF)-1. Maternal IGF-1 levels in plasma correlate with hPGH levels, not with hPL. hPGH seems to be a paracrine growth factor, which through insulin growth factors, may partially regulate the metabolic and growth needs of the fetus. Barbour et al. recently demonstrated in transgenic mice that hPGH, at levels similar to the third trimester of human pregnancy, causes severe insulin resistance, exhibited by both fasting and postprandial hyperinsulinaemia; these mice require insulin levels that are five to seven times higher in order to maintain euglycemia. They also demonstrate a marked decrease in insulin-induced GLUT-4 translocation to the plasma membrane. Additionally, Barbour et al. found that the skeletal muscle tissue of these mice demonstrates abnormalities in insulin signaling, which bear a remarkable similarity to the tissue found in normal pregnant women and in pregnant women with gestational diabetes. These data suggest that hPGH may be a significant mediator of insulin resistance in normal pregnancy (26,27).

The insulin resistance of normal pregnancy has been well described. Nevertheless, the hormonal mechanisms by which insulin resistance is triggered remain a subject of debate. Normal pregnancy is characterized by an approx 50% decrease in insulin-mediated glucose disposal and by a 200–250% increase in insulin secretion in humans (20,28). Hepatic gluconeogenesis is not normally suppressed by insulin. This procedure occurs in order to meet the metabolic demands of the fetus, the energy of which is 80% glucose, yet it maintains euglycemia in the mother (29). In normal pregnancy there is a decreased expression of the GLUT-4 glucose transporter protein in maternal adipose tissue (30) but not in skeletal muscle. Skeletal muscle is the main site of insulin-mediated glucose disposal in vivo, suggesting that the mechanisms behind insulin resistance lie in the skeletal muscle either in the pathways for insulin signaling, or in the abnormal translocation of GLUT-4 (31).

It has been demonstrated that in human incubated muscle fibers obtained at term by caesarean section from normal obese pregnant women, maximal insulin-stimulated 2-deoxyglucose transport was significantly reduced by 32% (31). In these skeletal muscle fibers, normal pregnancy caused reduced insulin receptor tyrosine kinase activity toward insulin receptor substrate (IRS)-1, as well as reduced expression of IRS-1 (32). Recent data in pregnancy also demonstrate increases in serine phosphorylation of the insulin receptor, which may prevent optimal binding of IRS-1 to phosphotidylinositol (PI) 3-kinase, resulting in inhibition of GLUT-4 translocation (32).

INSULIN RESISTANCE IN GESTATIONAL DIABETES

In pregnancies complicated by gestational diabetes mellitus (GDM), further insulin resistance and inability to a compensatory increase in insulin secretion occurs (20,28,33). The pancreatic β-cell secretory defect is present in both obese and lean women with GDM. It has been demonstrated that overweight women who will develop GDM present insulin resistance prior to pregnancy as measured by a hyperinsulinemic–euglycemic clamp (20). Insulin-mediated glucose disposal continues to decrease in the second and third trimester of pregnancy and is about two-thirds that of normal pregnant women matched for weight. Moreover, women with GDM improve their insulin resistance postpartum; however, they never achieve the same degree of insulin-mediated glucose disposal as normal pregnant women do.

Studies on muscle fibers from pregnant women undergoing Cesarean section demonstrated that the mechanisms for skeletal insulin resistance in obese women with GDM involve impaired insulin receptor β-subunit tyrosine-phosphorylation and decreased IRS-1-phosphorylation and expression (31,32). A significant decrease in maximal insulin receptor tyrosine-phosphorylation was demonstrated in muscle from obese women with GDM compared with obese pregnant women (30,31). This insulin-receptor tyrosine kinase activity (IRTK) catalyzes the phosphorylation of various insulin receptor substrates, particularly IRS-1, to undergo tyrosine-phosphorylation. Whereas insulin receptor tyrosine-phosphorylation is impaired in patients with GDM only, IRTK is significantly reduced by 23% in pregnant patients and by 41% in the muscle fibers of patients with GDM compared with obese, nonpregnant controls. Conclusively, these data suggest a possible insulin receptor defect that may exacerbate the physiological effects of normal pregnancy.

GDM IN WOMEN WITH PCOS

GDM is detected in 3–4% of pregnancies in women aged 15–49 years, and is associated with an increased later risk for type 2 diabetes. Risk factors for gestational diabetes include obesity, age, genetic background, PCOS, and ethnicity *(34)*. Fetal macrosomia in gestational diabetes increases the rates of birth trauma and Cesarean section *(35)*. Diagnosis and management of gestational diabetes may reduce perinatal, neonatal, and long-term pediatric complications *(34,35)*.

Insulin resistance and hyperinsulinemia, both of which are risk factors for gestational diabetes, characterize women with PCOS. These women—46% of whom develop GDM *(36)*—enter pregnancy with higher insulin resistance than normal women *(36–41)*. Women with PCOS probably develop GDM when pancreatic β-cells cannot overcome the superimposition of the physiological insulin resistance of pregnancy on their high preconception insulin resistance *(9–14,36)*. Women in whom gestational diabetes develops are likely to have underlying polycystic ovaries *(42)*, and women with PCOS are likely to develop gestational diabetes *(5,9,10,39)*.

Obesity, which characterizes a great percentage of patients with PCOS, has a deleterious additive effect on carbohydrate homeostasis and increases insulin resistance during gestation *(43)*. In normal women, high maternal insulin in early pregnancy promotes gestational weight-gain and weight-retention postpartum, increasing the risk of GDM and, later, of type 2 diabetes mellitus *(44)*. Body mass index (BMI) higher than 25 kg/m^2 is a major predictor of GDM *(45)*.

Women with PCOS often present with infertility *(46,47)*. Therefore, women with PCOS are older than the general population at conception, which is another risk factor for gestational diabetes *(15)*.

The association among insulin resistance, metabolic syndrome, and androgen excess in PCOS has led to the use of insulin-sensitizing agents, such as metformin, with reported improvements in hyperinsulinemia and hyperandrogenemia. Treatment with metformin only produced a modest reduction in weight and hirsutism in women with PCOS *(48)*. Metformin administration throughout pregnancy in women with PCOS reduces GDM from 26–31% to 3–4% *(13,49,50)*. Thus, the frequency of GDM in women with PCOS who are taking metformin does not differ from normal pregnant controls *(15)*.

Metformin administration during pregnancy leads to a modification of the observed changes in insulin resistance during gestation. In women on metformin, serum insulin levels did not rise significantly during the first and the second trimesters of pregnancy compared with the last preconception visit. Moreover, while taking metformin, there was no difference in fasting serum insulin levels between the third trimester (increase only 10%) and the last preconception visit, with insulin levels also lower in the third trimester than before metformin initiation *(17)*. Consequently, the expected changes during pregnancy, namely a significant increase in insulin and insulin resistance, were abated and blunted by metformin, suggesting that metformin improves the "natural" insulin resistance changes during gestation in hyperinsulinemic women with PCOS *(10,17,19,20,36)*.

A second benefit of metformin treatment in women with PCOS is weight maintenance before conception and weight loss throughout pregnancy, particularly evident in women with BMI of 30–40 and 40 kg/m^2 or higher. These actions probably contribute to insulin resistance reduction and to the development of GDM *(11–14)*.

A third effect of metformin treatment during pregnancy in women with PCOS is serum testosterone lowering, which, like the prevention of weight gain, is probably mediated through its insulin-sensitizing action *(51,52)*. It has been proposed that high androgen levels during pregnancy in untreated women with PCOS could provide a potential source of androgen excess for the fetus, without leading to fetal virilization *(53)*. Metformin treatment throughout pregnancy in PCOS should reduce any putative risk of fetal virilization conferred through androgen excess *(17)*.

The efficacy of the drug, as well as the first reports on metformin used in pregnancy, has encouraged the continued use of the drug after conception. It appears that its use throughout pregnancy is safe, as no increased frequency of congenital anomalies or teratogenicity have been reported so far *(54,55)*. In a study that had prospectively assessed growth and motor–social development during the first 18 months of life in 126 live births (122 pregnancies) to 109 women with PCOS who conceived on and continued taking metformin (1.5–2.55 g/day) through pregnancy, the use of metformin was not teratogenic and did not adversely affect birth length and weight, growth, or motor–social development in the first 18 months of life *(56)*.

HYPERTENSIVE DISORDERS OF PREGNANCY

Five to 10% of pregnancies are complicated by pregnancy-induced hypertension. This disorder is a major cause of maternal, fetal, and neonatal morbidity and mortality. Although complications of hypertensive disorders of pregnancy (HDP) have been recognized for centuries, the causes of these disorders remain poorly understood. Various data indicating associations of features of the insulin resistance syndrome and these disorders suggest that additional research is needed to elucidate the potential role of insulin resistance in the pathogenesis of pregnancy-induced hypertension.

HDPs include the following:

1. New onset of hypertension during pregnancy (gestational hypertension or preeclampsia).
2. Preexisting hypertension.
3. Exacerbation of preexisting hypertension *(57)*.

New-onset hypertension develops during the second half of pregnancy, usually in the third trimester in 3–5% of women who were previously normotensive. Preeclampsia is a multisystem syndrome mainly characterized by proteinuria (300 mg protein or more over 24 hours). Proteinuria caused by glomerular endotheliosis and edema secondary to increased vascular permeability represent only the tip of the iceberg of a widespread pathology arising from endothelial dysfunction and damage *(18)*. Other systemic manifestations include generalized intravascular coagulation, hemolysis, elevated liver function tests, and, rarely, seizures (eclampsia). Gestational hypertension, a generally more benign disorder, is diagnosed when blood pressure is elevated in the absence of the previously described findings. When other systemic manifestations of disease are absent, the distinction between preeclampsia and gestational hypertension is based on the presence and magnitude of proteinuria. It is not clear whether gestational hypertension and preeclampsia are different disease entities or different manifestations of the same disease process. It is possible that insulin resistance may play an important role in both of them. Twenty percent of women with preexisting hypertension develop superimposed preeclampsia with its attendant risks.

The etiology of hypertensive pregnancy is uncertain and includes immune, genetic, and placental abnormalities. Three main hypotheses have been proposed regarding the metabolic alterations involved in the etiology of hypertensive disorders in pregnancy: endothelial dysfunction and activation, oxidative stress, and insulin resistance. All may contribute to the characteristic endothelial dysfunction of hypertensive disorders in pregnancy. Endothelial dysfunction may, in turn, underlie several critical features of preeclampsia, including vasoconstriction, hypertension, loss of the usual pregnancy-associated refractoriness to pressor effects of angiotensin II, increased platelet aggregation, and proteinuria *(57)*.

It has been postulated that abnormalities of the placenta are the primary cause of preeclampsia. However, the observations that several metabolic abnormalities are predispositions to the development of preeclampsia, and that these abnormalities are also observed in the non-pregnant state in women who have had preeclampsia, suggest that maternal features must also be considered.

All cases of new-onset HDP are unlikely to be attributable to a single cause. Rather, different etiologies may lead to the same phenotype in different women.

Endothelial Dysfunction and Activation

Many markers of endothelial dysfunction have been observed in HDP. Coagulation activation proceeds the clinical onset by weeks to months. The damaged endothelium of HDP is reflected by elevated levels of plasminogen activator inhibitor (PAI)-1 and von Willebrand factor *(18)*. Endothelial dysfunction is indicated by the elevated plasma levels of soluble adhesion molecules, which may be manifested before the clinical onset *(58)*. Although the increased serum levels of cytokines (TNF-α, interleukin [IL]-6 and IL-8), observed only in the HDP group, indicated that endothelial activation is a consequence of abnormal trophoblast invasion, still additional factors are involved in its manifestation, which might be related to cytokine release.

Endothelial activation in HDP results in an enormous release of endothelin, thromboxane and superoxide, as well as an increased vascular sensitivity to the pressor effects of angiotensin II and a decreased formation of vasodilators, such as nitric oxide and prostacyclin, by the damaged endothelium *(59)*. This may lead to an increase in total peripheral resistance, despite the increasing plasma volume of pregnancy, and thus to vasospasm and hypertension. However, a case–control study of nonpregnant, normotensive pregnant, and HDP pregnant women showed that nitric oxide (NO) and endothelin-1 production were increased in the HDP group compared with the other groups *(60)*. The increased formation of the vasodilator NO was considered to be a compensatory response to the vasoconstriction and hypertension.

Oxidative Stress

Oxidative stress is a component of HDP. The oxidative stress theory of HDP involves the hypothesis that the abnormal placentation and dyslipidemia result in a release of free radicals, particularly superoxide anions, and lipid hydroperoxides, which damage the vascular endothelium *(61)*. Oxidative stress may link the decreased placental perfusion in HDP to the maternal response via direct vascular damage and endothelial dysfunction.

Data from the literature support the view that antioxidant supplementation was associated with an improvement in biochemical indices of the disease. Evidently, these findings need further investigation via large randomized, controlled trials, but raise the exciting possibility that antioxidants, either dietary or pharmaceutical, may have a role in the prevention of HDP in high-risk patients. It has been hypothesized that regular exercise enhances antioxidant enzymes in pregnant women, reduces oxidative stress and the incidence of HDP, and at the same time, promotes a healthy lifestyle *(62)*.

INSULIN RESISTANCE

In women with HDP, an exaggeration of insulin resistance and associated metabolic changes is noted. Although it is not clear to what extent these factors are pathogenic in hypertensive pregnancy, the available data suggest that some may play a role in the evolution of the disease, whereas others may be markers of the underlying disease process. Exaggerated hyperinsulinemia relative to normal pregnancy is well described in women with established gestational hypertension or preeclampsia. Studies on insulin resistance have suggested differences between women with *de novo* hypertension in pregnancy and normotensive women as well.

Insulin resistance precedes the development of HDP. Various studies have documented hyperinsulinemia and/or hyperglycemia in early or midpregnancy, before the development of preeclampsia, gestational hypertension, or both *(63,64)*. Hyperinsulinemia may directly predispose to hypertension by increased renal sodium reabsorption and stimulation of the sympathetic nervous system *(65)*. Insulin resistance and/or associated hyperglycemia may impair endothelial function *(66)*.

Two other factors, obesity and physical inactivity, are closely associated with insulin resistance and are predictive of hypertensive pregnancy. A higher body mass index before pregnancy or early in pregnancy is associated with increased risk for both gestational hypertension and preeclampsia *(63,67,68)*. Moreover, increased gestational weight gain has also predicted risk for gestational hypertension *(67)* or preeclampsia *(63)* between 6 and 16 weeks. Additional factors, such as diet composition, may explain the association between gestational hypertension and gestational weight gain. Furthermore, it has been suggested that gestational diabetes, which itself is associated with underlying insulin resistance, is a risk factor for the development of hypertensive pregnancy. This association persists even after adjusting for obesity and maternal age *(69)*.

Other Putative Factors Associated With Hypertensive Disorders in Pregnancy

LIPIDS

In women with established preeclampsia, serum triglyceride and free fatty acid levels have been found to be higher, and high-density lipoprotein cholesterol levels lower, than those in women with normotensive pregnancy *(70)*. Elevated total serum cholesterol, triglyceride, and free fatty acid levels have been reported to predate the development of either gestational hypertension or preeclampsia *(71)*. Oxidized lipids may impair endothelial function directly or indirectly by effects on prostaglandins, including increased synthesis of thromboxane and inhibited synthesis of prostacyclin *(72)*.

Increases in small, dense low-density lipoproteins and triglycerides may also contribute to impaired endothelial function.

LEPTIN

It has been reported that leptin levels at as early as 20 weeks of gestation may predict the development of preeclampsia in a high-risk population *(71)*. Increased leptin levels may in part reflect maternal adiposity and have also been hypothesized to reflect placental insufficiency. Leptin might also contribute to endothelial dysfunction by increasing free fatty acid oxidation *(73)*.

TUMOR NECROSIS FACTOR-α

It has been referred that TNF-α or its receptor are elevated in women with established preeclampsia compared with normotensive controls *(74)*. Elevated TNF-α levels in the early third trimester may predict the development of preeclampsia *(75)*. TNF-α may promote hypercoagulability and increased lipolysis, with resulting impairment of endothelial relaxation.

PLASMINOGEN ACTIVATOR INHIBITOR-1

PAI-1 is elevated in established preeclampsia and its increase is related to the severity of the disease. Among women at high risk for preeclampsia, the ratio of PAI-1 to PAI-2, the latter primarily produced by the placenta, was increased before the development of the disease. Increased PAI-1 may reflect impaired fibrinolytic function, which might predispose to the coagulopathy associated with preeclampsia *(71)*.

TESTOSTERONE AND SEX HORMONE-BINDING GLOBULIN

Total and free testosterone serum levels are higher in women with established preeclampsia compared with normotensive women *(76)*. In the first trimester, lower sex hormone-binding globulin (SHBG), but neither total nor free testosterone serum levels, predicted the later development of preeclampsia *(77)*. On the contrary, in a recent study, maternal androgen levels (androstcncdione, total and free testosterone) were already elevated in the early second trimester among women who eventually develop preeclampsia *(78)*.

PCOS, which is associated with insulin resistance, elevated testosterone, and low SHBG levels, has been linked to increased risk for pregnancy-induced hypertension, even in the absence of associated obesity *(79)*. Androgens increase vasoconstriction in response to pressors *(80)*. Androgens also affect the prostaglandin balance, decreasing the synthesis of prostacyclin *(81)* and leading to increased platelet aggregation, which are both characteristics of preeclampsia.

Clinical Implications and Future Directions

Although a cause-and-effect relationship between the insulin resistance syndrome and GDM and new-onset hypertension in pregnancy has not been proven, the associations between these conditions raise the possibility that interventions, which improve insulin sensitivity, may reduce the likelihood of these pregnancy complications. Because obesity is both a major contributor to insulin resistance and a well-established risk factor for preeclampsia, interventions that are scheduled to reduce weight before pregnancy and/or to avoid excessive weight gain during pregnancy may be proven effective.

Moreover, increased exercise, which improves insulin sensitivity, may also reduce risk. Given the well-recognized adverse effects of obesity on many pregnancy outcomes, including gestational diabetes and pregnancy-induced hypertension, these approaches might be worthwhile in women at high risk of these complications. Studies of pharmacological interventions, such as the use of metformin, may also warrant study in women at high risk for preeclampsia.

Multiple studies have demonstrated associations between markers of insulin resistance on one hand and GDM and hypertensive pregnancy on the other. Findings consistent with the insulin resistance syndrome have been observed before, during, and after these pregnancy complications. However, further work is needed in several areas. More data are needed to determine whether insulin resistance plays a causal role in the development of GDM, gestational hypertension, and preeclampsia. To improve our ability to identify women at risk for GDM and hypertensive pregnancy who might benefit from closer monitoring and intervention, large prospective longitudinal studies are needed to determine whether there are markers of insulin resistance with sufficient sensitivity and specificity to be clinically relevant. Studies should be designed to assess the effects of specific interventions directed to the insulin resistance syndrome on the risk of developing these complications in pregnancy.

KEY POINTS

- In normal pregnancy, insulin resistance and compensatory hyperinsulinemia occur in the second and maximize in the third trimester of pregnancy.
- The insulin resistance of normal pregnancy is mediated by several hormonal changes, including increases in serum levels of estradiol, progesterone, prolactin, cortisol, human chorionic gonadotropin, placental growth hormone, and human placental lactogen.
- GDM is detected in 3–4% of pregnancies in women aged 15–49 years.
- In pregnancies complicated by GDM, further insulin resistance and inability to a compensatory increase in insulin secretion occurs.
- Insulin resistance and hyperinsulinemia, all of which are risk factors for gestational diabetes, characterize women with PCOS. Women with PCOS enter pregnancy with higher insulin resistance than normal women.
- GDM is detected in 20–46% of pregnancies in women with PCOS.
- Obesity and older age at conception are factors contributing to the increased incidence of GDM in women with PCOS.
- Metformin administration during pregnancy is not teratogenic and leads to a modification of the observed changes in insulin resistance during gestation, to a reduction in body weight and to a decrease in androgen levels.
- Five to 10% of pregnancies are complicated by pregnancy-induced hypertension.
- Hypertensive disorders of pregnancy (HDP) include new onset of hypertension during pregnancy (gestational hypertension or preeclampsia), preexisting hypertension, and exacerbation of preexisting hypertension.
- Three main hypotheses have been proposed regarding the metabolic alterations involved in the etiology of HDP, namely endothelial dysfunction and activation, oxidative stress, and insulin resistance.
- HDP are increased in women with PCOS. Hyperandrogenism may be considered as an early risk marker of preeclampsia and it might be involved in the pathogenesis of preeclampsia.
- Additional clinical studies are needed to determine whether insulin resistance plays a causal role in the development of GDM, gestational hypertension, and preeclampsia.

REFERENCES

1. Diamanti-Kandarakis E, Kouli CR, Bergiele AT, et al. A survey of the polycystic ovary syndrome in the Greek island of Lesbos: hormonal and metabolic profile. J Clin Endocrinol Metab 1999;84:4006–4011.
2. Dunaif A. Insulin resistance and the polycystic ovary syndrome: mechanism and implications for pathogenesis. Endocr Rev 1997;18:774–800.
3. Carmina E, Lobo RA. Polycystic ovary syndrome (PCOS): arguably the most common endocrinopathy is associated with significant morbidity in women. J Clin Endocrinol Metab 2001;84:1897–1899.
4. Franks S, Gharani N, McCarthy M. Candidate genes in polycystic ovary syndrome. Hum Reprod Update 2001;47:405–410.
5. Radon PA, McMahon MJ, Meyer WR. Impaired glucose tolerance in pregnant women with polycystic ovary syndrome. Obstet Gynecol 1999;94:194–197.
6. Arslanian SA, Lewy VD, Danadian K. Glucose intolerance in obese adolescents with polycystic ovary syndrome: roles of insulin resistance and β-cell dysfunction and risk of cardiovascular disease. J Clin Endocrinol Metab 2001;86:66–71.
7. Executive summary of the third report of the national cholesterol education program (NCEP) expert panel on the detection, evaluation and treatment of high blood cholesterol in adults (Adult treatment panel III). JAMA 2001;285:2486–2497.
8. Diamanti-Kandarakis E, Baillargeon J-P, Iurno MJ, Jakubowicz DJ, Nestler JE. A modern medical quandary: polycystic ovary syndrome, insulin resistance and oral contraceptive pills. J Clin Endocrinol Metab 2003;88:1927–1932.
9. Lanzone A, Caruso A, Di Simone N, De Carolis S, Fulghesu AM, Mancuso S. Polycystic ovary disease. A risk factor for gestational diabetes? J Reprod Med 1995;40:312–316.
10. Paradisi G, Fulghesu AM, Ferrazzani S, et al. Endocrino-metabolic features in women with polycystic ovary syndrome during pregnancy. Hum Reprod 1998:13;542–546.
11. Glueck CJ, Goldenberg N, Streicher P, Wang P. The contentious nature of gestational diabetes: diet, insulin, glyburide and metformin. Expert Opin Pharmacother 2002;3:1557–1568.
12. Glueck CJ, Streicher P, Wang P. Treatment of polycystic ovary syndrome with insulin-lowering agents. Expert Opin Pharmacother 2002;3:1177–1189.
13. Glueck CJ, Wang P, Goldenberg N, Sieve-Smith L. Pregnancy outcomes among women with polycystic ovary syndrome treated with metformin. Hum Reprod 2002;17:2858–2864.
14. Glueck CJ, Wang P, Kobayashi S, Phillips H, Sieve-Smith L. Metformin therapy throughout pregnancy reduces the development of gestational diabetes in women with polycystic ovary syndrome. Fertil Steril 2002;77:520–525.
15. Glueck CJ, Bornovali S, Pranikoff J, Goldenberg N, Dharashivkar S, Wang P. Metformin, pre-eclampsia, and pregnancy outcomes in women with polycystic ovary syndrome. Diabet Med 2004;21: 829–836.
16. Seely EW, Solomon CG. Insulin resistance and its potential role in pregnancy-induced hypertension. J Clin Endocrinol Metab 2003;88:2393–2398.
17. Glueck CJ, Goldenberg N, Wang P, Loftspring M, Sherman A. Metformin during pregnancy reduces insulin, insulin resistance, insulin secretion, weight, testosterone and development of gestational diabetes: prospective longitudinal assessment of women with polycystic ovary syndrome from preconception throughout pregnancy. Hum Reprod 2004;9:510–521.
18. Rodie VA, Freeman DJ, Sattar N, Greer IA. Pre-eclampsia and cardiovascular disease: metabolic syndrome of pregnancy? Atherosclerosis 2004;175:189–202.
19. Buchanan TA, Metzger BE, Freinkel N, Bergman RN. Insulin sensitivity and β-cell responsiveness to glucose during late pregnancy in lean and moderately obese women with normal glucose tolerance or mild gestational diabetes. Am J Obstet Gynecol 1990;162:1008–1014.
20. Catalano PM, Huston L, Amini SB, Kalhan SC. Longitudinal changes in glucose metabolism during pregnancy in obese women with normal glucose tolerance and gestational diabetes mellitus. Am J Obstet Gynecol 1999;180:903–916.
21. Kirwan JP, Huston-Presley L, Kalhan SC, Catalano PM. Clinically useful estimates of insulin sensitivity during pregnancy: validation studies in women with normal glucose tolerance and gestational diabetes mellitus. Diabetes Care 2001;24:1602–1607.
22. Catalano PM, Kirwan JP, Haugel-de Mouzon S, King J. Gestational diabetes and insulin resistance: role in short- and long-term implications for mother and fetus. J Nutr 2003;133:1674–1683.

23. Handwerger S, Freemark M. The roles of placental growth hormone and placental lactogen in the regulation of human fetal growth and development. J Pediatr Endocrinol Metab 2000;13:343–356.

24. Kirwan JP, Hauguel-De Mouzon S, Lepercq J, et al. TNF-alpha is a predictor of insulin resistance in human pregnancy. Diabetes 2002;51:2207–2213.

25. Alsat E, Guibourdenche J, Couturier A, Evain-Brion D. Physiological role of human placental growth hormone. Mol Cell Endocrinol 1998;140:121–127.

26. Barbour LA, Shao J, Qiao L, et al. Human placental growth hormone causes severe insulin resistance in transgenic mice. Am J Obstet Gynecol 2002;186:512–517.

27. Barbour LA. New concepts in insulin resistance of pregnancy and gestational diabetes: long-term implications for mother and offspring. J Obstet Gynaecol 2003;23:545–549.

28. Yamashita H, Shao J, Friedman JE. Physiologic and molecular alterations in carbohydrate metabolism during pregnancy and gestational diabetes mellitus. Clin Obstet Gynecol 2000;43:87–98.

29. Aldoretta PW, Hay WW Jr. Metabolic substrates for fetal energy metabolism and growth. Clin Perinatol 1995;22:15–36.

30. Okuno S, Akazawa S, Yasuhi I, et al. Decreased expression of the GLUT4 glucose transporter protein in adipose tissue during pregnancy. Horm Metab Res 1995;27:231–234.

31. Friedman JE, Ishizuka T, Shao J, Huston L, Highman T, Catalano P. Impaired glucose transport and insulin receptor tyrosine phosphorylation in skeletal muscle from obese women with gestational diabetes. Diabetes 1999;48:1807–1814.

32. Shao J, Catalano PM, Yamashita H, et al. Decreased insulin receptor tyrosine kinase activity and plasma cell membrane glycoprotein-1 overexpression in skeletal muscle from obese women with gestational diabetes mellitus (GDM): evidence for increased serine/threonine phosphorylation in pregnancy and GDM. Diabetes 2000;49:603–610.

33. Kuhl C. Etiology and pathogenesis of gestational diabetes. Diabetes Care 1998;21(Suppl 2):B19–B26.

34. Butte NF. Carbohydrate and lipid metabolism in pregnancy: normal compared with gestational diabetes mellitus. Am J Clin Nutr 2000;71:S1256–S1261.

35. Persson B, Hanson U. Neonatal morbidities in gestational diabetes mellitus. Diabetes Care 1998; 21(Suppl 2):B79–B84.

36. Lanzone A, Fulghesu AM, Cucinelli F, et al. Preconceptional and gestational evaluation of insulin secretion in patients with polycystic ovary syndrome. Hum Reprod 1996;11:2382–2386.

37. Legro RS, Finegood D, Dunaif A. A fasting glucose to insulin ratio is a useful measure of insulin sensitivity in women with polycystic ovary syndrome. J Clin Endocrinol Metab 1998;83:2694–2698.

38. Lewy VD, Danadian K, Witchel SF, Arslanian S. Early metabolic abnormalities in adolescent girls with polycystic ovarian syndrome. J Pediatr 2001;138:38–44.

39. Mikola M, Hiilesmaa V, Halttunen M, Suhonen L, Tiitinen A. Obstetric outcome in women with polycystic ovarian syndrome. Hum Reprod 2001;16:226–229.

40. Vrbikova J, Bendlova B, Hill M, Vankova M, Vondra K, Starka L. Insulin sensitivity and beta-cell function in women with polycystic ovary syndrome. Diabetes Care 2002;25:1217–1222.

41. Schachter M, Raziel A, Friedler S, Strassburger D, Bern O, Ron-El R. Insulin resistance in patients with polycystic ovary syndrome is associated with elevated plasma homocysteine. Hum Reprod 2003;18:721–727.

42. Kousta E, Cela E, Lawrence N, et al. The prevalence of polycystic ovaries in women with a history of gestational diabetes. Clin Endocrinol (Oxf) 2000;53:501–507.

43. Galtier-Dereure F, Boegner C, Bringer J. Obesity and pregnancy: complications and cost. Am J Clin Nutr 2000;71:1242S–1248S.

44. Scholl TO, Chen X. Insulin and the 'thrifty' woman: the influence of insulin during pregnancy on gestational weight gain and postpartum weight retention. Matern Child Health 2002;6:255–261.

45. Turhan NO, Seckin NC, Aybar F, Inegol I. Assessment of glucose tolerance and pregnancy outcome of polycystic ovary patients. Int J Gynaecol Obstet 2003;81:163–168.

46. Panidis D, Balaris C, Farmakiotis D, et al. Serum parathyroid hormone concentrations are increased in women with polycystic ovary syndrome. Clin Chem 2005;51:1691–1697.

47. Panidis D, Farmakiotis D, Koliakos G, et al. Comparative study of plasma ghrelin levels in women with polycystic ovary syndrome, in hyperandrogenic women and in normal controls. Hum Reprod 2005;20:2127–2132.

48. Jayapogopal V, Kilpatrick ES, Holding S, Jennings PE, Atkin SL. Orlistat is as beneficial as metformin in the treatment of polycystic ovarian syndrome. J Clin Endocrinol Metab 2005;90:729–733.

49. Engelgau MM, Herman WH, Smith PJ, German RR, Aubert RE. The epidemiology of diabetes and pregnancy in the U.S., 1988. Diabetes Care 1995;18:1029–1033.
50. Checa MA, Requena A, Salvador C, et al. Insulin-sensitizing agents: use in pregnancy and as therapy in polycystic ovary syndrome. Hum Reprod Update 2005;11:375–390.
51. Velazquez EM, Mendoza S, Hamer T, Sosa F, Glueck CJ. Metformin therapy in polycystic ovary syndrome reduces hyperinsulinemia, insulin resistance, hyperandrogenemia, and systolic blood pressure, while facilitating normal menses and pregnancy. Metabolism 1994;43:647–654.
52. Velazquez EM, Mendoza SG, Wang P, Glueck CJ. Metformin therapy is associated with a decrease in plasma plasminogen activator inhibitor-1, lipoprotein(a), and immunoreactive insulin levels in patients with the polycystic ovary syndrome. Metabolism 1997;46:454–457.
53. Sir-Petermann T, Maliqueo M, Angel B, Lara HE, Perez-Bravo F, Recabarren SE. Maternal serum androgens in pregnant women with polycystic ovarian syndrome: possible implications in prenatal androgenization. Hum Reprod 2002;17:2573–2579.
54. Coetzee EJ, Jackson WP. Oral hypoglycaemics in the first trimester and fetal outcome. S Afr Med J 1984;65(16):635–637.
55. Brock B, Smidt K, Ovesen P, Schmitz O, Rungby J. Is metformin therapy for polycystic ovary syndrome safe during pregnancy? Basic Clin Pharmacol Toxicol 2005;96(6):410–412.
56. Glueck CJ, Goldenberg N, Pranikoff J, Loftspring M, Sieve L, Wang P. Height, weight, and motor–social development during the first 18 months of life in 126 infants born to 109 mothers with polycystic ovary syndrome who conceived on and continued metformin through pregnancy. Hum Reprod 2004;19(6):1323–1330.
57. National High Blood Pressure Education Program. Working group report on high blood pressure in pregnancy. Bethesda: NIH; NIH publication 00-3029, 2000.
58. Chaiworapongsa T, Romero R, Yoshimatsu J, et al. Soluble adhesion molecule profile in normal pregnancy and pre–eclampsia. J Matern Fetal Neonatal Med 2002;12:19–27.
59. Granger JP, Alexander BT, Llinas MT, Bennett WA, Khalil RA. Pathophysiology of preeclampsia: linking placental ischemia/hypoxia with microvascular dysfunction. Microcirculation 2002;9:147–160.
60. Vural P. Nitric oxide/endothelin-1 in preeclampsia. Clin Chim Acta 2002;317:65–70.
61. Hubel CA. Oxidative stress in the pathogenesis of preeclampsia. Proc Soc Exp Biol Med 1999;222:222–235.
62. Chambers JC, Fusi L, Malik IS, Haskard DO, De Swiet M, Kooner JS. Association of maternal endothelial dysfunction with preeclampsia. JAMA 2001;285:1607–1612.
63. Solomon CG, Graves SW, Greene MF, Seely EW. Glucose intolerance as a predictor of hypertension in pregnancy. Hypertension 1994;23:717 721.
64. Innes KE, Wimsatt JH, McDuffie R. Relative glucose tolerance and subsequent development of hypertension in pregnancy. Obstet Gynecol 2001;97:905–910.
65. Reaven GM. Pathophysiology of insulin resistance in human disease. Physiol Rev 1995;75:473–486.
66. Cales-Escandon J, Cipolla M. Diabetes and endothelial dysfunction: a clinical perspective. Endocr Rev 2001;22:36–52.
67. Saftlas A, Wang W, Risch H, Woolson R, Hsu C, Bracken M. Pre-pregnancy body mass index and gestational weight gain as risk factors for preeclampsia and transient hypertension. Ann Epidemiol 2000;10:475.
68. Sattar N, Clark P, Holmes A, Lean ME, Walker I, Greer IA. Antenatal waist circumference and hypertension risk. Obstet Gynecol 2001;97:268–271.
69. Vambergue A, Nuttens MC, Goeusse P, Biausque S, Lepeut M, Fontaine P. Pregnancy induced hypertension in women with gestational carbohydrate intolerance: the diagest study. Eur J Obstet Gynecol Reprod Biol 2002;102:31–35.
70. Kaaje R, Laivuori H, Laasko M, Tikkanen MJ, Ylikorkaia O. Evidence of a state of increased insulin resistance in preeclampsia. Metabolism 1999;48:892–896.
71. Chappell LC, Seed PT, Briley A, et al. A longitudinal study of biochemical variables in women at risk of preeclampsia. Am J Obstet Gynecol 2002;187:127–136.
72. Bruckdorfer KR. Antioxidants, lipoprotein oxidation, and arterial function. Lipids 1996;31:S83–S85.
73. Yamagishi SI, Edelstein D, Du XL, Kaneda Y, Guzman M, Brownlee M. Leptin induces mitochondrial superoxide production and monocyte chemoattractant protein-1 expression in aortic endothelial cells by increasing fatty acid oxidation via protein kinase A. J Biol Chem 2001;276:25,096–25,100.

74. Visser W, Beckmann I, Knook MA, Wallenburg HC. Soluble tumor necrosis factor receptor II and soluble cell adhesion molecule 1 as markers of tumor necrosis factor-α release in preeclampsia. Acta Obstet Gynecol Scand 2002;81:713–719.

75. Serin YS, Ozcelik B, Bapbou M, Kylyc H, Okur D, Erez R. Predictive value of tumor necrosis factor-α (TNF-α) in preeclampsia. Eur J Obstet Gynecol Reprod Biol 2002;100:143–145.

76. Serin IS, Kula M, Basbug M, Unluhizarci K, Gucer S, Tayyar M. Androgen levels of preeclamptic patients in the third trimester of pregnancy and six weeks after delivery. Acta Obstet Gynecol Scand 2001;80:1009–1013.

77. Wolf M, Sandler L, Muniz K, Hsu K, Ecker JL, Thadhani R. First trimester insulin resistance and subsequent preeclampsia: prospective study. J Clin Endocrinol Metab 2002;87:1563–1568.

78. Carlsen SM, Romundstad P, Jacobsen G. Early second-trimester maternal hyperandrogenemia and subsequent preeclampsia: a prospective study. Acta Obstet Gynecol Scand 2005;84:117–121.

79. Urman B, Sarac E, Dogan L, Gurgan T. Pregnancy in infertile PCOD patients: complications and outcome. J Reprod Med 1997;42:501–505.

80. Baker PJ, Ramey ER, Ramwell PW. Androgen-mediated sex differences in cardiovascular responses in rats. Am J Physiol 1978;235:H242–H246.

81. Wakasugi M, Noguchi T, Kazama YI, Kanemaru Y, Onaya T. The effects of sex hormones on the synthesis of prostacyclin (PGI2) by vascular tissues. Prostaglandins 1989;37:401–409.

V CHRONIC TREATMENT OF PCOS AND ITS RELATIONSHIP TO INSULIN RESISTANCE

25 Lifestyle Intervention in Polycystic Ovarian Syndrome

Onno E. Janssen, MD, Susanne Tan, MD, and Susanne Hahn, MD

Summary

From humble beginnings, lifestyle intervention has become one of the catchwords of the century. Necessitated by the obesity and diabetes pandemic, both prevention and treatment studies have proven that a combination of dietary changes and physical activity can reduce weight, cardiovascular risk, and progression of insulin resistance to manifest diabetes in high-risk subjects. Through its association with the metabolic syndrome, polycystic ovarian syndrome (PCOS) is a logical target for lifestyle intervention. Although several studies have now provided proof of principle of lifestyle intervention for obese PCOS patients, general implementation of appropriate programs awaits realization.

Key Words: Polycystic ovarian syndrome; PCOS; insulin resistance; lifestyle changes; diet; physical activity; obesity; hyperandrogenism; hirsutism; sedentary lifestyle; cardiovascular risk.

INTRODUCTION

The pandemic increase in obesity is the Pandora's box of industrialized nations. Currently, more than half of southern Europeans, more than two-thirds of central Europeans and more than four out of five North Americans are at least overweight, with an ever increasing prevalence of overt obesity. The increase in body weight is the main reason for the increase in the prevalence of both the metabolic syndrome (MBS)

From: *Contemporary Endocrinology: Insulin Resistance and Polycystic Ovarian Syndrome:
Pathogenesis, Evaluation, and Treatment*
Edited by: E. Diamanti-Kandarakis, J. E. Nestler, D. Panidis, and R. Pasquali © Humana Press Inc., Totowa, NJ

and type 2 diabetes mellitus (T2DM) in men *(1)* and women *(2)*. Apart from a genetic predisposition, the main culprit of this development is the modern, sedantary lifestyle with too little physical activity and constant availability of high-energy food.

Benefits From Successful Lifestyle Intervention

Randomized controlled trials (RCTs) have unequivocally proven that preventing T2DM is possible. A recent meta-analysis identified eight RCTs showing a reduction of 2-hour plasma glucose of almost 1 mmol/L and five RCTs showing a 50% reduction in 1-year diabetes incidence *(3)*. Lifestyle intervention varied from general dietary advice to regular individual counselling from a nutritionist and from no exercise education to regular circuit-type resistance training sessions.

A cost-effectiveness estimation of the Diabetes Prevention Program *(4)* found that lifestyle intervention would delay the development of T2DM by 11 years and reduce the absolute incidence by 22%, whereas metformin treatment would delay by only 3 years and reduce the incidence by 9% *(5)*. The Finnish Diabetes Prevention Study showed that 21% of the participants achieved at least four of the five lifestyle goals and only 6% did not reach any goal *(6)*. However, the Multiple Risk Factor Intervention Trial showed that although intervention worked in nonsmokers, reducing the 6-year diabetes incidence by 18%, it failed in smokers, who even had an increase in diabetes incidence *(7)*.

Rather than absolute weight, it is the distribution of fat that is important, with visceral fat (android or central obesity) being more of a risk factor than subcutaneous fat (gynaecoid obesity) *(8,9)*. Visceral adipose tissue is more metabolically active than subcutaneous fat and the amount of visceral fat correlates with insulin resistance and hyperinsulinaemia. Weight reduction of 5–10% may result in up to 30% loss of visceral adipose tissue *(10)* and this may explain why a modest weight loss can significantly improve metabolic and reproductive function. One of the key factors appears to be the reduction of lipid stores in muscle rather than fat tissues *(11)*. Waist circumference has been shown to correlate better with visceral fat than waist:hip ratio *(9)*, and a waist circumference in women >88 cm is indicative of an increased metabolic risk *(10)*. In at-risk subjects, characterized either by insulin resistance, prediabetes or the MBS, a weight loss of 10 kg is estimated to results in a reduction of overall mortality by more than 20% *(12)*, of diabetes-associated mortality by more than 30% *(13)*, and of obesity-related mortality from cancer by more than 40% *(12)*.

Caveats of Lifestyle Intervention

Some precautions are necessary to prevent unwanted side effects of lifestyle interventions. Physical activity has to be individualized to avoid mechanical overload resulting in arthrosis or congestive heart disease. Weight reduction also increases the risk of gallstone formation, with a higher risk from rapid or pronounced weight loss *(14)*. Furthermore, a low body mass index (BMI) or drastic weight loss can result in loss of bone density and osteoporotic fractures *(15)*. However, there is no evidence that "weight cycling" by itself has adverse health consequences *(16)*. Also, there is no evidence that dieting or weight reduction programs cause eating disorders *(17)*.

POLYCYSTIC OVARIAN SYNDROME, OBESITY, AND THE METABOLIC SYNDROME

Polycystic ovarian syndrome (PCOS) is a common endocrine disorder characterized by hyperandrogenism and chronic anovulation. The prevalence among women of reproductive age is at least 6% *(18)*. Its pathophysiology, most likely a combination of genetic disposition and environmental factors, is not completely understood *(19,20)*. PCOS is one of the leading causes of infertility and also characterized by hirsutism, cystic acne, seborrhoea, hair loss, and obesity *(21,22)*. A significant proportion of PCOS-patients have been found to suffer from defective insulin secretion and insulin resistance *(23)*. Accordingly, PCOS patients may be expected to have a higher morbidity and mortality from the sequelae of the MBS *(24,25)*.

Obesity frequently accompanies PCOS and preliminary estimates in the United States were that 50% of women with PCOS were obese *(26)*. A recent multicenter trial at 22 sites in the United States recruited PCOS patients with a BMI range from 35 to 38 kg/m^2 *(27)*. In the largest prevalence study of PCOS in the United States, which examined 400 unselected females applying for employment at a university hospital in Alabama, 24% were found to be overweight (BMI 25.0–29.9 kg/m^2) and 42% were obese (BMI >30 kg/m^2) *(18)*. However, in other countries, women with PCOS tend to be leaner, with mean BMIs of 25 kg/m^2 in England *(28)*, 28 kg/m^2 in Finland *(29)*, 31 kg/m^2 in Germany *(22)*, and 29 kg/m^2 in Italy *(30)*. In a study of blood donors in Spain, 30% of the women were overweight, but only 10% were obese *(31)*. The differences in the prevalence in obesity most likely reflect differences in physical activity and diet, and especially the composition of diet *(32)*. Nonetheless, weight gain after adolescence and abdominal obesity are associated with an increased prevalence of PCOS symptoms in non-US population studies *(33)*.

Obesity further exacerbates metabolic and reproductive abnormalities in women with PCOS and may bring out the PCOS phenotype in a susceptible population as family studies suggest *(34)*. For example, risk factors for glucose intolerance in women with PCOS include a family history of diabetes, age, obesity, and especially a centripetal fat distribution *(35–37)*. One mechanism for this is that elevated insulin levels suppress hepatic production of sex hormone-binding globulin (SHBG) levels. Thus both obesity and insulin resistance lead to lower SHBG levels and higher bioavailable levels of androgens *(38)*. Adipose tissue also is a source of aromatase, and may convert androgens into estrogens, leading to inappropriate gonadotropin secretion and unopposed estrogen effects on the endometrium *(39)*.

Concurrent with the increase in PCOS patients with obesity, the prevalence of the MBS, a disorder highly associated with insulin resistance, is substantially higher in women with PCOS, ranging in the United States from 33% to more than 50% *(40)*. Likewise for the prevalence of T2DM, which appears to affect 4–10% of young women with PCOS, respectively *(35–37)*. However, in some other countries, the prevalence of the metabolic syndrome and of T2DM between patients with PCOS is lower than that observed in the United States *(22,30)*, again most likely because of differences in body weight and environmental factors affecting the prevalence of metabolic disturbances in PCOS.

However, although the prevalence of obesity in PCOS varies according to ethnicity and geographic location, and appears to be increasing, it must be pointed out that even in the United States, in the midst of an obesity crisis, up to 50% of PCOS patients are not obese.

LIFESTYLE INTERVENTION IN PCOS

Treatment of a patient with PCOS should be tailored to her symptoms and special needs. In obese patients, there is worldwide agreement that dietary-induced weight loss should always represent the first-line therapeutic advice (41,42). Hypocaloric diet has shown to improve the endocrine profile, facilitate weight loss, normalize menstrual cycles, and increase the likelihood of ovulation and a healthy pregnancy (42–46) (see also Table 1).

Treatment options with insulin sensitizers (27,47,48) and antiandrogens (49–51) or their combination (52,53) have shown to be effective in the treatment of all aspects of PCOS. However, in dieting obese PCOS women, improvement of insulin sensitivity and hyperinsulinemia were mostly dependent on hypocaloric diet, rather than on pharmacological treatment (42,52,53). Furthermore, the effect of metformin in women with PCOS is apparently reduced by increasing obesity (54–57), although this could simply be owing to an inappropriate low metformin dose for obese patients (42,58).

Studies by Clark et al. (59,60), demonstrated that weight loss achieved by an exercise schedule, combined with a hypocaloric diet over a 6-month period, improved insulin sensitivity, endocrine parameters, menstrual regularity, the frequency of spontaneous ovulation, and the chance of pregnancy. Even a modest weight loss of 2–5% of total body weight can restore ovulation in overweight women with PCOS as well as achieving a reduction of central fat and an improvement in insulin sensitivity (46). The study by Crosignani et al. also found that women with anovulatory PCOS who lost weight experienced an improvement in ovarian function, ovulation, and anthropometric indices (61). However, Kiddy et al. found that insulin sensitivity and androgen concentrations were unlikely to improve in patients who lost less than 5% of their initial weight (44).

Pasquali et al. studied 20 obese women with PCOS with a control group of 20 obese women without PCOS who were comparable for age and pattern of body fat distribution. All were given a low-calorie diet (1200–1400 kcal/day) for 1 month, after which they were randomized to receive metformin 850 mg twice daily) or placebo for 6 months. Metformin treatment reduced body weight and BMI significantly more than placebo in both PCOS and control women. Fasting insulin decreased significantly in both PCOS women and controls and testosterone concentrations decreased only in PCOS women treated with metformin. SHBG concentrations remained unchanged in all PCOS women, although in the control group, they significantly increased after both metformin and placebo (52).

A recent study randomizing 38 women with a mean BMI of >39 kg/m^2 to receive either advice on lifestyle modification aiming for 500–1000 calorie deficit per day combined with exercise or no advice with either metformin (850 mg twice daily) or placebo found the greatest effect in the combination group with respect both to reduction of weight and hyperandrogenism, yet irrespective of treatment the greatest improvement in the ovulation rate was achieved by those who lost weight *(62)*.

Lifestyle modification is thus a key component for the improvement of reproductive function for overweight, anovulatory women with PCOS *(41,63–65)*. Weight loss should therefore be encouraged prior to ovulation induction treatments, because these are less effective when BMI is >28–30 kg/m^2 *(66)*. Monitoring treatment is also harder in the obese as visualization of the ovaries is more difficult which raises the risk of multiple ovulation and multiple pregnancy. Furthermore, pregnancy carries greater risks in the obese, for example: miscarriage, gestational diabetes, hypertension, and problems with delivery *(67–70)*. The main component of diet should be calorie restriction *(71,72)*, with an additional effect from diet composition *(32)*.

The importance of obesity in PCOS is also supported by the finding that obesity can profoundly affect quality-of-life (QoL) independent of the presence of other clinical symptoms in otherwise healthy subjects *(73)*. Interestingly, obesity is linked strongly to the physical dimension of quality of life, rather than with psychosocial status *(74)* and social adjustment *(75)*. A variety of studies demonstrated that BMI and hirsutism are the primary mediators in the relationship between PCOS and the reductions in QoL *(76–79)*. Additionally, in obese patients the impact of weight reduction on QoL has been well established *(75)*. Based on data documenting the psychological and emotional consequences of changes in outer appearance, clinical interventions in PCOS women that influence obesity, hirsutism, acne, menstrual disturbances, or infertility would be expected to improve overall QoL *(80)*. Independent of PCOS, any kind of weight loss achieved by either dietary modification, physical activity, pharmacotherapy, surgery, or combinations thereof yields significant improvement of physical and social functioning in obese patients *(81–84)*.

FUTURE AVENUES

The cardiometabolic risk of obese PCOS patients is not likely to be different from other prediabetic women. Although good data as to the prevention of hard endpoints of cardiovascular risk, namely myocardial infarction, stroke, the need for intervention, and, ultimately, death, is available for prediabetic and diabetic patients, such long-term, prospective multicenter studies need to be undertaken to find out whether, and how, PCOS modifies these risks. To this end, the effects of different components of lifestyle intervention would also need to be evaluated in prospective, long-term studies aimed to assess morbidity and mortality of cardiovascular risk in PCOS.

KEY POINTS

Large diabetes prevention studies have shown that lifestyle intervention is an effective tool to fight obesity and diabetes. Lifestyle intervention has also effectively reduced weight and androgen levels, improved insulin sensitivity and menstrual cycles, and facilitated pregnancies in PCOS patients. Thus, lifestyle changes, both by increasing physical activity and improving diet are considered mandatory first steps in any treatment plan for obese PCOS patients. Strategies need to be developed to motivate patients to maintain long-term improvement.

Table 1
Lifestyle Intervention in PCOS

Authors	Year	Subjects	Intervention	Time course	Findings
Bates and Whitworth (85)	1982	18 obese PCOS + 20 controls	Dietary calorie restriction	3 months	Weight loss of >15% bodyweight in 13 patients, 10 pregnancies
Harlass et al. (86)	1984	6 obese PCOS	500 kcal/d diet	4–6 months	Weight loss (7–18%); decreased total and free T, increased SHBG
Pasquali et al. (43)	1989	20 obese anovulatory women, 14 of whom had PCOS	1000–1500 kcal/d (20% protein, 30% lipids, 50% carbohydrates) diet	6–12 months	Mean 9.7 kg weight loss; decreasd mean glucose-stimulated insulin; decreased T, no modifications in A and DHEAS; 14/20 ovulated, 4 pregnant
Kiddy et al. (44)	1992	24 obese PCOS	1000 kcal/d, low fat (20 g fat) diet	7 months	Decreased both fasting and glucose-stimulated insulin; decreased free T, increased SHBG; 3 resumed regular cycles; 6 pregnant
Guzick et al. (87)	1994	6 obese PCOS	400 kcal/d during the first 8 weeks, followed by a 1000–1200 kcal/d diet	12 weeks	Mean 16.2 kg weight loss; decreased fasting insulin; decreased non-SHBG bound T, increased SHBG; 4/6 ovulated
Hamilton-Fairley et al. (88)	1993	6 obese PCOS	350 kcal/d diet	1 month	Mean 5.6 kg weight loss; decreased fasting insulin; increased SHBG
Holte et al. (89)	1995	13 obese PCOS + 23 obese controls	1200 kcal/d diet	15 months	Improved insulin sensitivity; decreased T, increased SHBG, no modifications in A; 7/13 ovulated
Clark et al. (59)	1995	13 obese PCOS + drop-out controls	Exercise and diet	6 months	Mean weight loss of 6.3 kg, improved ovulation and pregnancy rate, lower miscarriage rate, drop in insulin and testosterone, rise in SHBG
Andersen et al. (90)	1995	9 obese PCOS	Diet 421 kcal/d containing 51 g protein for 4 weeks, followed by 1000–1500 kcal/d (22% protein, 59% carbohydrates, 20% fat)	24 weeks	Improved insulin sensitivity; no changes in T and SHBG; decreased cholesterol and triglycerides at 4 weeks; 2/9 achieved regular menstruation and became pregnant

342

Reference	Year	Subjects	Intervention	Duration	Results
Jackubowicz and Nestler (45)	1997	12 obese PCOS + 11 obese controls	Diet 1000–1200 kcal/d (134 g carbohydrates, 68 g protein, 47 g fat)	8 weeks	Decreased basal and glucose-stimulated insulin; decreased total and free T, decreased basal and leuprolide-stimulated peak 170 HP; increased SHBG
Clark et al. (60)	1998	67 obese PCOS + 20 drop-out controls	Exercise and diet	6 months	Mean weight loss of 10.2 kg, improved ovulation and pregnancy rate, lower miscarriage rate, drop in insulin and testosterone, rise in SHBG
Wahrenberg et al. (91)	1999	20 obese PCOS divided between diet oral and contraceptive	Very low-calorie diet or oral contraceptives	3 months	Improved insulin sensitivity in the weight-loss group only; decreased T in weight-loss group (similar to oral contraceptive), decreased free T in the weight-loss group only
Huber-Buchholz et al. (46)	1999	18 obese PCOS	Minimal caloric decrease with exercise program modification	6 months	Decreased fasting insulin, improved insulin sensitivity; decreased free T index; 9/18 ovulated
Pasquali et al. (52)	2000	20 obese PCOS + 20 obese controls	Diet 1200–1400 kcal/d + metformin (M) or placebo (P)	7 months	Decreased fasting insulin in both treatments, decreased glucose-stimulated insulin levels in M group only; decreased total T in M group only; no modifications in DHEAS and SHBG in both treatments; 2 women treated with M pregnant
Moran et al. (92)	2003	28 obese PCOS; 14 HP + 14 LP	High protein (HP; 40% carbohydrate and 30% protein) or low protein (LP; 55% carbohydrate and 15% protein) diet	12 weeks of energy restriction followed by 4 weeks of weight maintenance	Improvement in menstrual cyclicity, lipid profile, and insulin resistance, decrease in weight (7.5%) and abdominal fat (12.5%) independently of diet composition
Hoeger et al. (62)	2004	38 overweight or obese PCOS	Metformin (M), lifestyle modification + M (LM), L + placebo (LP) or P	48 weeks	Modest weight loss in all groups, best in LM, drop in androgens only in LM

(Continued)

343

Table 1 (*Continued*)

Authors	Year	Subjects	Intervention	Time course	Findings
Moran et al. (93,94)	2005	43 overweight PCOS	Meal replacements	8 weeks weight loss followed by 6 months weight maintenance	Reduction in weight, waist circumference, body fat, insulin, and testosterone
Tang et al. (42)	2006	143 obese PCOS (mean BMI 38 kg/m^2)	Individualized dietary advice (carbohydrate 50%, fat 10% to reduce caloric intake by 500 kcal/day) and advice to increase physical activity + metformin (M) or placebo (P)	6 months	Improvement in menstrual frequency and weight loss in both M and P. Reduction in waist circumference, testosterone levels and free androgen index in M

BMI, body mass index; PCOS, polycystic ovarian syndrome; SHBG, sex hormone-binding globulin.

344

REFERENCES

1. Chan JM, Rimm EB, Colditz GA, Stampfer MJ, Willett WC. Obesity, fat distribution, and weight gain as risk factors for clinical diabetes in men. Diabetes Care 1994;17:961–969.
2. Colditz GA, Willett WC, Rotnitzky A, Manson JE. Weight gain as a risk factor for clinical diabetes mellitus in women. Ann Intern Med 1995;122:481–486.
3. Yamaoka K, Tango T. Efficacy of lifestyle education to prevent type 2 diabetes: a meta-analysis of randomized controlled trials. Diabetes Care 2005;28:2780–2786.
4. Knowler WC, Barrett-Connor E, Fowler SE, et al. Reduction in the incidence of type 2 diabetes with lifestyle intervention or metformin. N Engl J Med 2002;346:393–403.
5. Herman WH, Hoerger TJ, Brandle M, et al. The cost-effectiveness of lifestyle modification or metformin in preventing type 2 diabetes in adults with impaired glucose tolerance. Ann Intern Med 2005;142:323–332.
6. Tuomilehto J, Lindstrom J, Eriksson JG, et al. Prevention of type 2 diabetes mellitus by changes in lifestyle among subjects with impaired glucose tolerance. N Engl J Med 2001;344:1343–1350.
7. Davey Smith G, Bracha Y, Svendsen KH, Neaton JD, Haffner SM, Kuller LH. Incidence of type 2 diabetes in the randomized multiple risk factor intervention trial. Ann Intern Med 2005;142:313–322.
8. Despres JP. Health consequences of visceral obesity. Ann Med 2001;33:534–541.
9. Lord J, Wilkin T. Polycystic ovary syndrome and fat distribution: the central issue? Hum Fertil (Camb) 2002;5:67–71.
10. Despres JP, Lemieux I, Prud'homme D. Treatment of obesity: need to focus on high risk abdominally obese patients. BMJ 2001;322:716–720.
11. Perseghin G. Muscle lipid metabolism in the metabolic syndrome. Curr Opin Lipidol 2005;16: 416–420.
12. Williamson DF, Pamuk E, Thun M, Flanders D, Byers T, Heath C. Prospective study of intentional weight loss and mortality in never-smoking overweight US white women aged 40-64 years. Am J Epidemiol 1995;141:1128–1141.
13. Williamson DF, Thompson TJ, Thun M, Flanders D, Pamuk E, Byers T. Intentional weight loss and mortality among overweight individuals with diabetes. Diabetes Care 2000;23:1499–1504.
14. Everhart JE. Contributions of obesity and weight loss to gallstone disease. Ann Intern Med 1993;119: 1029–1035.
15. Langlois JA, Harris T, Looker AC, Madans J. Weight change between age 50 years and old age is associated with risk of hip fracture in white women aged 67 years and older. Arch Intern Med 1996; 156:989–994.
16. National Task Force on the Prevention and Treatment of Obesity. Weight cycling. JAMA 1994;272: 1196–1202.
17. National Task Force on the Prevention and Treatment of Obesity. Overweight, obesity, and health risk. Arch Intern Med 2000;160:898–904.
18. Azziz R, Woods KS, Reyna R, Key TJ, Knochenhauer ES, Yildiz BO. The prevalence and features of the polycystic ovary syndrome in an unselected population. J Clin Endocrinol Metab 2004;89: 2745–2749.
19. Dunaif A, Thomas A. Current concepts in the polycystic ovary syndrome. Annu Rev Med 2001;52: 401–419.
20. Escobar-Morreale HF, Luque-Ramirez M, San Millan JL. The molecular-genetic basis of functional hyperandrogenism and the polycystic ovary syndrome. Endocr Rev 2005;26:251–282.
21. Ehrmann DA. Polycystic ovary syndrome. N Engl J Med 2005;352:1223–1236.
22. Hahn S, Tan S, Elsenbruch S, et al. Clinical and biochemical characterization of women with polycystic ovary syndrome in North Rhine-Westphalia. Horm Metab Res 2005;37:438–444.
23. Venkatesan AM, Dunaif A, Corbould A. Insulin resistance in polycystic ovary syndrome: progress and paradoxes. Recent Prog Horm Res 2001;56:295–308.
24. Talbott EO, Zborowski JV, Sutton-Tyrrell K, McHugh-Pemu KP, Guzick DS. Cardiovascular risk in women with polycystic ovary syndrome. Obstet Gynecol Clin North Am 2001;28:111–133.
25. Christian RC, Dumesic DA, Behrenbeck T, Oberg AL, Sheedy PF, Fitzpatrick LA. Prevalence and predictors of coronary artery calcification in women with polycystic ovary syndrome. J Clin Endocrinol Metab 2003;88:2562–2568.
26. Yen SS. The polycystic ovary syndrome. Clin Endocrinol (Oxf) 1980;12:177–207.

27. Azziz R, Ehrmann D, Legro RS, et al. Troglitazone improves ovulation and hirsutism in the polycystic ovary syndrome: a multicenter, double blind, placebo-controlled trial. J Clin Endocrinol Metab 2001; 86:1626–1632.

28. Balen AH, Conway GS, Kaltsas G, et al. Polycystic ovary syndrome: the spectrum of the disorder in 1741 patients. Hum Reprod 1995;10:2107–2111.

29. Taponen S, Martikainen H, Jarvelin MR, et al. Metabolic cardiovascular disease risk factors in women with self-reported symptoms of oligomenorrhea and/or hirsutism: Northern Finland Birth Cohort 1966 Study. J Clin Endocrinol Metab 2004;89:2114–2118.

30. Carmina E, Chu MC, Longo RA, Rini GB, Lobo RA. Phenotypic variation in hyperandrogenic women influences the findings of abnormal metabolic and cardiovascular risk parameters. J Clin Endocrinol Metab 2005;90:2545–2549.

31. Asuncion M, Calvo RM, San Millan JL, Sancho J, Avila S, Escobar-Morreale HF. A prospective study of the prevalence of the polycystic ovary syndrome in unselected Caucasian women from Spain. J Clin Endocrinol Metab 2000;85:2434–2438.

32. Carmina E, Legro RS, Stamets K, Lowell J, Lobo RA. Difference in body weight between American and Italian women with polycystic ovary syndrome: influence of the diet. Hum Reprod 2003;18: 2289–2293.

33. Laitinen J, Taponen S, Martikainen H, et al. Body size from birth to adulthood as a predictor of self-reported polycystic ovary syndrome symptoms. Int J Obes Relat Metab Disord 2003;27:710–715.

34. Legro RS, Bentley-Lewis R, Driscoll D, Wang SC, Dunaif A. Insulin resistance in the sisters of women with polycystic ovary syndrome: association with hyperandrogenemia rather than menstrual irregularity. J Clin Endocrinol Metab 2002;87:2128–2133.

35. Legro RS, Kunselman AR, Dodson WC, Dunaif A. Prevalence and predictors of risk for type 2 diabetes mellitus and impaired glucose tolerance in polycystic ovary syndrome: a prospective, controlled study in 254 affected women. J Clin Endocrinol Metab 1999;84:165–169.

36. Ehrmann DA, Barnes RB, Rosenfield RL, Cavaghan MK, Imperial J. Prevalence of impaired glucose tolerance and diabetes in women with polycystic ovary syndrome. Diabetes Care 1999;22: 141–146.

37. Ehrmann DA, Kasza K, Azziz R, Legro RS, Ghazzi MN. Effects of race and family history of type 2 diabetes on metabolic status of women with polycystic ovary syndrome. J Clin Endocrinol Metab 2005;90:66–71.

38. Nestler JE, Powers LP, Matt DW, et al. A direct effect of hyperinsulinemia on serum sex hormone-binding globulin levels in obese women with the polycystic ovary syndrome. J Clin Endocrinol Metab 1991;72:83–89.

39. Bulun SE, Noble LS, Takayama K, et al. Endocrine disorders associated with inappropriately high aromatase expression. J Steroid Biochem Mol Biol 1997;61:133–139.

40. Apridonidze T, Essah PA, Iuorno MJ, Nestler JE. Prevalence and characteristics of the metabolic syndrome in women with polycystic ovary syndrome. J Clin Endocrinol Metab 2005;90:1929–1935.

41. Pasquali R, Gambineri A. Treatment of the polycystic ovary syndrome with lifestyle intervention. Curr Opin Endocrinol Diab 2002;9:459–468.

42. Tang T, Glanville J, Hayden CJ, White D, Barth JH, Balen AH. Combined lifestyle modification and metformin in obese patients with polycystic ovary syndrome. A randomized, placebo-controlled, double-blind multicentre study. Hum Reprod 2006;21:80–89.

43. Pasquali R, Antenucci D, Casimirri F, et al. Clinical and hormonal characteristics of obese amenorrheic hyperandrogenic women before and after weight loss. J Clin Endocrinol Metab 1989;68:173–179.

44. Kiddy DS, Hamilton-Fairley D, Bush A, et al. Improvement in endocrine and ovarian function during dietary treatment of obese women with polycystic ovary syndrome. Clin Endocrinol (Oxf) 1992;36: 105–111.

45. Jakubowicz DJ, Nestler JE. 17 alpha-Hydroxyprogesterone responses to leuprolide and serum androgens in obese women with and without polycystic ovary syndrome offer dietary weight loss. J Clin Endocrinol Metab 1997;82:556–560.

46. Huber-Buchholz MM, Carey DG, Norman RJ. Restoration of reproductive potential by lifestyle modification in obese polycystic ovary syndrome: role of insulin sensitivity and luteinizing hormone. J Clin Endocrinol Metab 1999;84:1470–1474.

47. Nestler JE, Jakubowicz DJ, Evans WS, Pasquali R. Effects of metformin on spontaneous and clomiphene-induced ovulation in the polycystic ovary syndrome. N Engl J Med 1998;338:1876–1880.

48. Moghetti P, Castello R, Negri C, et al. Metformin effects on clinical features, endocrine and metabolic profiles, and insulin sensitivity in polycystic ovary syndrome: a randomized, double-blind, placebo-controlled 6-month trial, followed by open, long-term clinical evaluation. J Clin Endocrinol Metab 2000;85:139–146.

49. De Leo V, Lanzetta D, D'Antona D, la Marca A, Morgante G. Hormonal effects of flutamide in young women with polycystic ovary syndrome. J Clin Endocrinol Metab 1998;83:99–102.

50. Eagleson CA, Gingrich MB, Pastor CL, et al. Polycystic ovarian syndrome: evidence that flutamide restores sensitivity of the gonadotropin-releasing hormone pulse generator to inhibition by estradiol and progesterone. J Clin Endocrinol Metab 2000;85:4047–4052.

51. Ibanez L, Potau N, Marcos MV, de Zegher F. Treatment of hirsutism, hyperandrogenism, oligomenorrhea, dyslipidemia, and hyperinsulinism in nonobese, adolescent girls: effect of flutamide. J Clin Endocrinol Metab 2000;85:3251–3255.

52. Pasquali R, Gambineri A, Biscotti D, et al. Effect of long-term treatment with metformin added to hypocaloric diet on body composition, fat distribution, and androgen and insulin levels in abdominally obese women with and without the polycystic ovary syndrome. J Clin Endocrinol Metab 2000; 85:2767–2774.

53. Gambineri A, Pelusi C, Genghini S, et al. Effect of flutamide and metformin administered alone or in combination in dieting obese women with polycystic ovary syndrome. Clin Endocrinol (Oxf) 2004;60: 241–249.

54. Crave JC, Fimbel S, Lejeune H, Cugnardey N, Dechaud H, Pugeat M. Effects of diet and metformin administration on sex hormone-binding globulin, androgens, and insulin in hirsute and obese women. J Clin Endocrinol Metab 1995;80:2057–2062.

55. Fleming R, Hopkinson ZE, Wallace AM, Greer IA, Sattar N. Ovarian function and metabolic factors in women with oligomenorrhea treated with metformin in a randomized double blind placebo-controlled trial. J Clin Endocrinol Metab 2002;87:569–574.

56. Maciel GA, Soares Junior JM, Alves da Motta EL, Abi Haidar M, de Lima GR, Baracat EC. Nonobese women with polycystic ovary syndrome respond better than obese women to treatment with metformin. Fertil Steril 2004;81:355–360.

57. Kumari AS, Haq A, Jayasundaram R, Abdel-Wareth LO, Al Haija SA, Alvares M. Metformin monotherapy in lean women with polycystic ovary syndrome. Reprod Biomed Online 2005;10:100–104.

58. Goldenberg N, Glueck CJ, Loftspring M, Sherman A, Wang P. Metformin-diet benefits in women with polycystic ovary syndrome in the bottom and top quintiles for insulin resistance. Metabolism 2005;54:113–121.

59. Clark AM, Ledger W, Galletly C, et al. Weight loss results in significant improvement in pregnancy and ovulation rates in anovulatory obese women. Hum Reprod 1995;10:2705–2712.

60. Clark AM, Thornley B, Tomlinson L, Galletley C, Norman RJ. Weight loss in obese infertile women results in improvement in reproductive outcome for all forms of fertility treatment. Hum Reprod 1998;13:1502–1505.

61. Crosignani PG, Colombo M, Vegetti W, Somigliana E, Gessati A, Ragni G. Overweight and obese anovulatory patients with polycystic ovaries: parallel improvements in anthropometric indices, ovarian physiology and fertility rate induced by diet. Hum Reprod 2003;18:1928–1932.

62. Hoeger KM, Kochman L, Wixom N, Craig K, Miller RK, Guzick DS. A randomized, 48-week, placebo-controlled trial of intensive lifestyle modification and/or metformin therapy in overweight women with polycystic ovary syndrome: a pilot study. Fertil Steril 2004;82:421–429.

63. Norman RJ, Davies MJ, Lord J, Moran LJ. The role of lifestyle modification in polycystic ovary syndrome. Trends Endocrinol Metab 2002;13:251–257.

64. Norman RJ, Noakes M, Wu R, Davies MJ, Moran L, Wang JX. Improving reproductive performance in overweight/obese women with effective weight management. Hum Reprod Update 2004;10: 267–280.

65. Pasquali R, Gambineri A. Role of changes in dietary habits in polycystic ovary syndrome. Reprod Biomed Online 2004;8:431–439.

66. Hamilton-Fairley D, Kiddy D, Watson H, Paterson C, Franks S. Association of moderate obesity with a poor pregnancy outcome in women with polycystic ovary syndrome treated with low dose gonadotrophin. Br J Obstet Gynaecol 1992;99:128–131.

67. Gjonnaess H. The course and outcome of pregnancy after ovarian electrocautery in women with polycystic ovarian syndrome: the influence of body-weight. Br J Obstet Gynaecol 1989;96:714–719.

68. Sebire NJ, Jolly M, Harris JP, et al. Maternal obesity and pregnancy outcome: a study of 287,213 pregnancies in London. Int J Obes Relat Metab Disord 2001;25:1175–1182.

69. Cedergren MI. Maternal morbid obesity and the risk of adverse pregnancy outcome. Obstet Gynecol 2004;103:219–224.

70. Linne Y. Effects of obesity on women's reproduction and complications during pregnancy. Obes Rev 2004;5:137–143.

71. Moran LJ, Noakes M, Clifton PM, Tomlinson L, Norman RJ. Dietary composition in restoring reproductive and metabolic physiology in overweight women with polycystic ovary syndrome. J Clin Endocrinol Metab 2003;88:812–819.

72. Stamets K, Taylor DS, Kunselman A, Demers LM, Pelkman CL, Legro RS. A randomized trial of the effects of two types of short-term hypocaloric diets on weight loss in women with polycystic ovary syndrome. Fertil Steril 2004;81:630–637.

73. Stunkard AJ, Faith MS, Allison KC. Depression and obesity. Biol Psychiatry 2003;54:330–337.

74. Mannucci E, Ricca V, Barciulli E, et al. Quality of life and overweight: the obesity related well-being (Orwell 97) questionnaire. Addict Behav 1999;24:345–357.

75. Swallen KC, Reither EN, Haas SA, Meier AM. Overweight, obesity, and health-related quality of life among adolescents: the National Longitudinal Study of Adolescent Health. Pediatrics 2005;115: 340–347.

76. Hashimoto DM, Schmid J, Martins FM, et al. The impact of the weight status on subjective symptomatology of the polycystic ovary syndrome: a cross-cultural comparison between Brazilian and Austrian women. Anthropol Anz 2003;61:297–310.

77. McCook JG, Reame NE, Thatcher SS. Health-related quality of life issues in women with polycystic ovary syndrome. J Obstet Gynecol Neonatal Nurs 2005;34:12–20.

78. Trent M, Austin SB, Rich M, Gordon CM. Overweight status of adolescent girls with polycystic ovary syndrome: body mass index as mediator of quality of life. Ambul Pediatr 2005;5:107–111.

79. Hahn S, Janssen OE, Tan S, et al. Clinical and psychological correlates of quality-of-life in polycystic ovary syndrome. Eur J Endocrinol 2005;153:853–860.

80. Elsenbruch S, Hahn S, Kowalsky D, et al. Quality of life, psychosocial well-being, and sexual satisfaction in women with polycystic ovary syndrome. J Clin Endocrinol Metab 2003;88:5801–5807.

81. Dittmar M, Heintz A, Hardt J, Egle UT, Kahaly GJ. Metabolic and psychosocial effects of minimal invasive gastric banding for morbid obesity. Metabolism 2003;52:1551–1557.

82. Jalil RA, Manan WA, Bebakar WM, Halim R, Ooi GS, Othman R. Assessing changes in quality of life among obese participants in Kelantan, Malaysia. Asia Pac J Clin Nutr 2004;13:S141.

83. Mathus-Vliegen EM, de Weerd S, de Wit LT. Health-related quality-of-life in patients with morbid obesity after gastric banding for surgically induced weight loss. Surgery 2004;135:489–497.

84. Ogden J, Clementi C, Aylwin S, Patel A. Exploring the impact of obesity surgery on patients' health status: a quantitative and qualitative study. Obes Surg 2005;15:266–272.

85. Bates GW, Whitworth NS. Effect of body weight reduction on plasma androgens in obese, infertile women. Fertil Steril 1982;38:406–409.

86. Harlass FE, Plymate SR, Fariss BL, Belts RP. Weight loss is associated with correction of gonadotropin and sex steroid abnormalities in the obese anovulatory female. Fertil Steril 1984;42: 649–652.

87. Guzick DS, Wing R, Smith D, Berga SL, Winters SJ. Endocrine consequences of weight loss in obese, hyperandrogenic, anovulatory women. Fertil Steril 1994;61:598–604.

88. Hamilton-Fairley D, Kiddy D, Anyaoku V, Koistinen R, Seppala M, Franks S. Response of sex hormone binding globulin and insulin-like growth factor binding protein-1 to an oral glucose tolerance test in obese women with polycystic ovary syndrome before and after calorie restriction. Clin Endocrinol (Oxf) 1993;39:363–367.

89. Holte J, Bergh T, Berne C, Wide L, Lithell H. Restored insulin sensitivity but persistently increased early insulin secretion after weight loss in obese women with polycystic ovary syndrome. J Clin Endocrinol Metab 1995;80:2586–2593.

90. Andersen P, Seljeflot I, Abdelnoor M, et al. Increased insulin sensitivity and fibrinolytic capacity after dietary intervention in obese women with polycystic ovary syndrome. Metabolism 1995;44:611–616.

91. Wahrenberg H, Ek I, Reynisdottir S, Carlstrom K, Bergqvist A, Arner P. Divergent effects of weight reduction and oral anticonception treatment on adrenergic lipolysis regulation in obese women with the polycystic ovary syndrome. J Clin Endocrinol Metab 1999;84:2182–2187.

92. Moran LJ, Noakes M, Clifton PM, Tomlinson L, Galletly C, Norman RJ. Dietary composition in restoring reproductive and metabolic physiology in overweight women with polycystic ovary syndrome. J Clin Endocrinol Metab 2003;88:812–819.

93. Moran LJ, Noakes M, Clifton PM, Wittert G, Norman RJ. Short term energy restriction (using meal replacements) improves reproductive parameters in polycystic ovary syndrome. Asia Pac J Clin Nutr 2004;13:S88.

94. Moran LJ, Noakes M, Clifton PM, Wittert G, Williams G, Norman RJ. Effective weight loss and maintenance strategies in polycystic ovary syndrome. Asia Pac J Clin Nutr 2005;14:S94.

26 Therapeutic Aspects of Polycystic Ovary Syndrome in Adolescence

George Mastorakos, MD,
Carolina Koliopoulos, MD,
and George Creatsas, MD

CONTENTS

Summary

Polycystic ovary syndrome (PCOS) is characterized by hyperandrogenism, chronic anovulation, and insulin resistance. The syndrome manifests with hirsutism, irregular menses, infertility, dyslipidemia, as well as a higher risk for type 2 diabetes mellitus, and cardiovascular disease. PCOS has a pubertal onset. The clinical signs and neuroendocrine features of adolescents with PCOS resemble those found in adult women with the syndrome. Early recognition and prompt treatment in adolescents is essential for preventing long-term consequences. This chapter reviews the clinical, hormonal, and metabolic features of PCOS in adolescence and current treatment options.

Key Words: Adolescence; polycystic ovary syndrome; obesity; insulin resistance; contraceptives; antiandrogens; cyproterone acetate; flutamide; spironolacone; finasteride; GnRH analogues; metformin; thiazolidinediones; roziglitazone; pioglitazone; sibutramine.

INTRODUCTION

Polycystic ovary syndrome (PCOS) is among the most common disorders of the premenopausal women. In a cross-sectional study of women of reproductive age from

From: *Contemporary Endocrinology: Insulin Resistance and Polycystic Ovarian Syndrome:*
Pathogenesis, Evaluation, and Treatment
Edited by: E. Diamanti-Kandarakis, J. E. Nestler, D. Panidis, and R. Pasquali © Humana Press Inc., Totowa, NJ

the Greek island Lesbos, the incidence of PCOS was found to be 6.8% *(1)*. PCOS is characterized by hyperandrogenism, chronic anovulation, and insulin resistance, which result in hirsutism, irregular menses, and infertility, as well as a higher risk for type 2 diabetes mellitus. Insulin resistance in PCOS is associated with dyslipidemia, central adiposity, and, in some cases, impaired glucose tolerance, factors that predispose to cardiovascular disease *(2)*. Some studies suggest a strong familial component in PCOS *(3)*. It is now proposed that PCOS is an oligogenic disorder in which a small number of key genes interact with environmental factors (notably dietary), resulting in the abnormalities associated with the syndrome *(4)*.

PCOS has a pubertal onset *(5)*. Therefore, early identification of women at risk for PCOS may lead to prevention of long-term complications associated with the syndrome.

PCOS IN ADOLESENCE

The first clinical signs of PCOS usually manifest soon after menarche. Adolescent girls affected by PCOS present with menstrual irregularity and often gain weight immediately or shortly after menarche. The diagnosis of PCOS, however, is delayed in many cases, because most of the signs of PCOS are interpreted as normal pubertal findings. Menstrual irregularities during the first reproductive years are considered by most clinicians as part of the maturation process of the hypothalamic–pituitary–ovarian axis. Similarly, acne is prevalent among adolescents. Recent data, however, indicate that oligomenorrhea in the first years after menarche may be indeed an early sign of PCOS *(6)*. Population surveys suggest that as many as 45–57% of oligomenorrheic girls had PCOS syndrome, as assessed by clinical and biochemical features of hyperandrogenism *(7,8)*. In another study, lean girls with menstrual irregularities during the first 3 years after menarche were found to have statistically significantly elevated serum levels of free testosterone and LH and an increased LH/FSH ratio *(9)*.

These girls develop signs of hyperandrogenism, associated with augmented LH pulse amplitude and frequency, increased LH/FSH ratio *(5)*, and increased ovarian volume because of increased ovarian stroma. Histologically, there are multiple atretic small follicles located peripherally in the ovary and a thickened sclerotic ovarian cortex *(10,11)*. These girls also present with hyperinsulinemia, reflecting insulin resistance, and reduced levels of insulin-like growth factor binding protein-1 and sex hormone-binding globulin (SHBG) *(12)*. In certain girls with premature adrenarche, hyperandrogenism may be the first sign of PCOS and/or insulin resistance *(13)*. The link between these disorders could be serine phosphorylation of the 17,20-lyase activity of P450c17 *(14)* and/or of the insulin receptor *(15)*.

In recent years PCOS has been transformed from a disorder of reproductive years to a clinical entity that begins *in utero* and ends in senescence, encompassing the whole life spectrum of a woman *(16)*. There are certain clinical findings that may help clinicians to identify and further investigate girls with increased risk for PCOS. PCOS and insulin resistance have been linked with reduced fetal growth, manifesting as low birth weight. Premature pubarche *(17)*, true sexual precocity, overgrowth caused by pseudoacromegaly, or childhood obesity are now viewed as early signs of PCOS later in life. During adolescence, the presence of persistent oligomenorrhea and/or amenorrhea, especially if accompanied by obesity should prompt further evaluation. PCOS has

Table 1
Clinical Features of PCOS in Adolescents

• Low birth weight
• Premature pubarche
• Menstrual irregularities (oligo-amenorrhea)
• Hyperandrogenism (hirsutism, acne, male type alopecia)
• Obesity
• Family history of PCOS, diabetes mellitus 2, premature
  cardiovascular disease.

a strong hereditary component: girls with a family history of PCOS, type 2 diabetes or premature cardiovascular disease warrant special attention. Finally, the presence of clinical signs of hyperandrogenism in pubertal years may also imply an underlying metabolic abnormality in the context of PCOS (Table 1).

Incidence of PCOS in Adolescence

In a random population, Brigdes et al. observed polycystic ovaries by ultrasound in 6% of girls who were 6 years old, in 18% of girls who were 10 years old and in 26% of adolescents who were 15 years old *(18)*. Dramusic et al. *(19)* reported that the incidence of PCOS in Singapore in a population of 1000 adolescent girls with irregular menses was 25.9%. As diagnostic criteria, they used the presence of irregular bleeding and/or clinical hyperandrogenism (hirsutism, acne), increased ratio of LH to FSH, hyperandrogenemia, and polycystic ovaries by ultrasound. In the same study it was reported that the incidence of acne and hirsutism in adolescence with PCOS was 55 and 51%, respectively, and that 27.4% of the girls were obese.

Diagnostic Approach of PCOS in Adolescense

Elevated serum free or bioavailable testosterone is an almost universal finding in adolescents with PCOS. SHBG is usually low, and total testosterone may therefore be within the normal range. Mean levels of DHEA-sulfate, Δ4-androstendione, LH, and LH/FSH ratio have been reported to be higher in adolescents with PCOS compared to age-matched normal controls *(20)*. Furthermore, ovarian as well as adrenal dynamics are reported to be deranged in girls with PCOS. Affected individuals are reported to have a male type androgen response to HCG stimulation, with earlier and higher peaks 17-OHProgesterone than normal controls *(21)*. Serum 17α-hydroxyprogsterone response to GnRH agonist stimulation is also augmented in patients with PCOS, indicating ovarian hyperactivity of P450c17α, a key enzyme in the biosynthesis of androgens *(22)*. Stimulated adrenal steroidogenesis is also reported as overactive, as evidenced by the exaggerated production of 17α-hydroxyprogesterone and Δ4-androstendione after stimulation with ACTH analogues *(23)*. The classic sonographic image of PCOS consists of enlarged ovaries with bright echogenic stroma and multiple small follicles located at the periphery, like a string of pearls *(24)*. The presence, however of polycystic morphology on ultrasound cannot establish the diagnosis of PCOS as a sole criterion, as it is a nonspecific finding in more than 20% of normal female population *(25)*.

Metabolic Disturbances in Adolescent Girls With PCOS

Recent studies indicate an increased prevalence of impaired glucose tolerance and β-cell dysfunction, similar to that seen in type 2 diabetes, is also present in adolescents with PCOS, independently of obesity *(26,27)*. By employing hyperinsulinemic-euglycemic and hyperglycemic clamp techniques, Lewy et al. *(28)* demonstrated that adolescent girls with PCOS manifest approximately a 50% reduction in peripheral tissue insulin sensitivity, evidence of hepatic insulin resistance, and compensatory hyperinsulinemia early in the course of the syndrome. When adolescents and young women with PCOS were followed for 10 years, a trend to worsening hyperinsulinism and insulin resistance was observed without accentuation of hyperandrogenism *(29)*.

Dyslipidemia is a primary aspect of the metabolic derangement encountered in PCOS and is invariably present independently of obesity. Affected women have lower HDL-cholesterol and higher triglyceride levels *(30,31)*. Furthermore, AI-apolipoprotein, the major apolipoprotein of HDL-cholesterol, is decreased in women with PCOS *(32)*. The severity of hypertriglyceridemia usually correlates with the degree of obesity and insulin resistance *(33)*. LDL-cholesterol may be elevated in PCOS *(17)*, but this is not a universal finding *(33)*. Dyslipidemia is considered one of the reasons for the increased incidence of cardiovascular disease in women with PCOS *(34)*.

Because adolescents with PCOS are at risk for dyslipidemia, cardiovascular disease, and diabetes mellitus, a fasting lipid profile, and an OGTT are indicated in the evaluation of girls with PCOS, especially for obese patients. In addition, it is recommended that primary relatives be evaluated for PCOS.

Obesity in Adolescents With PCOS

Although hormonal and metabolic derangements are inherent features of PCOS, obesity is found with increased prevalence in affected adolescents, aggravating the clinical course of the disease. Obesity *per se* is accompanied by insulin resistance and lipid-lipoprotein changes. Although a substantial percentage of girls with PCOS are of normal weight, many adolescents do not present with symptoms of the syndrome unless they gain weight. Furthermore, weight loss alone without medical therapy leads to marked improvement of menstrual cyclicity and hirsutism *(16,33)*.

Psychological and Social Consequences

Adolescents with PCOS suffer psychological stress which results from:

1. Problems related to the clinical signs of PCOS and their appearence (obesity, acne, hirsutism, alopecia). Dramusic et al. *(19)* asked PCOS adolescents to complete a special questionnaire, and 87.5% of the respondents reported that they were unhappy about their weight, 71% about their height, 86.6% did not have a boyfriend, 33.3% questioned whether they were attractive to the opposite sex, and 75% were disappointed with clinical signs that were attributable to PCOS.
2. Long-term effects of PCOS. In the same study by Dramusic et al. 75% of PCOS adolescents noted that they were worried about their future fertility. Moreover, other sources of stress for these adolescents and their parents may be the increased rate of abortion, diabetes mellitus, dyslipidemia, and cardiovascular disease.

Table 2
Overview of Therapeutic Options in the Treatment of PCOS in Adolescence

Inhibition of androgen production from the ovaries
  • Oral contraceptives
  • Gn-RH analogues
Inhibition of androgen action
  • Antiandrogens (cyproterone acetate, flutamide, spironolactone)
  • 5α-reductase inhibitors (finasteride)
Insulin sensitizers
  • Metformin
  • Thiazolidinediones

For all these reasons, it is imperative to diagnose PCOS as early as possible, to treat it appropriately and to continue to follow the patients to prevent any of the long-term effects of the syndrome.

THERAPEUTIC GOALS IN PCOS

The principal goals in the treatment of PCOS differ depending on the age of the woman and the priorities set by the patient and the doctor. Weight reduction applies to all obese women with PCOS. As mentioned earlier, this mode of intervention by itself reduces insulin resistance and in many cases ameliorates clinical signs of hyperandrogenism. In general, the ideal treatment should normalize menses, restore ovulation and fertility, reduce hirsutism and acne, improve the lipid profile and glucose tolerane, and thereby reduce cardiovascular risk. Most therapeutic modalities for PCOS have targeted excess androgen production from the ovaries and androgen action at the receptor level. Recently, insulin sensitizers have been increasingly used in the treatment of PCOS, with promising results in terms of both endocrine and metabolic aspects of the syndrome (Table 2).

CURRENT TREATMENT OPTIONS

Nonpharmacologic Treatment

WEIGHT REDUCTION: EXERCISE

The positive correlation between insulin values and BMI in women with PCOS suggests that obese teenage patients, along with psychological support, should also be encouraged to lose weight and exercise to improve the clinical and metabolic features of the syndrome. Weight reduction is one of the primary goals in the treatment of PCOS. Diet is the mainstay of PCOS treatment, and because the individual should acquire a lifelong healthy eating pattern, effective dietetic counselling is extremely important as first-line treatment of girls with PCOS. Physical exercise helps the adolescent girl both to increase energy expenditure and to improve self-esteem.

COSMETIC TREATMENT

Cosmetic treatment, although solely symptomatic, may help improve the self-image of patients with hirsutism, which is especially important for adolescents. Eflornithine

HCl topical cream retarded hair growth and reduced patient discomfort in placebo-controlled trials *(35)*. Cosmetic treatment of hirsutism includes depilation, such as shaving or chemical depilatories, epilation by plucking or waxing, and destruction of the dermal papilla with various methods such as laser therapy and electrolysis. Concerning PCOS-related alopecia it seems that combination therapy with an antiandrogen and oral contraceptive is superior to minoxidil *(36)*.

Hormonal Treatment

COMBINED ORAL CONTRACEPTIVES

Combined oral contraceptives (COC) have been the mainstay of treatment of menstrual and dermatologic problems associated with PCOS for many years. Beneficial effects are attributed to both their estrogenic and progestogenic components.

The ethinylestradiol contained in COC increases the levels of SHBG, resulting in lower free androgen levels *(37)*. The third generation of COC, such as those containing desogestrel, block the estrogen-mediated increase of SHBG to a lesser degree than older COC *(38)*. Furthermore, the progestogenic component inhibits LH-induced androgen production *(37–39)*.

The efficacy of COCs in reducing hyperandrogenemia and improving hirsutism and acne has been well documented *(40–43)*. Clinical effectiveness with respect to hirsutism and acne is evident by the sixth month. One of the most widely used COCs in Europe is the combination of ethinylestradiol 35 μg with the antiandrogen cyproterone acetate 2 mg (EE/CPA). This combination, wherein the progestin has antiandrogenic activity, is effective in reducing testosterone, Δ4-androstendione and the LH/FSH ratio after the 3rd cycle, and in improving hirsutism and acne after the 6th cycle, with most patients noting significant improvement between the 8th and the 12th cycles *(32,41,42)*.

Recently, newer COC combinations with third generation progestins, such desogestrel, have been used in the treatment of PCOS. These COCs are equally effective in reducing clinical and biochemical signs of PCOS. Adverse effects of minor importance occur in a small percentage of patients and include weight gain, breast tenderness, and mood changes *(42)*. Serious adverse effects such as venous thromboembolism are extremely rare in ambulatory young individuals. Recently, a new COC with 30 μg ethinylestradiol and drospirenone, a progestin with antimineralcorticoid and antiandrogen receptor activities, has been launched in the market. This COC is reported to improve androgen profile without the untoward effect of weight gain. Clinically, this preparation is effective in reducing acne by the sixth month of therapy, in reducing androgen levels and in increasing SHBG *(44–47)*, whereas its efficacy in reducing hirsutism has not been universally demonstrated *(44,48)*.

Obesity may sometimes diminish the positive effect of a COC on hyperandrogenism, as obese patients produce higher levels of androgens, because of both greater insulin resistance and increased steroidogenic enzyme activity *(49)*. On the other hand, COCs may increase body weight *(50)*.

Regarding the lipid profile, we recently found that total cholesterol as well as LDL cholesterol increased significantly in both users of the cyproterone acetate-containing COC and the desogestrel-containing COC, although the former combination caused a significant increase in triglyceride levels, a parameter already increased in PCOS subjects *(32,51,52)*.

The impact of COC on carbohydrate metabolism is variable. Some investigators report an increase in insulin resistance following COC use, as manifested by the increased fasting insulin levels or decreased glucose requirements during the hyperinsulinemic euglycemic clamp *(52–54)*, whereas other investigators did not observe any significant effect on glucose metabolism with newer COCs containing desogestrel or gestodene *(55,56)*. We recently found that the administration of two formulations of COC (desogestrel/ethinyl estradiol and cyproterone acetate/ethinyl estradiol) to adolescent girls with PCOS increased insulin resistance. Moreover, it seems that the cyproterone acetate-containing COC affects pancreatic β-cell function by increasing insulin secretion and producing marked hyperinsulinemia. The combination of ethinylestradiol/drospirenone is considered as neutral with respect to insulin resistance *(48,55)*.

As a general rule, COC treatment should be continued until the patient is gynecologically mature (5 years postmenarcheal) or has lost a substantial amount of excess weight *(57)*. At that point, it is advisable to withhold treatment for a few months to ascertain whether the menstrual abnormality persists.

GLUCOCORTICOIDS

Glucorticoids are indicated for those nonobese adolescents who have a prominent component of functional adrenal hyperplasia *(57)*. A modest bedtime dose (i.e., 5.0–7.5 mg prednisone) reduces secretion of adrenal androgens more than that of cortisol. It is recommended that DHEA should be suppressed to below the adult range without complete suppression. Significant glycocorticoid deficiency can be excluded by a cortisol level of 10 µg/dL or more at 8 AM or 18 µg/dL 30 minutes after administration of a low dose (1.0 µg) of ACTH.

ANTIANDROGENS

Antiandrogens act as competitive antagonists of steroid binding to the androgen receptor *(57)*.

1. *Cyproterone acetate.* Cyproterone acetate is a progestin with antiandrogenic activity and weak antiglucocorticoid effects. It is available in Europe as a COC containing ethinylestradiol. Usually is administered in combination with estrogen in the form of a COC, as mentioned earlier, at a low dose of 2 mg. In selected cases with severe hirsutism, high dose therapy consists of the EE/CPA COC administered for 21 days plus CPA 10–100 mg added for the first 10 days, to ensure CPA clearance from adipose tissue by the end of the cycle. Clinical studies, however, indicate that there is no dose-related effect of CPA and that the same clinical effects can be achieved by low doses of CPA *(58,59)*. Cyproterone acetate is not commercially available in the United States.

2. *Flutamide.* Flutamide is a pure antiandrogen, acting on the androgen receptor. At a daily dose of 250 mg, flutamide alone or in combination with COC has been shown to improve hirsutism and acne in PCOS *(58)*. Recent studies indicate that the lower dose of 125 mg daily is clinically equally effective, at least as maintenance therapy *(60)*. Flutamide is potentially hepatotoxic and may cause a rise in aminotransferase levels in as many as 10% of cases *(60)*. Frequent monitoring of liver function tests is therefore mandatory for patients treated with flutamide. Pregnancy should be avoided in women prescribed antiandrogen treatment. Because of the lack of information, its use in adolescents should be avoided.

3. *Spironolactone*. Spironolactone is an aldosterone antagonist and its primary use is as an anti-hypertensive. Spironolactone, however, also binds to the androgen receptor and, like CPA, has an antiandrogenic effect. It is also a weak progestin and weak glucocorticoid. This drug has been used in doses ranging from 50 to 200 mg daily with 40–71% improvement in hirsutism scores within 6 months of follow up *(61,62)*. A recommended protocol is to start with 100 mg twice daily until the maximal effect has been achieved, and then reducing the dose to 50 mg twice daily as maintenance therapy. Hyperkalemia may be a side effect, so serum potassium should be monitored. Prolonged use has been associated with menstrual irregularrities and breast tenderness, so the concomitant use of a COC may improve clinical effectiveness. Pregnancy should be avoided during treatment with spironolactone.

4. *Finasteride*. Finasteride inhibits 5α-reductase activity, the enzyme that converts testosterone to dihydrotestosterone. Therapy with 5 mg finasteride daily has been reported to reduce hirsutism within 3–6 months *(63)*. The addition of finasteride to EE/CPA COC may augment the clinical effectiveness on hirutism and may shorten the interval until a treatment effect becomes evident *(64)*. Nausea, breast tenderness, and weight gain are some of the reported side effects of finasteride. Pregnancy should be avoided during treatment with finasteride. Although many clinicians employ finasteride treatment in cases of severe hirsutism, we believe that owing to lack of evidence its use should be avoided in adolescents.

GnRH Analogues

Prolonged administration of GnRH analogues results in a down regulation of gonadotropin production and in subsequent hypogonadotrophic hypogonadism. This effectively reduces ovarian androgen production and clinical signs of hyperandrogenism *(65)*. Besides their high expense, these drugs need to be administered in conjunction with an COC or add-back estrogen therapy, as their prolonged use leads to signs and symptoms of ovarian failure *(65,66)*. In general, because of their cost and the resultant hypoestrogenism, their use in adolescents should be avoided.

Progestins

Adolescents whose main complaint is menstrual disturbance, without evident hirsutism or other manifestation of androgen excess, may be managed with progestins only, administered on a cyclical basis, for 14 days every month, in order to ensure regular withdrawal bleeding. Medroxyprogesterone acetate 5–10 mg, nortehisterone acetate 5 mg, dydrogesterone 10 mg, or micronized progesterone 100–200 mg daily may be used for this purpose. This therapy confers protection against endometrial hyperplasia and cancer as a result of prolonged estrogenic stimulation. The perimenarcheal girl can be maintained on a schedule of approx 6-week cycles to permit detection of spontaneous menses *(57)*. Adverse effects of progestins include depression, bloating, and breast tenderness. Hormonal disturbances, however, such as insulin resistance and hyperandrogenemia are not corrected by this mode of treatment *(67)*.

Insulin Sensitizers

Since it became evident that insulin resistance is a cardinal abnormality in PCOS, leading to hyperandrogenemia and metabolic abnormalities, efforts have been made to implement drugs that lower insulin resistance in the treatment of PCOS. Two pharmacologically distinct groups of drugs are currently available in the market: biguanides, with metformin as the principle agent, and thiazolidinediones, with roziglitazone and pioglitazone as the main representatives. Metformin has been increasingly used in the treatment of PCOS, whereas the latter compounds, being newer on the market, have not yet been extensively studied.

1. *Metformin.* Metformin has been widely used in women with PCOS. In the dose range of 500 to 2.550 mg daily, metformin reduces hyperandrogenemia, increases SHBG levels and improves hirsutism *(68–72)*. Metformin can also decrease the augmented response of steroidogenic enzymes to LH and ACTH in the ovaries and adrenals, respectively *(23)*. Clinically these effects translate into a reduction in the hirsutism score. Moreover, metformin is reported to reduce body weight in obese subjects with PCOS, an effect that adds to the primary effect of the drug on improving insulin resistance. Lean subjects also benefit from metformin therapy, as insulin resistance is an inherent characteristic in PCOS and is present independently of obesity *(23)*. In contrast to COC, metformin is reported to improve the deranged lipid profile commonly encountered in women with PCOS *(75)*. Finally, metformin reduces fasting insulin levels and the incidence of impaired glucose tolerance and type 2 diabetes, which are increased in patients with PCOS *(23,70)*. Direct comparison of metformin to COC containing EE/CPA has shown that although COC treatment may be more effective in reducing hyperandrogenic signs and symptoms, metformin treatment is superior with respect to weight reduction, restoration of waist-to-hip ratio and correction of hyper-insulinemia *(50,73)*.

   Metformin as a monotherapy is reported to restore ovulation and regular menses in a substantial proportion of treated women, a very important issue in cases where fertility is of primary interest *(70,74)*. Metformin can increase the rate of spontaneous pregnancies, either alone or in combination with clomiphene citrate *(75)*. Moreover metformin is reported to decrease the rate of first trimester miscarriages *(76)* and the incidence of gestational diabetes mellitus, conditions that frequently occur in women with PCOS. Metformin is classified as a category B drug, meaning that no teratogenic potential has been demonstrated in animal models, and thus it can be safely used throughout pregnancy *(77)*.

   During the past decade, metformin has also been used in adolescents with PCOS. Although the series are small and the follow-up intervals of short duration, all available data indicate that metformin in adolescents improves menstrual cyclicity, restores the ovulation rate, and reduces body weight in girls under hypocaloric diet *(78)*. In a small group of nonobese adolescent girls with premature pubarche and PCOS, metformin reduced hyperinsulinemia, hirsutism, and hyperandrogenism, attenuated the LH and 17-OH progesterone response to stimulation by GnRH agonists, improved the lipid profile and restored normal menses *(17)*. Recently, metformin was also shown to attenuate the augmented 17α-hydroxyprogesterone response to ACTH stimulation, reducing thus the functional adrenal hyperandrogenism present in PCOS *(23)*.

   Metformin therapy is generally well tolerated, and only in a minority of patients causes gastrointestinal discomfort and diarrhea. These symptoms usually are self-limited and can be avoided by starting with a low dose and gradually increasing the dosage. Lactic acidosis is an extremely rare condition and its occurrence is in large part limited to patients with liver or renal dysfunction; liver and function testing are therefore mandatory before the initiation of metformin therapy. Finally, the very low cost of metformin adds a practical advantage for the long-term treatment of PCOS.

2. *Thiazolidinediones.* Thiazolidinediones belong to a class of agents with insulin-sensitizing activity, acting through a postreceptor mechanism in muscles and adipose

tissue. Troglitazone, the first representative of this group was withdrawn from the market because of liver toxicity. The newer compounds, roziglitazone and pioglitazone, have not been associated with any significant toxicity. Thiazolidinediones are reported to lower androgen and insulin levels, improve hirsutism and restore ovulation in women with PCOS *(79–81)*. Recent reports suggest that both rozilglitazone and pioglitazone reduce baseline and stimulated insulin concentrations and normalize menstrual cyclicity *(82–85)*. Thiazolidinediones are classified as class C drugs with potential teratogenicity during the first trimester of pregnancy. Therefore, pregnancy should be avoided when using these drugs.

ANTIOBESITY DRUGS

When dietetic treatment is not sufficient, medical therapy aimed at reducing the amount of daily caloric intake may improve outcomes. Orlistat is a nonabsorbable drug that inhibits intestinal absorption of fatty acids. Compared with placebo, orlistat-treated patients displayed a 3% greater reduction in weight after 1 year of observation *(86)*. Sibutramine is a newer compound belonging to the selective serotonin reuptake inhibitors family. It acts in the central nervous system to reduce appetite. It has been recently used successfully in adolescents, leading to 8.5% weight reduction compared with 4% with diet alone *(87)*. More data are warranted to document the long-term safety of these drugs in adolescents.

CONCLUSION

Polycystic ovary disease is one of the most prevalent disorders with endocrine and metabolic implications. It usually presents with menstrual irregularities and signs of androgen excess such as hirsutism and acne. Its main endocrine abnormality is insulin resistance, which in the long term may lead to type 2 diabetes and cardiovascular morbidity. Early recognition and prompt treatment in adolescents is essential for preventing long-term sequellae. Menstrual irregularities during the first postmenarchal years should not be considered as benign, unless an endocrine-metabolic evaluation is normal. The reduction of insulin resistance should be one of the main therapeutic goals. Weight reduction and life style modification are essential and should always accompany any treatment modality, especially in the critical life period of adolescence. Metformin is the most widely used insulin reducing agent, with good results and few side effects.

FUTURE AVENUES

PCOS is most probably due to more than one genetic defects associated to environmental disturbances. Thus, knowing the specific involvement of the etiology-related genes will lead to specific cause-targeting medical interventions by employing new techniques such as proteomics to a vast extent. Therapeutic interventions should target the early life of the affected individuals starting eventually *in utero* or even preconceptually.

KEY POINTS

- Metabolic disturbances in adolescent with PCOS. There is increased prevalence of impaired glucose tolerance and β-cell dysfunction in adolescents with PCOS independently of obesity. Because adolescents with PCOS are at risk for dyslipedemia, cardiovascular disease, and diabetes mellitus, a fasting lipid profile and an OGTT would be necessary, especially for the obese patients.

- Therapeutic goals in PCOS. Weight reduction applies to all obese women with PCOS. In general, the ideal treatment should normalize menses, restore ovulation and fertility, reduce hirsutism and acne, improve lipid profile and glucose utilization, and, thus, reduce the cardiovascular risk. Most therapeutic modalities target at reducing androgen production from the ovaries and androgen action at the receptor level. During the last years, insulin sensitizers have been increasingly used in the treatment of PCOS with promising results in both endocrine and metabolic aspects of the syndrome.
- Nonpharmacological treatment. It includes weight reduction, exercise, and cosmetic treatment.
- COCs. COCs have been the mainstay of treatment of menstrual and dermatological problems associated with PCOS for many years. In mild or moderate cases of PCOS, as it is the case in most of adolescent PCOS girls, COC combinations with third generation progestins, such as desogestrel, have been used in the treatment of PCOS. These COC are equally effective in reducing clinical and biochemical signs of PCOS as compared to antiandrogen (cyproterone acetate)-containing COC.
- Flutamide, finasteride. Although many clinicians employ these pharmaceutical agents as antiandrogen treatment in cases of severe hirsutism, we believe that because of lack of evidence their use should be avoided in adolescents.
- GnRH analogues. In general, because of their cost and the resulting hypoestrogenism, their use in adolescents should be avoided.

REFERENCES

1. Diamanti-Kandarakis E, Kouli CR, Bergiele AT, et al. A survey of the polycystic ovary syndrome in the greek island of Lesbos: hormonal and metabolic pofile. J Clin Endocrinol Metab 1999;84:4006–4011.
2. Ehrmann DA. Obesity and glucose intolerance in androgen excess. In: Azziz R, Nestler JE, Dewailley D, eds. Androgen Excess Disorders in Women. Philadelphia, PA: Lipincott-Raven, 1997, pp. 705–712.
3. Legro RS. Polycystic ovary syndrome. Phenotype to genotype. Endocrinol Metab Clin North Am 1999;28:379–396.
4. Franks S, Gharani N, McCarthy M. Genetic abnormalities in polycystic ovary syndrome. Ann Endocrinol (Paris) 1999;60:131–133.
5. Apter D, Butzow T, Laughlin GA, Yen SS. Accelerated 24-hour LH pulsatile activity in adolescent girls with ovarian hyperandrogenism: relevance to the developmental phase of polycystic ovarian syndrome. J Clin Endocrinol Metab 1994;79:119–125.
6. Homburg R, Lambalk CB. Polycystic ovary syndrome in adolescence: a therapeutic conundrum. Hum Reprod 2004;19:1–4.
7. van Hooff MH, Voorhorst FJ, Kaptein MB, Hirasing RA, Koppenaal C, Schoemaker J. Polycystic ovaries in adolescents and the relationship with menstrual cycle patterns, luteninizing hormone, androgens, and insulin. Fertil Steril 2000;74:49–58.
8. van Hooff MH, Voorhorst FJ, Kaptein MB, Hirasing RA, Koppenaal C, Schoemaker J. Endocrine features of polycystic ovary syndrome in a random population sample of 14-16 year old adolescents. Hum Reprod 1999;14:2223–2239.
9. Avvad CK, Holeuwerger R, Silva VCG, Bordallo MAN, Breitenbach MMD. Menstrual irregularity in the first postmenarchal years: an early clinical sign of polycystic ovary syndrome in adolescence. Gynecol Endocrinol 2001;15:170–177.
10. Herter LD, Magalhaes JA, Spritzer PM. Relevance of the determination of ovarian volume in adolescent girls with menstrual disorders. J Clin Ultrasound 1996;24:243–248.
11. Venturoli S, Porcu E, Fabbri R, et al. Longitudinal change of sonographic ovarian aspects and endocrine parameters in irregular cycles of adolescence. Pediatr Res 1995;38:974–980.
12. Apter D, Butzow T, Laughlin GA, Yen SS. Metabolic features of polycystic ovary syndrome are found in adolescent girls with hyperandrogenism. J Clin Endocrinol Metab 1995;80:2966–2973.

13. Miller WL. The molecular basis of premature adrenarche: an hypothesis. Acta Paediatr Suppl 1999; 88:60–66.

14. Zhang LH, Rodriguez H, Ohno S, Miller WL. Serine phosphorylation of human P450c17 increases 17,20-lyase activity: implications for adrenarche and the polycystic ovary syndrome. Proc Natl Acad Sci USA 1995;92:10,619–10,623.

15. Dunaif A, Xia J, Book CB, Schenker E, Tang Z. Excessive insulin receptor serine phosphorylation in cultured fibroblasts and in skeletal muscle. A potential mechanism for insulin resistance in the polycystic ovary syndrome. J Clin Invest 1995;96:801–810.

16. Kent SC, Legro RS. Polycystic ovary syndrome in adolescents. Adolesc Med 2002;13:73–88.

17. Ibanez L, Vall C, Potau N, Marcus MV, de Zegher F. Sensitization to insulin in adolescent girls to normalize hirsutism, hyperandrogenism, oligomenorrhea and hyperinsulinism after precocious pubarche. J Clin Endocrinol Metab 2000;85:3526–3530.

18. Brigdes NA, Cooke A, Healy MR, Hindmarsh PC, Brook CGD. Standards of ovarian volume in childhood and puberty. Fertil Steril 1993;60:456–460.

19. Dramusic V, Rajan U, Chan P, Ratnam SS, Wong YC. Adolescent polycystic ovary syndrome. Ann N Y Acad Sci 1997;816:194–208.

20. Silfen ME, Denburg MR, Manibo AM, et al. Early endocrine, metabolic, and sonographic characteristics of polycystic ovary syndrome (PCOS): comparison between nonobese and obese adolescents. J Clin Endocrinol Metab 2003;88:4682–4688.

21. Koivunen RM, Morin-Papunen LC, Ruokonen A, Tapanainen JS, Martikainen HK. Ovarian steroidogenic response to human chorionic gonadotrophin in obese women with polycystic ovary syndrome. Hum Reprod 2001;16:2546–2551.

22. Nestler JE, Jakubowicz DJ. Lean women with polycystic ovary syndrome respond to isulin reduction with decreases in ovarian P450c17α activity and serum androgens. J Clin Endocrinol Metab 1997; 82:4075–4079.

23. Arslanian SA, Lewy V, Danadian K, Saad R. Metformin therapy in obese adolescents with polycystic ovary syndrome and impaird glucose tolerance: amelioration of exaggerated adrenal response to adrenocorticotropin with reduction of insulinemia/insulin resistance. J Clin Endocrinol Metab 2002;87:1555–1559.

24. Adams J, Polson DW, Abdulwahid N. Multifollicular ovaries: clinical and endocrine features and response to gonadotropin releasing hormone. Lancet 1985;2:1375–1378.

25. Polson DW, Wadsworth J, Adams J. Polycystic ovaries – a common finding in normal women. Lancet 1988;1:870–872.

26. Palmert MR, Gordon CM, Kartashov AI, Legro RS, Emans SJ, Dunaif A. Screening for abnormal glucose tolerance in adolescents with polycystic ovary syndrome. J Clin Endocrinol Metab 2001;87: 1017–1023.

27. Arslanian SA, Lewy VD, Danadian K. Glucose intolerance in obese adolescents with polycystic ovary syndrome: roles of insulin resistance and β-cell dysfunction and risk of cardiovascular disease. J Clin Endocrinol Metab 2001;86:66–71.

28. Lewy VD, Danadian K, Witchel SF, Arslanian S. Early metabolic abnormalities in adolescent girls with polycystic ovarian syndrome. J Pediatr 2001;138:38–44.

29. Pasquali R, Gambineri A, Antocetani B, et al. The natural history of metabolic syndrome 18 and the effect of long-term oestrogen-progestogen treatment. Clin Endocrinol (Oxf) 1999;50:517–527.

30. Conway GS, Agrawal R, Betteridge DJ, Jacobs HS. Risk factors for coronary artery disease in lean and obese women with the polycystic ovary syndrome. Clin Endocrinol (Oxf)1992;37:119–125.

31. Robinson S, Henderson AD, Gelding SV, et al. Dyslipidemia is associated with insulin resistance in women with polycystic ovaries. Clin Endocrinol (Oxf) 1996;44:277–284.

32. Mastorakos G, Koliopoulos K, Creatsas G. Androgen and lipid profiles in adolescents with polycystic ovary syndrome who were treated with two forms of combined oral contraceptives. Fertil Steril 2002;77:919–927.

33. Norman RJ, Masters SC, Hague W, Beng C, Pannall P, Wang IX. Metabolic approaches to the subclassification of the polycystic ovary syndrome. Fertil Steril 1995;63:329–335.

34. Wild RA. Obesity, lipids, cardiovascular risk and androgen excess. Am J Med 1995;98:27S–32S.

35. Balfour JA, McClellan K. Topical eflornithine. Am J Clin Dermatol 2001;2:197–201.

36. Vexiau P, Chaspoux C, Boudou P, et al. Effects of minoxidil 2% vs. cyproterone acetate treatment on female androgenetic alopecia: a controlled, 12-month randomized trial. Br J Dermatol 2002;146:992.

37. Murphy AA, Cropp CS, Smith BS, Burkman RT, Zacar HA. Effect of low dose oral contraceptive on gonadotropins, androgens and sex hormone binding globulin in non-hirsute women. Fertil Steril 1990;53:35–39.
38. Dewis P, Petsos P, Newman M, Anderson DC. The treatment of hirsutism with a combination of desogestrel and ethinyl oestradiol. Clin Endocrinol 1985;22:29–36.
39. Miller JA, Jacobs HS. Treatment of hirsutism and acne with cyproterone acetate. Cin Endocrinol Metab 1986;15:373–389.
40. Falsetti L, Dordoni D, Gastaldi C, Gastaldi A. A new association of ethinylestradiol (0.035mg) cyproterone acetate (2mg) in the therapy of polycystic ovary syndrome. Acta Eur Fertil 1986;17:19–25.
41. Falsetti L, Gambera A, Tisi G. Efficacy of the combination ethinyl oestradiol and cyproterone acetate on endocrine, clinical and ultrasonographic profile in polycystic ovarian syndrome. Hum Reprod 2001;16:36–42.
42. Prelevic GM, Wurzburger MI, Balint-Peric L, Puzigaca Z. Effects of a low-dose estrogen-antiandrogen combination (Diane-35) on clinical signs of androgenization, hormone profile and ovarian size in patients with polycystic ovary syndrome. Gynecol Endocrinol 1989;3:269–280.
43. Creatsas G, Koliopoulos C, Mastorakos G. Combined oral contraceptive treatment of adolescent girls with polycystic ovary syndrome. Lipid profile. Ann NY Acad Sci 2000;900:245–252.
44. Guido M, Romualdi D, Giuliani M, et al. Drospirenone for the treatment of hirsute women with polycystic ovary syndrome: a clinical, endocrinological, metabolic pilot study. J Clin Endocrinol Metab 2004;89:2817–2823.
45. Thorneycroft H, Gollnick H, Schellschmidt I. Superiority of a combined contraceptive containing drospirenone to a triphasic preparation containing norgestimate in acne treatment. Cutis 2004;74: 123–130.
46. Thorneycroft IH. Evolution of progestins. Focus on the novel progestin drospirenone. J Reprod Med 2002;47:975–980.
47. van Vloten WA, van Haselen CW, van Zuuren EJ, Gerlinger C, Heithecker R. The effect of 2 combined oral Contraceptives containing either drospirenone or cyproterone acetate on acne and seborrhea. Cutis 2002;69:2–15.
48. Palep-Singh M, Mook K, Barth J, Balen A. An observational study of Yasmin in the management of women with polycystic ovary syndrome. J Fam Plann Reprod Health Care 2004;30:163–165.
49. Cibula D, Hill M, Fanta M, Sindelka G, Zinvy J. Does obesity diminish the positive effect of oral contraceptive treatment on hyperandrogenism in women with polycystic ovarian syndrome? Hum Reprod 2001;16:940–944.
50. Morin-Papunen L, Vauhkonen I, Koivunen R, Ruokonen A, Martikainen H, Tapanainen JS. Metformin versus ethinyl estradiol-cyproterone acetate in the treatment of nonobese women with polycystic ovary syndrome: a randomized study. J Clin Endocrinol Metab 2003;88:148–156.
51. Falsetti L, Pasinetti E. Effects of long: term administration of an oral contraceptive containing ethinylestrdiol and cyproterone acetate on lipid metabolism in women with polycystic ovary syndrome. Acta Obstet Gynecol Scand 1995;74:56–60.
52. Prelevic GM, Wurzburger MI, Trpkovic D, Balint-Peric L. Effects of a low-dose estrogen–antiandrogen combination (Diane-35) on lipid and carbohydrate metabolism in patients with polycystic ovary syndrome. Gynecol Endocrinol 1990;4:157–168.
53. Godsland IF, Crook D, Simpson R, et al. The effects of different formulations of oral contraceptive agents on lipid and carbohydrate metabolism. N Engl J Med 1990;323:1375–1381.
54. Korytkowski MT, Mokan M, Horwitz MJ, Berga SL. Metabolic effects of oral contraceptives in women with polycystic ovary syndrome. J Clin Endocrinol Metab 1995;80:3327–3334.
55. Gaspard U, Scheen A, Endrikat J, et al. A randomized study over 13 cycles to assess the influence of oral contraceptives containing ethinylestradiol combined with drospirenone or desogestrel on carbohydrate metabolism. Contraception 2003;67:423–429.
56. Ludicke F, Gaspard UJ, Demeyer F, Scheen A, Lefebvre P. Randomized controlled study of the influence of two low estrogen dose oral contraceptives containing gestodene or desogestrel on carbohydrate metabolism. Contraception 2002;66:411–415.
57. Buggs C, Rosenfield RL. Polycystic ovary syndrome in adolescence. Endocrinol Metab Clin N Am 2005;34:677–705.
58. Dawber RPR, Sinclair RD. Hirsuties. Clin Dermatol 2001;19:189–199.
59. Barth JH, Cherry CA, Wojnarowska F, Dawber RP. Cyproterone acteate for severe hirsutism. J Clin Endocrinol Metab 1991;35:5–10.

60. Venturoli S, Paradisi R, Bagnoli A, et al. Low-dose flutamide (125mg/day) as maintenance therapy in the treatment of hirsutism. Horm Res 2001;56:25–31.
61. Spritzer PM, Lisboa KO, Mattielo S, Lhullier F. Spironolactone as a single agent for long-term therapy of hirsute patients. Clin Endocrinol (Oxf) 2000;52:587–594.
62. Barth JH, Cherry CA, Wojnaroswka F, Dawber RP. Spironolactone is an effective and well tolerated systemic antiandrogen therapy for hirsute women. J Clin Endocrinol Metab 1989;68:966–970.
63. Wong IL, Morris RS, Chang L, Spahn MA, Stanczyk FZ, Lobo RA. A prospective randomized trial comparing finasteride to spironolactone in the treatment of hirsute women. J Clin Endocrinol Metab 1995;80:233–238.
64. Tartagni M, Schonauer LM, De Salvia MA, Cicinelli E, De Pergola G, D´Addario V. Comparison of Diane 35 and Diane 35 plus finasteride in the treatment of hirsutism. Fertil Steril 2000;73:718–723.
65. De Leo V, Fulghesu AM, la Marca A, et al. Hormonal and clinical effects of GnRH agonist alone, or in combination with a combined oral contraceptive or flutamide in women with severe hirsutism. Gynecol Endocrinol 2000;14:411–416.
66. Castelo-Branco C, Martinez de Osaba MJ, Pons F, Fortuny A. Gonadotropin-releasing hormone analog plus an oral contraceptive containing desogestrel in women with severe hirsutism: effects on hair, bone, and hormone profile after 1-year use. Metabolism 1997;46:437–440.
67. Kahn JA, Gordon CM. Polycystic ovary syndrome. Adolesc Med 1999;10:321–336.
68. Armstrong VL, Wiggam MI, Ennis CN, et al. Insulin action and insulin secretion in polycystic ovary syndrome treated with ethinyl oestradiol / cyproterone acetate. QJM 2001;94:31–37.
69. Diamanti-Kandarakis E, Zapanti E. Insulin sensitizers and antiandrogens in the treatment of polycystic ovary syndrome. Ann NY Acad Sci 2000;900:203–212.
70. Pasquali R, Gambineri A, Biscotti D, et al. Effect of long-term treatment with metformin added to hypocaloric diet on body composition, fat distribution and androgen and insulin levels in abdominally obese women with and without the polycystic ovary syndrome. J Clin Endocrinol Metab 2000;85: 2767–2774.
71. Moghetti P, Castello R, Negri C, et al. Metformin effects on clinical features, endocrine and metabolic profiles, and insulin sensitivity in polycystic ovary syndrome: a randomized, double-blind, placebo-controlled 6-month trial, followed by open, long-term clinical evaluation. J Clin Endocrinol Metab 2000;85:139–146.
72. Loverro G, Lorusso F, De Pergola G, Nicolardi V, Mei L, Selvaggi L. Clinical and endocrinological effects of 6 months of metformin treatment in young hyperinsulinemic patients affected by polycystic ovary syndrome. Gynecol Endocrinol 2002;16:217–224.
73. Harborne L, Fleming R, Lyall H, Sattar N, Norman J. Metformin or antiandrogen in the treatment of hirsutism in polycystic ovary syndrome. J Clin Endocrinol Metab 2003;88:4116–4123.
74. Heard MJ, Pierce A, Carson SA, Buster JE. Pregnancies following use of metformin for ovulation induction in patients with polycystic ovary syndrome. Fertil Steril 2002;77:669–673.
75. Vandermolen DT, Ratts VS, Evans WS, Stovall DW, Kauma SW, Nestler JE. Metformin increases the ovulatory rate and pregnancy rate from clomiphene citrate in patients with polycystic ovary syndrome who are resistant to clomiphene citrate alone. Fertil Steril 2001;75:310–315.
76. Glueck CJ, Wang P, Kobayashi S, Phillips H, Sieve-Smith L. Metformin therapy throughout pregnancy reduces the development of gestational diabetes in women with polycystic ovary syndrome. Fertil Steril 2002;77:520–525.
77. Glueck CJ, Philips H, Cameron D, Sieve Smith L, Wang P. Continuing metformin throughout pregnancy in women with polycystic ovary syndrome appears to safely reduce first-trimester spontaneous abortion: a pilot study. Fertil Steril 2001;75:46–52.
78. Glueck CCJ, Wang P, Fontaine R, Tracy T, Sieve-Smith L. Metformin to restore normal menses in oligo-amenorrheic teenage girls with polycystic ovary syndrome (PCOS). J Adolesc Health 2001;29:160–169.
79. Azziz R, Ehrman D, Legro R, et al. Troglitazone improves ovulation and hirsutism in the polycystic ovary syndrome: a multicenter, double blind, placebo-controlled trial. J Clin Endocrinol Metab 2001;86:1626–1632.
80. Cataldo NA, Abbasi F, McLaughlin TL, Lamendola C, Reaven GM. Improvement in insulin sensitivity followed by ovulation and pregnancy in a woman with polycystic ovary syndrome who was treated with rosiglitazone. Fertil Steril 2001;76:1057–1059.
81. Ehrmann DA, Schneider DJ, Sobel BE, Cavaghan MK, Imperial J, Rosenfield RL, et al. Troglitazone improves defects in insulin action, insulin secretion, ovarian steroidogenesis and fibriolysis in women with polycystic ovary syndrome. J Clin Endocrinol Metab 1997;82:2108–2116.

82. Belli SH, Graffigna MN, Oneto A, Otero P, Schurman L, Levalle OA. Effect of rosiglitazone on insulin resistance, growth factors, and reproductive disturbances in women with polycystic ovary syndrome. Fertil Steril 2004;81:624–629.

83. Sepilian V, Nagamani M. Effects of rosiglitazone in obese women with polycystic ovary syndrome and severe insulin resistance. J Clin Endocrinol Metab 2005;90:60–65.

84. Baillargeon JP, Jakubowicz DJ, Iuorno MJ, Jakubowicz S, Nestler JE. Effects of metformin and rosiglitazone, alone and in combination, in nonobese women with polycystic ovary syndrome and normal indices of insulin sensitivity. Fertil Steril 2004;82:893–902.

85. Brettenthaler N, De Geyter C, Huber PR, Keller U. Effect of the insulin sensitizer pioglitazone on insulin resistance, hyperandrogenism, and ovulatory dysfunction in women with polycystic ovary syndrome. J Clin Endocrinol Metab 2004;89:3835–3840.

86. Padwal R, Li SK, Lau DC. Long-term pharmacotherapy for overweight and obesity: a systematic review and meta-analysis of randomized controlled trials. Int J Obes Relat Metab Disord 2003;27:1437–1446.

87. Berkowitz RI, Wadden TA, Tershakovec AM, Cronquist JL. Behavior Therapy and sibutramine for the treatment of adolescent obesity. JAMA 2003;289:1805–1812.

27 Pharmaceutical Intervention in Metabolic and Cardiovascular Risk Factors in Polycystic Ovary Syndrome

Evanthia Diamanti-Kandarakis, MD, PhD

CONTENTS

INTRODUCTION
INSULIN SENSITIZING AGENTS
ANTIANDROGENS
PHARMACEUTICAL INTERVENTION IN WEIGHT REDUCTION
 AND ITS EFFECT IN METABOLIC AND CARDIOVASCULAR RISKS
ORAL CONTRACEPTIVE PILLS
SUMMARY AND CONCLUSIONS
FUTURE AVENUES OF INVESTIGATION
KEY POINTS
REFERENCES

Summary

Polycystic ovary syndrome (PCOS) is the most common endocrinopathy of women in reproductive age, its prevalence internationally ranges between 6 and 8%. This syndrome is characterized by anovulation, hyperandrogenism, and frequently, insulin resistance (IR).

The past decade, the central importance of IR in the pathogenesis of this syndrome has been established, by pioneering elegant studies. Subsequently, in addition to the known hormonal and reproductive abnormalities characterizing this disorder, morbidities such as the enhanced risk for type 2 diabetes and an increased number of cardiovascular risk factors were revealed.

Therefore, current therapeutic approaches justifiably include insulin sensitising agents, promising to comfort women with PCOS from some of their sorrows, because the role of IR and hyperinsulinemia appear to contribute to the whole clinical spectrum of this multifaceted disorder. In comparison to oral contraceptives and antiandrogens, which are the widely accepted therapeutic modalities, the management with insulin sensitizers appears to embrace beneficially, in a global way several aspects of the syndrome and in particular the metabolic, vascular and cardiovascular aberrations.

Key Words: Insulin sensitizers; PCOS; metformin; thiazolinediones; orlistat; sibutramine.

From: *Contemporary Endocrinology: Insulin Resistance and Polycystic Ovarian Syndrome:
Pathogenesis, Evaluation, and Treatment*
Edited by: E. Diamanti-Kandarakis, J. E. Nestler, D. Panidis, and R. Pasquali © Humana Press Inc., Totowa, NJ

INTRODUCTION

The syndrome was initially described in 1935 by Stein and Levental as an infertility disorder in obese women. The etiology of polycystic ovary syndrome (PCOS) is unknown but current knowledge support the notion that there is interaction between environmental and genetic factors. Its pathogenesis remains controversial. It seems to implicate enzymatic abnormalities in ovarian and adrenal steroidogenesis as well as abnormalities in insulin secretion and action.

For many decades, infertility was the major concern between scientists and patients but the metabolic aberrations, apart from obesity, had received very little attention. Since insulin receptors were discovered on ovarian components and it was shown that hyperandrogenemia was positively correlated with hyperinsulinemia (1), the syndrome revealed the hidden multifaceted sides of its metabolic characteristics.

It is of particular clinical significance that in PCOS, the most common endocrinopathy (2,3), the metabolic syndrome, is several folds more common than in women of the same age and body weight (4).

There are studies suggesting that women with PCOS have a higher risk for development of type 2 diabetes mellitus (T2DM) and cardiovascular disease (CVD) (5). Prospective studies in United States revealed a 31–35% prevalence of impaired glucose tolerance and a 7.5–10% prevalence of T2DM in obese PCOS women by their fourth decade (5,6). These findings may even be present in younger women with PCOS (7), as it has been published recently in a Cohort study in Europe, from Mediterranean region. A 15.7 and 2.5% prevalence of impaired glucose tolerance and T2DM, respectively, was demonstrated in relatively young PCOS women (8). Furthermore, several investigators have shown that, in PCOS women, without intervention there is a substantial rate of conversion from normoglycaemia to impaired glucose tolerance or to T2DM over the time (9).

Women with the syndrome have also an increased prevalence of several cardiovascular risk factors including hyperinsulinemia, hypertension (10,11), and dyslipidemia (low high-density lipoproteins [HDL], high TG, high low-density lipoproteins [LDL]) (12).

Endothelial dysfunction, an early step in atherosclerotic process, is also present manifested by increased levels of endothelin-1 (13) and decreased vasodilatory capacity (14,15). Furthermore, imaging studies identified increased carotid intimal media thickness in middle and young aged women (16) and increased coronary artery calcification (17).

PCOS is also associated with dysfibrinolisis, elevated plasma levels of plasminogen activator inhibitor (PAI)-1 (18,19), and increased markers of chronic inflammation such as C-reactive protein (CRP) (20), interleukin (IL)-18, and homocysteine levels.

All these findings are indicative of an underling vascular dysfunction, but the definite risk of CVD is not known yet, because no prospective longitudinal studies have been conducted. However, it has been estimated that PCOS women have four- to sevenfold greater risk of myocardial infraction than normal women (10).

It is widely accepted that PCOS is not only a cosmetic annoyance or an infertility disorder, but also a metabolic problem with, probably, long-term consequences on women's health. The following chapter will focus on the pharmaceutical interventions, single agents as well as in combination, in the metabolic abnormalities and cardiovascular risk factors.

In PCOS management regarding the metabolic abnormalities, new therapeutic tools, such as insulin sensitizing, and weight reduction agents have been tried and shown to have beneficial effects on several metabolic aspects of the syndrome, although the classical treatment such as oral contraceptives with or without antiandrogens, appear to have contradictory effects on these parameters and are not considered primarily for the management of these abnormalities.

INSULIN SENSITIZING AGENTS

Insulin sensitizers are the group of therapeutic agents, promising to comfort women with PCOS from some of their sorrows, because the role of insulin resistance (IR) and hyperinsulinemia appear to be major contributors to the pathophysiology of the syndrome. It is a new therapeutic approach targeting to improve IR and aiming to modify the effect of hyperinsulinemia not only on classical insulin sensitive tissues but in the ovarian tissue as well.

In this chapter, we will focus only on the metabolic aspects of the syndrome, which although they are not universally present, they possibly play a significant role in the short as well as in the long term sequelae of the syndrome.

There are two families of insulin sensitizing agents that have been used in clinical trials for the management of PCOS. One is the family of biguanides and in particular metformin and the other one the family of thiazolidinediones (TZDs): troglitazone, rosiglitazone, and pioglitazone, for which the data are less but steadily increasing.

Metformin

PHARMACOLOGY

Metformin is a biguanide agent that has been used in the treatment of T2DM. It lowers blood glucose levels by reducing significantly the hepatic glucose production and by increasing peripheral glucose utilization. It lowers serum insulin levels and improves insulin sensitivity not only by its glucose lowering effect but also by increasing insulin binding to its receptor. Moreover, the drug appears to enter in the cells and enhance the tyrosine phosphorylation of the intracellular portion of β-subunit of the insulin receptor and of insulin receptor substrate proteins *(21)*.

Recently, it has been suggested that insulin receptor substrate proteins genotype may modulate the response to metformin treatment in PCOS women *(22)*.

EFFECTS ON CARBOHYDRATE METABOLISM

A number of studies have been published investigating the effect of metformin on IR in women with PCOS. The first study was by Velazquez et al. *(23)* published in United States. In this study it was found that metformin treatment in 26 obese PCOS women for 2 months reduced hyperinsulinemia, systolic blood pressure, and improved hormonal and reproductive abnormalities as well. In Europe, the first study was in 1998 and confirmed the increase in insulin sensitivity (glucose utilization rate) using the euglycemic clamp, irrespectively of the changes in body weight, after administration of 1700 mg metformin for 6 months in 13 obese PCOS women *(24)*. A reduction in fasting glucose and insulin levels after treatment with metformin was reported by investigators in both obese *(25)* and non-obese PCOS women.

More recently, it has been reported a significant improvement in insulin levels in non-obese PCOS women treated with metformin compared with obese ones *(26)*. In a meta-analysis of 13 controlled studies, in different ethnic populations, it was confirmed that metformin has a significant effect in reducing fasting insulin levels, associated with a small reduction of fasting glucose *(27)*. However, some studies did not report beneficial results *(28)*.

It has been suggested that the administration of metformin in extremely obese PCOS women has no effect on IR. The reason for the partly conflicting results is not known, but is possible that severe obesity is a confounding factor and that only certain PCOS groups respond, predicting factors have not as yet been identified.

Women with PCOS commonly have IR are older and more obese than the general population at conception, which are known risk factors for gestational diabetes. In some studies, it has been shown that women with PCOS develop gestational diabetes more often than healthy women, 20 vs 8.9%. Interestingly, Glueck et al. showed that metformin therapy in PCOS women during pregnancy (2.55 g/d), reduces the rate of gestational diabetes mellitus by 10-fold *(29)*.

The previously listed findings remain to be confirmed by other investigators, because no randomized prospective trial has established the effectiveness of metformin for reducing the risk of gestational diabetes.

EFFECTS ON LIPIDS

Metformin has been shown to improve the lipid profile, mainly by increasing serum HDL cholesterol concentrations *(30,31)*. On the other hand, some other studies have shown only a negligible or no effect on lipids in women with PCOS *(23,28)*.

The mechanisms by which metformin improves the lipid profile are not clear. Metformin has been suggested to reduce lipid uptake or synthesis in the intestine and in the hepatocytes. The improvement of obesity and especially abdominal obesity with a subsequent decreased release of free fatty acids (FFAs) from adipose tissue observed during metformin therapy could also partly explain the improvement of lipid profile during metformin treatment, at least in obese women *(32)*.

EFFECTS ON ENDOTHELIUM

The presence of abnormal vascular function has been shown in PCOS by several investigators, the syndrome is associated with surrogate cardiovascular markers such as: increased serum levels of PAI-1 *(19)*, increased endothelin-1 levels *(13,15)*, elevated serum levels of CRP *(33)*, elevated plasma advanced glycation end-products levels (AGEs) *(34)*, endothelial dysfunction *(15,35)*, and echocardiographic abnormalities.

The pathophysiology remains unclear but a number of mechanisms could be implicated to link endothelial dysfunction with IR, including disturbances of subcellular signalling pathways to insulin action, or other potential unifying links such as oxidant stress, ET-1, renin–angiotensin system, and the secretion of hormones and cytokines by adipose tissue. Insulin sensitizers, therefore, have justifiably been tried in this group of abnormalities.

In a recent study *(15)*, the administration of 1700 mg metformin daily for 6 months in PCOS women normalized Endothelium-dependent FMD of the brachial artery (method for measurement of endothelial function) and at the same time decreased significantly ET-1 plasma levels.

The first study to examine the presence of low-grade chronic inflammatory markers in women with PCOS was by Kelly et al. in 2001. They showed for the first time that women with PCOS have significantly increased CRP concentrations relative to those in healthy women with normal menstrual cycle and normal androgens (20).

Metformin treatment, in addition to its beneficial effects on hormonal and metabolic parameters in obese and nonobese women with PCOS, has been associated with a significant decrease of serum CRP levels, indicating a decrease of the degree of low-grade inflammation.

Papunen et al. (36) in a randomized study administered metformin in both obese and lean PCOS women demonstrated a significant reduction in serum CRP levels by 31% in nonobese subjects and 56% in obese ones.

Diamanti et al. (37) showed in addition to other inflammatory factors, a significant reduction of CRP levels after 6 months of metformin administration (850 mg twice daily), an effect independent of body weight changes.

The levels of the adhesion molecules (AM), sIVAM-1, sVCAM-1, and sE-selectin in serum, reflect low-grade chronic inflammation of the endothelium. They independently predict coronary heart disease, T2D (38) and have been implicated as major contributors in atherogenic process.

The mechanisms of metformin's beneficial effect on CRP and AM are unknown but they could be direct or indirect via modification of insulin action.

An other interesting recent finding is that young women with PCOS have elevated potent atherogenic molecules such as AGEs. These molecules constitute a complex and heterogeneous group of compounds with diverse molecular structure and biological function. The most well-characterized AGE are N-ε-(carboxymethyl)lysine, pentosidine, 3-deoxyglucosone, and methylglyoxal, which are elevated in diabetes and have been correlated with molecular damage, oxidative stress, endothelial cell activation, and they have been implicated in long-term vascular sequelae in diabetics (39).

Recently, increased serum levels of AGES and their receptors (RAGE) have been found in young women with PCOS (34). Although the mechanism of this finding is not clear, it could be because of defected insulin action, via decreased PI3K activity induced clearence but also dietary composition may contribute to it, because they are also absorbed from food. Metformin administration, for 6 months, reduced but not normalized the AGE levels compared to pretreatment levels, this effect of metformin, if confirmed, could be of clinical significance in long-term sequelae of the syndrome (40).

COMBINED TREATMENT METFORMIN AND LIFESTYLE MODIFICATION

The combination of metformin with lifestyle modification has been advocated clinically as a more effective way of management in several aspects of the syndrome, however long-term studies are lacking. In a recent randomized, 48-week, placebo-controlled trial by Hoeger (41), 38 overweight or obese women with PCOS were randomly assigned to one of four groups: metformin, a lifestyle modification program with placebo, lifestyle modification with metformin, or placebo only. Weight loss continued in both lifestyle groups over the second half of the study, thus suggesting continued compliance with the lifestyle goals over the long term. The amount of weight loss with metformin alone approached that seen in the group that received specific lifestyle management instruction with placebo. Additionally, weight reduction seemed to be enhanced in the guided lifestyle intervention group when metformin was used in combination. Weight loss was approx 30% greater overall in the combined group than in the lifestyle modification group alone. They did not demonstrate group differences in AUC_{ins} after oral glucose load, although a general trend toward reduction was noted across time. Regarding glucose metabolism, however, either improvement or no deterioration in overall glucose metabolism was noted in all the subjects completing the treatment arms, whereas a deterioration of glucose status occurred in two subjects in the placebo group. This is one of the longest studies of combined therapy of modification in lifestyle and metformin in PCOS women, showing clearly that the combination is a more promising approach in the management of metabolic aspects of the syndrome.

In another trial, metformin (850 mg twice daily) plus a low-calorie diet was superior to a low-calorie diet alone in facilitating weight loss in both women with PCOS and obese women *(32)*.

SIDE EFFECTS OF METFORMIN

To assess the incidence of fatal and nonfatal lactic acidosis with metformin use compared to placebo and other glucose-lowering treatments in patients with T2DM, a search was performed of the Cochrane Controlled Trials Register and the Database of Abstracts of Reviews of Effectiveness, Medline (up to 11/2000), to identify all studies of metformin treatment from 1966 to November 2000 *(42)*. Pooled data from 176 comparative trials and cohort studies revealed no cases of fatal or nonfatal lactic acidosis in 35,619 patient-years of metformin use or in 30,002 patients-years in the non-metformin group.

About 10% of cases of lactic acidosis owing to metformin have occurred in patients after the intravenous administration of iodinated contrast agents. Therefore, the recommendation should be followed is that metformin should be discontin-ued 48 hours prior to any radiological procedure that involves intravenous administration of iodinated contrast material *(42)*.

CONCLUSION ON METFORMIN

The majority of studies controlled and uncontrolled in different ethnical groups, agree that metformin has a beneficial effect on IR, and on several cardiovascular risk factors in PCOS, regardless of the body weight changes. The effects of metformin, however are not universal in every woman with the syndrome and further more, there are not known as yet predicting factors of their response. Additionally the documentation of the presence of IR by different methods, does not appear to be a prerequisite for the treatment with metformin in PCOS, probably because the methods are not adequately sensitive to detect it *(43)* and because it is very likely that metformin works on several pathways besides insulin sensitization.

Interestingly, regarding metformin's effect on metabolism, the evidence that metformin may alter the outcome of gestation diabetes is an important one. One study has shown that metformin therapy throughout pregnancy prevents the development of gestational diabetes in women with PCOS *(29)*.

Finally, there are no long-term studies focusing specifically on the effects of metformin on lipid profile and other cardiovascular factors and our knowledge comes as complementary information from studies on other IR syndromes.

Thiazolidinediones

Pharmacology

TZDs include three drugs, troglitazone, rosiglitazone, and pioglitazone. They act by enhancing glucose uptake in adipose and muscle tissues. In comparison to the effect observed by metformin, TZDs increase more peripheral glucose uptake and decrease lesser hepatic glucose output. They improve insulin sensitivity and they decrease not only circulating insulin levels but also the release of FFA and TNF-α from adipose tissue. At cellular level they bind and activate the peroxisome proliferator activated receptor-γ and they induce transcription of genes that are involved in the glucose and lipid metabolism.

In PCOS women, the therapeutic effect of insulin sensitisers is mediated by the reduction of hyperinsulinemia, IR, and, consequently, by alteration of ovarian steroidogenesis. Moreover, an inhibitory effect in steroidogenesis has been demonstrated on humanized yeast cells and recently TZDs (rosiglitazone and pioglitazone) inhibited estradiol and testosterone production in cultured human ovarian cells *(44)*.

Effects of TZDs on Carbohydrate Metabolism

Troglitazone was the first of TZDs to become available for IR treatment in diabetes. However, because acute liver failure was linked to troglitazone in numerous reports, the drug was withdrawn from the market.

In 1996, Dunaif *(45)* was the first who studied the effects of troglitazone on metabolic profile in women with PCOS. Twenty-five women with PCOS were enrolled in a double-blind randomized 3-month trial of two doses (200 and 400 mg) of the insulin-sensitizing agent, troglitazone. Fasting and 2-hour post-75-g glucose load insulin levels, as well as integrated insulin responses to the glucose load, decreased significantly and insulin sensitivity assessed by a frequently sampled iv glucose tolerance test increased significantly.

The beneficial effects of troglitazone on glucose metabolism in PCOS women were also confirmed by Ehrmann a year later *(46)*. In 13 obese women with PCOS with impaired glucose tolerance, troglitazone (400 mg daily) was administrated for 12 weeks. An improvement in OGTT with concordant reduction in glycosylated hemoglobin and IR were observed.

Azziz et al. *(47)* in the largest prospective double blind trial, studied 410 women with PCOS, randomly assigned in placebo or troglitazone (150, 300, or 600 mg/day), for 44 weeks of treatment and showed that troglitazone improved IR in PCOS in a dose-related fashion, with a minimum of adverse effects.

The other two TZDs, rosiglitazone and pioglitazone, did not demonstrate a similar hepatotoxicity and their administration improved insulin sensitivity in PCOS women in the four studies conducted, since 2003 for rosiglitazone and in a few with pioglitazone *(48)*.

Effects on Lipids

It could be hypothesized that the administration of an insulin-sensitizing agent of the thiazolidinedione class, would improve dyslipidemia associated with decrease of IR in PCOS. This claim, at least regarding troglitazone, was recently rejected by the results of a multicenter, double-blind trial *(49)* of 398 women with PCOS who were randomly assigned to a 44-week treatment with: placebo or troglitazone (150, 300, or 600 mg/day).

There was a high prevalence of abnormal baseline lipid parameters, as defined by National Cholesterol Education Program guidelines. No significant response of any of the circulating lipids to treatment with either placebo or one of the troglitazone arms (after correction for multiple analyses) was reported. Baseline models showed that parameters of insulin action had poor predictive power on lipid parameters, partially explaining the lack of beneficial effect on lipid profile and suggesting that other mechanisms participate as well.

To investigate the effectiveness and safety of pioglitazone (45 mg/day) on clinical and endocrine-metabolic features of PCOS, Romualdi et al. *(48)* studied 18 obese PCOS patients, classified as normoinsulinaemic and hyperinsulinaemic. A trend toward improvement was observed in lipid assessment of both groups. The therapy was well tolerated. Reported data suggested that there was a selective effect, partially independent of insulin secretion, of pioglitazone on the clinical and hormonal disturbances of PCOS including the lipid profile.

Conclusions regarding the TZDs effects on lipid or other parameters in the PCOS, should not been drawn as a group but in each TZD separately, because it appears that their effects are differentiated in various metabolic or reproductive pathways.

EFFECTS ON ENDOTHELIUM AND ON CARDIOVASCULAR RISK FACTORS

TZDs have been reported to decrease PAI-1 levels *(46)* and to improve in endothelial-dependent vasodilatation *(50)* suggesting reduction of cardiovascular risk. In fact, Paradisi et al. *(50)* were the first who demonstrated a normalization of endothelial function in a clinical state of IR with troglitazone treatment. They studied blood flow responses to graded intrafemoral artery infusion of the endothelium-dependent vasodilator in 10 PCOS women, before and after 3 months treatment with troglitazone (600 mg/day) and compared them with 13 obese women matched for age, weight, body fat, blood pressure, and total cholesterol. Troglitazone restored endothelium-dependent vasodilation to control levels.

Combined Studies

TZDS AND METFORMIN

Consequently, there are studies that compared metformin to TZDs treatment (Table 1). In a recent one *(51)*, pioglitazone has been compared with metformin in obese PCOS women. It has been shown that pioglitazone is as effective as metformin in improving insulin sensitivity and hyperandrogenemia despite an increase in weight and waist to hip ratio with pioglitazone. Moreover, in another study *(52)* the combined therapy, and more precisely the addition of pioglitazone 45 mg/day to metformin treatment, in women resistant to metformin, improvement in insulin resisstance and glucose utilization were observed.

CONCLUSION

Large long-term trials are needed to confirm the beneficial effects of TZDs on the metabolic abnormalities in PCOS. However, there are two limitations in using these drugs. One is regarding weight gain (0.5–3.5 kg) which is undesirable in already obese PCOS women and the second one is that they are pregnancy category C drugs, which means that in animal studies they retard fetal development. This potential embryotoxicity

Table 1
Studies Comparing Metformin With Thiazolidinediones

Authors	No. of PCOS patients	Duration	Medication	BMI	W/H	Insulin levels	Insulin sensitivity	Hcy	LDL	HDL	Triglycerides	Blood pressure
Ortega-Gonzalez et al. (2005) (51)	35 Obese	6 months	metf (2250 mg)	↑	↑	→	←		↑	↑	→	
			piogl (30 mg)	←	←	→	←		↑	↑	↑	
Kilicdag et al. (2005) (71)	30 Obese	3 months	metf (1700 mg)	↑			↑	←	↑	↑	↑	
			rosigl (4 mg)	↑			↑	←	→	→	↑	
Baillargeon et al. (2004) (77)	100 Non-obese normo-insulinemic	6 months	metf (850 mg)	↑	→	→	←					→
			rosigl (4 mg)	←	→	↑	↑					→
			metf + rosigl (4 mg)	↑→	→	→→	←←					→→
Glueck et al. (2003) (52)	39 Obese (26 resp, 13 non-resp)	12 months	metf resp (2250 mg)	↑ (weight)		→	↑			↑		↑
			metf non-resp	↑		↑				↑		
		12 months + 10 months	metf non-resp +piogl (45 mg)	↑		→	←			←		↑

→, no significant change; ↓, significant decrease; ↑, significant increase; BMI, body mass index; metf, metformin; piogl, pioglitazone; rosigl, rosiglitazone; resp, women responders to metformin treatment; non-resp, women non-responders to metformin treatment; Hcy, homocystein levels.

would limit their use in women who desire pregnancy. Therefore, TZDs should be considered a second-line treatment, alternative to metformin, for management of PCOS and regular monitoring of liver enzyme levels should be kept in mind.

D-Chiro-*Inositol*

Other insulin-sensitising agents such as D-*chiro*-inositol (DCI), which mediates the action of insulin, are also being trialled. Evidence suggests that some actions of insulin are mediated by inositolphosphoglycans (IPG). A deficiency in DCI and/or a specific DCI-containing IPG (DCI-IPG) may contribute to IR in humans. In a very recent study, it was demonstrated that in PCOS women there is a defect in tissue availability or utilization of DCI that may contribute to the IR of the syndrome *(53)*. Nestler *(54)* and others have shown that oral administration of DCI to women with PCOS improves glucose tolerance while reducing insulin levels in both obese and lean women with PCOS, and also decreases serum androgens and improves ovulatory function. The evidence that a deficiency in DCI-IPG, contributes to the IR of PCOS is further supported by evidence that administration of metformin to PCOS women enhances insulin-stimulated release of DCI-IPG *(55)*. Currently, there are no data regarding the effect of DCI-IPG on other metabolic or cardiovascular risk factors in PCOS.

In conclusion, oral administration of DCI to women with PCOS, is under investigation and has not been used in clinical practice as yet.

ANTIANDROGENS

Antiandrogens as monotherapy have found very limited therapeutic application in the management of clinical features in PCOS, because of feminizing effects on male fetuses. Therefore, they are used in clinical practice in combination with OCs as adjuvant therapy in skin manifestations of the syndrome. Since the establishment of the presence of the metabolic abnormalities of the syndrome, the antiandrogenic properties on the metabolic profile have received more attention.

The most widely used antiandrogens are either androgen receptor blockers or 5α-reductase inhibitors. The aim of this section will be to focus on the effects of these agents on the common metabolic aberrations present in women with PCOS.

Receptor Blockers

SPIRONOLACTONE

Spironolactone is an aldosterone antagonist used originally to treat hypertension. It is also a weak inhibitor of testosterone binding with intracellular receptor and of androgens biosynthesis.

Effects of Spironolactone on Lipid Profile. The effects on lipid profile and insulin sensitivity of spironolactone in PCOS women were studied recently *(56)*. Twenty-five patients were studied at baseline and then received oral spironolactone (100 mg/day) for 12 months and advised to lose weight. The therapy was associated with a significant average decline of triglycerides in overweight subjects and with increased HDL-cholesterol levels in lean patients.

Effects of Spironolactone on IR. The insulin levels during OGTT, and area under curve of insulin were significantly decreased in overweight women after 12 months on spironolactone *(56)*, but no changes in insulin secretion and sensitivity were observed.

Effects of Spironolactone on Cardiovascular Risk Factors. No data are available regarding the effects of spironolactone on other cardiovascular risk factors in PCOS women. However, from studies in other populations it has been shown that in hypertensive subjects, PAI-1 antigen was significantly decreased.

Flutamide

Flutamide is a potent nonsteroidal antiandrogen. However its effects on the metabolic profile in PCOS are under investigation and in clinical practice are not established.

EFFECTS OF FLUTAMIDE ON LIPID PROFILE

In doses of 500 mg/day it has been shown to improve the lipid profile reducing total and LDL cholesterol levels and triglycerides as well *(57,58)*.

Contrasted results have been published recently showing no improvement. Vrbikova et al. *(59)* administered 250 mg flutamide daily in 12 obese PCOS women for 2 months and no significant change in basal blood glucose, insulin, total cholesterol, HDL cholesterol, LDL cholesterol, triglycerides, or in IR was observed. Another randomized controlled study by Sahin et al. *(60)* designed to evaluate the effects of metformin vs flutamide on metabolic parameters and IR in 30 non-obese women with PCOS. Flutamide failed to improve insulin sensitivity in the non-obese women with PCOS, a finding which is in agreement with previous studies.

EFFECTS OF FLUTAMIDE ON IR

In 1995, Diamanti et al. *(61)* used the hyperinsulinemic euglycemic clamp in groups of lean and obese PCOS women and weight-matched controls to determine IR, showed that 250 mg of flutamide twice daily did not significantly influence the insulin sensitivity. A year later, Moghetti et al. *(62)* used a slight modified hyperinsulinemic euglycemic clamp (two step 20 and 80 mU/m^2/minute) administered 125 mg of flutamide three times daily for 3 months to lean and obese PCOS women and observed an improvement in insulin sensitivity but these differences reach statistical significance, only in obese subjects and not in lean ones. There is still debate about whether flutamide may improve IR *(60)*.

No data are available regarding the effects of flutamide on other cardiovascular risk factors in PCOS women.

Cyproterone Acetate

Cyproterone acetate (CA) is a potent progestin causing a decrease of androgen production and also increase testosterone clearance. It is available in Europe and Canada but not in the United States, and is used either as an adjuvant to OCP (2 mg CA and 35 μg ethinyl estradiol) or alone as a 10- and 50-mg tablet.

EFFECTS OF CA ON LIPID PROFILE

The OCP–CA pill is associated with increased serum HDL cholesterol and triglyceride concentrations in both non-obese and obese subjects and it has been observed a reduction in the total cholesterol:HDL cholesterol ratio *(63)*. On the other hand, it causes a slight worsening of glucose tolerance with compensatory hyperinsulinemia and increases serum FFA levels, when compined with oral contraceptives (25,64).

5α-Reductase Inhibitor: Finasteride

Finasteride is a potent inhibitor of skin 5α-reductase and it has fewer side effects than the other antiandrogens. Regarding its action on the metabolic profile of PCOS women there are not available published data.

PHARMACEUTICAL INTERVENTION IN WEIGHT REDUCTION AND ITS EFFECT IN METABOLIC AND CARDIOVASCULAR RISKS

Whichever is the priority in the mind or the body of a woman with PCOS, the first step should always include lifestyle modification and body weight reduction. Studies indicated that changes in the lifestyle could improve IR better than any of the pharmaceutical agents alone and the addition of them to the lifestyle modification could further improve the outcome on the metabolic as well as to the other abnormalities of the syndrome (Table 2). This combined approach is more likely to prevent the development of diabetes in high-risk individuals like PCOS women (32).

However, adherence to the diet appears to be a major problem, therefore, the need of supplementation with pharmaceutical agents is a nessessary tool. There are two drugs available for the treatment of obesity, orlistat and sibutramine, both recently have been tried either alone or in combination to face the metabolic abnormalities of the syndrome. They both increase compliance to the diet and weight loss.

Orlistat

Orlistat, a synthetic derivative, binds to intestinal lipases and impairs digestion of dietary triglycerides and vitamin esters. Less than 1% of ingested orlistat is absorbed, so it has no effect on systemic lipases. At the current recommended dose of 120 mg three times a day with meals, orlistat blocks the absorption of almost one-third of ingested fat; higher doses of orlistat are unlikely to increase fat malabsorption.

Studies have shown that it produces significant and sustained weight loss with associated improvement in lipid parameters in patients with primary hyperlipidaemia. Additionally has been shown to augment the effects of lifestyle modification in reducing the incidence of type 2 diabetes and to improve glycemic control in individuals with type 2 diabetes.

So far, only one short term study has been conducted in PCOS women (10 obese) seeking the potential benefits of orlistat in metabolism (65). In the orlistat-treated group when compared with baseline, there was no significant reduction seen in fasting insulin or HOMA. Additionally, there was no significant improvement in any of the lipid parameters studied, despite a reduction in weight.

It is possible that the small number of patients enrolled in the study and the short duration of the study could have caused the lack of statistically significant improvement in any of the metabolic parameters studied.

Studies on the effects of orlistat in metabolic aspects of the syndrome are in process and recently it has been shown that PCOS women in an acute experiment, orlistat reduced AGEs levels, after ingestion of meals high in dietary AGEs. In this study however no

Table 2
Studies Concerning the Management With Combination of Diet/Lifestyle Modification and Pharmacological Agents

Authors	No. of PCOS patients	Duration	Medication	BMI	W/H	VAT	Insulin levels	Insulin sensitivity	Cholesterol	Triglycerides	HDL	Blood pressure
Pasquali et al. (2000) (32)	20, BMI >28	6 months	diet	↓	→	→	↓	→				
			diet + metf	↓	→	↓	↓	↑				
Glueck et al. (2003) (52)	50 obese with metabolic syndrome	6 months	diet + metf	↓ (weight)					↓	↓	↑	↓
Hoeger et al. (2004) (41)	23, BMI >30	12 months	metf	↓				→				
			lifestyle	↓				→				
			lifestyle + metf	↓				→				
Gambineri et al. (2004) (58)	40, BMI >28	6 months	diet	↓		→	↓	↑	→	→	→	
			diet + metf	↓		↓	↓	↑	→	→	→	
			diet + flut	↓		↓	→	↑	↓	→	→	
			diet + metf + flut	↓		↓	↓	↑	↓	→	↑	
Sabuncu et al. (2003) (67)	40, BMI >30	6 months	diet + OCP	↓	→			→	→	↑	↑	→
			diet + sibut	↓	↓			↑	→	↓	→	↓
			diet + OCP + sibut	↓	→			→	→	↑	↑	→
Jayagopal et al. (2005) (65)	21, BMI >30	3 months	diet + metf	→ (weight)		→	→	→	→	→	→	
			diet + orlistat	↓			→	→	→	→		

→, no significant change; ↓, significant decrease; ↑, significant increase; metf, metformin; flut, flutamide; OCP, oral contraceptives; sibut, sibutramine; BMI, body mass index; W/H, waist to hip ratio; VAT, visceral adipose tissue.

any significant effect on other metabolic parameters, was observed, acutely. These results seem to be confirmed in a 6-month trial with orlistat, by the same investigators (66).

Sibutramine

Sibutramine is an appetite regulator recommended in the treatment of obesity. It is a noradrenaline and 5-hydroxytryptamine reuptake inhibitor, which exerts its effects in vivo predominantly via its secondary and primary amine metabolites. It is indicated as an adjunctive therapy within a weight management program in patients with obesity (body mass index $\geq$ 30 kg/m^2) or in overweight subjects (body mass index $\geq$ 27 kg/m^2) if other risk factors are present (i.e., dyslipidaemias, diabetes mellitus).

There is one study (67) in which sibutramin was administrated in obese PCOS women. Sibutramine treatment alone and in combination with ethinyl oestradiol and CA in obese women with PCOS, has been found to have positive effects on clinical and metabolic risk factors for CVD (reduced body weight, WHR, diastolic blood pressure, triglyceride, AUC-glucose, and AUC-insulin, and increased insulin sensitivity). Sibutramine also increased the SHBG level, which is thought to indirectly reflect insulin sensitivity. However, it is difficult to assess long-term the clinical efficiency of the medications because literature is rather inconclusive (small number of patients and short-term studies).

ORAL CONTRACEPTIVE PILLS

For many years, oral contraceptives have been the mainstay of therapy in PCOS. Nevertheless, it has been argued whether they are appropriate treatment for all aspects of PCOS and in particular their effects on metabolic aberrations of the syndrome have been questioned. Their use has been postulated to cause deterioration in insulin sensitivity and to adversely affect circulating lipids. However, the published data is scant and controversial.

Effects of OCPs on Metabolic Profile and on the Risk of Diabetes Mellitus and CVD

Because IR appears to accompany the syndrome, the use of OCPs as first-line therapy in PCOS women, became controversial. Although these agents improve hirsutism and acne, studies suggested a decrease in insulin sensitivity (64,68). In non-obese PCOS women a significant deterioration in insulin sensitivity was suggested assessed by hyperglycemic or hyperinsulinemic-euglycemic clamp (68). Similarly, in obese PCOS women treated with OCPs for 3–6 months it was demonstrated deterioration in glucose tolerance, proved by the increase of plasma glucose levels during the oral glucose tolerance test (64). On the other hand, other reports in non-obese PCOS women did not demonstrate significant changes in glucose tolerance and in insulin sensitivity (69).

A recent study with drospirenone in non-obese PCOS women did not find changes in oral glucose tolerance (70). Possibly the metabolic effect of OCPs may depend on the group of PCOS women and especially on the degree of obesity. OCPs modify also the lipid profile by raising total cholesterol and triglycerides. Nevertheless, no changes in the total cholesterol:HDL cholesterol and LDL:HDL cholesterol has been found a fact that is likely to depend on the type of progestin used (63,70).

There have not been any cohort studies performed to assess the risk of T2DM in PCOS women who use OCPs. Nevertheless, in two Nurses' Health Cohort Studies it has been assessed the risk of T2DM in healthy women used OCPs. In the first study, it was observed an increase in the relative risk of developing T2DM, whereas in the second one, the relative risk did not attain statistically significance. The available data regarding the use of OCP in women with PCOS, are not conclusive regarding the increase of the relative risk for T2DM, because long term studies are lacking. There are also no studies to assess the risk of CVD in PCOS women who use OCPs. However, it is suggested that OCP use might increase the risk of myocardial infraction in healthy women. Their effect on cardiovascular risks in women with PCOS can not be predicted. Consequently, OCPs should be used with caution, in women with PCOS, particularly in those who carry increased of CVS factors and positive family history of DM, until more data are available.

SUMMARY AND CONCLUSIONS

In PCOS women the medical management remains a very complex issue because a single therapy for all aspects of the syndrome is not established. It is indispensable to carefully assess the predominant symptoms and the risk factors in the metabolic profile of each woman and consequently individualize the treatment.

Based on the pathophysiological role of the underling IR of the syndrome it is expected, by improving insulin sensitivity, several other interlinked metabolic abnormalities will improve. Metformin is the most widely used insulin sensitiser for the metabolic and reproductive abnormalities in PCOS, with minimal side effects. Regarding the cardio-vascular risk factors, in view of the lack of studies showing increased incidence of CVD, their use is under investigation. Short prospective studies with thizolinediones either alone or combined with metformin appear to be equally effective.

The metabolic effects of antiandrogens and oral contraceptives have not been studied extenxsively. These agents, although suitable for management of other aspects of the syndrome should not be used for the abnormalities in metabolism and the health care providers should be aware of possible adverse effects .

FUTURE AVENUES OF INVESTIGATION

One of the major difficulties in medical management of PCOS is that there are not specific diagnostic signs or characteristic phenotypes, which could preclude the response to different therapeutic modalities particularly on the metabolic parameters. In the future, the pharmaceutical intervention will be targeted to different phenotypes, aiming at the most beneficial outcome in metabolic as well as in the other aspects of the syndrome. Ideally, when the pathogenesis of the syndrome will be clearly established then the treatment will be less symptomatic and more aetiologically oriented. Until then, large, randomized controlled studies are needed to ascertain the medications safety and efficacy in reducing long-term metabolic sequellae.

KEY POINTS

- Any pharmaceutical intervention in the management of PCOS, should always be as adjuvant treatment in lifestyle modification.

- The pharmaceutical intervention in metabolic and cardiovascular risk factors in women suffering from PCOS appears to be a useful therapeutic tool not only in those with obesity and features of metabolic syndrome.
- Other pharnaceutical modalities, when indicated, should take into consideration aggravation of the metabolic abnormalities of the syndrome, i.e., IR, dyslipideamia, and so on.

REFERENCES

1. Burghen GA, Givens JR, Kitabchi AE. Correlation of hyperandrogenism with hyperinsulinism in polycystic ovarian disease. J Clin Endocrinol Metab 1980;50:113–116.
2. Diamanti-Kandarakis E, Kouli CR, Bergiele AT, et al. A survey of the polycystic ovary syndrome in the Greek island of Lesbos: hormonal and metabolic profile. J Clin Endocrinol Metab 1999;84: 4006–4011.
3. Asuncion M, Calvo RM, San Millan JL, Sancho J, Avila S, Escobar-Morreale HF. A prospective study of the prevalence of the polycystic ovary syndrome in unselected Caucasian women from Spain. J Clin Endocrinol Metab 2000;85:2434–2438.
4. Apridonidze T, Essah PA, Iuorno MJ, Nestler JE. Prevalaence and characteristics of the metabolic syndrome in women with polycystic ovary syndrome. J Clin Endocrinol Metab 2005;90:1929–1935.
5. Legro RS, Kunselman AR, Dodson WC, Dunaif A. Prevalence and predictors of risk for type 2 diabetes mellitus and impaired glucose tolerance in polycystic ovary syndrome: a prospective, controlled study in 254 affected women. J Clin Endocrinol Metab 1999;84:165–169.
6. Ehrmann DA, Barnes RB, Rosenfield RL, Cavaghan MK, Imperial J. Prevalence of impaired glucose tolerance and diabetes in women with polycystic ovary syndrome. Diabetes Care 1999;22:141–146.
7. Palmert MR, Gordon CM, Kartashov AI, Legro RS, Emans SJ, Dunaif A. Screening for abnormal glucose tolerance in adolescents with polycystic ovary syndrome. J Clin Endocrinol Metab 2002;87: 1017–1023.
8. Gambineri A, Pelusi C, Manicardi E, et al. Glucose intolerance in a large cohort of mediterranean women with polycystic ovary syndrome: phenotype and associated factors. Diabetes 2004;53:2353–2358.
9. Norman RJ, Masters L, Milner CR, Wang JX, Davies MJ. Relative risk of conversion from normoglycaemia to impaired glucose tolerance or non-insulin dependent diabetes mellitus in polycystic ovarian syndrome. Hum Reprod 2001;16:1995–1998.
10. Dahlgren E, Janson PO, Johansson S, Lapidus L, Oden A. Polycystic ovary syndrome and risk for myocardial infarction. Evaluated from a risk factor model based on a prospective population study of women. Acta Obstet Gynecol Scand 1992;71:599–604.
11. Wild S, Pierpoint T, McKeigue P, Jacobs H. Cardiovascular disease in women with polycystic ovary syndrome at long-term follow-up: a retrospective cohort study. Clin Endocrinol (Oxf) 2000;52: 595–600.
12. Legro RS, Kunselman AR, Dunaif A. Prevalence and predictors of dyslipidemia in women with polycystic ovary syndrome. Am J Med 2001;111:607–613.
13. Diamanti-Kandarakis E, Spina G, Kouli C, Migdalis I. Increased endothelin-1 levels in women with polycystic ovary syndrome and the beneficial effect of metformin therapy. J Clin Endocrinol Metab 2001;86:4666–4673.
14. Kelly CJ, Speirs A, Gould GW, Petrie JR, Lyall H, Connell JM. Altered vascular function in young women with polycystic ovary syndrome. J Clin Endocrinol Metab 2002;87:742–746.
15. Diamanti-Kandarakis E, Alexandraki K, Protogerou A, et al. Metformin administration improves endothelial function in women with polycystic ovary syndrome. Eur J Endocrinol 2005;152:749–756.
16. Talbott EO, Guzick DS, Sutton-Tyrrell K, et al. Evidence for association between polycystic ovary syndrome and premature carotid atherosclerosis in middle-aged women. Arterioscler Thromb Vasc Biol 2000;20:2414–2421.
17. Christian RC, Dumesic DA, Behrenbeck T, Oberg AL, Sheedy PF 2nd, Fitzpatrick LA. Prevalence and predictors of coronary artery calcification in women with polycystic ovary syndrome. J Clin Endocrinol Metab 2003;88:2562–2568.
18. Kelly C, Lyall H, Petrie JR, et al. A specific elevation in tissue plasminogen activator antigen in women with polycystic ovarian syndrome. J Clin Endocrinol Metab 2002;87:3287–3290.
19. Diamanti-Kandarakis E, Palioniko G, Alexandraki K, Bergiele A, Koutsouba T, Bartzis M. The prevalence of 4G5G polymorphism of plasminogen activator inhibitor-1 (PAI-1) gene in

polycystic ovarian syndrome and its association with plasma PAI-1 levels. Eur J Endocrinol 2004;150:793–798.

20. Kelly C, Lyall H, Petrie JR, Gould GW, Connell JM, Sattar N. Low grade chronic inflammation in women with polycystic ovarian syndrome. J Clin Endocrinol Metab 2001;86:2453–2455.

21. Wiernsperger NF, Bailey CJ. The antihyperglycaemic effect of metformin: therapeutic and cellular mechanisms. Drugs 1999;58:31–39.

22. Ertunc D, Tok EC, Aktas A, Erdal EM, Dilek S. The importance of IRS-1 Gly972Arg polymorphism in evaluating the response to metformin treatment in polycystic ovary syndrome. Hum Reprod 2005;20:1207–1212.

23. Velazquez EM, Mendoza S, Hamer T, Sosa F, Glueck CJ. Metformin therapy in polycystic ovary syndrome reduces hyperinsulinemia, insulin resistance, hyperandrogenemia, and systolic blood pressure, while facilitating normal menses and pregnancy. Metabolism 1994;43:647–654.

24. Diamanti-Kandarakis E, Kouli C, Tsianateli T, Bergiele A. Therapeutic effects of metformin on insulin resistance and hyperandrogenism in polycystic ovary syndrome. Eur J Endocrinol 1998;138:269–274.

25. Morin-Papunen LC, Vauhkonen I, Koivunen RM, Ruokonen A, Martikainen HK, Tapanainen JS. Endocrine and metabolic effects of metformin versus ethinyl estradiol-cyproterone acetate in obese women with polycystic ovary syndrome: a randomized study. J Clin Endocrinol Metab 2000;85:3161–3168.

26. Maciel GA, Soares Junior JM, Alves da Motta EL, Abi Haidar M, de Lima GR, Baracat EC. Nonobese women with polycystic ovary syndrome respond better than obese women to treatment with metformin. Fertil Steril 2004;81:355–360.

27. Lord JM, Flight IH, Norman RJ. Metformin in polycystic ovary syndrome: systematic review and meta-analysis. BMJ 2003;327:951–953.

28. Ehrmann DA, Cavaghan MK, Imperial J, Sturis J, Rosenfield RL, Polonsky KS. Effects of metformin on insulin secretion, insulin action, and ovarian steroidogenesis in women with polycystic ovary syndrome. J Clin Endocrinol Metab 1997;82:524–530.

29. Glueck CJ, Wang P, Kobayashi S, Phillips H, Sieve-Smith L. Metformin therapy throughout pregnancy reduces the development of gestational diabetes in women with polycystic ovary syndrome. Fertil Steril 2002;77:520–525.

30. Rautio K, Tapanainen JS, Ruokonen A, Morin-Papunen LC. Effects of metformin and ethinyl estradiol-cyproterone acetate on lipid levels in obese and non-obese women with polycystic ovary syndrome. Eur J Endocrinol 2005;152:269–275.

31. Moghetti P, Castello R, Negri C, et al. Metformin effects on clinical features, endocrine and metabolic profiles, and insulin sensitivity in polycystic ovary syndrome: a randomized, double-blind, placebo-controlled 6-month trial, followed by open, long-term clinical evaluation. J Clin Endocrinol Metab 2000;85:139–146.

32. Pasquali R, Gambineri A, Biscotti D, et al. Effect of long-term treatment with metformin added to hypocaloric diet on body composition, fat distribution, and androgen and insulin levels in abdominally obese women with and without the polycystic ovary syndrome. J Clin Endocrinol Metab 2000;85:2767–2774.

33. Boulman N, Levy Y, Leiba R, et al. Increased C-reactive protein levels in the polycystic ovary syndrome: a marker of cardiovascular disease. J Clin Endocrinol Metab 2004;89:2160–2165.

34. Diamanti-Kandarakis E, Piperi C, Kalofoutis A, Creatsas G. Increased levels of serum advanced glycation end-products in women with polycystic ovary syndrome. Clin Endocrinol (Oxf) 2005;62:37–43.

35. Paradisi G, Steinberg HO, Hempfling A, et al. Polycystic ovary syndrome is associated with endothelial dysfunction. Circulation 2001;103:1410–1405.

36. Morin-Papunen L, Rautio K, Ruokonen A, Hedberg P, Puukka M, Tapanainen JS. Metformin reduces serum C-reactive protein levels in women with polycystic ovary syndrome. J Clin Endocrinol Metab 2003;88:4649–4654.

37. Diamanti-Kandarakis E, Paterakis T, Alexandraki K, et al. Indices of low grade chronic inflammation in polycystic ovary syndrome and the beneficial effect of metformin. Hum Reprod 2006;21:1426–1431.

38. Roldan V, Marin F, Lip GY, Blann AD. Soluble E-selectin in cardiovascular disease and its risk factor. A review of the literature. Thromb Haemost 2003;90:1007–1020.

39. Vlassara H, Bucala R, Striker L. Pathogenic effects of advanced glycosylation: biochemical, biologic, and clinical implications for diabetes and aging. Lab Invest 1994;70:138–151.

40. Diamanti-Kandarakis E, Alexandraki K, Piperi C, et al. Effect of metformin administration on advanced glycation end products plasma levels in women with polycystic ovary syndrome. Metabolism 2007;56: 129–134.

41. Hoeger KM, Kochman L, Wixom N, Craig K, Miller RK, Guzick DS. A randomized, 48-week, placebo-controlled trial of intensive lifestyle modification and/or metformin therapy in overweight women with polycystic ovary syndrome: a pilot study. Fertil Steril 2004;82:421–429.

42. Salpeter S, Greyber E, Pasternak G, Salpeter E. Risk of fatal and nonfatal lactic acidosis with metformin use in type 2 diabetes mellitus. Cochrane Database Syst Rev 2003;2:CD002967.

43. Diamanti-Kandarakis E, Kouli C, Alexandraki K, Spina G. Failure of mathematical indices to accurately assess insulin resistance in lean, overweight, or obese women with polycystic ovary syndrome. J Clin Endocrinol Metab 2004;89:1273–1276.

44. Seto-Young D, Paliou M, Schlosser J, et al. Direct thiazolidinedione action in the human ovary: insulin-independent and insulin-sensitizing effects on steroidogenesis and insulin-like growth factor binding protein-1 production. J Clin Endocrinol Metab 2005;90:6099–6105.

45. Dunaif A, Scott D, Finegood D, Quintana B, Whitcomb R. The insulin-sensitizing agent troglitazone improves metabolic and reproductive abnormalities in the polycystic ovary syndrome. J Clin Endocrinol Metab 1996;81:3299–3306.

46. Ehrmann DA, Schneider DJ, Sobel BE, et al. Troglitazone improves defects in insulin action, insulin secretion, ovarian steroidogenesis, and fibrinolysis in women with polycystic ovary syndrome. J Clin Endocrinol Metab 1997;82:2108–2116.

47. Azziz R, Ehrmann D, Legro RS, et al. PCOS/Troglitazone Study Group. Troglitazone improves ovulation and hirsutism in the polycystic ovary syndrome: a multicenter, double blind, placebo-controlled trial. J Clin Endocrinol Metab 2001;86:1626–1632.

48. Romualdi D, Guido M, Ciampelli M, et al. Selective effects of pioglitazone on insulin and androgen abnormalities in normo- and hyperinsulinaemic obese patients with polycystic ovary syndrome. Hum Reprod 2003;18:1210–1218.

49. Legro RS, Azziz R, Ehrmann D, Fereshetian AG, O'Keefe M, Ghazzi MN. Minimal response of circulating lipids in women with polycystic ovary syndrome to improvement in insulin sensitivity with troglitazone. J Clin Endocrinol Metab 2003;88:5137–5144.

50. Paradisi G, Steinberg HO, Shepard MK, Hook G, Baron AD. Troglitazone therapy improves endothelial function to near normal levels in women with polycystic ovary syndrome. J Clin Endocrinol Metab 2003;88:576–580.

51. Ortega-Gonzalez C, Luna S, Hernandez L, et al. Responses of serum androgen and insulin resistance to metformin and pioglitazone in obese, insulin-resistant women with polycystic ovary syndrome. J Clin Endocrinol Metab 2005;90:1360–1365.

52. Glueck CJ, Moreira A, Goldenberg N, Sieve L, Wang P. Pioglitazone and metformin in obese women with polycystic ovary syndrome not optimally responsive to metformin. Hum Reprod 2003;18: 1618–1625.

53. Baillargeon JP, Diamanti-Kandarakis E, Ostlund R Jr., Apridonidze T, Iuorno M, Nestler JE. Altered D-chiro-inositol urinary clearance in women with polycystic ovary syndrome. Diabetes Care 2006;29:300–305.

54. Nestler JE, Jakubowicz DJ, Reamer P, Gunn RD, Allan G. Ovulatory and metabolic effects of D-chiro-inositol in the polycystic ovary syndrome. N Engl J Med 1999;340:1314–1320.

55. Baillargeon JP, Iuorno MJ, Jakubowicz DJ, Apridonidze T, He N, Nestler JE. Metformin therapy increases insulin-stimulated release of D-chiro-inositol-containing inositolphosphoglycan mediator in women with polycystic ovary syndrome. J Clin Endocrinol Metab 2004;89:242–249.

56. Zulian E, Sartorato P, Benedini S, et al. Spironolactone in the treatment of polycystic ovary syndrome: effects on clinical features, insulin sensitivity and lipid profile. J Endocrinol Invest 2005;28:49–53.

57. Diamanti-Kandarakis E, Mitrakou A, Raptis S, Tolis G, Duleba AJ. The effect of a pure antiandrogen receptor blocker, flutamide, on the lipid profile in the polycystic ovary syndrome. J Clin Endocrinol Metab 1998;83:2699–2705.

58. Gambineri A, Pelusi C, Genghini S, et al. Effect of flutamide and metformin administered alone or in combination in dieting obese women with polycystic ovary syndrome. Clin Endocrinol (Oxf) 2004;60:241–249.

59. Vrbikova J, Hill M, Dvorakova K, Stanicka S, Vondra K, Starka L. Flutamide suppresses adrenal steroidogenesis but has no effect on insulin resistance and secretion and lipid levels in overweight women with polycystic ovary syndrome. Gynecol Obstet Invest 2004;58:36–41.
60. Sahin I, Serter R, Karakurt F, et al. Metformin versus flutamide in the treatment of metabolic consequences of non-obese young women with polycystic ovary syndrome: a randomized prospective study. Gynecol Endocrinol 2004;19:115–124.
61. Diamanti-Kandarakis E, Mitrakou A, Hennes MM, et al. Insulin sensitivity and antiandrogenic therapy in women with polycystic ovary syndrome. Metabolism 1995;44:525–531.
62. Moghetti P, Tosi F, Castello R, et al. The insulin resistance in women with hyperandrogenism is partially reversed by antiandrogen treatment: evidence that androgens impair insulin action in women. J Clin Endocrinol Metab 1996;81:952–960.
63. Mastorakos G, Koliopoulos C, Deligeoroglou E, Diamanti-Kandarakis E, Creatsas G. Effects of two forms of combined oral contraceptives on carbohydrate metabolism in adolescents with polycystic ovary syndrome. Fertil Steril 2006;85:420–427.
64. Nader S, Riad-Gabriel MG, Saad MF. The effect of a desogestrel-containing oral contraceptive on glucose tolerance and leptin concentrations in hyperandrogenic women. J Clin Endocrinol Metab 1997;82: 3074–3077.
65. Jayagopal V, Kilpatrick ES, Holding S, Jennings PE, Atkin SL. Orlistat is as beneficial as metformin in the treatment of polycystic ovarian syndrome. J Clin Endocrinol Metab 2005;90:729–733.
66. Diamanti-Kandarakis E, Piperi C, Alexandraki K, et al. Short-term effect of orlistat on dietary glyco-toxins in healthy women and women with polycystic ovary syndrome. Metabolism 2006;55:494–500.
67. Sabuncu T, Harma M, Harma M, Nazligul Y, Kilic F. Sibutramine has a positive effect on clinical and metabolic parameters in obese patients with polycystic ovary syndrome. Fertil Steril 2003;80:1199–1204.
68. Korytkowski MT, Mokan M, Horwitz MJ, Berga SL. Metabolic effects of oral contraceptives in women with polycystic ovary syndrome. J Clin Endocrinol Metab 1995;80:3327–3334.
69. Cagnacci A, Paoletti AM, Renzi A, et al. Glucose metabolism and insulin resistance in women with polycystic ovary syndrome during therapy with oral contraceptives containing cyproterone acetate or desogestrel. J Clin Endocrinol Metab 2003;88:3621–3625.
70. Guido M, Romualdi D, Giuliani M, et al. Drospirenone for the treatment of hirsute women with polycystic ovary syndrome: a clinical, endocrinological, metabolic pilot study. J Clin Endocrinol Metab 2004;89:2817–2823.

28 Anti-Androgens

Kürşad Ünlühizarci, MD
and Fahrettin Keleştimur, MD

CONTENTS

Summary

Hirsutism is defined as an excess of body hair in the androgen-sensitive skin regions of women. The most important purpose for investigation is to identify patients with androgen-secreting tumors because they require different therapy. Androgen-secreting tumors should be suspected when the onset and the progression of hirsutism is rapid and/or when it is associated with virilization. In most of the patients, the underlying causes are benign, such as polycystic ovary syndrome and idiopathic hirsutism. Treatment of hirsutism depends on the patient's expectation and the underlying cause. Patients should be informed about the type and the duration of the therapy. The selection of the drug(s) depends on the severity of the hirsutism, associated conditions such as menstrual irregularities, systemic disorders such as diabetes mellitus, hypertension, and any contraindication to possible therapeutic agent. Peripheral blockade of androgen actions at the skin by using cyproterone acetate, spironolactone, finasteride, or flutamide, either alone or in combination with oral contraceptive pills is an effective in the treatment of hirsutism.

Key Words: Hirsutism; anti-androgen treatment; PCOS; androgen secreting tumors.

INTRODUCTION

Hirsutism is caused by increased androgen production and/or increased sensitivity of follicles to androgens, leading to the appearance of body hair in a male pattern. It is particularly distressing condition for women and a common reason to seek medical advice. Hirsutism affects 5–8% of the whole female population of fertile age, and it

From: *Contemporary Endocrinology: Insulin Resistance and Polycystic Ovarian Syndrome: Pathogenesis, Evaluation, and Treatment*
Edited by: E. Diamanti-Kandarakis, J. E. Nestler, D. Panidis, and R. Pasquali © Humana Press Inc., Totowa, NJ

may be associated with underlying endocrine and metabolic disturbances or, more importantly, it may be the initial manifestation of an androgen-secreting tumor *(1)*. Polycystic ovary syndrome (PCOS), nonclassic congenital adrenal hyperplasia (NCAH), Cushing's syndrome, acromegaly, and some drugs may be the underlying causes of hirsutism, or it may be idiopathic *(2)*. The management of hirsutism involves a range of diagnostic and therapeutic issues, and it is essential to identify the underlying cause of hirsutism.

DISEASES ASSOCIATED WITH HIRSUTISM

PCOS is by far the most common cause of hirsutism. It is characterized by oligo-amenorrhea, hyperandrogenemia/hyperandrogenism, and polycystic ovarian changes; however, diagnosing PCOS remains a matter of excluding specific disorders of the ovaries, adrenal glands, and the pituitary gland *(3)*. The pathogenesis of PCOS is hetero-geneous, but insulin resistance may have a central role in most of the patients *(4,5)* and in addition to insulin resistance, women with PCOS have metabolic derangements such as impaired glucose tolerance, dyslipidemia, and cardiovascular disease.

Some hirsute patients do not have evidence of detectable androgen excess or endocrine imbalance, as in women with "idiopathic hirsutism." Idiopathic hirsutism is defined as hirsutism associated with both normal circulating androgen and gonado-tropin concentrations, regular menses, and ovulatory cycles with normal ovarian morphology *(1,2)*. PCOS and idiopathic hirsutism constitute the majority of the patients with hirsutism.

In between 1 and 8% of women with hirsutism, the underlying cause of the disease is NCAH. It results from a defect in the enzymes necessary for the biosynthesis of cortisol and/or aldosterone *(6)*. The clinical picture is very similar to the clinical presentation of PCOS, and most of the patients demonstrate polycystic ovaries on ultrasound, which are secondary to hyperandrogenemia. It has been suggested that the most common form of NCAH is 21-hydroxylase (21-OH) deficiency *(7)*; however, it has been previously reported that NCAH caused by 11-β hydroxylase deficiency may be more common in some populations *(8)*.

A number of patients with hirsutism have hyperandrogenemia with normal ovaries and regular cycles. These patients present different features and other disorders, such as NCAH, androgen-secreting tumors, and Cushing's syndrome can be easily excluded. These patients also exhibit similar basal follicle-stimulating hormone (FSH), luteiniz-ing hormone (LH), free testosterone, androstenedione, and dehydroepiandrosterone sulfate (DHEAS) levels with PCOS subjects. The authors defined this group of patients as idiopathic hyperandrogenemia (IHA) *(9)*. Those patients may have functional ovar-ian and/or adrenal hyperandrogenism *(9,10)*.

Androgen-secreting tumors are very rare cause of hirsutism but should be excluded in every patient. These tumors usually arise from the ovaries or the adrenal glands. There is no clear-cut level of androgen concentrations for the differential diagnosis of benign vs malignant etiologies, therefore androgen-secreting tumors should be suspected when the onset and the progression of hirsutism is rapid and/or when it is associated with virilization.

Table 1
Pharmacological Agents Used in the Treatment of Hirsutism

1. Suppression of ovarian androgen production
        Oral contraceptive pills
        Gonadotropin-releasing hormone agonists
2. Suppression of adrenal androgen production
        Glucocorticoids
3. Anti-androgens
        Cyproterone acetate
        Spironolactone
        Drospirenone
        Flutamide
        Finasteride
4. Topical agents
        Eflornithine

GENERAL PRINCIPLES OF THE TREATMENT IN A HIRSUTE PATIENT

Specific causes of hirsutism, such as Cushing's syndrome or adrenal/ovarian tumors, should be treated by surgical excision. In the other patients, a pharmacological approach is the mainstay of the therapy (Table 1). Patients should be informed about the type and the duration of the therapy. Generally, at least 6 months are necessary to evaluate the success of the medical therapy. The goal of medical therapy is at least to prolong the intervals for removing unwanted hair. The treatment of hirsutism involves the reduction of excessive androgen secretion and/or the blockade of androgens. In addition, mechanical amelioration of the unwanted hairs may be adjunctive. The selection of the drug(s) depends on the severity of the hirsutism, associated conditions such as menstrual irregularities, systemic disorders such as diabetes mellitus, hypertension, and any contraindication to possible therapeutic agent. Patients should be made aware that most of the drugs used in the management of hirsutism are contraindicated if the patient desires pregnancy and that simultaneous treatment of infertility and hirsutism is difficult. Oral contraceptives (OCs) are commonly used drugs in the treatment of hirsutism, but they are out of scope of this paper and so we will not discuss them in more detail. The treatment of hirsutism is most effective when combination therapy used. Combination therapy includes the inhibition of androgen secretion and the peripheral blockade of androgens. In selected cases, combination of anti-androgens with different mechanisms of action may be used. Whatever the cause of hirsutism, anti-androgen drugs play a key role in the treament of hirsutism. In this chapter, anti-androgen drugs and their effects in the treatment of hirsutism are described.

ANTI-ANDROGENS

The most commonly used anti-androgens are cyproterone acetate, flutamide, and spironolactone, which act by inhibiting the binding of testosterone and dihydrotestosterone (DHT) to the androgen receptor. Another anti-androgen, bicatulamide, had been used in a limited number of patients but there is not enough data regarding its effect on hirsutism. The other important drug, finasteride, decreases the formation of potent DHT by its 5α reductase inhibitor activity (Table 2). In general, hirsutism responds better to medications that block androgen action rather than ovarian or adrenal suppression.

Cyproterone acetate (CPA) is a steroidal anti-androgen derived from 17-hydroxy-progesterone (1). CPA is one of the most widely used drugs in the management of hirsutism. CPA is a strong progestogen and causes a decrease in circulating testosterone levels through a decrease in the production of LH. It also antagonizes the effect of androgens at the peripheral level (11). CPA may also inhibit 5α-reductase activity (12). It has also been suggested that CPA may reduce adrenocorticotropic hormone (ACTH) secretion from the pituitary gland and thereby reduces androgen secretion from the adrenal glands (13). Diane 35 (which combines low-dose ethinyl estradiol with a small but therapeutic dose of cyproterone acetate) is one of the most commonly used first-line treatments for mild to moderate hirsutism. On the other hand, some authors recommend induction therapy of ethinyl estradiol combined with high-dose CPA (50–100 mg) followed by gradual reduction to a maintenance dose of 2 mg CPA (14). Barth et al. performed a dose-ranging study on the effects of CPA, which showed that patients who underwent 2 mg/day CPA saw results of a significant reduction in clinical hair growth scores, as did those with the addition of 20 or 100 mg/day CPA at 12 months (15). The combination of 30–35 μg ethinyl estradiol and 50–100 mg CPA was found as more effective than 100 mg/day spironolactone; the decrease in the Ferriman-Gallwey (F-G) score was 60 and 44%, respectively (16). In another study, the combination of ethynil estradiol and 2 mg/day CPA 21 days per month was found as significantly effective, and there was a remarkable improvement in 90% of hirsute patients; however, relapse occurred in 80% of these patients after the stopping of treatment at 6 months (17). Pazos et al. compared the long-acting gonadotropin-releasing hormone agonist triptorelin, flutamide, and CPA combined with an OC in the treatment of hirsutism and found that CPA was as effective as the other drugs at a lower cost (18). CPA may cause headache, weight gain, breast tenderness, nausea, loss of libido, edema, hepatotoxicity, fatigue, and mood changes and its use is associated with the risk of feminizing a male fetus, and for this reason, adequate contraception should be used (11,19). It has been demonstrated that the use of CPA/ethinyl estradiol in women with acne, hirsutism, or PCOS is associated with an increased risk of venous tromboembolism, although residual confounding by indication cannot be excluded (20). If the patient who is on CPA wishes to become pregnant, CPA should be stopped at least two cycles before the pregnancy to avoid the risk of feminizing a male fetus.

Spironolactone, a potassium-sparing agent, is a competitive inhibitor of aldosterone and has antiandrogenic effects by binding to the androgen receptors, thereby inhibiting testosterone from binding to its receptors. Spironolactone also increases the metabolic clearance of testosterone and inhibits the production of androgen by inhibiting cytochrome P450. Spironolactone inhibits the interaction of DHT with its intracellular androgen receptor (21). It was found that spironolactone and CPA were similarly effective, but spironolactone was more effective than finasteride in the treatment of hirsutism (22,23). Zulian et al. investigated the long-term effects of 100 mg/day of spironolactone on clinical features, lipid profile, and insulin levels in women with PCOS. They found that 12 months of treatment with spironolactone had no negative effects on

Table 2
Mechanisms of Actions of the Commonly Used Anti-Androgens

	Androgen receptor blockade	Clearance of androgens	Effect on LH secretion	Glucorticoid activity	5α-Reductase activity	Progestogenic activity
Cyproteronee acetate	+	+	+	+	–	+
Spironolactone	+	+	–	–	–	+
Drospirenone	+	+	+	–	–	–
Flutamide	+	–	–	–	–	–
Finasteride	–	–	–	–	+	–

lipoprotein profile and glucose metabolism. They also reported that spironolactone seemed to exert a direct effect on the increase of high-density lipoprotein cholesterol independenly from weight loss and diet *(24)*. Spironolactone is a safe drug and its tolerabilty is good. It has potentially mild side effects such as breast tenderness and enlarged breasts, transient diuresis, dizziness, headache, hyperkalemia (which would not occur in patients with normal kidney function), gastrointestinal discomfort, nausea, allergic reactions, fatigue, somnolance, vertigo, polyuria, and polydipsia, particularly in the first days of treatment *(25)*. Side effects can be prevented or minimized by increasing the doses of the drug gradually. Spironolactone is commonly used in doses of 100 mg/day and, rarely, 200 mg/day. The most common side effect of spironolactone is polymenorrhea and its frequency has been reported as 50–60% *(26,27)*. Addition of an OC to spironolactone improves irregular menstrual bleeding. At least theoretically, there is a risk of feminizing a male fetus if pregnancy occurs during spironolactone treatment. A Diane 35 plus spironolactone (100 mg) combination was compared in 50 women with hirsutism. Hirsutism scores were significantly decreased at the end of therapy in both groups, but the percentage change in the hirsutism score at 12 months was higher in the Diane 35 plus spironolactone group. Therefore, the addition of spironolactone to Diane 35 may have a synergistic effect on hirsutism score *(28)*.

A new progestin derived from 17α-spironolactone, drospirenone (DRSP), shares progesterone's anti-androgenic and antimineralocorticoid properties with no androgenic, estrogenic, glucocorticoid, or antiglucocorticoid activity. DSRP has been demonstrated to display anti-androgenic activity at the peripheral level by competetive binding to the androgen receptor that is intrinsic to its molecular structure. The blockade of androgen receptors in the skin represents an additional mechanism when combined with ethinyl estradiol. In addition to blocking androgen receptors, drospirenone inhibits ovarian androgen production *(29)*.

Finasteride, which is a 5α-reductase inhibitor blocks the conversion of testosterone to the more potent DHT. It does not bind to the androgen receptor, but rather binds to the 5α-reductase enzyme and interferes with its action. Therefore, it has no effect on androgen secretion. Finasteride treatment results in reduction in the DHT level, which is accompanied by a reduction in metabolites of DHT, such as 3α-diol glucuronide and a rise in plasma testosterone levels. 5α-Reductase has two isoenzymes, including

5α-reductase type 2, which is found predominantly in genital skin and the prostate in the male, and 5α-reductase type 1, which is found in the scalp, pubic skin, and non-sex skin. Finasteride is more effective against isoenzyme 5α-reductase type 2 than type 1, but the specificity for these two isoenzymes is incomplete *(30)*. In a study of 12 months, 5 mg/day of finasteride induced a statistically significant decrease in hirsutism score *(31)*. In another similar study, 2.5 mg/day of finasteride was given instead of 5 mg/day of finasteride, and it was also found effective in the treatment of hirsutism *(32)*. Low- (2.5 mg/day) and high-dose (5 mg/day) finasteride have been compared in hirsute patients to investigate whether low-dose finasteride can be used instead of high-dose finasteride, and both low- and high-dose finasteride have been found similarly effective in the treatment of hirsutism. Because of cost-effectiveness, low-dose finasteride may be used instead of high-dose finasteride *(33)*. Neither low- nor high-dose finasteride in those studies changed FSH, LH, testosterone, androstenedione, sex hormone-binding globulin (SHBG), 17-hydroxyprogesterone, or DHEAS levels. Because finasteride may cause feminization, pregnancy should be avoided in women taking finasteride. Moghetti et al. compared the effectiveness of finasteride, spironolactone, and flutamide in a randomized, double-blind, placebo-controlled study lasting 6 months and they found that all three drugs had similarly reduced hair diameter and F-G score compared with the placebo group *(26)*. Finasteride is a very safe drug and its very low side profile makes it a good therapeutic choice. However, its effectiveness is lower than the other antiandrogens. In a study of 12 months, Şahin et al. *(34)* compared the clinical efficacy and safety of the combination of Diane 35 (2 mg of CPA and 35 mg of ethinyl estradiol) plus finasteride (5 mg) and Diane 35 alone in the treatment of hirsutism. The percentage decrease in the hirsutism score at 12 months was higher in the Diane 35 plus finasteride group than in the Diane 35 group. The study included 40 unselected hirsute women with idiopathic hirsutism and PCOS. In this combination, three drugs (CPA, estrogen, and finasteride) with different mechanisms of action were administered. Diane 35 plus finasteride has been proposed as an effective and safe combination in the treatment of hirsutism *(34)*. It has been shown that the combination of spironolactone and finasteride may be used without any increased side effects *(27)*. Spironolactone was found better than metformin in the treatment of hirsutism in women with PCOS *(35)*. In a prospective study the efficacy of Diane 35 alone, Diane 35 plus spironolactone, and spironolactone alone were compared in women with hirsutism, and all treatment regimens were found to be effective and well tolerated *(36)*. Lumachi et al. compared the effectiveness of CPA (12.5 mg for the first 10 days of the cycle), finasteride (5 mg/day), and spironolactone (100 mg/day) in the treatment of idiopathic hirsutism in a prospective study of 12 months. Hirsutism was evaluated by F-G scoring. The androgenic profile did not change significantly during treatment. They have found that the short-term results of treatment with CPA, finasteride, and spironolactone were similar, but spironolactone was more effective for a longer time *(37)*.

Flutamide, which is a nonsteroidal selective anti-androgen, has been commonly used in the treatment of hirsutism, and it has no progestogenic, glucocorticoid, androgenic, estrogenic, or antigonadotropic action. It seems that flutamide works only at the androgen receptor. It is an inhibitor of testosterone binding to its receptor. Erenus et al. found that 500 mg/day of flutamide (250 mg twice a day) is similarly effective to 100 mg/day spironolactone in women with idiopathic hirsutism *(38)*. In a study of 12 months that included the hirsute women with PCOS and idiopathic hirsutism, the effectiveness of flutamide (250 mg twice a day) and finasteride (5 mg/day) were compared, and flutamide was found more effective *(39)*. Flutamide did not modify the hormonal profile in that study. Only two (3.6%) of the patients in flutamide group had abnormal transaminase levels after 6 months of treatment and 67.3% of the patients had dry skin. Cesur et al. also demonstrated the effectiveness of 500 mg/day of flutamide in the treatment of hirsutism *(40)*. In a study including the women with PCOS, flutamide was found to be effective in the treatment of hirsutism, and hormonal investigation showed a significant reduction in both total and free testosterone, androstenadione, and DHEAS levels only in women with PCOS; SHBG levels were increased in women with PCOS *(41)*. Ibanez et al. treated 18 non-obese adolescent girls with 250 mg/day of flutamide and found that significant decrease in hirsutism score was associated with significant decrease in free androgen index, free testosterone, testosterone, androstenedione, and DHEAS levels, and increase in SHBG levels *(42)*. Because of its potentially life-threatening side effects, relatively high-dose flutamide has not been widely used. Lower doses of flutamide, including 250 mg/day, 125 mg/day, and 62.5 mg/day in place of 500 mg/day, were equally effective in the treatment of hirsutism *(43–45)*. The low or ultra-low doses of flutamide (62.5–250 mg/day) have been shown to be as effective in the treatment of hirsutism, particularly when combined with metformin plus an OC pill, and were found to confer benefit on multiple PCOS markers, such as interleukin-6, adiponectin, and abdominal and total fat mass without any hepatotoxicity *(46)*. The most serious side effect of flutamide is liver toxicity, with an estimated frequency ranging from 0.36 to 5% . Fatal or non-fatal hepatotoxicity is a well-known side effect of flutamide. Liver function tests should be monitored regularly during the treatment period. It may be used in hirsute women when the other drugs fail to improve the hirsutism. The most common side effects of flutamide are increased appetite and dry skin, but it does not result in irregular menses.

A relatively uncommon problem is andogenic alopecia in some patients with hyperandrogenemia. Although isolated cases may be seen, in most of the patients it is associated with PCOS. Androgenic alopecia is also a therapeutic target for the antiandrogenic drugs. Finasteride may be a good alternative for the treatment and, actually, a 1-mg dose of finasteride has been used for male pattern baldness.

One of the most important issues in the treatment of hirsutism is the duration of remission after the treatment has been stopped, and studies addressing this subject are limited. Carmina and Lobo investigated the effectiveness of the addition of dexamethasone to antiandrogen therapy and they found that dexamethasone (0.37 mg/day) plus spironolactone (100 mg/day) for 1 year or dexamethasone (0.37 mg/day) plus spironolactone (100 mg/day) for 2 years were more effective than spironolactone alone in terms of the duration of remission *(47)*. In some patients, lifelong therapy may be necessary to prevent recurrences. One of the debated subjects is the timing of the treatment. It is reasonable that physicians should start anti-androgen therapy earlier in order to prevent worsening of hirsutism.

CONCLUSION

Hirsutism is a very common clinical problem during reproductive age and is also an associated psychological disturbance. Hirsutism is the result of either androgen excess caused by ovarian and/or adrenal disorders, increased sensitivity of the hair follicle to normal levels of androgens, or their combinations. On the other hand, it may also be a cutaneous sign of a systemic disorder. The underlying cause should be clarified before the treatment has been started. Treatment of hirsutism should be individualized and depends on the patients expectations and underlying cause. Anti-androgens may be combined with OCs or each other. The anti-androgen plus OC combination is a good choice for both to treat the hirsutism effectively and prevent pregnancy. Therefore, anti-androgen plus OC combination should be administered to women who are sexually active. If the patient desires pregnancy and discontinues the OC, anti-androgen therapy should be stopped in order to prevent feminization of the male fetus. Although there are some data, long-term safety of anti-androgen drugs in the treatment of hirsutism, the duration of the treatment, prevention of the recurrence, the effectiveness of the low-dose anti-androgens, and the effectiveness of the different anti-androgen combinations remains to be investigated. One of the most difficult questions is related to the duration of the study. The causes of hyperandrogenism are commonly ovarian and/or adrenal in origin, so permanent removal of the sources of hyperandrogenism is not usually the best course of action. For this reason, treatment of hirsutism may be long-term, and a logical approach is to decrease the dose of anti-androgens once an acceptable level of improvement is obtained.

FUTURE AVENUES OF INVESTIGATION

Most of the treatment strategies in hirsutism are symptomatic and the treatment should be directed at the cause of the problem. In this regard, clinical and experimental studies have been published for identifying the pathophysiological mechanisms of hirsutism, particularly in women with PCOS, and it has been shown that insulin resistance has a significant role. On the other hand, treatment with insulin sensitizers showed very limited effect or was ineffective in treating the hirsutism. Women with idiopathic hirsutism are another group of patients. The mechanisms of the disease are not clearly known, but our studies and experience suggest that, although those patients had normal serum androgen levels, they are hyperandrogenic at the tissue level. By establishing the pathogenetic mechanisms underlying the causes of hirsutism, new therapeutic strategies may play an important role in offering more effective therapies.

KEY POINTS

- Apart from patients with ovarian or adrenal androgen-secreting tumors, the clinical picture is very similar among patients with other causes.
- Because the treatment of androgen-secreting malignant tumors are absolutely different, it should be excluded in every patient with hirsutism.
- Most of the treatment strategies in hirsutism are symptomatic. Oral contraceptive pills and anti-androgen drugs either alone or combined may be given. Weight loss should be encouraged in obese women.

REFERENCES

1. Conn JJ, Jacobs HS. The clinical management of hirsutism. Eur J Endocrinol 1997;136:339–348.
2. Azziz R. The evaluation and management of hirsutism. Obstet Gynecol 2003;101:995–1007.
3. Rotterdam ESHRE/ASRM-Sponsored PCOS Consensus Workshop Group. Revised 2003 consensus on diagnostic criteria and long term health risks related to polycystic ovary syndrome. Fertil Steril 2004;81:19–25.

4. Dunaif A. Insulin resistance and the polycystic ovary syndrome: mechanisms and implications for pathogenesis. Endocrine Rev 1997;18:774–800.

5. Strauss JF, Dunaif F. Molecular mysteries of polycystic ovary syndrome. Mol Endocrinol 1999;13: 800–805.

6. Azziz R, Hincapie LA, Knochenhauer ES, Dewailly D, Fox L, Boots LR. Screening for 21-hydroxylase-deficient nonclassic adrenal hyperplasia among hyperandrogenic women: a prospective study. Fertil Steril 1999;72:915–925.

7. Azziz D, Dewailly D, Owerbach D. Nonclassic adrenal hyperplasia: current concepts. J Clin Endocrinol Metab 1994;78:810–815.

8. Kelestimur F, Sahin Y, Ayata D, Tutus A. The prevalence of non-classic adrenal hyperplasia due to 11b-hydroxylase deficiency among hirsute women in a Turkish population. Clin Endocrinol (Oxf) 1996;45:381–384.

9. Unluhizarci K, Gokce C, Atmaca H, Bayram F, Kelestimur F. A detailed investigation of hirsutism in a Turkish population: Idiopathic hyperandrogenemia as a perplexing issue. Exp Clin Endocrinol Diabetes 2004;112:504–509.

10. Carmina E, Chu MC, Longo RA, Rini GB, Lobo RA. Phenotypic variation in hyperandrogenic women influences the findings of abnormal metabolic and cardiovascular risk parameters. J Clin Endocrinol Metab 2005;90:2545–2549.

11. Raudrant D, Rabe T. Progestogens with antiandrogenic properties. Drugs 2003;63:463–492.

12. Fruzzetti F, Bersi C, Parrini D, Ricci C, Genazzani AR. Treatment of hirsutism: comparisons between different antiandrogens with central and peripheral effects. Fertil Steril 1999;71:445–451.

13. Girard J, Baumann JB, Buhler U, et al. Cyproterone acetate and ACTH: adrenal function. J Clin Endocrinol Metab 1978;47:581–586.

14. Miller JA, Jacobs HS. Treatment of hirsutism and acne with cyproterone acetate. Clin Endocrinol Metab 1986;15:373–389.

15. Barth JH, Cherry CA, Wojnarowska F, Dawber RP. Cyproterone acetate for severe hirsutism: results of a double-blind dose-ranging study. Clin Endocrinol 1991;35:5–10.

16. Venturoli S, Marescalchi O, Colombo FM, et al. A prospective randomized trial comparing low dose of flutamide, finasteride, ketoconazole, and cyproterone acetate-estogen regimens in the treatment of hirsutism. J Clin Endocrinol Metab 1999;84:1304–1310.

17. Kokaly W, McKenna TJ. Relapse of hirsutism following long-term successful treatment with oestrogen-progestogen combination. Clin Endocrinol 2000;52:379–382.

18. Pazos F, Escobar-Morreale HF, Balsa J, Sancho JM, Varela C. Prospective randomized study comparing the long-acting gonadotropin-releasing hormone agonist triptorelin, flutamide, and cyproterone acetate, used in combination with an oral contraceptive, in the treatment of hirsutism. Fertil Steril 1999;71:122–128.

19. Aziz R, Carmina E, Sawaya ME. Idiopathic hirsutism. Endocr Rev 2000;21:347–362.

20. Seaman HE, de Vries CS, Farmer RD. The risk of liver disorders in women prescribed Cyproteronee acetate in combination with ethinyloestradiole (Dianette): a nested case-control study using the GPRD. Pharmacoepidmiol Drug Safe 2003;12:541–550.

21. McMullen GR, Van Herle AJ. Hirsutism and the efectiveness of spironolactone in its management. J Endocrinol Invest 1993;16:925–932.

22. Erenus M, Yucelten D, Gurbuz O, Durmusoglu F, Pekin S. Comparison of spironolactone-oral contraceptive versus Cyproteronee acetate-estrogen regimens in the treatment of hirsutism. Fetil Steril 1996;66:216–219.

23. Erenus M, Yucelten D, Durmusoglu F, Gurbuz O. Comparison of finasteride versus spironolactone in the treatment of idiopathic hirsutism. Fertil Steril 1997;68:1000–1003.

24. Zulian E, Sartorato P, Benedini S, et al. Spironolactone in the treatment of polycystic ovary syndrome: effects on clinical features, insulin sensitivity and lipid profile. J Endocrinol Invest 2005;28: 49–53.

25. Sahin Y, Kelestimur F. Medical treatment regimens of hirsutism. Reprod BioMed Online 2004;8: 538–546.

26. Moghetti P, Tosi F, Tosti A, et al. Comparison of spironolactone, flutamide, and finasteride efficacy in the treatment of hirsutism: a randomized, double blind, placebo controlled trial. J Clin Endocrinol Metab 2000;85:89–94.

27. Kelestimur F, Everest H, Unluhizarci K, Bayram F, Sahin Y. A comparison between spironolactone plus finasteride and spironolactone in the treatment of hirsutism. Eur J Endocrinol 2004;150:351–354.

28. Kelestimur F, Sahin Y. Comparison of Diane 35 and Diane 35 plus spironolactone in the treatment of hirsutism. Fertil Steril 1998;69:66–69.

29. Guido M, Romualdi D, Giuliani M, et al. Drospirenone for the treatment of hirsute women with polycystic ovary syndrome: a clinical, endocrinological, metabolic pilot study. J Clin Endocrinol Metab 2004;89:2817–2823.

30. Dallob AL, Sadick NS, Unger W, et al. The effect of finasteride, a 5 alpha-reductase inhibitor on scalp skin testosterone and dihydrotestosterone concentrations in patients with male pattern baldness. J Clin Endocrinol Metab 1994;79:703–706.

31. Bayram F, Muderris II, Sahin Y, Kelestimur. Finasteride treatment for one year in 35 hirsute patients. Exp Clin Endocrinol and Diabetes 1999;107:195–197.

32. Bayram F, Muderris I, Guven M, Ozcelik B, Kelestimur F. Low dose (2.5 mg/day) finasteride treatment in hirsutism. Gynecol Endocrinol 2003;17:419–422.

33. Bayram F, Muderris II, Guven M, Kelestimur F. Comparison of high-dose finasteride (5 mg/day) versus low dose (2.5 mg/day) finasteride in the treatment of hirsutism. Eur J Endocrinol 2002;147:467–471.

34. Sahin Y, Dilber S, Kelestimur F. Comparison of Diane 35 and Diane 35 plus finasteride in the treatment of hirsutism. Fertil Steril 2001;75:496–500.

35. Ganie MA, Khurana ML, Eunice M, et al. Comparison of efficacy of spironolactone with metformin in the management of polycystic ovary syndrome: an open-labeled study. J Clin Endocrinol Metab 2004;89:2756–2762.

36. Sert M, Tetiker T, Kirim S. Comparison of the efficiency of anti-androgenic regimens consisting of spironolactone, Diane 35, and Cyproteronee acetate in hirsutism. Acta Med Okayama 2003;57:73–76.

37. Lumachi F, Rondinone R. Use of Cyproteronee acetate, finasteride, and spironolactone to treat idiopathic hirsutism. Fertil Steril 2003;79:942–946.

38. Erenus M, Gurbuz O, Durmusoglu F, Demircay Z, Pekin S. Comparison of the efficacy of spironolactone versus flutamide in the treatment of hirsutism. Fertil Steril 1994;61:613–616.

39. Falsetti L, Gambera A. Comparison of finaseride versus flutamide in the treatment of hirsutism. Eur J Endocrinol 1999;141:361–367.

40. Cesur V, Kamel N, Uysal AR, Erdogan G, Baskal N. The use of antiandrogen flutamide in the treatment of hirsutism. Endocr J 1994;41:573–577.

41. Marugo M, Bernasconi D, Meozzi M, et al. The use of flutamide in the management of hirsutism J Endocrinol Invest 1994;17:195–199.

42. Ibanez L, Potau N, Marcos MV, de Zegher F. Treatment of hirsutism, hyperandrogenism, oligomenorrhea, dyslipidemia, and hyperinsulinism in nonobese, adolescent girls: effect of flutamide. J Clin Endocrinol Metab 2000;85:3251–3255.

43. Muderris II, Bayram F, Sahin Y, Kelestimur F. A Comparison between two doses of flutamide (250 mg/d and 500 mg/d) in the treatment of hirsutism. Fertil Steril 1997;68:644–647.

44. Müderris II, Bayram F. Clinical efficacy of lower dose flutamide 125 mg/d in the treatment of hirsutism. J Endocrinol Invest 1999;22:165–168.

45. Müderris II, Bayram F, Güven M. Treatment of hirsutism with lowest-dose flutamide (62.5 mg/day). Gynecol Endocrinol 2000;14:38–41.

46. Ibanez L, Jaramillo A, Ferrer A, de Zegher F. Absence of hepatotoxicity after long-term, low-dose flutamide in hyperandrogenic girls and young women. Hum Reprod 2005;20:1833–1836.

47. Carmina E, Lobo RA. The addition of dexamethasone to antiandrogen therapy for hirsutism prolongs the duration of remission. Fertil Steril 1998;69:1075–1079.

29 Chronic Treatment of Polycystic Ovary Syndrome

Oral Contraceptive Pills

Shahla Nader, MD

CONTENTS

Summary

There is a long history of oral contraceptive pill (OCP) use in subjects with polycystic ovary syndrome (PCOS). The more immediate benefits have been amply demonstrated and include improvement in acne, hirsutism, alopecia, as well as regulation of abnormal cycles with the potential for preventing endometrial hyperplasia and, subsequently, cancer. In addition, OCPs provide protection against pregnancy, especially if other medications, such as anti-androgens, biguanides, or thiazo-lidinediones, are also given. Although epidemiological evidence of actual increased risk of coronary events in subjects with PCOS is lacking, surrogate markers are certainly consistent with an increased risk of cardiovascular disease in PCOS. The possibility that OCP may increase this risk adds urgency to the need for more systematic research in this field. It is in this context that knowledge of the effects of OCP on carbohydrate and lipid metabolism in normal and, particularly, in subjects with PCOS is so critical, given the well-known association of glucose intolerance, dyslipidemia, and cardiovascular events.

Evidence presented in this paper supports the following concepts:

1. Estrogen may impair carbohydrate tolerance and insulin sensitivity, and this may be dose-dependent. This effect may also be dependent on the endogenous insulin sensitivity of the individual.

From: *Contemporary Endocrinology: Insulin Resistance and Polycystic Ovarian Syndrome:*
Pathogenesis, Evaluation, and Treatment
Edited by: E. Diamanti-Kandarakis, J. E. Nestler, D. Panidis, and R. Pasquali © Humana Press Inc., Totowa, NJ

2. Progestins with intrinsic androgenic properties may also impair insulin sensitivity and glucose tolerance.

3. Lowering of free androgens may improve insulin sensitivity and glucose tolerance in some subjects.

4. The composite effect of OCP on glucose tolerance and insulin sensitivity may be determined by the interplay of the above with the endogenous insulin sensitivity of the individual, which is determined genetically, environmentally, and by other factors. The environmental influence may also vary over time.

5. The effect of OCP on lipid metabolism relates to estrogen-induced increases in high density lipoprotein cholesterol and triglycerides. The latter effect may be attenuated by pills of greater androgenicity.

Inasmuch as OCP have the potential for impairment of glucose tolerance and insulin sensitivity, in many subjects with PCOS, and given that this effect alone may increase the potential for cardiovascular disease (as may changes in lipid metabolism and coagulation parameters), OCPs should be used cautiously in at least some subgroups of patients with PCOS. These include the obese, those with strong family histories of diabetes, and perhaps adolescents, given the lower endogenous insulin sensitivity in these subgroups. Consideration should therefore be given to the concomitant use of agents that may modify these effects, such as biguanides, thiazolidinediones, and androgen blockers in appropriate individuals.

Key Words: Polycystic ovary syndrome; oral contraceptive pills; insulin resistance; metabolic syndrome; dyslipidemia; hyperandrogenism; acne; hirsutism; glucose intolerance; cardiovascular disease.

INTRODUCTION

Polycystic ovary syndrome (PCOS) is the most common endocrine disorder in women of reproductive age *(1)*. Although the specific manifestations and sequelae that lead patients to seek medical attention is varied *(2,3)*, the consensus of opinion is that the syndrome encompasses ovulatory dysfunction, presenting as oligomenorrhea or amenorrhea, signs, symptoms, and biochemical evidence of a hyperandrogenic state, and multicystic ovaries *(4)*. As is evident to most physicians involved in the care of these patients, these commonalities may mask significant differences among individuals *(5–7)*. For many women with PCOS, the initial encounter relates to their inability to achieve pregnancy and the overriding priority is induction of ovulation. However, for many others it is the sundry other complaints that are the presenting symptoms, such as hirsutism, acne, alopecia, irregular or abnormal menses, amenorrhea, the diagnosis of ovarian cysts, and often also obesity *(8)*. The purpose of this chapter is to review the role, benefits, and potential risks of oral contraceptive pills (OCPs) in the management of women with PCOS not desiring pregnancy.

Combined OCPs have had a long traditional role in the management of PCOS *(9,10)*. Although ovulation occurs infrequently, it may occur and for many, OCPs are the most acceptable method of contraception. In addition, the use of other agents, such as spironolactone, used as an androgen-blocker, makes contraception a priority. Unopposed estrogen stimulation of the endometrium, a consequence of the anovulatory state, is well recognized to be a predeterminant of endometrial hyperplasia and cancer *(11,12)*. The progestin component of the OCP protects the endometrium, prevents hyperplasia, and treats the erratic menses and meno-metrorrhagia, often seen in women with PCOS.

The estrogen component of OCP enhances hepatic production of sex hormone-binding globulin, thereby reducing *free* androgen availability. Oral contraceptive steroids also reduce luteinizing hormone concentrations, reducing the drive to ovarian androgen production and thus circulating androgens *(13–15)*. Even adrenal androgen secretion may be reduced by these pills *(11,12)*. However, many of the progestins used as components of OCP are 19-nortestosterone derivatives and thus have androgenic effects, thereby potentially negating the beneficial androgen-lowering effects of OCPs *(9)*. Norgestimate and desogestrel are virtually non-androgenic and drospirenone, an analog of spironolactone, has antiandrogenic properties *(16,17)*. In addition, norgestimate is an inhibitor of skin 5α-reductase in vitro. In Europe, Canada, and many other parts of the world, although not in the United States, OCPs containing the anti-androgen cyproterone acetate are also available. The choice of contraceptive pills may thus be determined by their properties as well as their side effect profiles. The estrogen in OCP is virtually always the synthetic estrogen ethinylestradiol (EE) and although high-dose pills were previously commonly used, the majority of women are currently on OCPs containing 20–35 μg of EE.

INDICATIONS AND BENEFITS OF OCP IN PCOS

Treatment of Acne, Hirsutism, and Alopecia

The effect of oral contraceptives on hirsutism was recently reviewed by Azziz *(18)*, Guzick *(19)*, and Ehrmann *(2)*. Overall, 70–80% of women with androgen excess demonstrate hirsutism, although this prevalence is less common in women of Asian origin. Androgens increase the growth rate of hair and transform vellus hair to terminal hair in androgen-sensitive areas. Reduction of serum androgens with OCP reduces new hair growth and slows the growth of terminal hair already present *(20,21)*. It may take six or more months for this effect to become manifest *(22)*. Treatment of acne is often most satisfactory, and several OCPs are approved by the Food and Drug Administration in the United States for such treatment. With 6–9 months of use, inflammatory-lesion counts are reduced by 30–60%, with improvements in 50–90% of patients *(23)*. Hormonal treatment may be especially useful in a subset of women with deep-seated nodules of the lower face *(24)*. Furthermore, adult women who relapse following isotretinoin therapy are likely to respond to hormonal therapy. Androgen blockers, such as spironolactone or flutamide, may be combined with OCPs, enhancing their effect *(25)*. Contraceptive pills containing 2 mg cyproterone acetate are also widely available in Europe and Canada for the treatment of symptomatic hyperandrogenism *(26)*.

Prevention and Treatment of Ovarian Cysts

Use of OCPs to treat functional ovarian cysts is a common practice. In a study of almost 1000 hospitalized women, the incidence of cysts among women 20–44 years old not using OCPs was 38 per 100,000 per year, whereas for women using OCPs, it was 3 per 100,0000 per year *(27)*. In a study of OCPs containing cyproterone, ovarian volume decreased following pill usage *(28)*. However, the dose of EE in the oral contraceptive may be important. Holt et al. *(29,30)* found that current use of low-dose monophasic oral contraceptives did not substantially reduce the risk of functional ovarian cysts in contrast to higher dose pills. This conclusion was supported by Lanes et al. *(31)*.

Cycle Control and Prevention of Endometrial Hyperplasia and Cancer

Regular menses can be achieved with the use of OCPs. Preference is often given to OCP containing progestins that are of low androgenicity or anti-androgenic. Unopposed estrogen stimulation of the endometrium in anovulatory subjects with PCOS is associated with an increased risk of endometrial cancer in these individuals *(32–34)*. OCP have been shown to protect against endometrial cancer in the general population *(35)*.

METABOLIC AND VASCULAR EFFECTS OF OCPs

The association of PCOS with adverse long-term metabolic consequences and markers of cardiovascular disease has generated a great deal of interest and concern in the interaction and possible potentiation of adverse outcomes with OCP use *(36)*. Even in the absence of PCOS, adverse long-term effects of OCPs have been under intense scrutiny *(37)*. Although the results are somewhat varied, broad conclusions are briefly summarized next.

Carbohydrate Metabolism and OCP Use

The effect of OCPs on carbohydrate metabolism in the general population is of paramount importance and interest in relation to PCOS. Several epidemiological studies, including two Nurses' Health Study cohort studies, have looked at this relationship. In the first *(38)*, with 12 years of follow-up, and a mean age of 58 years at follow-up, the relative risk of developing type 2 diabetes associated with past use of OCPs was 10% greater than in those who had never used OCPs. However, a large proportion used high-dose OCPs. In the second cohort study *(39)*, with the use of low-dose OCP for a mean of 4 years and a mean follow-up age of 38 years, the adjusted relative risk was increased in past (1.2) and current (1.6) users; these differences were not statistically significant, however. In a third study *(40)*, cross-sectional data from the Third National Health and Nutrition Examination Survey were assessed. Mean fasting glucose, insulin, C-peptide, and hemoglobin A1C were evaluated during the survey; past and present OCP users did not differ from never-users after adjusting for potential confounders.

Smaller studies on carbohydrate metabolism and glucose tolerance in oral contraceptive users have yielded varying results. Luyckx *(41)* reported mild deterioration of glucose tolerance of 7–12% as measured by area-under-the-glucose curve in 38 women using three different formulations. Plasma insulin responses to glucose were not increased. In the study of van den Ende *(42)* a 20-μg EE–desogestrel OCP was used in 16 healthy volunteers. A slight but significant deterioration in glucose tolerance and increased insulin responses were seen. In 1987, van der Vange *(43)* investigated the effects of seven low-dose (30–40 μg of EE) pills on carbohydrate metabolism in groups of healthy volunteers. The pills differed in content and type of progestin. The area-under-the-glucose and -insulin curves did not change, nor was there a significant change in glycosylated proteins. In a trial of triphasic preparations in 130 women, Bowes et al. *(44)* tested glucose tolerance orally and found small, but significant increases in plasma glucose levels; small increase in serum insulin was also found. Godsland *(45)* observed the metabolic effects of nine types of oral contraceptives in 1060 women, using oral glucose tolerance tests (GTTs). Two of these were progestin only pills. Depending on the dose and type of progestin, combination pills were associated with plasma glucoses that were 43–61% higher than in controls with insulin responses 12–40% higher. Progestin only pills or combinations containing desogestrel or low-dose norethindrone were associated with the most favorable profiles. Godsland et al. *(46)* also investigated the metabolic effects of four different OCP preparations, with similar estrogen but differing progestins, employing intravenous GTTs. They also tested one progestin-only pill. Incremental glucose, insulin, and C-peptide varied according to the progestin content with greater increase following levonorgestrel compared with desogestrel. The norethindrone-only pill actually reduced incremental C-peptide. Estrogen-containing pills caused similar degrees of insulin resistance, as reflected by glucose elimination. The progestin-only pill did not affect resistance to insulin. They concluded that the effects related to estrogen-induced insulin resistance and progestin-associated changes in insulin half-life. A similar conclusion, related to estrogen, was reached by Kojima et al. *(47)*; they used three different doses of EE and found reduced insulin sensitivity in the group as a whole, but this effect was seen mainly with use of the highest dose. Crook et al. *(48)* studied women on desogestrel (low androgenic) vs gestodene (more androgenic) OCPs and compared them with women who were not on OCPs. The use of OCPs leads to increased high-density lipoprotein (HDL; with higher HDL2 in desogestrel users) and triglycerides. Although fasting insulin and glucose were similar in the three groups, their responses to a glucose load were higher in OCP users. The late plasma insulin response to glucose was also higher in gestodene vs desogestrel users. They concluded that the metabolic profiles induced by OCPs were remarkably similar and suggested that these changes may be reflective of the estrogen component. In another study, Petersen et al. *(49)* studied insulin sensitivity index, glucose effectiveness, and insulin response in a group of young, healthy women given EE–norgestimate or EE–gestodene, using intravenous glucose GTTs. Both compounds increased fasting insulin and reduced the insulin sensitivity index, but only gestodene increased the insulin response to intravenous glucose. They, too, considered that insulin resistance might relate to the estrogenic component.

Indeed, in a comprehensive review of the influence of female sex steroids on glucose metabolism and insulin action, Godsland *(50)* again stated that OCPs were generally associated with reduced glucose tolerance, hyperinsulinemia, and insulin resistance and that the estrogen component was primarily responsible for these changes. It was also stated that the progestin component could modify these changes. Supporting evidence comes from a population-based sample of 380 young healthy Caucasians who had a combined intravenous GTT with the addition of tolbutamide *(51)*. About one-third of the variation in the insulin sensitivity index was related to body fat, maximum aerobic capacity, and OCP use (lower sensitivity with OCP).

Small sophisticated clamp studies have found variable effects. For example, in a study of seven healthy, young women using a cyproterone acetate-containing pill, Scheen et al. *(52)* performed euglycemic clamp studies before and at 6 and 12 months following therapy. No significant effect on insulin sensitivity was noted. However, in a euglycemic clamp study of normal, lean women using or not using OCP (20–30 µg EE with desogestrel or gestodene), Perseghin et al. *(53)* found a 40% reduction in insulin sensitivity, along with increased free fatty acids and triglycerides, in pill users.

Lipid Metabolism and OCP Use

In a review of lipid effects of oral contraceptives, Fotherby *(54)* concluded that preferred formulations should contain a low dose of EE and should not raise total or low-density lipoprotein (LDL) cholesterol or reduce HDL cholesterol. He reviewed progestin differences: certain OCPs, for example desogestrel, were favorable in raising HDL. He also stated that for women, the risk of OCPs with respect to cardiovascular disease was only a minor risk factor unless other risk factors were also present (relevant to PCOS). Other studies on OCPs and lipids have shown varied results. Godsland *(45)* found increased triglycerides in his cross-sectional study of 1060 women on various OCPs. Some found decreased LDL and increased HDL (desogestrel); others decreased HDL (levonorgestrel). Studies assessing the impact of 24 months of a 35 µg EE–norgestimate pill on lipid metabolism in 450 women reported a significant increase in HDL and a decrease in LDL/HDL ratio *(55)*. Crook et al. *(48)* found increased HDL and triglycerides in both gestodene and desogestrel users, with higher HDL2 in users of desogestrel. Van Rooije *(56)* did a crossover study using the same amount of EE with either desogestrel or levonorgestrel. The desogestrel pill increased HDL as compared with both baseline and levonorgestrel pills. Both increased triglycerides, but was more pronounced with desogestrel.

Myocardial Infarction, Stroke, Thromboembolic Disease, and OCP Use

The relationship of oral contraceptives and myocardial infarction and its surrogates has been the subject of numerous studies, and was recently reviewed by the Practice Committee of the American Society for Reproductive Medicine *(57)*. The baseline risk of myocardial infarction is low in young women and rises from 2 per million at age 30–34 years to 20 per million at age 40–44 years *(58)*. Low-dose oral contraceptives increase this risk twofold among users even after controlling for cardiovascular risk factors, such as smoking, hypertension, hypercholesterolemia, diabetes, and obesity *(59)*. Factors, such as smoking, significantly compound that risk, especially after age 35 years *(60)*, hence the recommendation to avoid OCP in smokers over age 35 years. Spitzer et al. *(61)* evaluated the findings of seven recent oral contraceptive studies on the risk of myocardial infarction among users of second- and third-generation OCPs. Compared with non-users, the aggregated odds ratio for third-generation OCPs was 1.13 (0.66–1.92), and for second-generation it was 2.18 (1.62–2.94). Thus, the overview suggested that third-generation OCPs do not convey harm as regards myocardial infarction compared with non-users. However, in a more recent meta-analysis of the association of current use of low-dose OCPs and cardiovascular arterial disease, the authors concluded that there was a significant increased risk of cardiac and vascular arterial events, including a significant increased risk of vascular arterial complications with third-generation OCPs *(37)*.

With regards to ischemic stroke, a summary of five epidemiological case–control studies concluded that the risk of ischemic stroke was 2.2-fold higher with current use of OCPs containing less than 50 µg EE and does not appear to be related to the progestin *(62)*. Again, the baseline risk is low, rising from 6 per million at age 20 years to 16 per million at age 40–44 years *(58,63)*. For hemorrhagic stroke, the risk is not increased by OCPs used by women under age 35. For those over age 35 using OCPs, the risk is 2.2-fold over that of non-users *(57,64)*.

Venous thromboembolic (VTE) risk in relation to OCP use has been the subject of intense investigation. Oral contraceptives are associated with a threefold increased risk of VTE and the risk appears to be proportional to estrogen dose *(58)*. The possibility of higher risk in relation to newer progestins (desogestrel and gestodene), as suggested by some studies, was the basis of a meta-analysis that included three cohort and nine case–control studies. An overall adjusted odds ratio for VTE in relation to the newer progestins was found to be 1.7, as compared with second-generation progestins *(65)*. Although significant, the occurrence of VTE is still a rare event, and the Food and Drug Administration suggested no change in prescribing *(57)*. The risk for VTE is, however, more substantial in women with prothrombotic mutations, such as Leiden factor V mutation, and these women should not receive OCPs *(66)*.

METABOLIC EFFECTS OF OCPs IN PCOS: CARBOHYDRATE METABOLISM

The metabolic effects of oral contraceptives in patients with PCOS have not been extensively or systematically studied and the literature is as varied as the patient population itself. Study variables have included age, body mass indices (BMI), methodology for determining the metabolic effects, use of different contraceptive preparations and the inclusion of otherwise healthy subjects. This literature is briefly reviewed in the following subheadings.

Carbohydrate Metabolism and OCP Use in PCOS: Results of Individual Studies

Falsetti and Pasinetti *(67)* administered a low-dose cyproterone OCP for 36 cycles to 72 women with PCOS and compared them with 39 healthy controls. There was no change in serum insulin and glucose values after 36 cycles of treatment in patients with PCOS. Twenty of the PCOS subjects were overweight (mean BMI of these women was 27 vs 22 for the whole group).

Korythowski et al. *(68)* performed hyperglycemic clamp studies in 9 PCOS and 10 controls, treated with a low-dose norethindrone pill. Both groups were overweight and the baseline androgens, triglycerides, and insulin responses to oral glucose were higher and the insulin sensitivity index lower in the PCOS subjects. There was a further decline in insulin sensitivity in the women with PCOS and also a decline in the controls. Nader et al. *(69)* performed oral GTTs in 16 nondiabetic, extremely obese women with PCOS (BMI 36.8 ± 1.8 kg/m^2) with acanthosis nigricans before and after six cycles of a desogestrel-containing pill. Despite a lack of change in weight, glucose tolerance deteriorated significantly and two women developed diabetes.

Pasquali et al. *(70)* reevaluated 37 women with PCOS approx 10 years after their initial assessment. The patients were advised to follow hypocaloric diets if obese and OCPs were offered. Sixteen women took OCPs for an average of 97 months, whereas 21 never took them. Glucose tolerance area-under-the-curve (AUC) improved and basal insulin declined significantly in users of OCPs, but not in non-users. Insulin AUC increased in non-users of OCP, but remained unchanged in users. Thus, there was a spontaneous worsening of hyperinsulinemia and insulin resistance in the non-pill users. At initial evaluation 10 women were normal weight (BMI ≤ 26) and 27 were overweight or obese (BMI ≥ 26). The pill users had mean BMIs of 28.8 and 27.9 before and after treatment. Non-users had values of 32.7 and 34.4, respectively.

Morin-Papunen *(71)* compared the effects of metformin with a cyproterone acetate pill in 32 obese women with PCOS. Oral GTT and euglycemic clamp studies were performed.

They observed the expected decline in insulin and improved glucose utilization with metformin, but noted an increased glucose AUC during the oral GTT on the pill, although insulin sensitivity as measured by the clamp studies did not change significantly. Escobar-Morreale et al. *(72)* evaluated 16 hirsute women (five oligomenorrheic) before and 6 months after a desogestrel-containing OCP (mean BMI 25.9). Fasting insulin and insulin resistance as measured by homeostatic model assessment (HOMA) significantly improved, as did biochemical and clinical markers of hyperandrogenism.

Armstrong et al. *(73)* utilized the euglycemic hyperinsulinemic clamp method to evaluate insulin action in 11 patients with PCOS and 13 controls (with BMI of 27.3 and 25.3, respectively). During clamp studies, the glucose infusion rate required to maintain euglycemia was lower in PCOS compared with controls but similar in PCOS before and after treatment with a cyproterone acetate OCP. In a study by Elter et al. *(74)*, 40 non-obese patients with PCOS were assigned either a cyproterone-containing OCP or to the same OCP plus metformin and treated for 4 months. Although the addition of metformin improved insulin sensitivity, as measured by the glucose/insulin ratio and reduced BMI, those receiving only OCPs had no significant change in BMI or insulin sensitivity after the 4 months. Cibula et al. *(75)* evaluate non-obese PCOS subjects (BMI ≤ 30) during treatment with OCP of low androgenicity (norgestimate) and compared 13 women with PCOS with 9 controls. Hyperinsulinemic euglycemic clamp studies showed no deterioration in glucose disposal rate, insulin sensitivity index, or metabolic clearance rate of glucose, after 6 months of treatment.

Morin-Papunen et al. *(71)* extended their original studies of obese patients with PCOS to the study of non-obese patients with PCOS who were treated with either metformin or cyproterone acetate OCP *(76)*. Seventeen non-obese patients with PCOS (BMI < 25) were randomized to treatment and euglycemic clamp studies were performed. Metformin did not affect glucose tolerance or insulin sensitivity but fasting insulin declined and menstrual cyclicity improved. The OCP did not significantly affect glucose tolerance, serum insulin, or insulin sensitivity but slightly increased the BMI. Cagnacci et al. *(77)* compared monophasic (35 µg EE) cyproterone acetate-containing pills with a biphasic (40/30 EE) desogestrel pill in lean women with PCOS (BMI < 25). Glucose tolerance was evaluated using an oral GTT and the minimal model intravenous GTT was also performed. The cyproterone pill improved insulin sensitivity that was impaired by the desogestrel pill.

Sabancu et al. *(78)* evaluated the use of a cyproterone OCP, along with sibutramine, in obese patients with PCOS. They were compared with PCOS given OCPs alone or sibutramine alone. All were advised to follow a calorie-restricted diet and had oral GTTs. All groups lost significant weight, even those on OCP alone. Waist-to-hip ratios, blood pressure, and triglycerides were significantly reduced only in the sibutramine group. Glucose and insulin AUC were unchanged before vs after OCP alone, but AUC insulin was lower in the sibutramine group than in the OCP group after treatment. The combination of OCPs and sibutramine resulted in lower BMI, decreased AUC for insulin, and glucose as compared with pretreatment values. Ibanez and Zegher *(79)* assessed the metabolic impact of the addition of a gestodene-containing OCP to metformin-flutamide in 24 non-obese young women (mean age 18.7 years) with PCOS (12 received OCP and 12 did not; all received flutamide and metformin). The beneficial effects of the flutamide–metformin combination on hyperinsulinemia were maintained in contraceptive-treated women, with an additional drop in the free androgen index.

Vrbikova et al. *(80)* compared oral vs transdermal estrogen, along with oral cyproterone acetate in 24 women with PCOS (BMI 24.5 ± 3.9). Euglycemic clamp studies were performed. In those on oral estrogen (OCP group), but not in the transdermal group, insulin sensitivity decreased significantly and total and HDL cholesterol increased significantly. Guido et al. *(81)* performed oral GTTs and euglycemic hyperinsulinemic clamp studies in 15 hirsute patients (mean BMI < 25) with PCOS given a drospirenone-containing OCP. Hirsutism significantly improved as did the free androgen index. The treatment did not affect glucose–insulin homeostasis. Palep-Singh *(82)* studied 13 subjects with PCOS treated with a drospirenone OCP. While acne improved, there was a significant increase in fasting insulin and triglycerides. Cibula et al. *(83)* evaluated the role of a combination of a norgestimate-containing OCP and metformin vs the OCP therapy alone in 28 patients with PCOS (mean BMI < 25). Euglycemic clamp studies were performed. There were no significant changes in anthropometric parameters, fasting glucose, or insulin sensitivity in either group. Androgens decreased significantly in both groups though a more pronounced effect on free androgen index was noted in the combination treatment group.

Carbohydrate Metabolism and OCP Use in PCOS: Discussion

The variable results of epidemiological studies of the effects of OCPs on carbohydrate metabolism in the general population, discussed in a previous section (Metabolic and Vascular Effects of OCP), highlight the potentially confounding effects of different doses of estrogen, differing progestins, different formulations, and the genetic and anthropometric make-up of the population studied. Existing evidence supports the notion that estrogen may impair insulin action *(50)*. This is supported by its use in postmenopausal women in whom higher doses of estrogen were associated with insulin resistance *(84)*. The progestin component may modify these effects, for example, by increasing insulin half-life, decreasing estrogen elimination, or other effects *(50,84)*.

A further and important confounding variable is also differences in androgenicity of different progestins. Existing evidence supports the concept of androgen mediated insulin resistance. This data comes not only from the study of subjects with PCOS, but also from studies on female-to-male transsexuals who were treated with testosterone, showing not only decreased insulin sensitivity *(85)* but accumulation of visceral fat *(86)*. Thus, it is not surprising that comparison of different OCPs in normal women, as well as PCOS, has found differing effects on carbohydrate metabolism. Finally, it appears highly likely that differences in the genetic and anthropometric make-up of the population studied may also affect the outcome. For example, in a study by Watanabe *(87)* high-dose estrogen OCP users of a norgestrel pill did not differ from controls, but low-dose estrogen users with the same progestin had lower insulin sensitivity and glucose effectiveness. They suggested that the high-dose users may have represented a special self-selected population.

In relation to PCOS and the effects of OCP on carbohydrate metabolism, all the previously described variables may apply, compounded by differences in the patient population studied. As is evident from the studies previously quoted, carbohydrate metabolism may deteriorate, improve, or remain unchanged. Different results have even been obtained by the same authors according to the patient population studied *(71,76)*. In addition, different preparations have yielded different outcomes, such as cyproterone acetate vs desogestrel in the study of Cagnacci *(77)* and gestodene vs drospirenone in the study of Ibanez and Zegher *(88)*, as have routes of administration of estrogen *(80)*. Importantly, even without OCP, the natural history of PCOS may lead to increasing insulin resistance, as was demonstrated in the study by Pasquali et al. *(70)*, after approx 10 years of follow-up and with weight gain in the interval.

In the ensuing discussion, reference will be made to an arbitrary scale of endogenous insulin sensitivity among subjects with PCOS, determined genetically, environmentally, and by other factors. Applying the hypothesis that the effect of OCPs on carbohydrate metabolism in PCOS relates to the interplay of the previously described factors, four hypothetical groups will be presented and are depicted in Table 1. The outcome, or effect, of OCPs on carbohydrate metabolism will be determined by the interplay of factors such as the women's androgenicity, the androgen-lowering effect of the OCPs, endogenous insulin sensitivity, and obesity/anthropometric differences. Even differences in androgenicity of the progestin may tip the balance one way or the other *(77,88)*.

- Group I: These subjects with PCOS have near normal insulin sensitivity. Their only adverse factor is their androgenicity. When OCPs lower their free androgen concentrations, their insulin sensitivity may improve. Typical examples are thin patients with PCOS. Despite the *potential* for estrogen-mediated insulin resistance, they improve when their androgens are lowered.
- Group II: These subjects with PCOS may have mild endogenous insulin resistance, perhaps aggravated by their androgenicity. In response to OCPs, their insulin sensitivity/glucose tolerance remains unchanged. It may be that estrogen-induced impairment is balanced by the lowering of circulating free androgens. Normal-weight patients with PCOS or mildly overweight patients, possibly with a genetic predisposition, would fall into this category.
- Group III: These subjects with PCOS will show deterioration of glucose tolerance or insulin sensitivity with OCPs. Despite the lowering of free androgens, estrogen-mediated insulin resistance, in the setting of lower endogenous insulin sensitivity, determined both genetically and environmentally (obesity), swings the individual toward increasing resistance. Puberty, which is a time of greater insulin resistance, even in normal-weight girls *(89)*, may also fall into this category.
- Group IV: These subjects with PCOS will show even greater deterioration with OCPs, sometimes leading to frank diabetes, even with short-term use, as in the study of Nader et al. *(69)*. Most of these will be severely obese; often there is a strong family history of diabetes. It may even be that the greater the endogenous insulin resistance, the greater the estrogen-induced deterioration, and there is support in the literature for this effect *(50)*.

As previously stated, the natural history of these groups, even in the absence of OCPs, may also be different, making it even more difficult to sort out these effects. The study of Pasquali et al. *(70)* demonstrated this phenomenon. In that study, follow-up of subjects with PCOS for a mean of 10 years showed the group who never took OCPs (who were obese with higher BMI and who gained significant weight) deteriorated, as regards their glucose tolerance, whereas the group who took OCPs actually improved (more normal in weight with lower BMI).

Further support for the previously described overall concept comes from the study of Dahlgren et al. *(90)*. The authors compared treatment with 50 μg EE plus 100 mg reverse sequential cyproterone acetate vs gonadotropin-releasing hormone analogs in

Table 1
Effects of OCP on Glucose Tolerance/Insulin Sensitivity in PCOS Subjects
Grouped According to a Hypothetical Scale of Endogenous Insulin Sensitivity,
Determined Genetically, Environmentally or by Other Factors (I highest, IV lowest)

| | Determinants of insulin sensitivity | | Carbohydrate metabolism: | |
Group	Genetic	Environmental/other	Outcome with OCP[†]	References
I	Normal	Impaired by androgens	Improvement	70,72,77[*]
II	Normal or mildly impaired	Impaired by androgens, mild obesity	No change	67,73,74,75, 76,78,81,83
III	Mild or moderately impaired	Impaired by androgens, moderate obesity, puberty	Deterioration	68,71,77[**] 80,82
IV	Moderate or severely impaired	Impaired by androgens, severe obesity	Deterioration leading to diabetes	69

[*]Cyproterone acetate containing pill.
[**]Desogestrel containing pill.
[†]See text for explanation.

overweight subjects with PCOS. Hyperinsulinemic euglycemic clamp studies were performed. There was a significant reduction in free androgens in both groups. However, whereas the group using gonadotropin-releasing hormone analogs had an improvement in insulin sensitivity, presumably because of lowering of androgens and possibly also endogenous estrogens, the EE–cyproterone group deteriorated (representing Group III in the previously listed schema). Weight loss itself may modify the grouping. In the study of Sabancu et al. *(78)*, patients received OCPs vs the weight-reducing drug sibutramine, or both. In the group receiving OCPs in addition to diet (leading to significant weight loss) there was no change in carbohydrate tolerance, whereas the subjects receiving both sibutramine and OCPs improved (they went up a group presumably because of more significant weight loss).

METABOLIC EFFECTS OF OCP IN PCOS: LIPID METABOLISM

Lipid Metabolism and OCP Use in PCOS: Results of Individual Studies

Cullberg et al. *(91)* compared lipid and lipoprotein effects in 20 patients with PCOS and 13 controls given a 30-µg EE pill containing desogestrel. Two-thirds of the patients with PCOS were overweight (but none of the controls) and had higher blood pressure. Treatment resulted in increase of cholesterol and triglycerides without changes in LDL or HDL in the subjects with PCOS, with an increase in HDL in the controls. There was a greater increase in triglycerides in the women with PCOS. The author concluded that a positive influence on lipids could not be considered an advantage of OCP treatment in women with PCOS. In the study by Falsetti and Pasinetti *(67)* a low-dose cyproterone

OCP was given to 72 women with PCOS and compared with healthy controls. A significant increase in triglycerides (greater than in controls) and HDL was seen, and LDL was reduced. Twenty-eight of the subjects were overweight. Dodin et al. *(92)* found that, whereas flutamide alone had no significant effect on lipoproteins, the addition of a triphasic OCP lead to increased concentrations of triglycerides and HDL. In Korythowski's study *(68)*, although subjects with PCOS had higher baseline triglycerides, there was no further increase with the norethindrone-containing OCP.

In the study by Pasquali et al. *(70)* that compared PCOS pill users vs non-users, HDL cholesterol increased in pill users. Escobar-Morreale et al. *(72)* evaluated 16 hirsute women (5 oligomenorrheic) before and 6 months after a desogestrel-containing OCP (mean BMI 25.9). HDL, LDL, and total cholesterol increased without a significant change in triglycerides. Although LDL remained within the normal range, low HDL concentrations were normalized in four out of seven patients. Cibula et al. *(93)* compared the effects of OCP in 28 lean and 15 obese subjects with PCOS, and noted no change in LDL/HDL ratio in either group, with greater clinical and biochemical improvement in androgenicity in lean subjects.

Mastorakos et al. *(94)* compared a desogestrel-containing OCP with one containing cyproterone and although both pills led to a significant decrease in hirsutism, the level of triglycerides increased significantly only in the cyproterone group. The ratios of LDL/HDL were unchanged.

Guido et al. *(81)* gave a drospirenone-containing OCP to 15 hirsute patients with PCOS (mean BMI <25). A trend toward increase in cholesterol (HDL and LDL cholesterol) and triglycerides was observed, although all parameters remained in the normal range. In the study of Vrbikova et al. *(80)*, total and HDL cholesterol increased significantly following a cyproterone containing OCP. Rautio et al. *(95)* reported on the lipid effects of a cyproterone-containing OCP in obese and non-obese women with PCOS. There were significant increases in total cholesterol, HDL cholesterol, and triglycerides and a decrease in the total cholesterol:HDL ratio in the treated women. Subgroup analysis of obese vs non-obese patients showed similar trends.

Lipid Metabolism and OCP Use in PCOS: Discussion

In general, the studies show an increase in HDL cholesterol, presumably related to the estrogen component of OCPs. The majority also show significant increases in triglycerides, especially in cyproterone acetate-containing pills, presumably related to their lower androgenicity.

METABOLIC EFFECTS OF OCP IN PCOS: OTHER EFFECTS

Ibanez and Zegher *(96)* observed body adiposity and effects on adipocytokines of an OCP containing drospirenone with and without a flutamide–metformin combination in adolescents. At the start, the proinflammatory marker levels were high (interleukin-6), whereas those of the anti-inflammatory marker adiponectin were low. Abnormal adipocytokine levels, hypertriglyceridemia, and body adiposity diverged further from the norm in the adolescents on OCPs, whereas girls receiving the flutamide–metformin combination reverted all study indices toward normal and lost part of their fat excess. They also looked at young women who were randomized to the OCPs with or without metformin–flutamide. Again, abnormal adipocytokines and adiposity were aggravated on OCP alone and improved in the women on OCPs with metformin and flutamide. They concluded that OCPs alone may not be a prime choice for PCOS. Ibanez et al. *(97)* also showed the pivotal role of adding low-dose flutamide to an OCP regimen containing drospirenone to help improve the hypoadiponectinemia and central adiposity of lean young women with PCOS, age approx 17 years. Finally, Ibanez and Zegher *(98)* studied the additive effects of metformin in young women (approximate age and BMI 19 and 22, respectively) given a drospirenone OCP and flutamide. The addition of metformin consistently had more normalizing effects on interleukin-6, adiponectin, abdominal fat excess, and lean body mass. In a separate study, they discontinued metformin in some patients receiving flutamide–metformin OCPs and continued it in others. Similar advantageous effects of continuing metformin were found.

CONCLUSIONS AND KEY POINTS

The literature previously reviewed generally supports the conclusion reached by Vrbikova and Cibula *(99)*, that therapy should be tailored to the individual. Furthermore, evidence presented in this chapter supports the following concepts:

1. Estrogen may impair carbohydrate tolerance and insulin sensitivity, and this may be dose dependent. This effect may also be dependent on the endogenous insulin sensitivity of the individual.
2. Progestins with intrinsic androgenic properties may also impair insulin sensitivity and glucose tolerance.
3. Lowering of free androgens may improve insulin sensitivity and glucose tolerance in some subjects.
4. The composite effect of OCPs on glucose tolerance and insulin sensitivity may be determined by the interplay of the above with the endogenous insulin sensitivity of the individual, which itself is determined genetically, environmentally, and by other factors. The environmental influence may also vary over time.
5. The effect of OCPs on lipid metabolism relate to estrogen induced increases in HDL and triglycerides. The latter effect may be attenuated by pills of greater androgenicity. The analysis of these composite effects on individual subjects will require the development of appropriate clinical and laboratory tools and provides a stimulus for future research endeavors.

Inasmuch as OCPs have the potential for impairment of glucose tolerance and insulin sensitivity in many subjects with PCOS and given that this effect alone may increase the potential risk for cardiovascular disease (as may changes in lipid metabolism and coagulation parameters), OCPs should be used cautiously in at least some subgroups of patients with PCOS. These include the obese, those with strong family histories of diabetes, and perhaps adolescents, given the lower endogenous insulin sensitivity in these subgroups. Consideration should, therefore, be given to the concomitant use of agents that may modify these effects, such as biguanides, thiazolidinediones, and androgen blockers in appropriate individuals.

FUTURE AVENUES

The hypothesis outlined in this chapter can be validated using appropriately designed clinical studies. Laboratory tools useful in the clinical setting need to be determined, developed, and validated. Finally, it is important to educate both physicians and the public about potentially adverse long-term effects of OCPs in patients with PCOS who are at-risk individuals, particularly during the adolescent to adult transition.

ACKNOWLEDGMENT

The author appreciates the excellent secretarial assistance of Ms. Kathryn Merceri in the preparation of this manuscript.

REFERENCES

1. Scarpitta AM, Sinegra D. Polycystic ovary syndrome: an endocrine and metabolic disease. Gynecol Endocrinol 2000;14:392–395.
2. Ehrmann DA. Polycystic ovary syndrome. N Engl J Med 2005;352:1223–1236.
3. Futterweit W, Dunar JA, Yeh C, Kingsley P. The prevalence of hyperandrogenism in 109 consecutive female patients with diffuse alopecia. J Am Acad Dermatol 1988;19:831–836.
4. Rotterdam ESHRE/ASRM-Sponsored PCOS Consensus Workshop Group. Revised 2003 consensus on diagnostic criteria and long-term health risks related to polycystic ovary syndrome. Fertil Steril 2004;81:19–25.
5. De Ugarte CM, Bartolucci AA, Azziz R. Prevalence of insulin resistance in the polycystic ovary syndrome using the homeostatic model assessment. Fertil Steril 2005;83:1454–1460.
6. Legro RS, Chiu P, Kunselman AR, Bentley CM, Dodson WC, Dunaif A. Polycystic ovaries are common in hyperandrogenic chronic anovulation but do not predict metabolic or reproductive phenotype. J Clin Endocrinol Metab 2005;90:2571–2579.
7. Carmina E, Chu MC, Longo RA, Rini GB, Lobo RA. Phenotypic variation in hyperandrogenic women influences the findings of abnormal metabolic and cardiovascular risk parameters. J Clin Endocrinol Metab 2005;90:2545–2549.
8. Smith S. Polycystic ovary syndrome. Postgrad Obstet Gynecol 2005;25:1–7.
9. Rittmaster RG. Evaluation and treatment of hirsutism. In: Pittaway DE, ed. Infertility and Reproductive Medicine Clinics of North American: Hyperandrogenism Vol 2(3) Philadelphia: Saunders, 1991, pp. 511–530.
10. American Association of Clinical Endocrinologists Position Statement on metabolic and cardiovascular consequences of PCOS. Endocrine Practice 2005;11:126–134.
11. Balen A. Polycystic ovary syndrome and cancer. Human Reprod Update 2001;7:522–525.
12. Hardiman P, Pillay OC, Altiomo W. Polycystic ovary syndrome and endometrial carcinoma. Lancet 2003;362:1810–1812.
13. Burkman RT Jr. The role of oral contraceptives in the treatment of hyperandrogenism disorders. Am J Med 1995;98(Suppl 1A):1305–1365.
14. Azziz R, Gay F. The treatment of hyperandrogenism with oral contraceptives. Semin Reprod Endocrinol 1989;7:246–254.
15. Wild RA, Demers LM, Applebaum-Bowden D, Lenker R. Hirsutism: metabolic effects of two commonly used oral contraceptives and spironolactone. Contraception 1991;44:113–124.
16. Kaunitz AM. Enhancing oral contraceptives success: the potential of new formulations. Am J Obstet Gynecol 2004;190:S23–S29.
17. Krattenmacher R. Drospirenone pharmacology and pharmakinetics of a unique progestogen. Contraception 2000;62:29–38.
18. Azziz R. The evaluation and management of hirsutism. Obstet Gynecol 2003;101:995–1007.
19. Guzick DS. Polycystic ovary syndrome. Obstet Gyecol 2004;103:181–193.
20. Cullberg G, Hamberger L, Mattsson LA, Mobacken H, Samsioe G. Effect of a low dose desogestrel-ethinyl/estradiol combination on hirsutism, androgens and sex hormone binding globulins in women with polycystic ovary syndrome. Acta Obstet Gynecol Scand 1985;64:195–202.
21. Falsetti L, Gambera A, Tisi G. Efficacy of the combination ethinyl estradiol and cyproterone acetate on endocrine clinical and ultrasonographic profile in polycystic ovarian syndrome. Human Reprod 2001;16:36–42.

22. Porcile A, Gallardo E. Long-term treatment of hirsutism: desogestrel compared with cyproterone acetate in oral contraceptives. Fertil Steril 1991;55:877–881.
23. James WD. Acne. N Engl J Med 2005;352:1463–1472.
24. Gollnick H, Cunliffe WJ, Berson D, et al. Management of acne: a report from a Global Alliance to Improve Outcomes in Acne. J Am Acad Dermatol 2003;49(Suppl):S1–S37.
25. Shaw J. Acne: effect of hormones on pathogenesis and management. Am J Clin Dermatol 2002;3: 571–578.
26. Lunde O, Djoseland O. A comparative study of Aldactone and Diane in the treatment of hirsutism. J Steroid Biochem Mol Biol 1987;28:161–165.
27. Should oral contraceptives be prescribed to prevent adnexal masses? Contracept Technol Update 1982;3:116–118.
28. Prelevic GM, Puzigaca Z, Balint-Peric LA. Effects of an oral contraceptive containing cyproterone acetate on the symptoms, hormone profile and ovarian volume of hirsute women with polycystic ovary syndrome. Ann NY Acad Sci 1993;687:255–262.
29. Holt VL, Daling JR, McKnight B, Moore D, Stergachis A, Weiss NS. Functional ovarian cysts in relation to the use of monophasic and triphasic oral contraceptives. Obstet Gynecol 1992;80:472–473.
30. Holt VL, Cushing-Haugen KL, Daling JR. Oral contraceptives, tubal sterilization and functional ovarian cyst risk. Obstet Gynecol 2003;102:252–258.
31. Lanes SF, Birmann F, Walker AM, Singer S. Oral contraceptive type and functional ovarian cysts. Am J Obstet Gynecol 1992;166:956–961.
32. Coulam CB, Annegers JF, Kranz JS. Chronic anovulation syndrome and associated neoplasia. Obstet Gynecol 1983;61:403–407.
33. Hardiman P, Pillay OC, Atiomo W. Polycystic ovary syndrome and endometrial carcinoma. Lancet 2003;362:1082–1084.
34. Balen A. Polycystic ovary syndrome and cancer. Human Reprod Update. 2001;7:522–525.
35. Schlessman JJ. Oral contraceptives and neoplasia of the uterine corpus. Contraception 1991;43: 557–559.
36. Diamanti-Kandarakis E, Baillargeon JP, Iuorno MJ, Jakubowicz DJ, Nestler JE. A modern medical quandary: polycystic ovary syndrome, insulin resistance and oral contraceptive pills. J Clin Endocrinol Metab 2003;88:1927–1932.
37. Baillargeon JP, McClish DK, Essah PA, Nestler JE. Association between the current use of low-dose oral contraceptives and cardiovascular arterial disease: a metaanalysis. J Clin Endocrinol Metab 2005;90:3863–3870.
38. Rimm EB, Manson JE, Stampfer MJ, et al. Oral contraception use and the risk of type 2 diabetes in a large prospective study of women. Diabetologia 1992;35:967–972.
39. Chasen-Taber L, Willett WC, Stampfer MJ, et al. A prospective study of oral contraceptives and NIDDM among U.S. women. Diabetes Care 1997;20:330–335.
40. Troisi RJ, Cowie CC, Harris MI. Oral contraceptive use and glucose metabolism in a national sample of women in the United States. Am J Obstet Gynecol 2000;183:389–395.
41. Luyckx AS, Gaspard UJ, Romus MA, Grigorescu F, De Meyts P, Labefvre PJ. Carbohydrate metabolism in women who used oral contraceptives containing levonorgestrel or desogestrel, a 6-month prospective study. Fertil Steril 1986;45:635–642.
42. van den Ende A, Lutjens RGA, van Wayjen RGA, Kloosterboer HJ. Effects of the oral contraceptive combination 0.150 mg desogestrel plus 0.020 mg ethinyl estradiol on carbohydrate metabolism in healthy female volunteers. Acta Obstet Gynecol Scand Suppl 1987;144:29–32.
43. van der Vange N, Kloosterboer HJ, Haspels AA. Effect of seven low-dose combined oral contraceptive preparations on carbohydrate metabolism. Am J Obstet Gynecol 1987;156:918–922.
44. Bowes WA, Katta LR, Droegmueller W, Bright TA. Triphasic randomized clinical trial: comparison of effects on carbohydrate metabolism. Am J Obstet Gynecol 1989;161:1402–1407.
45. Godsland IF, Crook D, Simpson R, et al. The effect of different formulations of oral contraceptive agents on lipid and carbohydrate metabolism. N Engl J Med 1990;323:1375–1381.
46. Godsland IF, Walton C, Felton C, Proudler A, Patel A, Wynn V. Insulin resistance, secretion and metabolism in users of oral contraceptives. J Clin Endocrinol Metab 1991;74:64–70.
47. Kojima T, Lindheim SR, Duffy DM, Vijod MA, Stanczyk FZ, Lobo RA. Insulin sensitivity is decreased in normal women by doses of ethinyl estradiol used in oral contraceptives. Am J Obstet Gynecol 1993;169:1540–1544.

48. Crook D, Godsland IF, Worthington M, Felton CV, Prudler AJ, Stevenson JC. A comparative study of two low-estrogen-dose oral contraceptives containing desogestrel or gestodene progestins. Am J Obstet Gynecol 1993;169:1183–1189.

49. Petersen KR, Christiansen E, Madsbad S, Skouby SO, Andersen LF, Jespersen J. Metabolic and fibrinolytic response to changed insulin sensitivity in users of oral contraceptives. Contraception 1999;60: 337–344.

50. Godsland IF. The influence of female sex steroids on glucose metabolism and insulin action. J Intern Med Suppl 1996;738:1–60.

51. Clausen JO, Borch-Johnsen K, Ibsen H, Bergman RN, Hougaard P, Winther K. Insulin sensitivity index, acute insulin response, and glucose effectiveness in a population-based sample of 380 young healthy Caucasians. J Clin Invest 1996;98:1195–1209.

52. Scheen AJ, Jandrain BJ, Humblet DMP, Jaminet CB, Gaspard UJ, Lefebvre PJ. Effects of a 1 year treatment with a low-dose combined oral contraceptive containing ethinyl estradiol and cyproterone acetate on glucose and insulin metabolism. Fertil Steril 1993;59:797–802.

53. Perseghin G, Scifo P, Pagliato E, et al. Gender factors affecting fatty acids-induced insulin resistance in non-obese humans: effects of oral steroidal contraception. J Clin Endocrinol Metab 2001;86:3188–3196.

54. Fotherby K. Oral contraceptives, lipids and cardiovascular disease. Contraception 1985;31:367–394.

55. Burkman RT, Kafrissen ME, Olson W, Osterman J. Lipid and carbohydrate effects of a new triphasic oral contraceptive containing norgestimate. Acta Obstet Gynecol Scand Suppl 1992;156:5–8.

56. Van Rooijen M, Schoultz BV, Silveira A, Hamsten A, Bremme K. Different effects of oral contraceptives containing levonorgestrel or desogestrel on plasma lipoproteins and coagulation factor VII. Am J Obstet Gynecol 2002;186:44–48.

57. Practice committee of the American Society for Reproductive Medicine. Hormone contraception: recent advances and controversies. Fertil Steril 2004;82:S26–S32.

58. Farley TM, Meirik O, Collins J. Cardiovascular disease and combined oral contraceptives receiving the evidence and balancing the risks. Human Reprod Update 1999;5:721–735.

59. Tanis BC, van den Bosch MA, Kemmeren JM, et al. Oral contraceptives and the risk of myocardial infarction. N Engl J Med 2001;345:1787–1793.

60. WHO Collaborative study of cardiovascular disease and steroid hormone contraception: acute myocardial infarction and combined oral contraceptives: results of an international multicenter case control study. Lancet 1997;349:1202–1209.

61. Spitzer WO, Faith JM, MacRae KD. Myocardial infarction and third generation oral contraceptives: aggregation of recent results. Human Repro 2002;17:2307–2314.

62. Kemmeren JM, Tanis BC, van den Bosch MA, et al. Risk of arterial thrombosis in relation to oral contraceptives (RATIO) study: oral contraceptives and the risk of ischemic stroke. Stroke 2002;33:1202–1208.

63. WHO Collaborative Study of Cardiovascular Disease and Steroid Hormone Contraception. Ischemic stroke and combined oral contraceptives: results of an international multicenter case control study. Lancet 1996;348:498–505.

64. WHO Collaborative Study of Cardiovascular Disease and Steroid Hormone Contraception. Haemorrhagic stroke, overall stroke risk and combined oral contraceptives: results of an international multicenter case-control study. Lancet 1996;348:505–510.

65. Kemmeren JM, Algra A, Grobbee DE. Third generation oral contraceptives and risk of venous thrombosis: meta-analysis. BMJ 2001;323:131–134.

66. van den Brouche JP, Rosing J, Bloemenkamp KW, et al. Oral contraceptives and the risk of venous thrombosis. N Engl J Med 2001;344:1527–1535.

67. Falsetti L, Pasinetti E. Effects of long-term administration of an oral contraceptive containing ethinylestradiol and cyproterone acetate on lipid metabolism in women with polycystic ovary syndrome. Acta Obstet Gynecol Scan 1995;74:56–60.

68. Korytkowski MT, Mokan M, Horwitz MJ, Berga SL. Metabolic effects of oral contraceptives in women with polycystic ovary syndrome. J Clin Endocrinol Metab 1995;80:3327–3334.

69. Nader S, Riad-Gabriel MG, Saad MF. The effect of desogestrel-containing oral contraceptives on glucose tolerance and leptin concentrations in hyperandrogenic women. J Clin Endocrinol Metab 1997;82:3074–3077.

70. Pasquali R, Gambineri A, Anconetani B, et al. The natural history of the metabolic syndrome in young women with polycystic ovary syndrome and the effect of long-term oestrogen-progestogen treatment. Clin Endocrinol 1999;50:517–527.

71. Morin-Papunen LC, Vauhkonen I, Koivunen RM, Puokonen A, Martikainen HK, Tapanainen JS. Endocrine and metabolic effects of metformin versus ethinyl/estradiol cyproterone acetate in obese women with polycystic ovary syndrome: a randomized study. J Clin Endocrinol Metab 2000;85: 3161–3168.

72. Escobar-Morreale H, Lasuncion MA, Sancho J. Treatment of hirsutism with ethinyl/estradiol– desogestal contraceptive pills has beneficial effects on the lipid profile and improves insulin sensitivity. Fertil Steril 2000;74:816–819.

73. Armstrong VL, Wiggam MI, Ennis CN, et al. Insulin action and insulin secretion in polycystic ovary syndrome treated with ethinyl/estradiol/cyproterone acetate. Q J Med 2001;94:31–37.

74. Elter K, Imir G, Durmusoglu F. Clinical, endocrine and metabolic effects of metformin added to ethinyl/estradiol-cyproterone acetate in non-obese women with polycystic ovary syndrome: a randomized control study. Hum Reprod 2002;17:1729–1737.

75. Cibula D, Fanta M, Hill M, Sindelka A, Skrha J, Zivny J. Insulin sensitivity in non-obese women with polycystic ovary syndrome during treatment with oral contraceptives containing low androgenic progestin. Hum Reprod 2002;17:76–82.

76. Morin-Papunen L, Vauhkonen I, Koivunen R, Ruokonen A, Martikainen H, Tapanainen JS. Metformin versus ethinyl/estradiol-cyproterone acetate in the treatment of non-obese women with polycystic ovary syndrome. J Clin Endocrinol Metab 2003;88:148–156.

77. Cagnacci A, Paoletti AM, Renzi A, et al. Glucose metabolism and insulin resistance in women with polycystic ovary syndrome during therapy with oral contraceptives containing cyproterone acetate or desogestrel. J Clin Endocrinol Metal 2003;88:3621–3625.

78. Sabuncu T, Harma M, Harma M, Nazligul Y, Kilic F. Sibutramine has a positive effect on clinical and metabolic parameters in obese patients with polycystic ovary syndrome. Fertil Steril 2003;80: 1199–1204.

79. Ibanez L, deZegher F. Low-dose combination of flutamide, metformin and an oral contraceptive for non-obese young women with polycystic ovary syndrome. Hum Reprod 2003;18:57–60.

80. Vrbikova J, Stanicka S, Dvorakova K. Metabolic and endocrine effects of treatment with peroral or transdermal oestrogen in conjunction with peroral cyproterone acetate in women with polycystic ovary syndrome. Eur J Endocrinol 2004;150:215–223.

81. Guido M, Romualdi D, Giuliani M, et al. Drospirenone for the treatment of hirsute women with polycystic ovary syndrome: a clinical, endocrinological, metabolic pilot study. J Clin Endocrinol Metab 2004;89:2817–2823.

82. Palep-Singh M, Barth JH, Mook K, Balen AH. An observation study of Yasmin in the management of polycystic ovary syndrome. J Fam Plan Repro Health Care 2004;30:163–165.

83. Cibula D, Fanta M, Vrbikova J, et al. The effect of combination therapy with metformin and combined oral contraceptives (COC) versus COC alone on insulin sensitivity, hyperandrogenemia, SHBG and lipids in PCOS patients. Hum Reprod 2005;20:180–184.

84. Lindheim SR, Presser SC, Ditkoff EC, Vijod MA, Stanczyk FZ, Lobo RA. A possible biomodal effect of estrogen on insulin sensitivity in post menopausal women and the attenuating effect of added progestin. Fertil Steril 1993;60:664–667.

85. Polderman KH, Gooren LJ, Asscheman H, Bakker A, Heine RJ. Induction of insulin resistance by androgens and estrogens. J Clin Endocrinol Metab 1994;79:265–271.

86. Elbers JM, Asscheman H, Seidell JC, Megens JA, Gooren LJ. Long term testosterone administration increases visceral fat in female to male transsexuals. J Clin Endocrinol Metab 1997;82: 2044–2047.

87. Watanabe RM, Azen CG, Roy S, Perlman JA, Bergman RN. Defects in carbohydrate metabolism in oral contraceptive users without apparent metabolic risk factors. J Clin Endocrinol Metab 1994;79:1277–1283.

88. Ibanez L, de Zegher R. Flutamide-metformin plus an oral contraceptive (OC) for young women with polycystic ovary syndrome: switch from third- to fourth-generation OC reduces body adiposity. Hum Reprod 2004;19:1725–1727.

89. Moran A, Jacobs DR, Steinberger J, et al. Insulin resistance during puberty: results from clamp studies in 357 children. Diabetes 1999;48:2039–2044.

90. Dahlgren E, Landin K, Krotkiewski M, Holm G, Janson PO. Effects of two antiandrogen treatments on hirsutism and insulin sensitivity in women with polycystic ovary syndrome. Hum Reprod 1998;13: 2706–2711.

91. Cullberg G, Hamberger L, Mattsson LA, Mobacken H, Samsioe G. Lipid metabolism studies in women with a polycystic ovary syndrome during treatment with a low-dose desogestrel ethinyl estradiol combination. Acta Obstet Gynecol Scand 1985;64:203–207.

92. Dodin S, Faure N, Cedrin I, et al. Clinical efficacy and safety of low dose flutamide alone and combined with an oral contraceptive for the treatment of idiopathic hirsutism. Clin Endocrinol 1995;43:575–592.

93. Cibula D, Hill M, Fanta M, Sindelka G, Zivny J. Does obesity diminish the positive effect of oral contraceptive treatment on hyperandrogenism in women with polycystic ovary syndrome? Hum Reprod 2001;16:940–944.

94. Mastorakos G, Koliopoulos C, Creatsas G. Androgen and lipid profiles in adolescents with polycystic ovary syndrome who were treated with two forms of combined oral contraceptives. Fertil Steril 2002;77:919–927.

95. Rautio K, Tapanainen JC, Ruokonen A, Morin-Papunen LC. Effects of metformin and ethinyl/estradiol-cyproterone acetate on lipid levels in obese and non-obese women with polycystic ovary syndrome. Eur J Endocrinol 2005;152:269–275.

96. Ibanez L, de Zegher R. Ethinylestradiol-drospirenone, flutamide-metformin, or both for adolescents and women with hyperinsulinemic hyperandrogenism: opposite effects on adipocytokines and body adiposity. J Clin Endocrinol Metab 2004;89:1592–1597.

97. Ibanez L, Vals C, Cabre S, de Zegher F. Flutamide-metformin plus ethinylestradiol-drospirenone for lipolysis and antiatherogenesis in young women with ovarian hyperandrogenism: the key role of early, low-dose flutamide. J Clin Endocrinol Metab 2004;89:4716–4720.

98. Ibanez L, de Zegher F. Flutamide-metformin plus ethinylestradiol-drospirenone for lipolysis and antiatherogenesis in young women with ovarian hyperandrogenism: the key role of metformin at the start and after more than one year of therapy. J Clin Endocrinol Metab 2005;90:39–43.

99. Vrbikova J, Cibula D. Combined oral contraceptives in the treatment of polycystic ovary syndrome. Hum Reprod Update 2005;11:277–291.

30 Statins, Oxidative Stress, and Polycystic Ovary Syndrome

Pinar H. Kodaman, MD, PhD
and Antoni J. Duleba, MD

CONTENTS

Summary

Polycystic ovary syndrome (PCOS) is typically characterized by hyperandrogenism, menstrual dysfunction, and altered ovarian morphology. Typically, women with PCOS also have a broad range of metabolic changes including hyperinsulinemia, increased oxidative stress, systemic inflammation, dyslipidemia, and elevation of several growth factors and cytokines. Oxidative stress, proinflammatory cytokines, and hyperinsulinemia may significantly contribute to excessive growth of the ovarian theca–interstitial compartment and to increased production of androgens.

It has become apparent that statins not only improve lipid profile, but may also have anti-inflammatory and antioxidant effects. Furthermore, statins may modify important signal transduction pathways involved in the regulation of cell proliferation. In vitro studies have demonstrated that statins inhibit growth and steroidogenesis of ovarian theca–interstitial cells. In these cells, statins may also limit oxidative stress by decreasing expression of subunits of NADPH oxidase.

A recent randomized prospective clinical trial evaluated the effects of simvastatin on women with PCOS. Simvastatin treatment reduced serum testosterone, normalized gonadotropins, and improved lipid profile.

In summary, inhibition of the mevalonate pathway by statins profoundly affects function and growth of ovarian mesenchyme and may result in both improved ovarian function and systemic cardiovascular benefits in women with PCOS.

From: *Contemporary Endocrinology: Insulin Resistance and Polycystic Ovarian Syndrome: Pathogenesis, Evaluation, and Treatment*
Edited by: E. Diamanti-Kandarakis, J. E. Nestler, D. Panidis, and R. Pasquali © Humana Press Inc., Totowa, NJ

Key Words: Polycystic ovary syndrome; theca cells; statins; oxidative stress; testosterone.

INTRODUCTION

Polycystic ovary syndrome (PCOS) is a common endocrinopathy that affects approx 5–7% of women of reproductive age *(1–3)*. According to a recent consensus statement, PCOS may be diagnosed in women demonstrating at least two of the following three criteria:

1. Oligo- or anovulation.
2. Hyperandrogenism and/or hyperandrogenemia.
3. Polycystic ovaries *(4)*.

Women with PCOS suffer from infertility, menstrual dysfunction, and hirsutism. Poor reproductive function is caused by anovulation and a high rate of early pregnancy loss *(5,6)*. These women also have increased cardiovascular risk factors including dyslipidemia, which typically consists of elevated total cholesterol and low-density lipoprotein (LDL) *(7–10)*, hypertension, increased carotid intima-media thickness, and a greater prevalence of subclinical atherosclerosis *(9,11)*. In the long term, many, but not all, studies indicate that women with PCOS may have significant cardiovascular morbidity and mortality *(8,12–16)*.

The ovaries of women with PCOS are usually enlarged with prominent hyperplasia of theca–interstitial cells that produce excessive amounts of androgens *(17–19)*. Most patients with PCOS have elevated plasma concentrations of luteinizing hormone (LH) and normal or relatively decreased levels of follicle-stimulating hormone (FSH) *(20)*. Increased LH promotes thecal steroidogenesis and thus contributes to the hyperandrogenism seen with the disorder.

Insulin resistance with consequent compensatory hyperinsulinemia, which is seen in both obese and nonobese women with PCOS *(21–23)*, is likely a major contributor to hyperandrogenism, as insulin stimulates the production of androgens by thecal and stromal cells *(24,25)*. Furthermore, free-bioavailable, insulin-like growth factor (IGF)-I levels are also elevated in women with PCOS *(26–29)*. Both insulin and IGF-I stimulate proliferation of rat and human theca–interstitial cells *(30–33)*, as well as protect these cells from apoptosis *(34)*. Insulin and IGF-I increase growth of steroidogenically active ovarian cells, while having little effect on nonsteroidogenic cells *(30)*, demonstrating the relationship between hyperinsulinemia, thecal hyperplasia, and hyperandrogenism.

More recently, dysregulation of theca–interstitial growth with resulting stimulation of steroidogenesis has been attributed to an increase in oxidative stress. PCOS is associated with excessive oxidative stress and increased systemic inflammation as shown by elevations of tumor necrosis factor (TNF)-α and C-reactive protein *(35–38)*. Reactive oxygen species (ROS) induce proliferation of various cell types, including fibroblasts and aortic endothelial cells *(39)*, whereas antioxidants, such as α-tocopherol, inhibit proliferation of vascular smooth muscle, fibroblasts, and many cancer cell lines *(40–43)*. It is also possible that the stimulatory effect of insulin and TNF-α on theca–interstitial cell growth may be mediated, at least in part, by ROS *(44)*.

Statins are selective inhibitors of 3-hydroxy-3-methylglutaryl-coenzyme A (HMG-CoA) reductase, the rate-limiting enzyme in the cholesterol biosynthetic pathway. They improve the lipid profile, primarily by decreasing total cholesterol and LDL levels *(45,46)* and therefore, also decrease both cardiovascular morbidity and mortality *(45,47)*. The competitive and reversible inhibition of HMG-CoA reductase by statins impairs hepatic cholesterol synthesis and induces a compensatory increase in the expression of LDL receptors in the liver *(48–50)*. This mechanism results in binding and subsequent removal of LDL and very low-density lipoprotein (VLDL) particles from the circulation, leading to a reduction of total cholesterol, LDL, and triglycerides. Yet recent studies have demonstrated that statins have many other favorable effects, including anti-inflammatory actions *(51)*, improved nitric oxide-mediated endothelial function *(52,53)*, and anti-proliferative actions on vascular smooth muscle *(54)*.

This chapter focuses on the role of oxidative stress in PCOS and the novel use of statins in the treatment of this endocrinopathy. This approach appears to have beneficial effects not only on the cardiovascular risk factors associated with PCOS, but it may also improve hyperthecosis and hyperandrogenism by a variety of mechanisms.

PCOS AND OXIDATIVE STRESS

PCOS is associated with increased oxidative stress, elevation of markers of systemic inflammation, such as C-reactive protein *(37,38)*, and TNF-α *(35,36)*, and decreased antioxidant reserve *(37)*. TNF-α and insulin stimulate theca–interstitial cell proliferation *(30,32,55)*. Several in vitro and in vivo studies have shown that insulin and TNF-α also induce oxidative stress *(56–58)*. For example, insulin and IGF-I increase LDL peroxidation *(58)*.

Oxidants and antioxidants are involved in the regulation of gene expression under both physiological and pathological conditions. For example, whereas high concentrations of ROS induce oxidative damage and are cytotoxic, at moderate concentrations, ROS can play a role in signal transduction mediating cell growth and differentiation and protection from apoptosis *(59–61)*. ROS appear to act as intra- and intercellular messengers capable of producing these cellular responses *(62–64)*.

The biphasic effect of ROS has been demonstrated in rat theca–interstitial cell cultures *(44)*. Specifically, modest oxidative stress induced by hypoxanthine and xanthine oxidase stimulated a twofold increase in theca–interstitial cell proliferation, whereas greater oxidative stress profoundly inhibited proliferation (Fig. 1). On the other hand, antioxidants, such as vitamin E succinate, the glutathione peroxidase mimetic ebselen, and superoxide dismutase, all inhibited the growth of ovarian theca–interstitial cells *(44)*. The inhibitory effects of antioxidants occurred under basal conditions, that is, in the absence of ROS induction, indicating that the source of ROS resides within theca–interstitial cells. Both oxidants and antioxidants had comparable effects on steroidogenically active and inactive cells *(44)*.

These findings raise the possibility that the increased oxidative stress associated with PCOS may contribute to ovarian mesenchymal hyperplasia in addition to the cardiovascular risk factors associated with the syndrome. Furthermore, apart from increasing the number of steroidogenically active cells, ROS induces the expression of steroidogenic enzymes, including cholesterol side-chain cleavage (P450scc), 17α-hydroxylase/17,20 lyase (P450c17), and 3-β-hydroxysteroid dehydrogenase (3βHSD), as well as the steroidogenic acute regulatory protein, which mediates the transport of

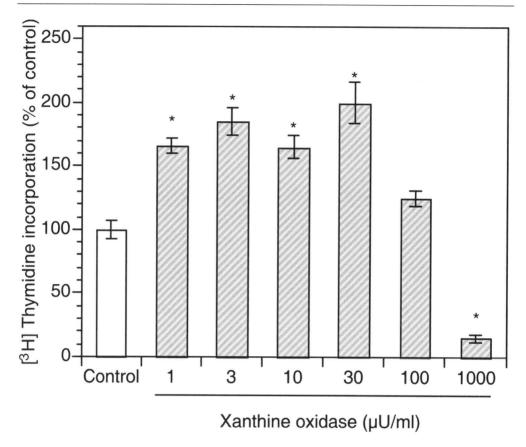

Fig. 1. Effect of hypoxanthine/xanthine oxidase on DNA synthesis of rat theca–interstitial cells. The cells were cultured for 48 hours under serum-free conditions with hypoxanthine (1 mmol/L) with and without xanthine oxidase (1–1000 μM/mL). Cultures were carried out in 96-well plates (35,000 cells/well). Each bar represents the mean ± SEM of eight replicates; *$p < 0.01$ compared with control. (Adapted from ref. *44*.)

cholesterol for steroid synthesis *(65)*. In this way, ROS may further exacerbate the hyperandrogenemia of PCOS. At present, the specific mechanisms involved in the generation of ROS in PCOS remain elusive; however, in intact cells, the major intracellular source of ROS is NADPH oxidase, a multisubunit enzyme.

THE MEVALONATE PATHWAY

In order to understand how statins produce their effects, it is essential to understand the mevalonate pathway (Fig. 2). This pathway consists of the reactions starting from acetyl-coenzyme A (acetyl-CoA) and leads to the formation of farnesyl pyrophosphate (FPP). This compound serves as a substrate for several biologically important agents, including cholesterol, isoprenylated proteins, coenzyme Q, and dolichol *(46,66)*. The rate-limiting step in the mevalonate pathway is conversion of HMG-CoA to mevalonate by HMG-CoA reductase. The resulting depletion of mevalonate leads to a decrease in downstream agents, including FPP and geranylgeranyl-pyrophosphate (GGPP). FPP

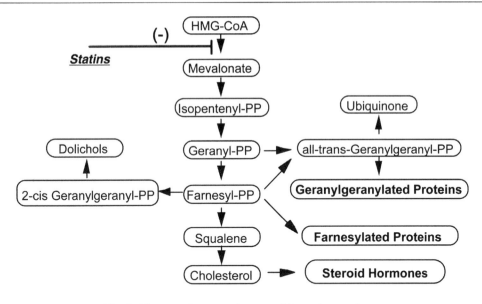

Fig. 2. The mevalonate pathway and its major products.

and GGPP farnesylate and geranylgeranylate proteins, respectively their post-translational modifications, known collectively as isoprenylation, have important consequences *(67)*.

Isoprenylation is important to membrane attachment and subsequent function of several families of proteins, including Ras, Ras-related GTP-binding proteins, and protein kinases *(67)*. Particularly relevant members of the Ras superfamily include Ras, Rho, Rac, and Cdc42. These small GTPases modulate proliferation, apoptosis, and other cellular functions, some of which are mediated by the mitogen activated protein kinase (MAPK) pathway. Actions of Ras depend on farnesylation, whereas Rho, Rac, and Cdc42 require geranylgeranylation. Isoprenylation also affects generation of ROS by NADPH oxidase, as the assembly of this enzyme requires the presence of isoprenylated Rac at the plasma cell membrane *(68)*. Two cytosolic components of NADPH oxidase— p47phox and p67phox—form a complex with Rac1 to induce NADPH oxidase activity *(69)*. Thus, disruption of isoprenylation can lead to profound disturbances in cellular function, including decreased generation of intracellular ROS.

MECHANISM OF STATIN ACTION

Like penicillin, the first statin mevastatin was identified in *Penicillium* mold *(70)*. Subsequently, more statins were developed, including lovastatin (Mevacor®), simvastatin (Zocor®), pravastatin (Pravachol®), atorvastatin (Lipitor®), and rosuvastatin (Crestor®). Statins significantly reduce both fatal and nonfatal cardiovascular disease events in primary and secondary prevention trials *(45,71,72)*. Atherosclerotic plaque rupture is the direct cause of most acute coronary events, and statins appear to stabilize plaques by decreasing the levels of metalloproteases and reducing oxidized-LDL levels *(49,73)*. In addition to improving the lipid profile, beneficial cardiovascular effects of statins include improvement of endothelial function, such as increased nitric oxide production and inhibition of endothelin *(74,75)*, enhanced cellular immunity, antioxidant effects, and anti-inflammatory actions *(49)*.

By inhibiting HMG-CoA reductase, statins block the mevalonate biosynthetic pathway, which results in many downstream effects, including decreased cholesterol synthesis, as previously described, and also a decrease in downstream agents involved in intracellular signaling. Specifically, blockade of HMG-CoA conversion to mevalonate by statins, which is the rate-limiting step in the pathway, results in depletion of mevalonate and, subsequently, decreased isoprenylation of proteins in the form of geranylgeranylation or farnesylation *(67)*.

Inhibition of HMG-CoA and the consequent decrease of isoprenylation of Ras and Rho may inactivate important signal transduction pathways regulating mitotic activity, as shown by a recent study in mesangial cells where statin-induced inhibition of proliferation was associated with suppression of Rho GTPase/p21 signaling *(76)*. Of note, this effect was independent of cholesterol-lowering actions. Statin-induced inhibition of proliferation is blocked by the addition of mevalonic acid and FPP, but not squalene, suggesting a central role of isoprenylation *(77)*. However, the antiproliferative actions of statins are not ubiquitous and depend on cell type. For example, statins induce proliferation in endothelial progenitor cells *(78)*.

The pleiotropic actions of statins also include their inhibitory effect on N-linked glycosylation *(79)*. Decreased N-linked glycosylation inhibits maturation of insulin and type I IGF-I receptors *(80)*. In addition, statins possess both indirect and direct antioxidant activity *(81)*. The antioxidant actions of statins include inhibition of NADPH oxidase activity, preservation of relative levels of vitamins C and E, as well as inhibition of the uptake and generation of oxidized LDL *(68,82)*. Statins have intrinsic antioxidant activity with both anti-hydroxyl and anti-peroxyl radical activity *(81)*. In vitro, simvastatin is the most effective anti-hydroxyl radical antioxidant, whereas fluvastatin is the most effective anti-peroxyl radical antioxidant *(81)*. In vivo, statins reduce plasma levels of nitrotyrosine and chlorotyrosine *(83)*. Statins also exert anti-inflammatory effects by lowering C-reactive protein levels and suppressing pro-inflammatory agents, such as TNF-α *(84)*.

RATIONALE FOR USAGE OF STATINS IN PCOS

Given the pleiotropic nature of the mechanism of statin action, the effect of statins on ovarian function, specifically in women with PCOS, is likely to involve multiple pathways (Fig. 3). First, by directly inhibiting production of cholesterol, the substrate for testosterone, statins can improve hyperandrogenemia. Second, by decreasing N-linked glycosylation, and thus maturation of insulin and type I IGF-I receptors, statins can block the actions of insulin and IGF-I on ovarian cells. Furthermore, their effects on the mevalonate pathway correlate with the sites of insulin action, as insulin stimulates ovarian steroidogenesis, protein isoprenylation, and ovarian theca–interstitial cell proliferation *(31,85–88)*. Thus, the blockade of the mevalonate pathway by statins can lead to an abrogation of the effects of hyperinsulinemia. In addition, by decreasing isoprenylation of small GTPases, such as Ras and Rac, statins can inhibit cellular proliferation and ROS generation by NADPH oxidase. The intrinsic antioxidant activities of statins can also

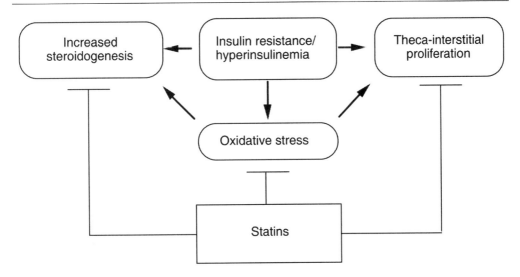

Fig. 3. Rationale for use of statins in polycystic ovary syndrome.

block cellular proliferation and decrease oxidative stress associated with PCOS. The latter, along with the statin-mediated improvement in lipid profile, can have a beneficial effect on the cardiovascular morbidity and mortality associated with this syndrome.

EFFECTS OF STATINS ON OVARIAN FUNCTION

The statin mevastatin inhibits proliferation of theca–interstitial cells in vitro *(89)*; specifically, mevastatin induces a dose-dependent inhibition of theca–interstitial DNA synthesis by 72–92% (Fig. 4) *(89)*. Furthermore, mevastatin inhibits LH-stimulated production of both progesterone and testosterone by these cells that is independent of its effect on cell number (Fig. 5) *(89)*. Inhibition of theca–interstitial cell proliferation by statins persists in the presence of 5% serum, indicating that statin-induced inhibition of proliferation is independent of the supply of cholesterol *(90)*. The inhibitory effects of mevastatin on ovarian cell proliferation are consistent with previous reports regarding other mesenchymal cell types, including vascular smooth muscle *(53,91,92)*, cardio-myocytes *(93)*, and mesangial cells *(76)*.

The effects of statins on ovarian steroidogenesis may be caused by several mechanisms. Besides impairing the availability of the substrate cholesterol, statins also decrease the expression of several key enzymes involved in testosterone production including P450scc, P450c17, and 3βHSD as demonstrated in adrenocortical cells *(94,95)*; similar findings have been observed in ovarian cells *(96)*. It has been previously established that oxidative stress increases the expression of these same steroidogenic enzymes in the ovary *(65)*.

As previously described, NADPH oxidase is a major source of intracellular ROS. Mevastatin and simvastatin, in the presence of LH, inhibit the expression of p22phox, a membrane-bound subunit essential for function of NADPH oxidase in theca–interstitial cells *(97)*. The expression of another NADPH oxidase subunit p47phox, which requires isoprenylated Rac for its activity, is also decreased by these statins *(97)*. In addition,

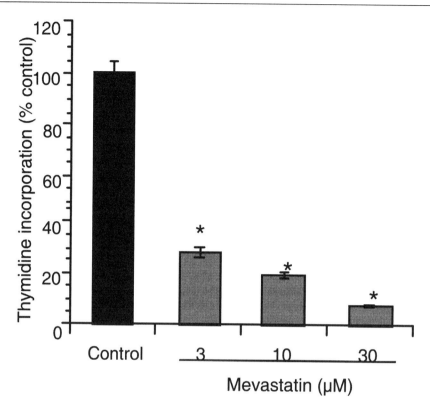

Fig. 4. Effect of mevastatin on DNA synthesis in theca–interstitial cell cultures. The cells were cultured for 48 hours under serum-free conditions without (control) or with mevastatin (3–30 µ*M*). Each bar represents the mean of eight replicates; *$p < 0.01$ significantly different from control. (Adapted from ref. *89*.)

mevastatin blocks basal and insulin-dependent activation of the MAPK pathway in vitro, as measured by phosphorylation of Erk1/2, a downstream kinase, which requires farnesylation of Ras *(90)*.

Thus, in summary, in vitro studies on ovarian theca–interstitial cells demonstrate that statins decrease cell proliferation and testosterone production, inhibit expression of steroidogenic enzymes, decrease expression of NADPH oxidase subunits, and block MAPK-dependent phosphorylation. Taken together, these findings raise the possibility that the use of statins in women with PCOS may decrease thecal hyperplasia, hyper-androgenism, and oxidative stress.

Recently, a randomized, prospective clinical trial investigated for the first time the effects of simvastatin on women with PCOS *(98)*. Specifically, 48 women with PCOS were randomized to one of two groups:

1. The Statin group (20 mg simvastatin daily plus oral contraceptive pill [OCP] containing 20 µg ethinyl estradiol and 150 µg desogestrel).
2. The OCP group (OCP alone).

After 12 weeks of treatment, testosterone levels declined by an average of 41% ($p < 0.0001$) in the Statin group and by 14% ($p = 0.1$) in the OCP group; the treatment

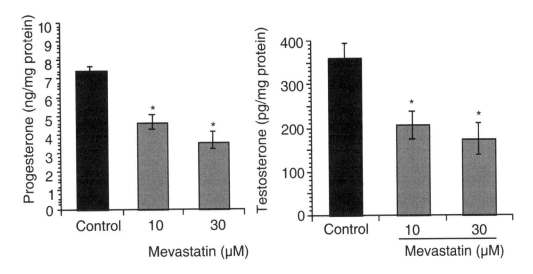

Fig. 5. Effect of mevastatin on progesterone and testosterone production by theca–interstitial cell cultures. The cells were cultured for 48 hours under serum-free conditions in the presence of luteinizing hormone (100 ng/mL) without (control) or with mevastatin (3–30 μM). Each bar represents the mean of four replicates; *p < 0.01 significantly different from control. (Adapted from ref. 89.)

effect (i.e., the effect of simvastatin) between groups was significant ($p < 0.006$) (Fig. 6). In contrast to the effects on testosterone, simvastatin had no effect on dehydroepiandrosterone sulfate (DHEAS) levels, suggesting that the actions of statins are selective and may not alter adrenal steroidogenesis.

However, simvastatin affected the hypothalamo–pituitary axis because between the groups, there were distinctly different responses noted with respect to gonadotropin levels. LH declined by 43% in the Statin group and only by 9% in the OCP group. As FSH levels did not change significantly, the net effect was a reduction in the LH:FSH ratio by approx 44% in the Statin group and a nonsignificant decrease by 12% in the OCP group. Neither of the treatments had a significant effect on body mass index (BMI). Improvements in testosterone and LH levels in the Statin group were not mediated by improved insulin sensitivity, as determined by fasting and postglucose challenge levels of insulin and glucose.

As would be expected, total cholesterol and LDL decreased in the Statin group by 10 and 24%, respectively, whereas there were small increases in these parameters in the OCP group (Fig. 7). There was a small, but significant increase in high-density lipoprotein in both groups, and triglyceride levels were not affected by simvastatin treatment. Improvement of the lipid profile by simvastatin is of particular value in PCOS, a condition characterized by dyslipidemia and other cardiovascular risk factors. Usage of statins in these patients is likely to offer significant protection from long-term cardiovascular morbidity.

Although the design of the previously described clinical trial did not allow direct dissociation of the effects of statins on the ovary from those on the hypothalamus and pituitary, it is likely that primary actions of statins are exerted at the ovarian level by decreasing testosterone, which in turn, may cause a decrease of LH. This is supported

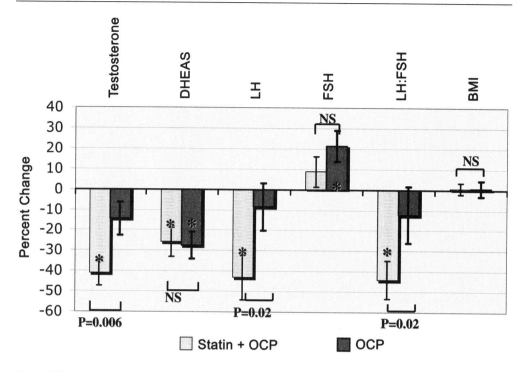

Fig. 6. Effect of statin (simvastatin 20 mg/day) and oral contraceptive pills (OCP) vs OCP alone on serum levels on androgens, gonadotropins, and body mass index in women with polycystic ovary syndrome after 12 weeks of treatment. Asterices denote significant effect of treatment vs baseline; brackets with *p*-values beneath refer to significant differences between treatment groups. NS, non-significant differences. (Modified from ref. *98*.)

by in vitro studies that show direct effects of statins on testosterone production by theca–interstitial cells *(89)* and also by the finding that ovarian wedge resection or laparoscopic diathermy, both of which decrease ovarian androgen production, also leading to a marked decline LH and the LH:FSH ratio *(99,100)*.

CONCLUSION

Prominent features of PCOS include hyperinsulinemia, increased oxidative stress, and elevation of growth factors and cytokines, including IGF-I and TNF-α. These alterations may contribute to the increased size of ovarian theca–interstitial compartment and to increased production of androgens. Furthermore, PCOS is associated with a broad range of cardiovascular risk factors including dyslipidemia, endothelial dysfunction, and systemic inflammation.

Growing evidence points to statins as agents capable of not only correcting dyslipidemia, but also improving systemic inflammation, endothelial function, and oxidative stress. It is likely that statins may block excessive growth of theca–interstitial cells and limit excessive steroidogenesis. In addition, by reducing oxidative stress, statins may also reduce steroidogenesis and cellular proliferation indirectly. Inhibition of N-glycosylation of insulin and IGF-I receptors along with inhibition of the mevalonate pathway by

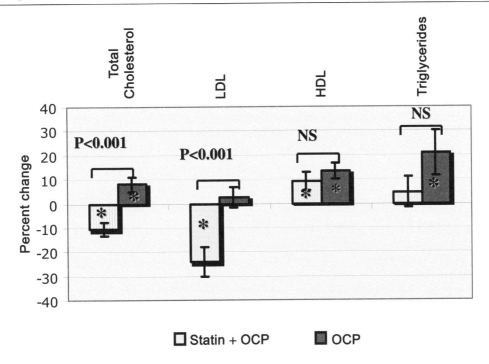

Fig. 7. Effect of statin (simvastatin 20 mg/day) and oral contraceptive pills (OCP) vs OCP alone on lipid profile in women with polycystic ovary syndrome after 12 weeks of treatment. Asterices denote significant effect of treatment vs baseline; brackets with *p*-values refer to significant differences between treatment groups. NS, nonsignificant differences. (Modified from ref. *98*.)

statins, can abrogate the actions of insulin, which otherwise would contribute to thecal hyperplasia and hyperandrogenemia that occurs in PCOS.

Taken together, the available evidence supports the hypothesis that mevalonate pathway plays a prominent role in the function of theca–intersitial cells and that modulation of this pathway by agents such as statins may provide both systemic cardiovascular benefits and improved local ovarian function in PCOS. Given the involvement of the mevalonate pathway in posttranslational modification of small GTPases involved in many signaling pathways, care must be taken to avoid usage of statins in women who are trying to conceive.

FUTURE AVENUES OF INVESTIGATION

Further efforts are needed to better characterize the effects of statins on ovarian function and on PCOS. More extensive in vitro studies should better evaluate the mechanisms of statins' actions on all cellular components of the ovary. Clinical trials should address both short- and long-term effects of statins in diverse populations of women with PCOS. Particularly important will be studies evaluating statins in the absence of concomitant therapies.

KEY POINTS

- Excessive growth and steroidogenesis of the ovarian theca–interstitial compartment in women with PCOS may be related to hyperinsulinemia and increased oxidative stress.

- Statins inhibit the mevalonate pathway. This action may have a broad range of consequences including inhibition of cholesterol synthesis, decreased maturation of insulin receptors, and decreased isoprenylation of several families of proteins. This latter action may interfere with important signal transduction pathways and may decrease intracellular generation of reactive oxygen species.
- In vitro, statins inhibit proliferation and steroidogenesis of ovarian theca–interstitial cells; mechanisms of action may involve blocking the mitogen-activated protein kinase pathway and decreasing expression of key enzymes involved in synthesis of ovarian steroids.
- The first clinical trial evaluating the effects of simvastatin on PCOS was carried out in women who were also receiving oral contraceptive pills. Simvastatin significantly reduced serum testosterone and luteinizing hormone.

REFERENCES

1. Diamanti-Kandaraki E, Kouli CR, Bergiele AT, et al. A survey of the polycystic ovary syndrome in the Greek island of Lesbos: hormonal and metabolic profile. J Clin Endocrinol Metab 1999;84: 4006–4011.
2. Azziz R, Woods KS, Reyna R, Key TJ, Knochenhauer ES, Yildiz BO. The prevalence and features of the polycystic ovary syndrome in an unselected population. J Clin Endocrinol Metab 2004;89: 2745–2749.
3. Asuncion M, Calvo RM, San Millan JL, Avila S, Escobar-Morreale HF. A prospective study of the prevalence of the polycystic ovary syndrome in unselected Caucasian women from Spain. J Clin Endocrinol Metab 2000;85:2434–2438.
4. Rotterdam ESHRE/ASRM-Sponsored PCOS Consensus Workshop Group. Revised 2003 consensus on diagnostic criteria and long-term health risks related to polycystic ovary syndrome. Fertil Steril 2004;81:19–25.
5. Homburg R, Armar NA, Eshel A, Adams J, Jacobs HS. Influence of serum luteinising hormone concentrations on ovulation, conception and early pregnancy loss in polycystic ovary syndrome. Br Med J 1988;297:1024–1026.
6. Sagle M, Bishop K, Ridley N, et al. Recurrent early miscarriage and polycystic ovaries. Br Med J 1988;297:1027–1028.
7. Wild RA, Painter PC, Coulson PB, Carruth KB, Ranney GB. Lipoprotein lipid concentrations and cardiovascular risk in women with polycystic ovary syndrome. J Clin Endocrinol Metab 1985;61: 946–951.
8. Mahabeer S, Naidoo C, Norman RJ, Jialal I, Reddi K, Joubert SM. Metabolic profiles and lipoprotein lipid concentrations in non-obese and obese patients with polycystic ovarian disease. Horm Metab Res 1990;22:537–540.
9. Guzick DS, Talbott EO, Sutton-Tyrrell K, Herzog HC, Kuller LH, Wolfson SKJ. Carotid atherosclerosis in women with polycystic ovary syndrome:initial results from a case-control study. Am J Obstet Gynecol 1996;174:1224–1229.
10. Talbott EO, Guzick DS, Clerici A, et al. Coronary heart disease risk factors in women with polycystic ovary syndrome. Arterioscler Thromb Vasc Biol 1995;15:821–826.
11. Talbott EO, Guzick DS, Sutton-Tyrrell K, et al. Evidence for association between polycystic ovary syndrome and premature carotid atherosclerosis in middle-aged women. Arterioscler Thromb Vasc Biol 2000;20:2414–2421.
12. Wild RA, Applebaum-Bowden D, Demers L, et al. Lipoprotein lipids in women with androgen excess: independent associations with increased insulin and androgens. Clin Chem 1990;36: 283–289.
13. Dahlgren E, Johansson S, Lindsted G, et al. Women with polycystic ovary syndrome wedge resected in 1956 to 1965: a long-term follow-up focusing on natural history and circulating hormones. Fertil Steril 1992;57:505–513.
14. Dahlgren E, Janson PO, Johansson S, Lapidus L, Oden A. Polycystic ovary syndrome and risk for myocardial infarction. Acta Obstet Gynecol Scand 1992;71:599–604.
15. Wild S, Pierpoint T, McKeigue P, Jacobs H. Cardiovascular disease in women with polycystic ovary syndrome at long-term follow-up: a retrospective cohort study. Clin Endocrinol 2000;52: 595–600.

16. Wild RA, Pierpoint T, Jacobs H, McKeigue P. Long-term consequences of polycystic ovary syndrome: results of a 31 year follow-up study. Hum Fertil (Camb) 2000;3(2):101–105.

17. Hughesdon PE. Morphology and morphogenesis of the Stein-Leventhal ovary and of so-called "hyperthecosis". Obstet Gynecol Surv 1982;37:59–77.

18. Wickenheisser JK, Quinn PG, Nelson VL, Legro RS, Strauss JF 3rd, McAllister JM. Differential activity of the cytochrome P450 17 alpha hydroxylase and steroidogenic acute regulatory protein gene promoters in normal and polycystic ovary syndrome theca cells. J Clin Endocrinol Metab 2000;85:2304–2311.

19. Nelson VL, Legro RS, Strauss JF 3rd, McAllister JM. Augmented androgen production is a stable steroidogenic phenotype of propageted theca cells from polycystic ovaries. Mol Endocrinol 1999;13:946–957.

20. Yen SS, Vela P, Rankin J. Inappropriate secretion of follicle-stimulating hormone and luteinizing hormone in polycystic ovarian disease. J Clin Endocrinol Metab 1970;30:435–442.

21. Burghen GA, Givens JR, Kitabchi AE. Correlation of hyperandrogenism with hyperinsulinism in polycystic ovarian disease. J Clin Endocrinol Metab 1980;50:113–116.

22. Chang RJ, Nakamura RM, Judd HL, Kaplan SA. Insulin resistance in non-obese patients with polycystic ovarian disease. J Clin Endocrinol Metab 1983;57:356–359.

23. Dunaif A, Graf M, Mandell J, Laumas V, Dobrjansky A. Characterization of groups of hyperandrogenic women with acanthosis nigricans, impaired glucose tolerance, and/or hyperinsulinemia. J Clin Endocrinol Metab 1987;65:499–507.

24. Barbieri RL, Makris A, Ryan KJ. Insulin stimulates androgen accumulation in incubations of human ovarian stroma and theca. Obstet Gynecol 1984;64:74S–80S.

25. Barbieri RL, Makris A, Randall RW, Daniels G, Kistner RW, Ryan KJ. Insulin stimulates androgen accumulation in incubations of ovarian stroma obtained from women with hyperandrogenism. J Clin Endocrinol Metab 1986;62:904–910.

26. Iwashita M, Mimuro T, Watanabe M, et al. Plasma levels of insulin-like growth factor-I and its binding protein in polycystic ovary syndrome. Horm Res 1990;33:21–26.

27. Homburg R, Pariente C, Lunenfeld B, Jacobs HS. The role of insulin-like growth factor-I (IGF-I) and IGF binding protein in patients with polycystic ovarian disease. Hum Reprod 1992;7: 1379–1383.

28. Suikkari AM, Ruutiainen K, Erkkola R, Seppala M. Low levels of low molecular weight insulin like growth factor binding proteon in patients with polycystic ovarian disease. Hum Reprod 1989;4: 136–139.

29. Thierry van Dessel HJ, Lee PD, Faessen G, Fauser BC, Giudice L. Elevated serum levels of free insulin-like growth factor I in polycystic ovary syndrome. J Clin Endocrinol Metab 1999;84: 3030–3035.

30. Duleba AJ, Spaczynski RZ, Olive DL, Behrman HR. Effects of insulin and insulin-like growth factors on proliferation of rat ovarian theca-interstitial cells. Biol Reprod 1997;56:891–897.

31. Duleba AJ, Spaczynski RZ, Olive DL. Insulin and insulin-like growth factor I stimulate the proliferation of human ovarian theca-interstitial cells. Fertil Steril 1998;69:335–340.

32. Duleba AJ, Spaczynski RZ, Arici A, Carbone R, Behrman HR. Proliferation and differentiation of rat theca-interstitial cells: comparison of effects induced by platelet-derived growth factor and insulin-like growth factor-I. Biol Reprod 1999;60:546–550.

33. Duleba AJ, Spaczynski RZ, Olive DL, Behrman HR. Divergent mechanism regulate proliferation/survival and sterodiogenesis of theca-interstitial cells. Mol Hum Reprod 1999;5: 193–198.

34. Duleba AJ, Spaczynski RZ, Tilly JL, Olive DL. Insulin and insulin-like growth factors protect ovarian theca-interstitial cells from apoptosis. 45th Annual Meeting of the Society of Gynecologic Investigation, 1998, Atlanta, GA.

35. Naz RK, Thurston D, Santoro N. Circulating tumor necrosis factor (TNF)-alpha in normally cycling women and patients with premature ovarian failure and polycystic ovaries. Am J Reprod Immunol 1995;34:170–175.

36. Gonzalez F, Thusu K, Abdel-Rahman E, Prabhala A, Tomani M, Dandona P. Elevated serum levels of tumor necrosis factor alpha in normal-weight women with polycystic ovary syndrome. Metab Clin Exp 1999;48:437–441.

37. Sabuncu T, Vural H, Harma M. Oxidative stress in polycystic ovary syndrome and its contribution to the risk of cardiovascular disease. Clin Biochem 2001;34:407–413.

38. Kelly CC, Lyall H, Petrie JR, Gould GW, Connell JM, Sattar N. Low grade chronic inflammation in women with polycystic ovarian syndrome. J Clin Endocrinol Metab 2001;86:2453–2455.
39. Ruiz-Gines JA, Lopez-Ongil S, Gonzalez-Rubio M, Gonzalez-Santiago L, Rodriguez-Puyol M, Rodriguez-Puyol D. Reactive oxygen species induce proliferation of bovine aortic endothelial cells. J Cardiovasc Pharmacol 2000;35:109–113.
40. Ivanov VO, Ivanova SV, Niedzwiecki A. Ascorbate affects proliferation of guinea pig vascular smooth muscle cells by direct and extracellular matrix-mediated effects. J Mol Cell Cardiol 1997;29:3293–3303.
41. Azzi A, Aratri E, Boscoboinik D, et al. Molecular basis of alpha-tocopherol control of smooth muscle cell proliferation. Biofactors 1998;7:3–14.
42. Nesaretnam K, Stephen R, Dils R, Darbre P. Tocotrienols inhibit the growth of human breast cancer cells irrespective of estrogen receptor status. Lipids 1998;33:461–469.
43. Onat D, Boscoboinik D, Azzi A, Basaga H. Effects of alpha-tocopherol and silibin dihemisuccinate on the proliferation of human skin fibroblasts. Biotechnol Appl Biochem 1999;29:213–215.
44. Duleba AJ, Foyouzi N, Karaca M, Pehlivan T, Kwintkiewicz J, Behrman HR. Proliferation of ovarian theca-interstitial cells is modulated by antioxidants and oxidative stress. Hum Reprod 2004;19(7):1519–1524.
45. Anonymous. Randomised trial of cholesterol lowering in 4444 patients with coronary heart disease: the Scandinavian Simvastatin Survival Study (4S). Lancet 1994;344:1383–1389.
46. Goldstein JL, Brown MS. Regulation of the mevalonate pathway. Nature 1990;343:425–430.
47. Sacks FM, Pfeffer MA, Moye LA, et al. The effect of pravastatin on coronary events after myocardial infarction in patients with average cholesterol levels. N Engl J Med 1996;335:1001–1009.
48. Clearfield M. Evolution of cholesterol management therapies exploiting potential for further improvement. Am J Ther 2003;10:275–281.
49. McFarlane SI, Muniyappa R, Francisco R, Sowers JR. Clinical review 145: Pleiotropic effects of statins: lipid reduction and beyond. J Clin Endocrinol Metab 2002;87:1451–1458.
50. Corsini A, Bellosta S, Baetta R, Fumagalli R, Paoletti R, Bernini F. New insignts into the pharmacodynamic and pharmacokinetic properties of statins. Pharmacol Ther 1999;84:413–428.
51. Albert MA, Staggers J, Chew P, Ridker PM. The pravastatin inflammation CRP evaluation (PRINCE): rationale and design. Am Heart J 2001;141:893–898.
52. Trochu JN, Mital S, Zhang X, et al. Preservation of NO production by statins in the treatment of heart failure. Cardiovasc Res 2003;60:250–258.
53. O'Driscoll G, Green D, Taylor RR. Simvastatin, an HMG coenzyme A reductase inhibitor, improves endothelial function within 1 month. Circulation 1997;95:1126–1131.
54. Porter KE, Naik J, Turner NA, Dickinson T, Thompson MM, London NJ. Simvastatin inhibits human saphenous vein neointima formation via inhibition of smooth muscle cell proliferation and migration. J Vasc Surg 2002;36:150–157.
55. Spaczynski RZ, Arici A, Duleba AJ. Tumor necrosis factor-alpha stimulates proliferation of rat ovarian theca-interstitial cells. Biol Reprod 1999;61:993–998.
56. Adamson GM, Billings RE. Tumor necrosis factor induced oxidative stress in isolated mouse hepatocytes. Arch Biochem Biophys 1992;294:223–229.
57. Krieger-Brauer HI, Kather H. Human fat cells possess a plasma membrane-bound H2O2 generating system that is activated by insulin via a mechanism bypassing the receptor kinase. J Clin Invest 1992;89:1006–1013.
58. Rifici VA, Schneider SH, Khachadurian AK. Stimulation of low-density lipoprotein oxidation by insulin and insulin like growth factor I. Atherosclerosis 1994;107:99–108.
59. Clement MV, Pervaiz S. Reactive oxygen intermediates regulate cellular response to apoptotic stimuli: a hypothesis. Free Radical Res 1999;30:247–252.
60. Kamata H, Hirata H. Redox regulation of cellular signalling. Cell Signal 1999;11:1–14.
61. Kunsch C, Medford RM. Oxidative stress as a regulator of gene expression in the vasculature. Circulation Res 1999;85:753–766.
62. Burdon RH, Alliangana D, Gill V. Hydrogen peroxide and the proliferation of BHK-2 cells. Free Radical Res 1995;23:471–486.
63. Burdon RH, Gill V, Alliangana D. Hydrogen peroxide in relation to proliferation and apoptosis in BHK-21 hamster fibroblasts. Free Radical Res 1996;24:81–93.

64. delBello B, Paolicchi A, Comporti M, Pompella A, Maellaro E. Hydrogen peroxide produced during gamma-glutamyl transpeptidase activity is involved in prevention of apoptosis and maintainance of proliferation in U937 cells. FASEB J 1999;13:69–79.

65. Piotrowski P, Rzepczynska I, Kwintkiewicz J, Duleba AJ. Oxidative stress induces expression of CYP11A, CYP17, StAR and 3bHSD in rat theca-interstitial cells. 52nd Annual Meeting of the Society for Gynecologic Investigation, March 23–26, 2005; Los Angeles, CA.

66. Turunen M, Olsson J, Dallner G. Metabolism and function of coenzyme Q. Biochem Biophys Acta 2004;1660:171–199.

67. Zhang FL, Casey PJ. Protein preynlation: molecular mechanism and functional consequences. Ann Rev Biochem 1996;65:241–269.

68. Wassmann S, Laufs U, Muller K, et al. Cellular antioxidant effects of atorvastatin in vitro and in vivo. Arterioscler Thromb Vasc Biol 2002;22:300–305.

69. Gregg D, Rauscher FM, Goldschmidt-Clermont PJ. Rac regulates cardiovascular superoxide through diverse molecular interactions: more than a binary GTP switch. Am J Cell Physiol 2003;285: C723–C734.

70. Endo A, Kuroda M, Tsujita Y. ML-236A, ML-236B, and ML236C, new inhibitors of cholesterogenesis produced by Penicillium citrinium. J Antibiot 1976;29:1346–1348.

71. Shepard J, Cobbe SM, Ford I, et al. Prevention of coronary heart disease with pravastatin in men with hypercholesterolemia. West of Scotland Coronary Prevention Study Group. N Engl J Med 1995;333:1301–1307.

72. Downs JR, Clearfield M, Weis S, et al. Primary prevention of acute coronary events with lovastatin in men and women with average cholesterol levels: results of AFCAPS/TexCAPS. Air Force/Texas Coronary Atherosclerosis Prevention Study. JAMA 1998;279:1615–1622.

73. Crisby M, Nordin-Fredriksson G, Shah PK, Yano J, Zhu J, Nilsson J. Pravastatin treatment increases collagen content and decreases lipid content, inflammation, metalloproteinases, and cell death in human carotid plaques: implications for plaque stabilization. Circulation 2001;103: 926–933.

74. Petricone F, Ceravolo R, Maio R, et al. Effects of atorvastatin and vitamin C on endothelial function of hypercholesterolemic patients. Atherosclerosis 2000;152:512–518.

75. Alvarez De Sotomayor M, Herrera MD, Marhuenda E, Andriantsitohaina R. Characterization of endothelial factors involved in the vasodilatory effect of simvastatin in aorta and small mesenteric artery of the rat. Br J Clin Pharmacol 2000;131:1179–1187.

76. Danesh FR, Sadeghi MM, Amro N, et al. 3-Hydroxy-3-methylglutaryl CoA reductase inhibitors prevent high glucose-induced proliferation of mesangial cells via modulation of Rho GTPase/p21 signaling pathway: implications for diabetic nephropathy. Proc Natl Acad Sci USA 2002;99: 8301–8305.

77. Raiteri M, Arnaboldi L, McGeady P, et al. Pharmacological control of the mevalonate pathway:effect on arterial smooth muscle cell proliferation. J Pharmacol Exp Ther 1997;281:1144–1153.

78. Assmus B, Urbich C, Aicher A, et al. HMG-CoA reductase inhibitors reduce senescence and increase proliferation of endothelial progenitor cells via regulation of cell cycle regulatory genes. Circ Res 2003; 92:1049–1055.

79. Siddals KW, Marshman E, Westwood M, Gibson JM. Abrogation of insulin-like growth factor-I (IGF-I) and insulin action by mevalonic acid depletion; synergy between protein prenylation and receptor glycosylation pathways. J Biol Chem 2004;279:38,353–38,359.

80. Carlberg M, Dricu A, Blegen H, et al. Mevalonic acid is limiting for N-linked glycosylation and translocaion of the insulin-like growth factor-I receptor to the cell surface. Evidence for a new link between 3-hydroxy-3-methylglutaryl coenzyme A reductase and cell growth. J Biol Chem 1996;271: 17,453–17,462.

81. Franzoni F, Quinones-Galvan A, Regoli F, Ferrannini E, Galetta F. A comparative study of the in vitro antioxidant activity of statins. Int J Cardiol 2003;90:317–321.

82. Avram M, Dankner G, Cogan U, Hochgraf E, Brook JGW. Lovastatin inhibits low-density lipoprotein oxidation and alters its fluidity and uptake by macrophages: in vitro and in vivo studies. Metabolism 1992;41:229–235.

83. Shishehbor MH, Brennan ML, Aviles RJ, et al. Statins promote potent systemic antioxidant effects through specific inflammatory pathways. Circulation 2003;108:426–431.

84. Ando H, Takamura T, Ota T, Nagai Y, Kobayashi K. Cerivastatin improves survival of mice with lipopolysaccharide-induced sepsis. J Pharmacol Exp Ther 2000;294:1043–1046.

85. Goalstone ML, Leitner JW, Wall K, et al. Effect of insulin on farnesyltransferase. Specificity of insulin action and potentiation of nuclear effects of insulin-like growth factor-1, epidermal growth factor, and platelet-derived growth factor. J Biol Chem 1998;273:23,892–23,896.

86. Goalstone ML, Draznin B. Effect of insulin on farnesyltransferase activity in 3T3-L1 adipocytes. J Biol Chem 1996;271:27,585–27,589.

87. Goalstone ML, Leitner JW, Golovchenko I, et al. Insulin promotes phosphorylation and activation of geranylgeranyltransferase II. Studies with geranylgeraylation of rab-3 and rab-4. J Biol Chem 1999; 274:2880–2884.

88. Barbieri RL, Makris A, Ryan KJ. Effects of insulin on steroidogenesis in cultured porcine ovarian theca. Fertil Steril 1983;40:237–241.

89. Izquierdo D, Foyouzi N, Kwintkiewicz J, Duleba AJ. Mevastatin inhibits ovarian theca-interstitial cell proliferation and steroidogenesis. Fertil Steril 2004;82:1193–1197.

90. Kwintkiewicz J, Foyouzi N, Piotrowski P, Rzepczynska I, Duleba AJ. Mevastatin inhibits proliferation of rat ovarian theca-interstitial cells by blocking the mitogen activated protein kinase pathway. Fertil Steril 2006;86(Suppl 4):1053–1058.

91. Axel DI, Riessen R, Runge H, Viebahn R, Karsch KR. Effects of cerivastatin on human arterial smooth muscle cell proliferation and migration in transfilter cocultures. J Cardiovasc Pharmacol 2000;35: 619–629.

92. Buemi M, Allegra A, Senatore M, et al. Pro-apoptotic effect of fluvastatin on human smooth muscle cells. Eur J Pharmacol 1999;370:201–203.

93. El-Ani D, Zimlichman R. Simvastatin induces apoptosis of cultured rat cardiomyocytes. J Basic Clin Physiol Pharmacol 2001;12:325–338.

94. Wu CH, Lee SC, Chiu HH, et al. Morphologic change and elevation of cortisol secretion in cultured human normal adrenocortical cells caused by mutant p21K-ras protein. DNA Cell Biol 2002;21: 21–29.

95. Dobs AS, Schrott H, Davidson MH, et al. Effects of high-dose simvastatin on adrenal and gonadal steroidogenesis in men with hypercholesterolemia. Metab Clin Exp 2000;49:1234–1238.

96. Rzepczynska I, Piotrowski P, Kwintkiewicz J, Duleba AJ. Effect of mevastatin on expression of CYP17, 3bHSD, CYP11A and StAR in rat theca-interstitial cells. 52nd Annual Meeting of the Society for Gynecologic Investigation, March 23–26, 2005; Los Angeles, CA.

97. Piotrowski P, Kwintkiewicz J, Rzepczynska I, Duleba AJ. Simvastatin and mevastatin inhibit expression of NADPH oxidase subunits: p22phox and p47phox in rat theca-interstitial cells. 52nd Annual Meeting of the Society for Gynecologic Investigation, March 23–26, 2005; Los Angeles, CA.

98. Duleba AJ, Banaszeweska B, Spaczynski RZ, Pawelczyk L. Simvastatin improves biochemical parameters of polycystic ovary syndrome: results of a prospective randomized trial. Fertil Steril 2006;85:996–1001.

99. Duleba AJ, Banaszewska B, Spaczynski RZ, Pawelczyk L. Success of laparoscopic ovarian wedge resection is related to obesity, lipid profile, and insulin levels. Fertil Steril 2003;79:1008–1014.

100. Amer SA, Li TC, Cooke ID. A prospective dose-finding study of the amount of thermal energy required for laparoscopic ovarian diathermy. Hum Reprod 2003;18:1693–1698.

VI   TREATMENT OF INFERTILITY IN PCOS

31 Insulin-Sensitizing Drugs for the Treatment of Infertility in Polycystic Ovary Syndrome

Cynthia S. Ryan, MD and John E. Nestler, MD

CONTENTS

INTRODUCTION
PHARMACOLOGY OF INSULIN-SENSITIZING AGENTS
INSULIN-SENSITIZING AGENTS AS MONOTHERAPY
INSULIN-SENSITIZING DRUGS WITH CLOMIPHENE CITRATE
INSULIN-SENSITIZING DRUGS WITH FSH INDUCTION
INSULIN SENSITIZERS AND EARLY PREGNANCY LOSS
CONCLUSION
FUTURE AVENUES
KEY POINTS
REFERENCES

Summary

Infertility in polycystic ovary syndrome (PCOS) is characterized by anovulation and early pregnancy loss. A key component of PCOS is the presence of insulin resistance and compensatory hyperinsulinemia, which has an important role in the pathogenesis of infertility. As a result, insulin-sensitizing agents such as metformin and thiazolinediones have been studied in women with PCOS with the goal of improving ovulation.

Multiple studies have demonstrated the effectiveness of metformin in improving ovulatory rates as a single agent and in combination with clomiphene citrate. Pregnancy rates are also increased when metformin is added to clomiphene. In addition, metformin with follicle-stimulating hormone induction may minimize ovarian hyperstimulation, although studies are limited. Recent data suggests metformin improves the endometrial environment during the peri-implantation period, thereby decreasing the rate of early miscarriage.

Rosiglitazone and pioglitazone monotherapy increase ovulatory rates, as well as the combination of clomiphene and rosiglitazone. Preliminary studies suggest that thiazolinediones may be more effective in obese women with PCOS compared with metformin in improving ovulation. However, with the thiazolinediones as category C pregnancy drugs, their use as fertility agents is less clear than metformin.

Key Words: Polycystic ovary syndrome; insulin sensitizers; ovulation; fertility; metformin; thiazolinediones; clomiphene citrate.

From: *Contemporary Endocrinology: Insulin Resistance and Polycystic Ovarian Syndrome: Pathogenesis, Evaluation, and Treatment*
Edited by: E. Diamanti-Kandarakis, J. E. Nestler, D. Panidis, and R. Pasquali © Humana Press Inc., Totowa, NJ

INTRODUCTION

Polycystic ovary syndrome (PCOS) is the most common cause of infertility among premenopausal women, affecting 6–10% in their reproductive years *(1,2)*. The infertility is primarily anovulatory, and 75% of women with oligo-amenorrhea have PCOS *(3)*. PCOS is also characterized by increased early pregnancy loss. In the past, medical options for the treatment and management of anovulation included anti-estrogens, such as clomiphene citrate or gonadotropins, for induction of ovulation. More recently, insight into the pathogenesis of PCOS has linked insulin resistance and compensatory hyperinsulinemia with hyperandrogenism, which in turn may impair ovulation *(4–6)*. As a result, researchers have increasingly focused on evaluating insulin-sensitizing agents as therapeutic alternatives for managing women with PCOS desiring fertility.

PHARMACOLOGY OF INSULIN-SENSITIZING AGENTS

Metformin

Metformin is in the class of biguanides, the only one available in the United States, and has been on the market worldwide for the treatment of type 2 diabetes since 1957. Its primary action is to increase insulin sensitivity in peripheral tissues, particularly the liver and muscle. In the liver, metformin decreases basal glucose output by enhancing insulin's action to suppress gluconeogenesis. In addition, insulin-mediated glucose uptake in the muscle is increased by metformin as well. Because it does not enhance insulin release, metformin does not cause hypoglycemia in nondiabetic patients *(7)*. It is a category B drug for use in pregnancy.

Side effects of metformin most commonly involve the gastrointestinal tract, such as cramping, nausea, and diarrhea, and occur in 5–20% of patients *(8)*. These are reversible or minimized by taking the drug with food and starting at a low dose of 500 mg daily and slowly titrating upward to a maximum dose of 2000 mg daily. The most serious adverse reaction of metformin is lactic acidosis. This adverse reaction is rare, and it is more common in individuals with cardiac and renal insufficiency *(9)*.

Thiazolinediones

A second class of insulin-sensitizing agents includes the thiazolinediones, to which three drugs belong: troglitazone, rosiglitazone, and pioglitazone. These are synthetic agonists of the nuclear peroxisome proliferator-activated receptor-γ (PPARγ) that is predominantly expressed in adipose tissue, but also in muscle and the liver. Activation of PPARγ increases gene transcription that ultimately increases insulin sensitivity in the liver, muscle, and adipose tissue. As a result, glucose uptake is enhanced and insulin levels are decreased in insulin-resistant nondiabetic individuals. Like metformin, hypoglycemia does not occur.

In 1997, troglitazone was approved for treatment of type 2 diabetes; however, the US Food and Drug Administration (FDA) withdrew it from the market in 2000 because of hepatotoxicity. Since then, both rosiglitazone and pioglitazone, introduced in 1999, are available for treatment of type 2 diabetes *(10)*. Pioglitazone binds to the PPARγ receptor with 10- to 15-fold greater affinity than troglitazone, whereas rosiglitazone is the most potent, with an affinity 100-fold greater than troglitazone *(11,12)*. Both rosiglitazone and pioglitazone are category C drugs for pregnancy.

INSULIN-SENSITIZING AGENTS AS MONOTHERAPY

Metformin

The most extensively studied insulin-sensitizing agent in PCOS is metformin. Metformin was first used in 1994 in an uncontrolled observational study, where 26 women with PCOS received metformin for 8 weeks, resulting in improvements in insulin sensitivity and decreases in serum androgens. During that time, menstrual cyclicity normalized in seven women, and three spontaneous pregnancies occurred (13). Nestler et al. performed the first randomized and placebo-controlled trial assessing ovulation in response to metformin in an unselected group of women with PCOS. Twelve of 35 women (34%) treated with 500 mg metformin three times daily spontaneously ovulated after 5 weeks, with a mean serum progesterone higher than 13 ng/mL compared with 1 of 26 women (4%) given placebo ($p < 0.001$) (14).

Because of many studies containing small numbers of patients and variable durations of treatment, a meta-analysis for the Cochrane review was published in 2003 that included only randomized, controlled trials to determine if a true benefit occurred with metformin (15). Among the seven studies included in the analysis of metformin monotherapy, study subjects were both clomiphene-resistant and sensitive. The study did not show any heterogeneity or bias. As seen in Fig. 1, the ovulation rate was 46% when subjects were treated with metformin alone compared with 24% when subjects were treated with placebo. Therefore, this analysis demonstrated that metformin induced ovulation significantly more often than placebo ($p < 0.0001$). The number needed to treat was 4.4, indicating that the use of metformin in doses of at least 1500 mg daily is very effective for managing anovulatory patients with PCOS.

When the authors of this analysis reviewed the data on pregnancy rates in five trials, there was no evidence of benefit of metformin over placebo. However, none of the trials targeted pregnancy as a primary outcome variable, and all of them were of short duration, i.e., less than 4 months.

Most recently, metformin was directly compared with clomiphene citrate in a randomized double-blinded crossover trial of 100 nonobese women with PCOS who desired pregnancy (16). After 6 months, the ovulation rate was similar between the two groups (63% with metformin and 67% with clomiphene). The pregnancy rate per ovulatory cycle, however, was significantly higher in the metformin group. In addition, the cumulative pregnancy rate in the metformin group (69%) was significantly greater than the clomiphene group (34%). In other words, administering metformin to three women with PCOS will lead to one pregnancy. Over the 6-month period, metformin continued to be effective, whereas clomiphene's success in inducing ovulation decreased after multiple cycles. This suggests that metformin alone is superior to placebo and clomiphene for treatment of anovulatory infertility associated with PCOS.

Troglitazone

Although troglitazone has been withdrawn from the market, it will be discussed briefly for historical reasons. Five trials studied the treatment of women who had PCOS with troglitazone (17–21). Three of these studies specifically evaluated ovulation (17,20,21). These studies showed that treatment with troglitazone increased the ovulatory rate in unselected and clomiphene citrate-resistant women. The largest double-blind,

Comparison: Metformin versus placebo or no treatment (clinical outcomes)
Outcome: Ovulation rate

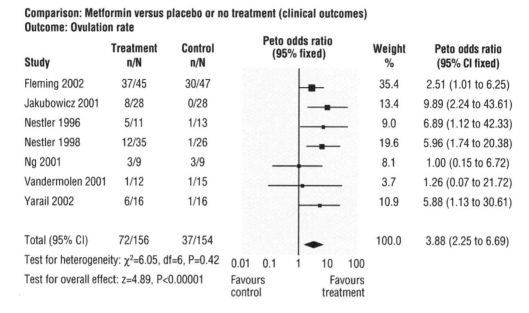

Study	Treatment n/N	Control n/N	Peto odds ratio (95% fixed)	Weight %	Peto odds ratio (95% CI fixed)
Fleming 2002	37/45	30/47		35.4	2.51 (1.01 to 6.25)
Jakubowicz 2001	8/28	0/28		13.4	9.89 (2.24 to 43.61)
Nestler 1996	5/11	1/13		9.0	6.89 (1.12 to 42.33)
Nestler 1998	12/35	1/26		19.6	5.96 (1.74 to 20.38)
Ng 2001	3/9	3/9		8.1	1.00 (0.15 to 6.72)
Vandermolen 2001	1/12	1/15		3.7	1.26 (0.07 to 21.72)
Yarail 2002	6/16	1/16		10.9	5.88 (1.13 to 30.61)
Total (95% CI)	72/156	37/154		100.0	3.88 (2.25 to 6.69)

Test for heterogeneity: χ^2=6.05, df=6, P=0.42
Test for overall effect: z=4.89, P<0.00001

0.01   0.1   1   10   100
Favours control   Favours treatment

Fig. 1. Metformin compared with placebo or no treatment-ovulation rate. (Lord JM, Flight IH, Norman RJ. Metformin in polycystic ovary syndrome: systematic review and meta-analysis. BMJ 2003;327[7421]:951 953. Reproduced with permission from the BMJ Publishing Group.)

placebo controlled trial evaluated the effects of 44 weeks of escalating doses of troglitazone on ovulatory function in 305 women with PCOS *(17)*, and a clear dose–response was observed with increasing doses of troglitazone. With the intake of 600 mg of troglitazone daily, 57% of the subjects ovulated 50% of the time. In addition, the average time to resumption of ovulation in the subjects with PCOS taking 600 mg of troglitazone was briefer (53 days) as compared with the subjects with PCOS taking 150 mg or a placebo daily (88 and 107 days, respectively). The unplanned pregnancy rate was also significantly higher in the troglitazone-treated group (5.9%) compared with the placebo group (1.4%).

Rosiglitazone

Four studies since 2003 have evaluated the effect of rosiglitazone in women with PCOS. Three studies examined obese women with PCOS and one study examined nonobese women with PCOS *(22–25)*. The first prospective, uncontrolled study included 24 obese women with PCOS who were treated daily with 4 mg of rosiglitazone for 3 months *(23)*. By the second month, one patient became pregnant despite the request of the investigators to use barrier contraception. Menstrual cycles were restored in 22 of the 23 remaining participants (95%). Progesterone was not measured in this study to confirm ovulation.

More recently, Sepilian et al. prospectively assessed 12 obese patients with PCOS with an average body mass index (BMI) higher than 40 mg/m^2 and severe insulin resistance as defined by acanthosis nigricans on examination *(25)*. The subjects were treated with 4 mg of rosiglitazone daily for 6 months. Within 3 months, spontaneous menstruation occurred in 11 of the 12 women (91%), and ovulation was confirmed with a serum progesterone greater than 5 ng/mL on day 21.

In a randomized control trial, Ghazeeri et al. compared rosiglitazone with or without clomiphene citrate in previously clomiphene-resistant women with PCOS (24). Patients were treated with rosiglitazone at a dose of 4 mg twice daily for 2 months. Among the subjects receiving rosiglitazone monotherapy, 4 of the 12 subjects ovulated (33%), as defined by a serum progesterone higher than 5 ng/mL. One of the subjects became pregnant, which resulted in a successful live birth. The ovulation rate in this study was low compared to the first two discussed, and the discrepancy was most likely related to the difference in duration of treatment. Ovulation occurred at 3 months in the majority of the patients in the prospective studies previously discussed.

Unlike the prior studies, Baillergeon et al. assessed the frequency of ovulation in 100 nonobese women with PCOS who had normal indices of insulin sensitivity in a randomized, controlled trial (22). These subjects were treated with either rosiglitazone (4 mg bid), metformin (850 mg bid), a combination of rosiglitazone and metformin, or placebo. After 6 months, the ovulation rates were 100% in subjects treated with metformin or with the combination, 91% in subjects treated with rosiglitazone, and 37% in subjects treated with placebo ($p < 0.001$). The difference in ovulation rates between the metformin and combination group compared with rosiglitazone was statistically significant ($p < 0.05$). Figure 2 shows that ovulation rates increased every month in each group until months 5 and 6.

These studies indicate the rosiglitazone is effective in inducing spontaneous ovulation in both obese and nonobese patients with PCOS. In nonobese patients, it is less effective than metformin and there is no benefit in combining the two drugs. There may be a greater benefit of combination therapy in obese patients, but no randomized control trial comparing rosiglitazone to metformin in this population has been performed.

Pioglitazone

Few studies have examined the effectiveness of pioglitazone in the treatment of PCOS. One randomized, controlled trial compared 30 mg of pioglitazone daily to placebo in 35 women with PCOS (26). After 3 months, pioglitazone significantly decreased insulin resistance and the free androgen index, and increased serum sex hormone-binding globulin. Forty-one percent of women on pioglitazone experienced normalization of menstrual cycles and ovulation compared with 5.6% of women on placebo ($p < 0.02$).

Glueck et al. have studied the effect of adding pioglitazone on ovulation rates in women with PCOS who had failed to ovulate while on metformin therapy (27). Prior studies (13,28–30) had showed a failure rate of up to 23% for menstrual cycle normalization in patients with PCOS who were treated with metformin. Eleven obese patients with PCOS who were considered nonresponders to metformin after 1 year (defined as a 3-month menses rate of 46% compared with 78% in responders) started 45 mg of pioglitazone daily for 10 months while remaining on metformin. During the first 3 months, 67% of expected menses occurred and over 9 months, the percentage increased twofold compared with metformin alone.

One study compared pioglitazone to metformin head-to-head in a randomized control trial (31). Twenty-five obese women with PCOS, all with acanthosis nigricans, received 30 mg of pioglitazone daily and 27 women received 850 mg of metformin three times

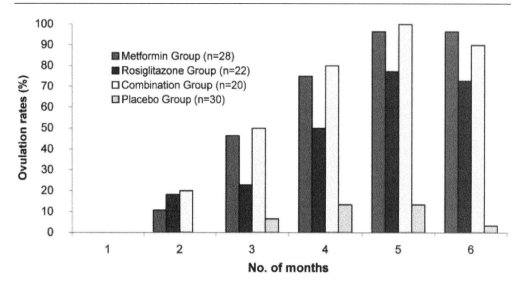

Fig. 2. Monthly ovulation rates in nonobese women with the polycystic ovary syndrome and normal indices of insulin sensitivity after administration of insulin-sensitizing drugs or placebo for 6 months. Values are the number of women who ovulated during each month in a group, divided by the total number of subjects in that group. $p < 0.001$ for differences among months using mixed-model repeated-measures logistic regression. (Adapted from ref. 22.)

daily for 6 months. The primary end point was metabolic parameters of insulin resistance; however, 29% (five) of women on pioglitazone and 17% (three) on metformin became pregnant during the trial. Ovulatory rates were not assessed in this study.

INSULIN-SENSITIZING DRUGS WITH CLOMIPHENE CITRATE

Clomiphene citrate induces ovulation because of its anti-estrogenic effects on the pituitary leading to increased production of luteinizing hormone and follicle-stimulating hormone (FSH). It has been the primary therapy for management of infertility in patients with PCOS. The success rate is reported as 70–80% for ovulation induction, but a pregnancy rate of only 30–40% *(32)*. Obese women with PCOS are more resistant to the ovulation effects of clomiphene, and these patients require higher doses to induce ovulation *(33)*. Twenty-five percent of patients with PCOS fail to respond to clomiphene and are called CC-resistant. CC-resistance appears to vary proportionately with insulin resistance in women with PCOS *(34)*. Thus, multiple studies have used insulin-sensitizing agents in conjunction with clomiphene to evaluate the effect on fertility.

Metformin

Two meta-analyses have assessed the effectiveness of metformin with clomiphene *(15,35)*. Both used different studies in their analysis but yielded similar results. Lord et al. included three trials, two of which included CC-resistant patients *(36,37)*. The ovulation rate was significantly improved when metformin was added to clomiphene (76%) compared with clomiphene alone (42%). The third trial included patients sensitive to clomiphene, and did not show evidence of an added benefit of metformin compared with clomiphene alone. However, the pregnancy rate in the three trials did show a significant treatment effect for the combination of metformin and clomiphene ($p = 0.0003$).

Similarly, Kayshap et al. analyzed the ovulation rates in four studies and the pregnancy rates in two studies that compared combination metformin and clomiphene treatment to clomiphene alone (35). Combination treatment resulted in a three- to fourfold increased rate of ovulation and pregnancy compared with clomiphene alone, as seen in Fig. 3. These studies support the theory that insulin-sensitizing agents improve the insulin resistance seen in previously CC-resistant women.

Rosiglitazone

Two randomized, controlled studies have examined the effect of rosiglitazone with clomiphene on ovulation. Ghazeeri et al. evaluated the ovulation rate as a primary outcome in previously clomiphene-resistant women. Subjects were randomized to treatment with 4 mg of rosiglitazone twice daily and either 50 mg of clomiphene citrate or placebo on days 5–9 of their cycle (24). Seventy-seven percent of women (10 of 13) treated with rosiglitazone and clomiphene ovulated after 2 months, compared with 33% on rosiglitazone alone. This suggests that when rosiglitazone is added to a low dose of clomiphene citrate, ovulation is improved within a short period of time. As prior studies showed, ovulatory rates with rosiglitazone monotherapy are higher after 3–6 months of treatment. Only one study has compared clomiphene with rosiglitazone to clomiphene monotherapy for ovulation induction (38). Clomiphene citrate, in doses of 100 mg, was given to 25 patients taking 4 mg of rosiglitazone or placebo for 3 months. Recovery of ovulatory menstrual cycles occurred in 72% of patients in the combination group compared with 48% receiving clomiphene monotherapy.

INSULIN-SENSITIZING DRUGS WITH FSH INDUCTION

In women who have failed clomiphene, a non-surgical next step to restore ovulation is administration of exogenous gonadotropins. One of the main risks of this procedure is ovarian hyperstimulation, which can lead to multiple gestations. DeLeo evaluated the effect of metformin in patients with PCOS undergoing FSH stimulation (39). Twenty women were randomized into two groups. The first group received 500 mg of metformin three times daily for 1 month prior to undergoing stimulation with urinary FSH for one cycle. The second group received two cycles of FSH alone, followed by a 1-month treatment with metformin combined with FSH for the third cycle. At baseline, no significant differences existed between the two groups. However, the group treated with metformin prior to receiving gonadotropins had significantly fewer follicles greater than 15 mm on the day hCG was administered. In addition, no cycles in the combined metformin–FSH group had hCG withheld because of excessive follicular development compared with 31.5% of cycles in the FSH-alone group. A similar effect was observed when the patients in the FSH-alone group received metformin prior to their third cycle with FSH. This suggested that pretreatment with metformin allowed for a decrease in follicular hyperstimulation and more orderly induction of ovulation with FSH in patients with PCOS.

Yarali et al. reported the only randomized placebo-controlled trial of metformin with FSH in patients with CC-resistant PCOS (40). These investigators evaluated the low-dose

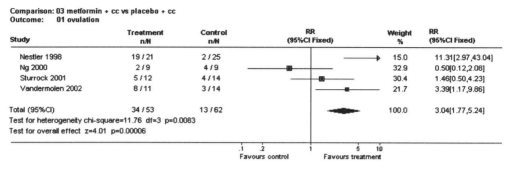

Fig. 3. Comparison of metformin + clomiphene citrate (CC) versus placebo + CC in infertile patients. The upper panel shows the outcome ovulation and the lower panel the outcome pregnancy. RR = relative risk. Generated from Meta-view 4.0. (Adapted from ref. *35*.)

step-up protocol with recombinant FSH, which improved monofollicular development and minimized ovarian hyperstimulation. Thirty-two women were randomized to placebo or 850 mg metformin twice daily for 6 weeks. Patients with spontaneous ovulation, six in the metformin group and one in the placebo group ($p < 0.05$), were excluded from treatment with recombinant (rFSH). After completion of the low-dose protocol, there was no difference between monofollicular or multifollicular development, estradiol level, endometrial thickness, or total dose of rFSH. Ovulatory rates (90% metformin and 73% placebo) and pregnancy rates per cycle (three in the metformin group and one in the placebo group) did not differ significantly between the two groups. This study suggests that metformin does not influence FSH-induced ovulation. However, De Leo and Yarali were limited by their small sample sizes. Additional research in this area is needed before making recommendations for or against the adjuvant use of metformin with gonadotropin induction.

INSULIN SENSITIZERS AND EARLY PREGNANCY LOSS

Women with PCOS are not only faced with difficulties conceiving, they also have an increased risk of miscarriage once they do become pregnant, either spontaneously or through induction. Within the first trimester, rates of early pregnancy loss of clinically recognized pregnancies are reported to be 30–50% *(41–43)*, approximately threefold higher than the rates for normal women *(44)*.

Hyperinsulinemia has been shown to be an independent risk factor for early pregnancy loss in obese insulin-resistant women (45). Recent evidence suggests that hyperinsulinemia may contribute to an inhospitable endometrial environment and promote early pregnancy loss. Two endometrial secretory proteins, glycodelin, and insulin-like growth factor binding protein (IGFBP)-1, are decreased in women with PCOS during the first trimester of pregnancy (46). Glycodelin, produced during the luteal phase by endometrial glands, may assist in implantation and maintenance of pregnancy through inhibition of the maternal immune response to the embryo (47,48). IGFBP-1 is produced by the endometrium during pregnancy and facilitates adhesion during implantation (49). One study demonstrated that insulin reduction by metformin in women with PCOS was associated with improvements in the circulating levels of glycodelin and IGFBP-1 during the luteal phase, presumably reflecting an improvement in the endometrial milieu throughout the implantation period and suggesting that hyperinsulinemia inhibits expression of glycodelin and IGFBP-1 in PCOS (50). In addition, treatment with metformin improved uterine vascularity. This latter effect was recently confirmed in women with PCOS by Palomba et al. as well (51).

Two studies have specifically assessed the effect of metformin on early pregnancy loss in women with PCOS. Glueck et al. studied 19 women prospectively during conception and throughout gestation on metformin (52). Normal live births occurred in 11 patients (58%), 2 had first-trimester spontaneous abortions (10.5%), and 6 had ongoing pregnancies. Glueck et al. evaluated prior miscarriage history and found that 10 of these women had 22 previous pregnancies while not taking metformin. Six (27%) of these previous pregnancies resulted in normal live births and 16 (73%) resulted in first-trimester spontaneous abortions. The rate of miscarriage in these women with PCOS while taking metformin was 10%. Thus, metformin appeared to reduce the rate of miscarriage to that seen in the normal population.

This is consistent with the results reported in a controlled, retrospective study by Jakubowicz et al. (53). A total of 65 women with PCOS had been treated with metformin throughout their pregnancies and compared with 31 women with PCOS who had not received metformin and served as the control group. As shown in Table 1, 6 of 68 (8%) pregnancies resulted in miscarriage in the metformin treated group, whereas 13 of 31 (42%) pregnancies resulted in miscarriage in the untreated group ($p < 0.001$). The decrease in miscarriage rate was significant regardless of the patient's history of prior pregnancy loss. These studies suggest that use of metformin during pregnancy decreases the rate of early pregnancy loss in women with PCOS, including those who have experienced prior miscarriages.

More recently, two head-to-head studies comparing metformin to other methods of ovulation induction, clomiphene citrate, and laparoscopic ovarian diathermy (LAD), further support the probability of hyperinsulinemia as a contributing cause for the early pregnancy loss in women with PCOS (16,54). Sixty women with PCOS were treated with metformin vs LAD in a 6-month, randomized, double-blind, controlled trial (54). Although the ovulation rate was similar in both groups, the pregnancy rate was significantly higher (18.6 vs 13.4%), and the miscarriage rate was significantly lower in the metformin treated group than in the LAD group (15.4 vs 29%). Hence, the live birth rate was significantly higher (82.1 vs 64.5%; $p < 0.05$) for those treated with metformin compared with those treated with LAD.

Table 1
Rates of Early Pregnancy Loss Among Women With Polycystic
Ovary Syndrome Who Either Received (Metformin Group)
or Did Not Receive (Control Group) Metformin During Pregnancy

| | Early pregnancy loss rate | | |
Cohort	Metformin group (n = 65)	Control group (n = 31)	p-value
All women	8.8% (6/68)	41.9% (13/31)	<0.001
EPL + women	11.1% (4/36)	58.3% (7/12)	0.002
EPL − women	6.3% (2/32)	31.6% (6/19)	0.04

[a]EPL−, women with no prior history of miscarriage (either nulliparous women or women with pregnancies completed to term).

[b]Among the 65 women in the metformin group, there were a total of 68 pregnancies. Of these, 36 pregnancies occurred in the context of a history of prior miscarriage, and 32 pregnancies occurred in the context of no previous miscarriage.

(From ref. 53.)

Similarly, in another study where metformin was compared with clomiphene citrate in 100 nonobese women with PCOS for 6 months, the ovulation rates during the treatment period did not differ (16). However, the subjects treated with clomiphene had an early pregnancy loss rate of 37.5% compared with 9.7% in women on metformin ($p = 0.045$). In both studies outlined previously (16,54), once pregnancy was confirmed in the women treated with metformin, the drug was discontinued. Thus, this suggests that metformin's salutary impact on reducing early pregnancy loss appears to occur primarily around the peri-implantation time, most likely because of an improvement of the endometrial milieu.

CONCLUSION

During the past decade, accumulating evidence for the treatment of infertility associated with PCOS favors the use of insulin-sensitizing agents. Metformin increases the ovulatory rate when administered alone and when combined with clomiphene citrate, improves the pregnancy rate, and appears to reduce early pregnancy loss. Although thiazolinediones show promise in improving ovulation and fertility, they are currently category C pregnancy drugs and caution is advised in patients desiring pregnancy. In conclusion, using metformin to treat the infertility of women with PCOS is a reasonable first step.

FUTURE AVENUES

Although the current studies have established improvements in ovulation with insulin sensitizers in women with PCOS, additional research is needed in the form of large randomized, controlled trials to answer several questions. First, how does the use of insulin sensitizers with or without clomiphene citrate affect live birth rates? Evidence is suggestive of metformin improving the endometrial milieu at peri-implantation. Is the benefit of metformin only in the first few weeks or does it extend throughout the pregnancy, when insulin resistance is increased in the third trimester? Further data on the safety and efficacy of both metformin and thiazolinediones need defining if they are used not only for ovulation but for prevention of miscarriage. In addition, the early pregnancy loss in women with PCOS should be understood at both a basic science as well as clinical level, as this will guide future therapies.

KEY POINTS

- PCOS is associated with insulin resistance.
- Insulin resistance may contribute to anovulation in PCOS.
- Ovulation is improved with the use of insulin-sensitizing agents with or without clomiphene citrate.
- PCOS is associated with early pregnancy loss.
- Metformin treatment may increase the pregnancy rate and decrease the miscarriage rate in women with PCOS.

REFERENCES

1. Franks S. Polycystic ovary syndrome. N Engl J Med 1995;333(13):853–861.
2. Knochenhauer ES, Key TJ, Kahsar-Miller M, Waggoner W, Boots LR, Azziz R. Prevalence of the polycystic ovary syndrome in unselected black and white women of the southeastern United States: a prospective study. J Clin Endocrinol Metab 1998;83(9):3078–3082.
3. Hull MG. Epidemiology of infertility and polycystic ovarian disease: endocrinological and demographic studies. Gynecol Endocrinol 1987;1(3):235–245.
4. Burghen GA, Givens JR, Kitabchi AE. Correlation of hyperandrogenism with hyperinsulinism in polycystic ovarian disease. J Clin Endocrinol Metab 1980;50(1):113–116.
5. Dunaif A, Segal KR, Futterweit W, Dobrjansky A. Profound peripheral insulin resistance, independent of obesity, in polycystic ovary syndrome. Diabetes 1989;38(9):1165–1174.
6. Dunaif A. Insulin resistance and the polycystic ovary syndrome: mechanism and implications for pathogenesis. Endocr Rev 1997;18(6):774–800.
7. Bailey CJ, Turner RC. Metformin. N Engl J Med 1996;334(9):574–579.
8. Krentz AJ, Ferner RE, Bailey CJ. Comparative tolerability profiles of oral antidiabetic agents. Drug Saf 1994;11(4):223–241.
9. Lalau JD, Race JM. Metformin and lactic acidosis in diabetic humans. Diabetes Obes Metab 2000;2(3):131–137.
10. Diamant M, Heine RJ. Thiazolidinediones in type 2 diabetes mellitus: current clinical evidence. Drugs 2003;63(13):1373–1405.
11. Balfour JA, Plosker GL. Rosiglitazone. Drugs 1999;57(6):921–930.
12. Gillies PS, Dunn CJ. Pioglitazone. Drugs 2000;60(2):333–343.
13. Velazquez EM, Mendoza S, Hamer T, Sosa F, Glueck CJ. Metformin therapy in polycystic ovary syndrome reduces hyperinsulinemia, insulin resistance, hyperandrogenemia, and systolic blood pressure, while facilitating normal menses and pregnancy. Metabolism 1994;43(5):647–654.
14. Nestler JE, Jakubowicz DJ, Evans WS, Pasquali R. Effects of metformin on spontaneous and clomiphene-induced ovulation in the polycystic ovary syndrome. N Engl J Med 1998;338(26):1876–1880.
15. Lord JM, Flight IH, Norman RJ. Metformin in polycystic ovary syndrome: systematic review and meta-analysis. BMJ 2003;327(7421):951–953.
16. Palomba S, Orio F Jr., Falbo A, et al. Prospective parallel randomized, double-blind, double-dummy controlled clinical trial comparing clomiphene citrate and metformin as the first-line treatment for ovulation induction in nonobese anovulatory women with polycystic ovary syndrome. J Clin Endocrinol Metab 2005;90(7):4068–4074.
17. Azziz R, Ehrmann D, Legro RS, et al. Troglitazone improves ovulation and hirsutism in the polycystic ovary syndrome: a multicenter, double blind, placebo-controlled trial. J Clin Endocrinol Metab 2001;86(4):1626–1632.
18. Dunaif A, Scott D, Finegood D, Quintana B, Whitcomb R. The insulin-sensitizing agent troglitazone improves metabolic and reproductive abnormalities in the polycystic ovary syndrome. J Clin Endocrinol Metab 1996;81(9):3299–3306.

19. Ehrmann DA, Schneider DJ, Sobel BE, et al. Troglitazone improves defects in insulin action, insulin secretion, ovarian steroidogenesis, and fibrinolysis in women with polycystic ovary syndrome. J Clin Endocrinol Metab 1997;82(7):2108–2116.

20. Hasegawa I, Murakawa H, Suzuki M, Yamamoto Y, Kurabayashi T, Tanaka K. Effect of troglitazone on endocrine and ovulatory performance in women with insulin resistance-related polycystic ovary syndrome. Fertil Steril 1999;71(2):323–327.

21. Mitwally MF, Kuscu NK, Yalcinkaya TM. High ovulatory rates with use of troglitazone in clomiphene-resistant women with polycystic ovary syndrome. Hum Reprod 1999;14(11):2700–2703.

22. Baillargeon JP, Jakubowicz DJ, Iuorno MJ, Jakubowicz S, Nestler JE. Effects of metformin and rosiglitazone, alone and in combination, in nonobese women with polycystic ovary syndrome and normal indices of insulin sensitivity. Fertil Steril 2004;82(4):893–902.

23. Belli SH, Graffigna MN, Oneto A, Otero P, Schurman L, Levalle OA. Effect of rosiglitazone on insulin resistance, growth factors, and reproductive disturbances in women with polycystic ovary syndrome. Fertil Steril 2004;81(3):624–629.

24. Ghazeeri G, Kutteh WH, Bryer-Ash M, Haas D, Ke RW. Effect of rosiglitazone on spontaneous and clomiphene citrate-induced ovulation in women with polycystic ovary syndrome. Fertil Steril 2003;79(3):562–566.

25. Sepilian V, Nagamani M. Effects of rosiglitazone in obese women with polycystic ovary syndrome and severe insulin resistance. J Clin Endocrinol Metab 2005;90(1):60–65.

26. Brettenthaler N, De Geyter C, Huber PR, Keller U. Effect of the insulin sensitizer pioglitazone on insulin resistance, hyperandrogenism, and ovulatory dysfunction in women with polycystic ovary syndrome. J Clin Endocrinol Metab 2004;89(8):3835–3840.

27. Glueck CJ, Moreira A, Goldenberg N, Sieve L, Wang P. Pioglitazone and metformin in obese women with polycystic ovary syndrome not optimally responsive to metformin. Hum Reprod 2003;18(8): 1618–1625.

28. Fleming R, Hopkinson ZE, Wallace AM, Greer IA, Sattar N. Ovarian function and metabolic factors in women with oligomenorrhea treated with metformin in a randomized double blind placebo-controlled trial. J Clin Endocrinol Metab 2002;87(2):569–574.

29. Glueck CJ, Wang P, Fontaine R, Tracy T, Sieve-Smith L. Metformin-induced resumption of normal menses in 39 of 43 (91%) previously amenorrheic women with the polycystic ovary syndrome. Metabolism 1999;48(4):511–519.

30. Velazquez E, Acosta A, Mendoza SG. Menstrual cyclicity after metformin therapy in polycystic ovary syndrome. Obstet Gynecol 1997;90(3):392–395.

31. Ortega-Gonzalez C, Luna S, Hernandez L, et al. Responses of serum androgen and insulin resistance to metformin and pioglitazone in obese, insulin-resistant women with polycystic ovary syndrome. J Clin Endocrinol Metab 2005;90(3):1360–1365.

32. Hughes E, Collins J, Vandekerckhove P. Clomiphene citrate for ovulation induction in women with oligo-amenorrhoea. Cochrane Database Syst Rev 2000;2:CD000056.

33. Lobo RA, Gysler M, March CM, Goebelsmann U, Mishell DR Jr. Clinical and laboratory predictors of clomiphene response. Fertil Steril 1982;37(2):168–174.

34. Murakawa H, Hasegawa I, Kurabayashi T, Tanaka K. Polycystic ovary syndrome. Insulin resistance and ovulatory responses to clomiphene citrate. J Reprod Med 1999;44(1):23–27.

35. Kashyap S, Wells GA, Rosenwaks Z. Insulin-sensitizing agents as primary therapy for patients with polycystic ovarian syndrome. Hum Reprod 2004;19(11):2474–2483.

36. Kocak M, Caliskan E, Simsir C, Haberal A. Metformin therapy improves ovulatory rates, cervical scores, and pregnancy rates in clomiphene citrate-resistant women with polycystic ovary syndrome. Fertil Steril 2002;77(1):101–106.

37. Malkawi HY, Qublan HS. The effect of metformin plus clomiphene citrate on ovulation and pregnancy rates in clomiphene-resistant women with polycystic ovary syndrome. Saudi Med J 2002; 23(6):663–666.

38. Shobokshi A, Shaarawy M. Correction of insulin resistance and hyperandrogenism in polycystic ovary syndrome by combined rosiglitazone and clomiphene citrate therapy. J Soc Gynecol Investig 2003;10(2):99–104.

39. De Leo V, la Marca A, Ditto A, Morgante G, Cianci A. Effects of metformin on gonadotropin-induced ovulation in women with polycystic ovary syndrome. Fertil Steril 1999;72(2):282–285.

40. Yarali H, Yildiz BO, Demirol A, et al. Co-administration of metformin during rFSH treatment in patients with clomiphene citrate-resistant polycystic ovarian syndrome: a prospective randomized trial. Hum Reprod 2002;17(2):289–294.

41. Homburg R, Armar NA, Eshel A, Adams J, Jacobs HS. Influence of serum luteinising hormone concentrations on ovulation, conception, and early pregnancy loss in polycystic ovary syndrome. BMJ 1988;297(6655):1024–1026.

42. Regan L, Owen EJ, Jacobs HS. Hypersecretion of luteinising hormone, infertility, and miscarriage. Lancet 1990;336(8724):1141–1144.

43. Watson H, Kiddy DS, Hamilton-Fairley D, et al. Hypersecretion of luteinizing hormone and ovarian steroids in women with recurrent early miscarriage. Hum Reprod 1993;8(6):829–833.

44. Gray RH, Wu LY. Subfertility and risk of spontaneous abortion. Am J Public Health 2000;90(9):1452–1454.

45. Fedorcsak P, Storeng R, Dale PO, Tanbo T, Abyholm T. Obesity is a risk factor for early pregnancy loss after IVF or ICSI. Acta Obstet Gynecol Scand 2000;79(1):43–48.

46. Jakubowicz DJ, Essah PA, Seppala M, et al. Reduced serum glycodelin and insulin-like growth factor-binding protein-1 in women with polycystic ovary syndrome during first trimester of pregnancy. J Clin Endocrinol Metab 2004;89(2):833–839.

47. Bolton AE, Pockley AG, Clough KJ, et al. Identification of placental protein 14 as an immunosuppressive factor in human reproduction. Lancet 1987;1(8533):593–595.

48. Okamoto N, Uchida A, Takakura K, et al. Suppression by human placental protein 14 of natural killer cell activity. Am J Reprod Immunol 1991;26(4):137–142.

49. Giudice LC, Mark SP, Irwin JC. Paracrine actions of insulin-like growth factors and IGF binding protein-1 in non-pregnant human endometrium and at the decidual-trophoblast interface. J Reprod Immunol 1998;39(1–2):133–148.

50. Jakubowicz DJ, Seppala M, Jakubowicz S, et al. Insulin reduction with metformin increases luteal phase serum glycodelin and insulin-like growth factor-binding protein 1 concentrations and enhances uterine vascularity and blood flow in the polycystic ovary syndrome. J Clin Endocrinol Metab 2001;86(3):1126–1133.

51. Palomba S, Russo T, Orio F Jr., et al. Uterine effects of metformin administration in anovulatory women with polycystic ovary syndrome. Hum Reprod 2006;21(2):457–465.

52. Glueck CJ, Phillips H, Cameron D, Sieve-Smith L, Wang P. Continuing metformin throughout pregnancy in women with polycystic ovary syndrome appears to safely reduce first-trimester spontaneous abortion: a pilot study. Fertil Steril 2001;75(1):46–52.

53. Jakubowicz DJ, Iuorno MJ, Jakubowicz S, Roberts KA, Nestler JE. Effects of metformin on early pregnancy loss in the polycystic ovary syndrome. J Clin Endocrinol Metab 2002;87(2):524–529.

54. Palomba S, Orio F, Jr., Nardo LG, et al. Metformin administration versus laparoscopic ovarian diathermy in clomiphene citrate-resistant women with polycystic ovary syndrome: a prospective parallel randomized double-blind placebo-controlled trial. J Clin Endocrinol Metab 2004;89(10):4801–4809.

32 Treatment of Infertility in Polycystic Ovary Syndrome

Ovulation Induction

Deborah S. Wachs, MD and R. Jeffery Chang, MD

Summary

Women with polycystic ovary syndrome (PCOS) suffer infertility primarily because of chronic anovulation, the basis for which has not been completely established. Fundamental to the problem is decreased follicle-stimulating hormone (FSH) secretion and arrest of follicle growth at the midantral stage of development. As a result, treatment methods that result in increased FSH release are associated with ovulatory responses in many individuals. In particular, clomiphene citrate has proven to be an effective means of ovulation induction. Failure to respond to clomiphene has led to the use of gonadotropin therapy with good results. However, the benefit of gonadotropin use is balanced against the increased risk for ovarian hyperstimulation syndrome. Insulin resistance is a common

From: *Contemporary Endocrinology: Insulin Resistance and Polycystic Ovarian Syndrome:
Pathogenesis, Evaluation, and Treatment*
Edited by: E. Diamanti-Kandarakis, J. E. Nestler, D. Panidis, and R. Pasquali © Humana Press Inc., Totowa, NJ

feature of PCOS and treatment with insulin-lowering drugs has provided an effective alternative for individuals that are clomiphene-resistant and reluctant to advance to gonadotropin therapy. Ovulatory responses to metformin and thiazolidinediones have been variable, as judged by published studies, although in general, they appear to be at least as effective as clomiphene citrate. Whether the combination of an insulin-lowering drug and clomiphene citrate holds greater benefit compared with either method alone remains to be established.

Key Words: Anovulation; clomiphene; gonadotropins; metformin; thiazolidinediones; aromatase inhibitors.

INTRODUCTION

It has been estimated that 80% of women with polycystic ovary syndrome (PCOS) exhibit irregular and infrequent menstrual bleeding as a result of anovulation *(1–3)*. The failure of ovulation leads to infertility, which is often the presenting complaint in these women. The precise mechanism responsible for anovulation in PCOS is unknown, although decreased follicle-stimulating hormone (FSH) secretion and follicle arrest at the midantral stage of development have been well documented. Based on these findings, primary treatment has been directed toward follicle stimulation and ovulation induction. However, ovulation induction in PCOS has proven to be a particular challenge to practicing physicians because of varied ovarian responses that range from a lack of initial follicle stimulation to an increased risk for ovarian hyperstimulation syndrome. In addition, common features of PCOS, such as insulin resistance and obesity, can adversely influence clinical responses to commonly used regimens for ovulation induction. The various treatment options for ovulation induction in women with PCOS will be discussed in this chapter.

WEIGHT LOSS

For obese women with PCOS, it has been well-recognized that weight loss alone may result in the initiation of regular ovulatory cycles, and in some cases, spontaneous pregnancy *(3–6)*. In these reports, weight loss was also associated with decreases in abdominal adiposity, insulin resistance, circulating insulin levels, and serum androgen concentrations, while improving adverse lipid profiles. Recently, it was demonstrated that dietary restriction combined with exercise in modestly overweight individuals reduced the risk of diabetes by 58% compared with a control group *(7)*. The potential benefit of lifestyle modification has been examined in obese women with PCOS, who exhibit many of the risk factors for diabetes *(8)*. Of 15 anovulatory women with PCOS who sustained lifestyle adjustment for 6 months, 9 resumed ovulation and 2 became pregnant. The body mass index (BMI) and waist circumference was lower in the responders compared with the six women who failed to ovulate. In addition, there were significant decreases in luteinizing hormone (LH) and fasting insulin levels in the ovulatory women, whereas no differences were detected for leptin, testosterone, free testosterone, and sex hormone-binding globulin (SHBG) levels between groups. Mean weight loss was between 2 and 5% of starting weight over the program. These findings suggest an effective role for lifestyle modification in women with PCOS burdened with anovulation irrespective of weight loss, as the percentage of body weight reduction was small.

Use of lifestyle modification in combination with metformin has been studied in anovulatory obese women with PCOS *(9)*. Ovulation rates were not significantly different among those treated with lifestyle modification and metformin compared with either therapy alone. However, a subgroup analysis based on the presence or absence of weight loss, independent of intervention group, showed that the odds ratio for weight loss was 9.0 with respect to regular ovulation. Thus, the women with PCOS who lost weight were estimated to be nine times more likely to ovulate than those who did not lose weight. Moreover, the group treated with metformin who experienced weight loss was estimated to be 16 times more likely to regularly ovulate. There was no difference in the amount of weight reduction among the treatment groups.

Although it is often perceived that women with PCOS have difficulty achieving weight loss, few studies have examined this particular issue. It has been theorized that differences may exist in energy expenditure or appetite regulation *(10,11)*, but further research is needed to elucidate the mechanisms involved. Weight loss should be the first line of treatment in obese women with PCOS with anovulatory infertility for improvements in both reproductive and metabolic health and associated physiological morbidities *(12)*. Although weight reduction may benefit women with PCOS in their effort to achieve pregnancy, it must be cautioned that maintenance of weight loss is difficult and dedication to lifestyle modification is essential to ensure any long-term health benefit.

CLOMIPHENE CITRATE

Clomiphene citrate (CC) was initially introduced for clinical trials in 1960 and received Food and Drug Administration (FDA) approval in 1967. In women with PCOS, its antiestrogenic action in blocking estrogen receptors inhibits the negative feedback effect of persistent estrogen exposure, which leads to increased FSH release and subsequent follicle stimulation. CC is given in an oral dose of 50–150 mg daily for 5 days, starting with the lowest dose, progressively increasing the dose by 50-mg increments if ovulation does not occur *(13)*. Treatment is commenced in the early follicular phase, usually on day 2 or 3. If the woman has not recently menstruated, CC may be initiated after progesterone-induced withdrawal bleeding. Approximately 80% of patients will ovulate on a dose of 150 mg or less *(14)*, as documented by midluteal phase serum progesterone, urine ovulation kits, or biphasic temperature change. The majority of pregnancies will occur within the first three cycles of treatment *(15)* and in women 35 years of age or younger *(16)*. In some instances, CC has been administered at greater doses (up to 250 mg/day and for more than 5 days) in an effort to achieve ovulation *(17,18)*. Although the total duration of CC treatment depends on several factors including age, BMI, cycle history, and androgen levels *(19)*, we generally limit use to 3–6 months depending on the ovulatory response. In has been reported that most patients treated with CC experience ovulation, although pregnancy occurs in only approx 40% *(15,19)*. This may be the result of several factors, including the antiestrogenic effects of CC on the endometrium and cervical mucus. In patients whom endometrial and/or cervical factors appear to be detrimental to the desired outcome of pregnancy, progression to an alternative therapy is recommended *(14)*.

GONADOTROPINS

Beginning in 1961, gonadotropins extracted from urine of postmenopausal women became available for use in clinical practice through intramuscular injection. In 1996, recombinant human FSH became available and had the added benefit of subcutaneous administration *(13)*. Although gonadotropins are often the next step in ovulation induction following failed CC therapy, women with PCOS pose a particularly precarious dilemma. In particular, the baseline antral follicle count in women with PCOS is markedly higher than in women without PCOS. The greater number of follicles relates to an increased risk of exaggerated ovarian responsiveness to progressively higher doses of gonadotropin therapy, thus making women with PCOS particularly prone to ovarian hyperstimulation syndrome and multiple pregnancies. Conversely, the onset of ovulation induction in women with PCOS is commonly fraught with a lack of follicle response to gonadotropin administration. This reduced follicle responsiveness may be overcome with progressive increases in the dose or duration of FSH. Low-dose administration of FSH has been particularly useful, as the risk of ovarian hyperstimulation syndrome is considerably diminished with this method of ovulation induction *(20)*. The gradual accumulation of constant low-dose FSH over time is preferred to an escalation of the daily dose because of an apparent FSH threshold beyond which the risk of ovarian hyperstimulation syndrome increases *(21)*. In summary, women with PCOS exhibit initial suboptimal ovarian responsiveness to FSH stimulation during the onset of ovulation induction, which is responsive to daily, low-dose gonadotropin therapy. Once follicle stimulation has been achieved, these women are predisposed to excessive follicle growth associated with continued FSH stimulation, which increases the risk of ovarian hyperstimulation syndrome.

The low-dose FSH regimens for women with PCOS have become standard practice and involve a daily dose of 50–75 IU of FSH for up to 14 days followed by small-dose increments where necessary at intervals of not less than 7 days. This is continued with close ultrasound and/or estradiol monitoring until criteria for human chorionic gonadotropin trigger are reached. Mono-ovulation is achieved in more than 70% of cycles and pregnancy rates are slightly improved over conventional dose therapy *(22,23)*. Using this regimen, the incidence of ovarian hyperstimulation syndrome is almost completely eliminated and the rate of multiple pregnancies is less than 6%.

CLOMIPHENE CITRATE WITH GONADOTROPINS

In women who are unresponsive or poorly responsive to CC, combined use with gonadotropin therapy has been described previously *(25–28)*. Notably and not surprisingly, the specific regimens contained within these reports differ in sequence and duration of CC and gonadotropin administration. Although none of these studies have focused specifically on women with PCOS, parameters for safety, cost, and potential pregnancy rates can be applied to this patient population. In a large retrospective study that compared outcomes of various stimulation protocol in a total of 770 cycles, the per-cycle fecundity for sequential CC/gonadotropin therapy was twice that of CC alone and equivalent to those of gonadotropins alone or a combined regimen of CC/gonadotropin *(27)*. A subsequent study tracked 416 treatment cycles of sequential CC/gonadotropins in women previously unable to conceive with CC therapy *(28)*. The pregnancy rate and live birth rate were 23.1 and 12.8%, respectively, in women younger than 35 years of age, and 10.3 and 8.6%, respectively, in women 35–40 years of age. These findings indicate that sequential administration of CC and gonadotropins may prove to be effective in PCOS women that have failed CC therapy.

Whether CC plus gonadotropins afford greater efficacy over that of gonadotropins alone is less clear. In a prospective randomized trial of women who had not responded to CC, gonadotropin administration resulted in a statistically significant higher pregnancy rate compared with the rate achieved in women treated with a combination of CC and gonadotropins *(29)*. In contrast, a greater response to sequential CC and gonadotropin therapy was not observed in two studies that failed to demonstrate different pregnancy rates between the sequential regimen and gonadotropin treatment alone *(30,31)*. In light of apparent higher or, at least, comparable pregnancy rates with CC and gonadotropin therapy, a potential benefit is a lower dose with less cost compared with that of gonadotropin employed alone.

INSULIN-LOWERING AGENTS

Insulin resistance probably exists in the majority of women with PCOS, which increases their risk for developing impaired glucose tolerance and type 2 diabetes. The prevalence of insulin resistance is exacerbated by the high rate of obesity in women with PCOS *(32)*. The introduction of the biguanide, metformin, and the thiazolididiones to the treatment of PCOS has modified our approach to anovulation by virtue of improved ovulatory rates following administration of these drugs *(33,34)*. The mechanism by which insulin-lowering agents act to enhance ovulation is not completely understood, although reductions in serum levels of insulin, LH, androgens, and increases in SHBG have been associated with their use. In addition, studies have demonstrated that these compounds appear to exert a direct effect on ovarian function, at least, in vitro *(35–41)*.

METFORMIN ALONE

Metformin is an oral biguanide that was developed for the treatment of diabetes more than 50 years ago. The primary mechanism of action involves inhibition of hepatic glucose production without causing hypoglycemia. In women with type 2 diabetes, metformin improves insulin sensitivity, reduces fasting glucose, and lowers insulin concentrations. In a study to determine the beneficial effects of metformin on endocrine–metabolic function in women with PCOS, it was observed that some women ovulated in association with treatment *(42)*. There followed several published reports demonstrating the restoration of ovulatory function in PCOS treated with metformin at a usual daily dose of 1500–2550 mg/day. The literature was summarized in a systematic review in 2003, which calculated that 56–61% of women with PCOS ovulate on metformin alone *(43)*. Consistent with these findings, a Cochrane review published that same year showed that metformin therapy increased the ovulation rate by a factor of 3.9 compared with the placebo response *(44)*. This data was corroborated by recent review, which concluded that metformin was 50% more effective than placebo for ovulation induction in infertile patients with PCOS *(45)*.

METFORMIN WITH CLOMIPHENE CITRATE

The use of combination metformin and CC in PCOS has provided additional benefit with regard to resumption of ovulation. In obese women with PCOS who failed to ovulate in response to metformin for 35 days, subsequent CC administration to 21 individuals was associated with a 90% ovulatory rate compared with 25 women in the placebo-treated group with a rate of 4% (46). The clinical benefit of combining metformin with CC in women with PCOS resistant to CC has also been studied. In a recent randomized, placebo-controlled trial, CC-resistant women receiving metformin for 7 weeks followed by CC exhibited a 79% (9 of 12) ovulation rate, whereas those treated with placebo and CC had a 27% (4 of 15) ovulatory response (47). Similar results were reported the following year in a study that compared metformin or placebo for one cycle followed by the addition of CC in the second cycle. Ovulation occurred in 77% of women in the metformin plus CC group compared with 14% in the placebo group (48).

METFORMIN WITH GONADOTROPINS

Women with PCOS who fail CC treatment are usually prescribed gonadotropins as the next line of therapy. However, the risk of ovarian hyperstimulation syndrome and higher order multiple pregnancies has always been a problematic concern. Pretreatment with metformin prior to FSH stimulation may lessen this risk compared with a regimen of FSH alone. In a small series that examined two groups of 10 women with PCOS, one group was administered 1500 mg of metformin daily for a minimum of 1 month prior to FSH stimulation (49). The other group did not receive metformin, but two cycles of FSH. In the metformin-treated group the number of follicles greater than 15 mm in diameter and the plasma estradiol levels were nearly twofold lower than in the group without metformin. In addition, the number of cycles cancelled in the metformin-treated group was significantly lower. In contrast, a significant benefit of metformin pretreatment was not found in 10 women with PCOS given a single cycle of FSH following 6 weeks of metformin compared with results observed in 15 placebo-treated women (50). Serum estradiol levels, mono- and multifollicular development, and ovulation rates were not different, although three pregnancies were observed in the metformin group vs one that occurred in the placebo group. Clearly, more studies are necessary in this area to determine whether metformin provides additional benefit to ovulation induction with gonadotropin therapy.

METFORMIN DURING PREGNANCY

Improved ovulation rates have led to an increased number of pregnancies in women taking metformin. The logical issue raised by patients and physicians alike is whether or not metformin should be continued during pregnancy. Metformin is a pregnancy class B medication. Continued use of metformin initially focused on the potential increased risk of first trimester miscarriage in women with PCOS. Although ascertainment of this risk has been controversial, some reports have indicated a 30–50% miscarriage rate in these women (51–53). Several case series and retrospective studies have described a reduced miscarriage rate of 9–17% in PCOS women taking metformin throughout the first trimester (54–57). This possible lower rate of miscarriage, however, has not been supported by a large, prospective, randomized clinical trial. Furthermore, although continued use of metformin has been advocated in women with PCOS who become pregnant to reduce the development of gestational diabetes, appropriate prospective studies have not been performed (57–59). In summary, the efficacy of metformin with respect to early pregnancy loss and protection from gestational diabetes has not been definitively established and warrants further study.

THIAZOLIDINEDIONES

The thiazolidinediones (TZDs) are widely available for the treatment of type 2 diabetes mellitus. These compounds increase insulin sensitivity by binding to the nuclear transcription factor peroxisome-proliferator-activated receptor to enhance glucose transport. In addition, this class of agents may have a role in treating patients with nondiabetic insulin-resistant conditions, such as PCOS. Similar to metformin, TZDs lower insulin levels without changing blood sugar levels (60). Clinical use with an early formulation, troglitazone, was associated with an unacceptable rate of liver abnormalities, including hepatic failure and, as a result, was withdrawn from the market in 2000. Currently, second-generation preparations, rosiglitzaone (Avandia) and pioglitazone (Actos), have not resulted in significant liver abnormalities and are available by prescription with recommended monitoring of liver enzyme levels. These drugs are rated as class C and, therefore, are not recommended in pregnancy.

Early reports indicated that TZDs were effective in stimulating or enhancing ovulation induction (61,62). In 2001, a large multicenter clinical trial of 410 women with PCOS demonstrated that treatment with troglitazone increased rates of ovulation compared with rates observed in individuals receiving placebo (63). The beneficial effects of troglitazone on ovulation were both dose- and duration-dependent and were associated with improvement of hirsutism, hyperandrogenemia, and insult resistance. Consistent with these results, a recent randomized, double-blind, controlled study of 40 women with PCOS revealed that pioglitazone administration significantly improved ovulation rates, hyperandrogenism, and insulin sensitivity compared with a group of individuals treated with placebo (64). More specifically, 41% of patients treated with pioglitazone had signs of ovulation during the study period compared with 6% of those treated with placebo.

To determine whether combined treatment with metformin and TZD offered greater reproductive–metabolic benefit, the effects of combination therapy in nonobese women with PCOS were compared with those resulting from either drug alone (65). Ovulation rates were statistically higher in women receiving metformin than those treated with rosiglitazone, and the combination of the two was not more effective. Serum-free testosterone levels were also lower in the treatment groups over placebo, although mean levels were comparable among all treatment regimens. Last, insulin levels and sensitivity improved significantly after metformin or combination therapies, but not after rosiglitazone. These findings indicated that metformin was more effective than rosiglitazone in improving ovulation, serum insulin levels, and insulin-sensitivity indices. Importantly, the addition of rosiglitazone to metformin did not provide any benefit beyond that of metformin alone. A caveat of this study was that all subjects with PCOS were nonobese and not clinically insulin resistant, which may represent a subset of individuals less receptive to TZD benefit.

AROMATASE INHIBITORS

Aromatase inhibitors interrupt the conversion of androgen to estrogen and cause a dramatic reduction of estrogen production. Letrozole and anastrazole are nonsteroidal aromatase inhibitors that act by competitively binding with the heme group of the cytochrome P-450 component of aromatase. The onset of action is rapid as demonstrated by a 50% reduction in circulating estradiol level following a 0.1-mg dose of letrozole *(66)*. The estimated half-life of letrozole is about 40 hours. In women with PCOS, administration of letrozole markedly lowers serum estradiol, which is believed to interrupt estrogen-negative feedback resulting in increased FSH secretion. The rise in FSH appears to be sufficient to initiate follicle growth as several studies have reported increased ovulatory function following letrozole treatment *(67–70)*. In a prospective study of 12 anovulatory PCOS, initial CC treatment was associated with a 44% ovulatory rate (8 of 18 cycles), whereas subsequent administration of 2.5 mg of letrozole a day for 5 days, resulted in 75% ovulation (9 of 12 cycles) *(67)*. Additionally, there was a statistically significant improvement in endometrial thickness on the day of human chorionic gonadotropin with letrozole compared with that observed with CC. In an extension of these studies, normal ovulatory women were examined during a spontaneous cycle and a cycle in which either CC or letrozole was used during the early follicular phase *(71)*. In both treatment groups the number of matures follicles was greater than the number occurring in spontaneous cycles. Between treatment groups there was no difference in endometrial thickness or follicle profiles, although serum estradiol levels were higher in CC-treated women compared with levels seen in the letrozole group. Thus, letrozole was as effective as CC in stimulating follicle growth, but did not exhibit any adverse effect on endometrial thickness. Recently, it was reported in normal women that ovarian and hormonal responses to the nonsteroidal aromatase inhibitor anastrozole were similar to those of letrozole *(72)*. The advantage of anastrozole is the lack of teratogenicity in mice as compared with that of letrozole.

Despite the relative paucity of reported experiences with letrozole, there have been several studies exploring the potential additive benefit in combination with other ovarian stimulation regimens, including CC, gonadotropins, and in vitro fertilization outcomes. As an adjunct to ovulation induction, letrozole use was associated with a lowered FSH dose requirement and in one study may have increased ovarian responsiveness in poor responders *(73–75)*. In addition, clinical outcomes have been examined in women treated with letrozole, either alone or in combination with other stimulation protocols vs regimens not involving letrozole (CC, gonadotropins, and spontaneous pregnancies). Of 394 pregnancies from three tertiary referral centers, miscarriage and ectopic pregnancy rates were not significantly different between women receiving letrozole compared with those not given letrozole *(76)*. Notably, letrozole use was associated with significantly fewer multiple gestations compared with the other regimens not involving letrozole.

Recently one report described an increased prevalence of fetal anomalies in women conceiving on letrozole over that of women conceiving spontaneously. However, in a subsequent review of a large experience of letrozole-induced pregnancies, the occurrence of fetal anomalies was not greater than that of the general population.

DEXAMETHASONE

Dexamethasone has been reported to facilitate ovulation induction in hirsute women with anovulation *(77,78)*. Dexamethasone (0.5 mg) given at bedtime blunts the early morning peak of adrenocorticotropic hormone (ACTH) release and causes a decrease in adrenal dehydroepiandrosterone sulfate (DHEA-S) and testosterone. As an adjunct to CC, dexamethasone appeared to benefit primarily those hyperandrogenic individuals with elevated levels of DHEA-S *(78)*. In a randomized study of anovulatory women who had not previously received CC, the effectiveness of dexamethasone plus CC was compared with that of CC alone *(79)*. Those treated with combination therapy exhibited a higher ovulatory and conception rate than the group given CC alone, provided that their DHEA-S levels were elevated. In the absence of increased DHEA-S, the two regimens produced similar rates of ovulation and pregnancy. In these studies, dexamethasone was administered daily until pregnancy was achieved. However, long-term therapy is not recommended as potential side effects may outweigh the benefits in this patient population.

CONCLUSION

Ovulation induction in women with PCOS can be a challenging and sometimes precarious endeavor for physicians treating this patient population. No single treatment regimen has proven to be uniformly successful in achieving ovulation in this disorder, which has spawned a variety of innovative and, occasionally novel, therapeutic protocols to promote follicle development while simultaneously minimizing risk of ovarian hyperstimulation. As is true with many of the practices within the field of infertility, additional prospective randomized trials are needed to continue the evolution of treatment options for ovulation induction in women with polycystic ovary syndrome.

FUTURE AVENUES

In women with PCOS:

1. Determine the efficacy of insulin-lowering drugs compared with clomiphene citrate for ovulation induction.
2. Assess the role of insulin-lowering drugs during ovulation induction with gonadotropin therapy.
3. Elucidate the basis for initial ovarian resistance to gonadotropin stimulation.
4. Identify the mechanism for ovarian hyperstimulation syndrome.

KEY POINTS

- Behavioral modification with weight loss is associated with resumption of ovulation in women with PCOS and should be the first line of therapy.
- Clomiphene citrate is an effective agent for ovulation induction in women with PCOS.
- Insulin-lowering drugs are effective for ovulation induction in women with PCOS, although efficacy compared with that of clomiphene citrate remains to be established.
- The demonstrated success of gonadotropin therapy is tempered by the increased risk of ovarian hyperstimulation in women with PCOS.

REFERENCES

1. Franks S. Polycystic ovary syndrome: a changing perspective. Clin Endocrinol 1989;31:87–120.
2. Conway GS, Honour JW, Jacobs HS. Heterogeneity of the polycystic ovary syndrome: clinical, endocrine and ultrasound features in 556 patients. Clin Endocrinol 1989;30:459–470.
3. Goldzieher JW, Green JA. The polycystic ovary. I. Clinical and histologic features. J Clin Endocrinol Metab 1962;22:325–338.
4. Bates GW, Whitworth NS. Effect of body weight reduction on plasma androgens in obese, infertile women. Fertil Steril 1982;38:406–409.
5. Kiddy DS, Hamilton-Fairley D, Bush A, et al. Improvement in endocrine and ovarian function during dietary treatment of obese women with polycystic ovary syndrome. Clin Endocrinol 1992;36:105–111.
6. Holte J, Bergh T, Berne C, Wide L, Lithell H. Restored insulin sensitivity but persistently increased early insulin secretion after weight loss in obese women with polycystic ovary syndrome. J Clin Endocrinol Metab 1995;80:2586–2593.
7. Tuomilehto J, Lindstrom J, Eriksson JG, et al. Finnish Diabetes Prevention Study Group. Prevention of type 2 diabetes mellitus by changes in lifestyle among subjects with impaired glucose tolerance. N Engl J Med 2001;344:1343–1350.
8. Huber-Buchholz MM, Carey DG, Norman RJ. Restoration of reproductive potential by lifestyle modification in obese polycystic ovary syndrome: role of insulin sensitivity and luteinizing hormone. J Clin Endocrinol Metab 1999;84:1470–1474.
9. Hoeger KM, Kochman L, Wixom N, Craig K, Miller RK, Guzick DS. A randomized, 48-week, placebo-controlled trial of intensive lifestyle modification and/or metformin therapy in overweight women with polycystic ovary syndrome: a pilot study. Fertil Steril 2004;82:421–429.
10. Robinson S, Chan SP, Spacey S, Anyaoku V, Johnston DG, Franks S. Postprandial thermogenesis is reduced in polycystic ovary syndrome and is associated with increased insulin resistance. Clin Endocrinol (Oxf) 1992;36:537–543.
11. Schofl C, Horn R, Schill T, Schlosser HW, Muller MJ, Brabant G. Circulating ghrelin levels in patients with polycystic ovary syndrome. J Clin Endocrinol Metab 2002;87:4607–4610.
12. Moran L, Norman RJ. Understanding and managing disturbances in insulin metabolism and body weight in women with polycystic ovary syndrome. In: Fraser I, Kovacs G, eds. Best Practices and Research: Clinical Obstetrics and Gynaecology, Vol. 18, No. 5, Philadelphia, PA: Elsevier, 2004, pp. 719–736.
13. Speroff L, Glass RH, Kase NG. Induction of ovulation. In: Clinical Gynecologic Endocrinology and Infertility, 6th Edition, Baltimore, MD: Lippincott Williams and Wilkins, 1999, pp. 1097–1132.
14. Homburg R. Management of infertility and prevention of ovarian hyperstimulation in women with polycystic ovary syndrome. In: Fraser I, Kovacs G, eds. Best Practices and Research: Clinical Obstetrics and Gynaecology, Vol. 18, No. 5, Philadelphia, PA: Elsevier, 2004, pp. 773–788.
15. Gysler M, March CM, Mishell DR, Bailey EJ. A decade's experience with an individualized clomiphene treatment regimen including its effect on the postcoital test. Fertil Steril 1982;37:161–167.
16. Agarwal SK, Buyalos RP. Clomiphene citrate with intrauterine insemination: is it effective therapy in women above the age of 35 years? Fertil Steril 1996;65:759–763.
17. Lobo RA, Granger LR, Davajan V, Mishell DR Jr. An extended regimen of clomiphene citrate in women unresponsive to standard therapy. Fertil Steril 1982;37:762–766.
18. O'Herlihy C, Pepperell RJ, Brown JB, Smith MA, Sandri L, McBain JC. Incremental clomiphene therapy: a new method for treating persistent anovulation. Obstet Gynecol 1981;58: 535–542.
19. Imani B, Eijkemans MJ, te Velde ER, Habbema JD, Fauser BC. A nomogram to predict the probability of live birth after clomiphene citrate induction of ovulation in normogonadotropic oligoamenorrheic infertility. Fertil Steril 2002;77:91–97.
20. White DM, Polson DW, Kiddy D, et al. Induction of ovulation with low-dose gonadotropins in polycystic ovary syndrome: an analysis of 109 pregnancies in 225 women. J Clin Endocrinol Metab 1996;81:3821–3824.
21. Van Der Meer M, Hompes PG, De Boer JA, Schats R, Schoemaker J. Cohort size rather than follicle-stimulating hormone threshold level determines ovarian sensitivity in polycystic ovary syndrome. J Clin Endocrinol Metab 1998;83:423–426.
22. Polson DW, Mason HD, Saldahna MB, Franks S. Ovulation of a single dominant follicle during treatment with low-dose pulsatile follicle stimulating hormone in women with polycystic ovary syndrome. Clin Endocrinol (Oxf) 1987;26:205–212.

23. Hedon B, Hugues JN, Emperaire JC, et al. A comparative prospective study of a chronic low dose versus a conventional ovulation stimulation regimen using recombinant human follicle stimulating hormone in anovulatory infertile women. Hum Reprod 1998;13:2688–2692.

24. Homburg R, Howles CM. Low-dose FSH therapy for anovulatory infertility associated with polycystic ovary syndrome: rationale, results, reflections and refinements. Hum Reprod Update 1999;5:493–499.

25. Kistner RW. Sequential use of clomiphene citrate and human menopausal gonadotropins in ovulation induction. Fertil Steril 1976;27:72–82.

26. Kemmann E, Jones JR. Sequential clomiphene citrate-menotropin therapy for induction or enhancement of ovulation. Fertil Steril 1983;39:772–779.

27. Dickey RP, Olar TT, Taylor SN, Curole DN, Rye PH. Sequential clomiphene citrate and human menopausal gonadotropin for ovulation induction: comparison to clomiphene citrate alone and human menopausal gonadotropins alone. Hum Reprod 1993;8:56–59.

28. Brzechff PR, Daneshmand S, Buyalos RP. Sequential clomiphene citrate and human menopausal gonadotropins with intrauterine insemination: the effect of patient age on clinical outcome. Hum Reprod 1998;13:2110–2114.

29. Ransom MX, Doughman NC, Garcia AJ. Menotropins alone are superior to a clomiphene citrate and menotropin combination for superovulation induction among clomiphene citrate failures. Fertil Steril 1996;65:1169–1174.

30. Jarrell J, McInnes R, Cooke R, Arronet G. Observations on the combination of clomiphene citrate-human menopausal gonadotropins-human chorionic gonadotropins in the management of anovulation. Fertil Steril 1981;35:634–637.

31. Lu PY, Chen AL, Atkinson EJ, Lee SH, Erickson LD, Ory SJ. Minimal stimulation achieves pregnancy rates comparable to human menopausal gonadotropins in the treatment of infertility. Fertil Steril 1996;65:583–587.

32. Carmina E, Lobo RA. Polycystic ovary syndrome (PCOS): arguably the most common endocrinopathy is associated with significant morbidity in women. J Clin Endocrinol Metab 1999;84:1897–1899.

33. Ibanez L, Valls C, Potau N, Marcos MV, de Zegher F. Sensitization to insulin in adolescent girls to normalize hirsutism, hyperandrogenism, oligomenorrhea, dyslipidemia, and hyperinsulinism after precocious pubarche. J Clin Endocrinol Metab 2000;85:3526–3530.

34. Moghetti P, Castello R, Negri C, et al. Metformin effects on clinical features, endocrine and metabolic profiles, and insulin sensitivity in polycystic ovary syndrome: a randomized, double-blind, placebo-controlled 6-month trial, followed by open, long-term clinical evaluation. J Clin Endocrinol Metab 2000;85:139–146.

35. Stuart CA, Prince MJ, Peters EJ, Meyer WJ 3rd. Hyperinsulinemia and hyperandrogenemia: in vivo androgen response to insulin infusion. Obstet Gynecol 1987;69:921–925.

36. Arlt W, Auchus RJ, Miller WL. Thiazolidindiones but not metformin directly inhibit the steroidogenic enzymes P450c17 and 3beta-hydorxysteroid dehydrogenase. J Biol Chem 2002;276:16,767–16,771.

37. Mu Y-M, Yanase T, Nishi Y, et al. Insulin sensitizer, troglitazone, directly inhibits aromatase activity in human ovarian granulosa cells. Biochem Biophys Res Commun 2000;271:710–713.

38. Gasic S, Bodenberg Y, Nagamani M, Green A, Urban RJ. Troglitazone inhibits progesterone production in porcine granulosa cells. Endocrinology 1998;139:4962–4966.

39. Gasic S, Nagamani M, Green A, Randall J. Urban RJ. Troglitazone is a competitive inhibitor of 3beta-hydroxysteroid dehydrogenase enzyme in the ovary. Am J Obstet Gynecol 2001;184:575–579.

40. Mansfield R, Galea R, Brincat M, Hole D, Mason H. Metformin has direct effects on human ovarian steroidogenesis. Fertil Steril 2003;79:956–962.

41. Attia GR, Rainey WE, Carr BR. Metformin directly inhibits androgen production in human thecal cells. Fertil Steril 2001;76:517–524.

42. Velazquez EM, Mendoza S, Hamer T, Sosa F, Glueck CJ. Metformin therapy in polycystic ovary syndrome reduces hyperinsulinemia, insulin resistance, hyperandrogenemia, and systolic blood pressure, while facilitating normal menses and pregnancy. Metabolism 1994;43:647–654.

43. Costello MF, Eden JA. A systematic review of the reproductive system effects of metformin in patients with polycystic ovary syndrome. Fertil Steril 2003;79:1–13.

44. Lord JM, Flight IH, Norman RJ. Metformin in polycystic ovary syndrome: systematic review and meta-analysis. BMJ 2003;327:951–953.

45. Kashyap S, Wells GA, Rosenwaks Z. Insulin-sensitizing agents as primary therapy for patients with polycystic ovary syndrome. Hum Reprod 2004;19:2474–2483.

46. Nestler JE, Jakubowicz DJ, Evans WS, Pasquali R. Effects of metformin on spontaneous and clomiphene-induced ovulation in the polycystic ovary syndrome. N Engl J Med 1998;338:1876–1880.

47. Vandermolen DT, Ratts VS, Evans WS, Stovall DW, Kauma SW, Nestler JE. Metformin increases the ovulatory rate and pregnancy rate from clomiphene citrate in patients with polycystic ovary syndrome who are resistant to clomiphene citrate alone. Fertil Steril 2001;75:310–315.

48. Kocak M, Caliskan E, Simsir C, Haberal A. Metformin therapy improves ovulatory rates, cervical scores, and pregnancy rates in clomiphene citrate-resistant women with polycystic ovary syndrome. Fertil Steril 2002;77:101–106.

49. De Leo V, la Marca A, Ditto A, Morgante G, Cianci A. Effects of metformin on gonadotropin-induced ovulation in women with polycystic ovary syndrome. Fertil Steril 1999;72:282–285.

50. Yarali H, Yildiz BO, Demirol A, Zeyneloglu HB, Yigit N, Bukulmez O, Koray Z. Co-administration of metformin during rFSH treatment in patients with clomiphene citrate-resistant polycystic ovarian syndrome: a prospective randomized trial. Hum Reprod 2002;17:289–294.

51. Balen AH, Tan SL, MacDougall J, Jacobs HS. Miscarriage rates following in-vitro fertilization are increased in women with polycystic ovaries and reduced by pituitary desensitization with buserelin. Hum Reprod 1993;8:959–964.

52. Homburg R, Eshel A, Armar NA, et al. One hundred pregnancies after treatment with pulsatile luteinising hormone releasing hormone to induce ovulation. BMJ 1989;298:809–812.

53. Filicori M, Flamigni C, Meriggiola MC, et al. Endocrine response determines the clinical outcome of pulsatile gonadotropin-releasing hormone ovulation induction in different ovulatory disorders. J Clin Endocrinol Metab 1991;72:965–972.

54. Glueck CJ, Phillips H, Cameron D, Sieve-Smith L, Wang P. Continuing metformin throughout pregnancy in women with polycystic ovary syndrome appears to safely reduce first-trimester spontaneous abortion: a pilot study. Fertil Steril 2001;75:46–52.

55. Jakubowitz DJ, Iuorno MJ, Jakubowicz S, Roberts KA, Nestler JE. Effects of metformin on early pregnancy loss in the polycystic ovary syndrome. J Clin Endocrinol Metab 2002;87:524–529.

56. Heard MJ, Pierce A, Carson SA, Buster JE. Pregnancies following use of metformin for ovulation induction in patients with polycystic ovary syndrome. Fertil Steril 2002;77:669–673.

57. Glueck CJ, Wang P, Goldenberg N, Sieve-Smith L. Pregnancy outcomes among women with polycystic ovary syndrome treated with metformin. Hum Reprod 2002;17:2858–2864.

58. Glueck CJ, Wang P, Kobayashi S, Phillips H, Sieve-Smith L. Metformin therapy throughout pregnancy reduces the development of gestational diabetes in women with polycystic ovary syndrome. Fertil Steril 2002;77:520–525.

59. Glueck CJ, Bornovali S, Pranikoff J, Goldenberg N, Dharashivkar S, Wang P. Metformin, preeclampsia, and pregnancy outcomes in women with polycystic ovary syndrome. Diabet Med 2004;21:829–836.

60. Lord JM, Flight IHK, Norman RJ. Insulin-sensitizing drugs (metformin, troglitazone, rosiglitazone, pioglitazone, D-chiro-inositol) for polycystic ovary syndrome. The Cochrane Database of Systematic Reviews 2003, Issue 2. Art. No.: CD003053.

61. Hasegawa I, Murakawa H, Suzuki M, Yamamoto Y, Kurabayashi T, Tanaka K. Effect of troglitazone on endocrine and ovulatory performance in women with insulin resistance-related polycystic ovary syndrome. Fertil Steril 1999;71:323–327.

62. Mitwally MF, Kuscu NK, Yalcinkaya TM. High ovulatory rates with use of troglitazone in clomiphene-resistant women with polycystic ovary syndrome. Hum Reprod 1999;14:2700–2703.

63. Azziz R, Ehrmann D, Legro RS, et al. PCOS/Troglitazone Study Group. Troglitazone improves ovulation and hirsutism in the polycystic ovary syndrome: a multicenter, double blind, placebo-controlled trial. J Clin Endocrinol Meta 2000;86:1626–632.

64. Brettenthaler N, de Geyter C, Huber PR, Keller U. Effect of insulin sensitizer pioglitazone on insulin resistance, hyperandrogenism, and ovulatory dysfunction in women with polycystic ovary syndrome. J Clin Endocrinol Metab 2004;89:3835–3840.

65. Baillargeon JP, Jakubowicz DJ, Iuorno MJ, Jakubowicz S, Nestler JE. Effects of metformin and rosiglitazone, alone and in combination, in nonobese women with polycystic ovary syndrome and normal indices of insulin sensitivity. Fertil Steril 2004;82:893–902.

66. Haynes BP, Dowsett M, Miller WR, Dixon JM, Bhatnagar AS. The pharmacology of letrozole. J Steroid Biochem Mol Biol 2003;87:35–45.

67. Mitwally M, Casper RF. Use of an aromatase inhibitor for induction of ovulation in patients with an inadequate response to clomiphene citrate. Fertil Steril 2001;75:305–309.

68. Healey S, Tan SL, Tulandi T, Biljan MM. Effects of letrozole on superovulation with gonadotropins in women undergoing intrauterine insemination. Fertil Steril 2003;80:1325–1329.
69. Fatemi HM, Kolibianakis E, Tournaye H, Camus M, Van Steirteghem AC, Devroey P. Clomiphene citrate versus letrozole for ovarian stimulation: a pilot study. Reprod Biomed 2003;7:543–546.
70. Al-Omari WR, Sulaiman WR, Al-Hadithi N. Comparison of two aromatase inhibitors in women with clomiphene-resistant polycystic ovary syndrome. Int J Gynaecol Obstet 2004;85:289–291.
71. Fisher SA, Reid RL, Van Vugt DA, Casper RF. A randomized double-blind comparison of the effects of clomiphene citrate and the aromatase inhibitor letrozole on ovulatory function in normal women. Fertil Steril 2002;78:280–285.
72. Tredway DR, Buraglio M, Hemsey G, Denton G. A phase I study of the pharmacokinetics, pharmacodynamics, and safety of single- and multiple-dose anastrozole in healthy, premenopausal female volunteers. Fertil Steril 2004;82:1587–1593.
73. Mitwally MF, Casper RF. Aromatase inhibition improves ovarian response to follicle-stimulating hormone in poor responders. Fertil Steril 2002;77:776–780.
74. Mitwally MF, Casper RF. Aromatase inhibition reduces gonadotrophin dose required for controlled ovarian stimulation in women with unexplained infertility. Hum Reprod 2003;18:1588–1597.
75. Goswami SK, Das T, Chattopadhyay R, et al. A randomized single-blind controlled trial of letrozole as a low-cost IVF protocol in women with poor ovarian response: a preliminary report. Hum Reprod 2004;19:2031–2035.
76. Mitwally M, Biljan MM, Casper RF. Pregnancy outcome after the use of an aromatase inhibitor for ovarian stimulation. Am J Obstet Gynecol 2005;192:381–386.
77. Chang RJ, Abraham GE. Effect of dexamethasone and clomiphene citrate on peripheral steroid levels and ovarian function in a hirsute amenorrheic patient. Fertil Steril 1976;27:640–646.
78. Lobo RA, Paul W, March CM, Granger L, Kletzky OA. Clomiphene and dexamethasone in women unresponsive to clomiphene alone. Obstet Gynecol 1982;60:497–501.
79. Daly DC, Walters CA, Soto-Albors CE, Tohan N, Riddick DH. A randomized study of dexamethasone in ovulation induction with clomiphene citrate. Fertil Steril 1984;41:844–848.

33 Surgery and Laser Diathermy

Stefano Palomba, MD, Fulvio Zullo, MD,
Evanthia Diamanti-Kandarakis, MD,
and Francesco Orio, Jr., MD, PhD

Summary

During the past decades, the surgical approach to ovulation induction in women with polycystic ovary syndrome has been continuously evaluated, criticized, reevaluated, and compared with newer medical treatments. This chapter presents an overview of the different techniques for surgical induction of ovulation, data on efficacy using clinical and metabolic end points, and unresolved questions and issues for future investigation.

Key Words: Anovulation; drilling; infertility; laparoscopy; PCOS.

INTRODUCTION

The new surgical techniques of ovulation induction using laparoscopic access are considered the first choice for the treatment of clomiphene citrate (CC)-resistant women with polycystic ovary syndrome (PCOS) by several scientific societies *(1)*. These are day-surgery procedures and are characterized not only by effectiveness in inducing ovulation and improving reproductive outcomes, but also by few side effects and no need for ongoing monitoring. In addition, ovarian drilling corrects the main endocrine abnormalities associated with PCOS *(2)*, and the benefits achieved appear to be maintained for several years after the procedure.

Despite these favorable aspects, ovarian drilling is an invasive procedure that can be associated with the formation of postoperative pelvic adhesions and other rare complications, including premature ovarian failure.

From: *Contemporary Endocrinology: Insulin Resistance and Polycystic Ovarian Syndrome:*
Pathogenesis, Evaluation, and Treatment
Edited by: E. Diamanti-Kandarakis, J. E. Nestler, D. Panidis, and R. Pasquali © Humana Press Inc., Totowa, NJ

AN HISTORICAL OVERVIEW

In 1935, Stein and Leventhal first described the surgical treatment of seven women with polycystic ovaries (PCOs) by wedge resection of the ovaries. In all the women, a normal menstrual pattern was restored, and two of them later conceived (3). Subsequently, Stein reported the efficacy of bilateral ovarian wedge resection (OWR) in terms of restoration of menstrual cyclicity and improved fertility in a larger sample of women (4).

In 1961, CC became available for the treatment of anovulatory infertility associated with PCOS (5), simplifying therapy for ovulation induction. Some years later, Kistner (6) stated that the positive results obtained by medical treatment of patients with PCOS were clear, and that surgical approaches should assume a minor role because of their association with adhesion formation, chronic pelvic pain, and iatrogenic infertility. Toaff et al. (7) supported these views in 1976 after performing laparoscopy on seven women with infertility persisting after bilateral OWR, and finding all patients to have extensive tubal and ovarian adhesions. During the course of this decade, surgical approaches to anovulatory infertility were convincingly replaced by developing medical therapies.

In 1972, Cohen et al. (8) reported 21 pregnancies obtained after 51 laparoscopic ovarian biopsies with cauterization using the Palmer forceps, not an easy procedure that seemed to confer no benefit over other methods of inflicting injury on the ovary.

Interest in the surgical approach was restored by the work of Gjönnaess in 1984, who reported ovulation and conception rates of 92 and 80%, respectively, in following laparoscopic electrosurgical drilling of the ovaries in CC-resistant patients (9,10). This was despite the fact that Campo's results in the previous year (11), obtained on a small sample of 12 patients alone with laparoscopic multiple biopsies, had been less encouraging, and reported ovulation and pregnancy rates of 45 and 42%, respectively. Gjönnaess's report established the impetus for exploration of surgical approaches to the treatment of this disease.

At present, after the return to a surgical approach for PCOS was reestablished, a large number of methods and techniques have been introduced, and a debate on the optimal surgical procedure persists.

SURGICAL PROCEDURES TO INDUCE OVULATION

Essentially, there are two surgical procedures that have been used for treating infertile PCOS patients:

1. Laparotomic/laparoscopic OWR.
2. Laparoscopic ovarian drilling (LOD).

Ovarian Wedge Resection

As noted previously, the technique of OWR was proposed by Stein and Leventhal in 1935, along with the first description of the syndrome. Originally, the procedure was performed by excising approximately one-third of the ovaries by laparotomy (3). In an initial series of 108 patients, restoration of normal menstrual cycles was reported in approx 94% of cases, and conception occurred in approx 87% of those who desired pregnancy (4).

Subsequent studies confirmed the benefits of the procedure, with varying rates of success (mean 58.8% pregnancy rate); however, a high rate of complications was also reported (7,12).

OWR has also been performed by laparoscopic access with the use of microlaser surgery *(13)*. This approach induced a low rate of pelvic adhesions (36.7% of cases laparoscopically reevaluated) and yielded a cumulative pregnancy rate of 60%. The most frequently reported complication of OWR (apart from complications caused by laparotomic access, i.e., wound infection, fever, long hospital stay, and so on) was periadnexal adhesions, with a reported incidence ranging from 30 to 100% *(14)*. Cases of premature ovarian failure have also been described *(10,14,15)*. This complication is probably the result of the substantial amount of tissue loss associated with the procedure.

For a long time, OWR was the only treatment for PCOs. When medical treatment with anti-estrogens was introduced and yielded excellent results, OWR was still used, but only primarily after failure of medical therapy for the induction of ovulation. The efficiency of OWR has been questioned, with lower pregnancy rates reported in many series because of formation of periovarian adhesions, which converted hormonal subfertility to mechanical subfertility because of scarring *(16,17)*. As a result, this technique was progressively abandoned in the 1970s *(14)*. After introduction of LOD, OWR became an obsolete procedure.

Laparoscopic Ovarian Drilling

The LOD is a less-invasive modification of OWR. Other terms have been used to describe the procedure, such as laparoscopic ovarian electrocautery, laparoscopic ovarian diathermy, laparoscopic electrocoagulation, and so on, but the term "LOD" has gained popularity and is more frequently used *(18)*.

SURGICAL TECHNIQUE

For the laparoscopic approach, a pneumo-peritoneum is generally attained using a Verres needle; a 10-mm video-laparoscope should be inserted umbilically, and two 5-mm ancillary lateral trocars in the left and right iliac fossae should be sufficient to perform the procedure. Careful inspection of the pelvic cavity should always be performed. The ovary is immobilized with laparoscopic forceps, and drilling is performed using different modalities and sources of energy as described in the following paragraphs.

Care should be taken to avoid inadvertent injury, such as energy application to the hilum of the ovary and excessive heating of the ovaries. Each of the holes created is approx 3 mm in diameter and 4–5 mm in depth *(19)*. We prefer the use of unipolar insulated needle cautery of 36 mm as described by Tulandi *(20)*. The whole length of the needle is inserted as perpendicularly as possible to the ovarian surface, after setting the electrosurgical device at a cutting current of 100 W power. The monopolar coagulating current is then set at 40 W power, and the needle is activated for 2–3 seconds at each point. We generally perform three to six punctures on each ovary depending on its size, and at the end of the procedure, the ovarian surface is washed with a crystalloid solution, and the injured areas are completely covered with hyaluronic acid gel.

Descriptions of the LOD techniques can vary in the literature, primarily in the source of energy used and the number of punctures performed.

Source of Energy Used. Although several different drilling techniques and modalities (laser, monopolar, and bipolar cautery) have been used, there are no randomized clinical trials establishing the superiority of any single technique over the others. In addition, most investigators have reported on small series of patients treated with a given technique or instrument, and the patient populations have been heterogeneous. Therefore, currently there is no standardization of the technique among different reproductive surgeons *(21)*.

In 1984, Gjonnaess *(9)* first reported the use of ovarian multielectrocauterization by laparoscopy in the treatment of infertile patients with PCOS. Using a unipolar electrode, he created 8–15 craters 2–4 mm deep in the capsule of each ovary. The procedure resulted in an ovulation rate of 92% and pregnancy rate of 69%. After 10 years of follow-up, the abortion rate in 89 women who conceived after electrocauterization was reported to be 15% *(22)*. In 1994, the results of a long follow-up of 252 women reported an ovulation and pregnancy rates of 92 and 84%, respectively *(10)*.

After this first description by Gjonnaess, other authors reported various similar techniques of ovarian electrocauterization using mono- or bipolar electrodes *(8,19)*.

In 1988, Huber et al. *(23)* proposed advantages in the use of CO_2 laser, and Daniell and Miller *(24)* reported on 85 women treated by either CO_2 laser or potassium-titanyl-phosphate (KTP) laser with favorable results. Argon and Nd:YAG lasers have also been used *(8)*.

Laser LOD was introduced with the purpose of obtaining better control of the power density, a desirable depth of penetration, less thermodamage of surrounding tissues, and a reduction in the risk of adhesions. However, although the use of laser provides greater control over the type of damage induced in the ovary, it has not been reported to have any clinical advantages. In addition, the impact of the different laser techniques on reducing adhesion formation remains theoretical *(8,25)*.

The CO_2 laser was the first to be used for ovarian drilling *(23)*. This can be introduced through a coaxial operating laparoscope or through a second puncture system. A further delivery system known as a waveguide may be used, where the laser beam is internally reflected through a fine ceramic-lined tube directly to the ovarian surface. Nd:YAG laser can be used in both noncontact and contact modes. Specifically, contact mode applications require sculptured quartz fibers or sapphire tips. Even if there is less smoke and improved hemostasis, Nd:YAG seems to offer no major advantage over electrosurgical drilling. Finally, KTP and Argon lasers have the advantage of using cheaper bare fibers in contact mode *(8,23,25,68)*.

When laser LOD is performed, all the same principles of electrosurgical energy application should also be followed and applied, such as avoiding inadvertent injury, irrigation and cooling of the ovary, and avoiding energy application to the hilum of the ovary. On the contrary, because of the reduced lateral thermal damage, a larger number of drills may be required when using laser compared with electrosurgery *(8)*.

In conclusion, even if lasers are theoretically more precise, there is no evidence that this translates into any clinical advantage over electrosurgery *(8)*.

Number of Ovarian Punctures. The number of punctures that the surgeon should apply to the ovary for achieving the optimal result with minimal complications is both an important and controversial issue.

Initially, about 20–25 drills per ovary were used *(9)*. In 1989, Dabirashrafi *(26)* suggested that the number of punctures should be as low as possible and tailored to the individual ovary in each patient, whereas Kovacs *(27)* and Gjonnaess *(10)* successively recommended a minimum of 10 and 8 drills per ovary, respectively. However, during the same time period, Balen and Jacobs *(28)* demonstrated that four drills may be sufficient, and that unilateral drilling may be as effective as bilateral treatment.

Amer et al. *(29)* published a retrospective study on the dose–response relationship of LOD. The hospital records of 161 women with PCOS who underwent LOD were reviewed and the clinical data before and after LOD were obtained. The authors concluded the following: two punctures per ovary are associated with poor results; three punctures per ovary seem to represent the plateau dose; and seven or more punctures per ovary may result in excessive destruction to the ovary without any improvement in the results and should therefore be discouraged.

More recently, patients with PCOS were treated with LOD and assigned to receive 5 or 10 ovarian punctures *(30)*. Because no difference in any biochemical and/or clinical outcome was detected between the two groups, the use of five punctures for each ovary has been considered sufficient for the treatment of patients with PCOS *(30)*.

According to our personal experience and that of most authors, however, we feel that the minimum number of drills to be performed should be decided based on ovarian dimensions.

COMPLICATIONS

LOD carries the usual risks of laparoscopy and general anesthesia, along with the risks associated with the drilling procedure itself, which includes the use of energy.

Recently, the use of other surgical approaches has been explored to improve the feasibility and reduce the invasiveness of the surgical procedure. In fact, although almost all described that surgical procedures to induce ovulation are typically performed under general anesthesia, some reports *(31)* have assessed the feasibility of the mini-laparoscopic approach under local anesthesia and conscious sedation.

An important complication associated with drilling is the formation of postoperative peri-adnexial adhesions, which may in turn be a cause of infertility or other problems, i.e., chronic pelvic pain. The incidence of postoperative adhesion formation is estimated to be 19–43% *(18)*, but reported rates vary from 0 to 100% *(8)*. The great diversity in the reported rate of adhesion formation may be partly because of variation of technique, partly to the surgical procedure performed for the second-look, and partly to varying systems applied by the surgeon to grade the adhesions. On the contrary, it seems well-defined that most adhesions following ovarian drilling are filmy *(32)*. Unfortunately, actually, it is not known neither the severity nor the exact type of the pelvic adhesion able to reduce fertility or induce pelvic pain.

A comparative study between laser and electrocoagulation LOD showed that the formation of postoperative pelvic adhesions occurs more frequently after the laser procedure *(33)*. In addition, it is common practice to use anti-adhesion agents during LOD, even if data supporting this procedure are few and inconclusive. In fact, two studies on an absorbable adhesion barrier, used to cover the ovary at the end of a procedure to reduce the rate of adhesion formation, showed no significant benefit *(32,34)*.

Because there is not clear data available, we feel it is not justified to routinely use anti-adhesion agents and/or to perform a laparoscopic second-look *(25)* for possible adhesiolysis.

Other complications associated with drilling are bleeding from the drilling site and/or the laceration of the utero-ovarian ligament, which is frequently grasped to immobilize the ovary. Further, excessive drilling or excessive amounts of energy will destroy a large number of follicles, resulting in decreased ovarian reserve. Similarly, an electrode introduced too deeply into the ovary may cause desiccation of hilar vessels, which in turn may result in ovarian necrosis and premature ovarian failure. Although most authors agree that the probability of premature ovarian failure is very low and almost only theoretical, it is also possible that gonad atrophy and/or premature ovarian failure caused by excessive ovarian destruction are more common than believed but observed only in unpublished series, i.e., in the "gray literature" *(8)*.

MECHANISM OF ACTION

A schematic summary of the mechanism(s) underlying the effects of surgical procedures for ovulation induction on hormonal, metabolic, and clinical events is shown in Fig. 1.

There is general agreement that LOD techniques have a mode of action similar to OWR, but destruction of ovarian tissue is less severe than that of the latter procedure *(8)*. Furthermore, the exact mechanisms for the beneficial effects of ovarian drilling remain unclear. However, it may be explained, in part, by the destruction of androgen-producing stroma. In fact, intraovarian androgen production and circulating androgen levels decrease after the procedure *(35,36)*. This, in turn, is responsible for a series of changes in endocrine and paracrine signaling that are thought to convert the adverse androgen-dominant intrafollicular environment to an estrogenic one *(37)*, restoring the hormonal environment to normal by correcting disturbances in ovarian–pituitary feedback *(38)*. These endocrine changes occur rapidly, and result in the recruitment of a new cohort of follicles and thus in the restoration of ovulation in most subjects *(19)*. Finally, the beneficial changes in endocrine milieu occurring after LOD seem sustained for several years *(2)*.

The decline in serum testosterone is associated with a decrease in pituitary responsiveness to stimulation by GnRH *(39)*, and ovarian drilling has an indirect modulating effect on the pituitary–ovary axis *(36)*. Although LH pulse frequencies are unchanged, LH pulse amplitudes are markedly reduced after ovarian surgery. Specifically, the serum concentration of LH increases immediately after the procedure and then decreases in a dose-dependent manner (the highest reduction is achieved if seven or more punctures are preformed per ovary). This could be explained by the greater reduction in serum androgen concentrations, which in turn results in reduced peripheral aromatization of androgens to estrone. The decline in estrone may be responsible for decreased positive feedback on LH and decreased negative feedback on FSH at the level of the pituitary. However, the greater reduction of serum LH levels was not associated with increases in rates of ovulation and pregnancy *(29)*.

The effect of LOD on FSH is variable and less pronounced *(40)*. The FSH concentration generally increases rapidly and thereafter demonstrates a cyclical rise in keeping with restoration of ovulation. After the procedure, normal inhibin pulsatility is also restored, in association with the onset of regular cycles *(41)*.

The postoperative endocrine alterations of LOD were first described by Grenblatt and Casper in 1987 *(42)* and 1 year later by Sumioki *(39)*. These investigators observed

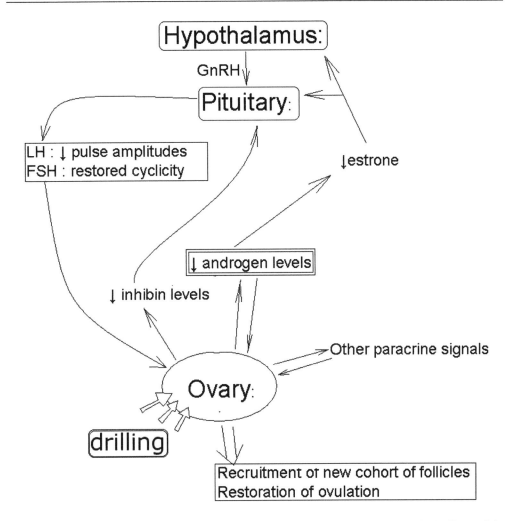

Fig. 1. Mechanism of action involved to explain the hormonal, metabolic, and clinical effects of the surgical procedures of ovulation induction.

significant decreases in LH and serum androgen concentrations during the days immediately following surgery. The decreases persisted for 6 weeks, and were considered sufficient to explain the correction of associated endocrine disorders and the occurrence of pregnancies. These authors agreed that the trauma incurred on the ovary was sufficient to induce a decrease in the production of local androgens, followed by a fall in estradiol and a decrease in positive feedback on LH secretion (39,42).

Sakata et al. (43) studied the activity of bioactive LH, FSH, androstenedione, and testosterone before and after LOD in nine anovulatory patients with PCO who underwent laparoscopic cauterization of the ovaries. They were the first to note a decrease in bioactive LH. Pellicer and Remohi (44) studied 131 anovulatory patients after cauterization, and confirmed the decrease in serum concentrations of LH, testosterone, and androstenedione, but demonstrated no change in serum insulin and insulin-like growth factor-1. Campo et al. (45) also confirmed the rapid postoperative decrease in serum androstenedione and testosterone concentrations in all subjects studied, but changes in these hormones were not linked to clinical success. On the contrary, no variation in LH concentrations was detected.

All authors appeared to agree on the fact that ovarian trauma causes a significant and immediate decrease in circulating androgens and a secondary increase in FSH, which could be related to a decrease in intraovarian inhibin as suggested by Grenblatt et al. *(41)*. On the other hand, it is more difficult to explain how a physical trauma induces endocrine modifications. It is feasible that the volume of tissue injury is not a key factor, considering that all authors used different techniques with similar results *(8)*. In 1983, Cohen formulated the hypothesis that ovarian stromal blood flow, which is significantly lower in women with PCOS than in healthy women, increases after LOD. In fact, the burning of the ovary during laparoscopy causes a secondary local hyperemia, inducing an increase in the gonadotropin concentration by surface unity *(8)*. In addition, eletrocoagulation stimulates the ovarian nerves, which transmit the excitation to the superior centers *(8)*. However, to date, little data has been produced to support this theory.

Recently it was suggested that the ovary produces a number of growth factors, such as insulin-like growth factor-1, in response to tissue injury, which sensitize the ovary to circulating FSH, resulting in stimulation of follicular growth *(29)*. It has also been hypothesized that minimal ovarian injury leads to production of nonsteroidal factors that affect ovarian feedback to the pituitary, resulting in an attenuated response of LH secretion to stimulation by GnRH, and, hence, to a decrease in serum LH concentrations *(36)*.

Another hypothesis is that drainage of androgens and inhibin from surface follicles could prevent the excessive collagenization of overlaying ovarian cortex. Neighboring follicles that are not undergoing atresia may then mature and gain access to the ovarian surface, facilitating normal ovulation *(46)*.

EFFICACY DATA

The goal of treatment with LOD is to yield an optimal pregnancy rate with a minimum of complications and an improvement in the endocrine milieu.

Before considering the outcomes of LOD, it is important to emphasize that there are considerable disparity in the reported results of LOD. Moreover, it is difficult to find in the literature well-designed studies that report data on large sample sizes. Variations of technique may explain the variability in results, but another important feature that should be considered is the heterogeneity of the patients enrolled. First, the definition and duration of infertility or subfertility are always lacking. Second, although there is general consensus that CC should be first-line treatment of anovulatory patients with PCOS *(47)*, most studies report also on patients with PCOS unselected for CC resistance. In addition, the definition of CC resistance varies widely, e.g., no ovulation after increasing doses to 250 mg daily or no ovulation after three cycles of 100–150 mg daily. Third, little attention has been given to anthropometric (body mass index [BMI] and/or weight-for-height index) and biochemical (hyperandrogenism and/or insulin resistance) characteristics of the patients. Finally, during the past few decades different criteria have been used for the definition and diagnosis of PCOS, especially between European and North American researchers.

Reproductive Outcomes. Many studies have claimed that LOD is followed, at least temporarily, by a high rate of spontaneous ovulation and conception, and/or that subsequent medical ovulation induction is rendered more successful *(10,21,24,37,45,48)*.

In reality, LOD restores menstrual regularity in a significant proportion (63–85%) of women, and its beneficial impact on menstrual cycle regularity is also observed after long-term follow-up *(10,21,33,45,48–50)*. In particular, Naether et al. *(51)* reported that, among the menstrual cycles examined after LOD, the proportion of regular cycles was approx 80% at 1–3 months, 82% at 6–24 months, and 92% at 36–72 months postoperatively. Amer et al. *(50)* reported comparable results, with significant differences (32 vs 82%) in the medium-term follow-up (1–3 years), suggesting that the beneficial effects of LOD wore off after 1 year in a high percentage of women. However, the reported increased frequency of menses with time may be a phenomenon related in part to the natural history of PCOS, in which the underlying endocrine abnormality becomes less pronounced with age and menstrual cycles become more regular *(52,53)*.

The reported rate of ovulation in CC-resistant patients with PCOS after drilling varies between 54 and 94% *(19)*; ovulation occurs spontaneously in most patients after surgery and the beneficial effect on ovulation is maintained over a long period. For example, in the series by Gjonnaess *(22)*, 74% of women were still ovulating 20 years after surgery.

Pregnancy and, more specifically, live births are considered the goals of treatment, and the reported rate of pregnancy is 43–84% *(19)*. After a period of 12 months from LOD, the spontaneous (without further treatment) pregnancy rate varies between 49 and 68%. Reported cumulative pregnancy rates, obtained using life-table analysis, at 18 and 24 months after surgery vary between 62–73% and 68–82%, respectively *(21,49,50,54)*.

The beneficial impact of LOD on reproductive performance appears to last for several years in a high proportion of women *(50)*, and patients who are not CC-resistant seem to obtain the best benefits *(24)*.

Most studies suggest an increase in miscarriage rate in patients with PCOS compared with healthy women *(55–57)*. In this regard, ovarian drilling appears to reduce the increased spontaneous miscarriage risk associated with PCOS. Abdel Gadir et al. *(58)* reported a miscarriage rate of 21% following LOD, which was significantly lower than those observed in the control group and in patients who received gonadotropins for ovulation induction. Amer et al. *(50)* also reported a reduction in miscarriage rate from 54 to 17% following LOD.

However, pretreatment with LOD does not appear to decrease the miscarriage rate after in vitro fertilization *(59)*. A systematic review of published studies could not reveal significant differences in miscarriage rates between women undergoing LOD and those receiving gonadotropins *(25)*.

Response to other treatments for infertility appears to be improved after LOD. Infertile and CC-resistant patients with PCOS may respond to this medication after surgery *(60,61)*. Different studies report an increased sensitivity to gonadotropin treatment, lower duration of stimulation, lower total dose, and higher pregnancy rate *(9,10,61–65)*. Tozer et al. *(66)* reported an improvement in reproductive outcomes in women undergoing in vitro fertilization after LOD. This seems to be associated with a more orderly growth of follicles, lower concentration of serum estradiol, reduced rate of cycle cancellation, and reduced incidence of ovarian hyperstimulation *(59,64–66)*.

Other Outcomes. As noted earlier ("Mechanism of Action" Subheading), LOD seems to also correct the primary endocrine abnormalities associated with PCOS. The immediate endocrine responses to LOD are similar to those previously described following OWR, indicating that the effects of all techniques of ovarian destruction are likely similar *(60)*.

After LOD, the main hormonal changes reported in many studies are a rapid and persistent decline in serum androgens, i.e., testosterone and androstenedione, with a transient increase in gonadotropins during the first 24–48 hours, followed later by a gradual decrease in gonadotropins *(37,42,67)*. Although the short-term endocrine effects of LOD have been extensively investigated, it is still uncertain how long these effects last. Some investigators have reported that the endocrine effects of LOD are rather transient *(63,68)*, whereas others have indicated that the treatment might have long-term beneficial effects *(10,51)*.

In a long-term follow-up study, Gjonnaess *(22)* reported on the late endocrine effects of LOD in 51 women with PCOS, and concluded that ovarian electrocautery normalizes serum levels of androgens and LH, and that the results are sustained for 18–20 years. Naether et al. *(51)* also demonstrated long-term effects of LOD on serum androgens (testosterone and dehydroepiandrosterone) levels in a wider population of 206 patients.

However, these studies did not include a control population, and it is, therefore, unclear to what extent the long-term observations could be attributed to the impact of LOD alone. A study by Elting et al. *(53)*, in fact, suggested that some women with PCOS have spontaneous improvement in their menstrual characteristics with increasing age.

In contrast, Amer et al. *(2)* studied the intermediate- and long-term endocrine changes in women who underwent LOD for PCOS, and compared the data with a control group of untreated women with PCOS. Serum concentrations of LH, FSH, testosterone, androstenedione, and sex hormone-binding globulin were assessed at different intervals after LOD. Biochemical data obtained at short- (<1 year), medium- (1–3 years), and long-term (4–9 years) were then compared. LH/FSH ratio, mean serum concentrations of LH and testosterone, and free androgen index decreased significantly after LOD and remained, during the medium- and long-term follow-up periods, lower in comparison with values obtained before treatment and on an untreated population. The authors concluded that the beneficial hormonal effects of LOD appear to be sustained for up to 9 years in most patients with PCOS *(2)*.

However, some disparities between hormonal improvement and ovulation rate have been reported *(58)*. Recently, Parsanezhad et al. *(69)* suggested that hyperprolactinemia after ovarian cauterization may be a possible cause of anovulation in women with PCO and improved gonadotropin and androgen levels.

Consistent with the reduction in androgens is the observation of a trend toward a modest improvement in acne and hirsutism in some of the women who reported these symptoms prior to LOD. This improvement seems to be sustained at follow-up after 9 years *(50)*. To date, LOD should not be considered as a treatment for symptoms because of hyperandrogenemia *(50)*.

Few clinical studies have examined the effect of LOD on insulin sensitivity and lipoprotein profile, concluding that LOD appears to have little or no effect on these parameters. These findings are in accord with classical studies showing that reduction of hyperandrogenism by GnRH analog therapy does not alter insulin sensitivity or circulating insulin concentrations. Rather, the reverse seems to be true. Improvement in insulin sensitivity is followed by an amelioration of hyperandrogenism *(18)*.

Studies on opioidergic and dopaminergic activity have concluded that there is no evidence that ovarian surgery affects the influence of opioidergic and dopaminergic activity on gonadotropin secretion *(70)*.

Finally, in one study, the short-term effect of LOD on ovarian volume, as measured by three-dimensional ultrasound, has been evaluated *(71)*. LOD induced a transient increase followed by a significant reduction in ovarian volume of about 50% (from 12.2 to 6.9 mL). Amer et al. *(2)* confirmed this reduction in ovarian volume after ovarian drilling (from 11 to 8.5 mL), and showed that the change is maintained with time.

PREDICTIVE FACTORS

Many factors have been assessed as predictors of success of LOD, such as LH levels, LH/FSH ratio, androgen levels, BMI, patient age, age at menarche, duration of infertility, ovarian size, and glucose level.

Van Wely, in a recent randomized controlled trial *(72)*, examined the predictors of failure of LOD in terms both of ovulation and pregnancy. From all clinical, endocrine, and ultrasonographic parameters evaluated in initial screening of CC-resistant women with PCOS, LH/FSH ratio results were the most predictive variable of ovarian response to surgery, followed by age at menarche and fasting glucose levels *(72)*. On the contrary, no significant predictor of failure for ongoing pregnancy has been identified *(72)*. These results are in agreement with previous reports that showed a higher success rate in patients with high preoperative LH levels *(49,73–75)*.

BMI seems to be a predictor factor influencing ovulation *(49,76–78)*, but not pregnancy success after LOD *(49,76)*.

Other authors showed that hyperandogenism *(10,76)*, duration of infertility *(49,76)*, and patient age *(77)* are predictors of response to LOD.

Our recent data *(79)* showed that LOD, such as for all infertility treatments, is less effective in women aged older than 35 years than in younger women, without any differences between them, even if categorized for groups of age. On the other hand, a basal FSH value higher than 10 UI/L seems to be a good predictive factor for LOD inefficacy.

INDICATIONS AND STRATEGIES FOR LOD USE

There is general consent that CC should be the first-line treatment in infertile patients with PCOS *(47)*, whereas different studies have concluded that LOD is an effective second-line treatment for anovulatory infertility associated with PCOS *(49,50)*.

However, to date, the place that LOD should take in the treatment of infertile patients with PCOS is debatable. In a descriptive review of this topic, Donesky and Adashi *(80)* concluded that: "Until it can be conclusively shown that laparoscopic ovulation induction does no harm to fertility potential or to long-term health, these procedures should be used when all available non-invasive options have been explored."

Data from comparative studies with gonadotropins and metformin are too poor and incomplete to evaluate the differences between the therapeutic options.

A recent meta-analysis stated that there was no evidence of a difference in live births or ongoing pregnancies between LOD and ovulation induction with gonadotropins.

Multiple pregnancy rates were lower with ovarian drilling than with gonadotropins, and there was no difference in miscarriage rates between the two treatments *(25)*. Considering the lower cost of LOD compared with gonadotropin use, Kovacs et al. *(81)* concluded that the use of LOD should be considered as the next line of treatment if CC fails to induce ovulation in patients with PCOS, and that LOD should precede gonadotropin therapy. The need for monitoring during ovulation induction with gonadotropins also makes surgery an attractive option. In addition, patient preference may favor LOD vs gonadotropins *(25)*.

In a recent randomized controlled trial, electrocautery was compared with recombinant FSH given in a low-dose step-up protocol *(82)*. After a diagnostic laparoscopy, patients were randomized to receive or not receive LOD. In the first arm, 83 women with PCOS were followed for a 6-month period after surgery without any treatment, and then the anovulatory patients were treated for three cycles with clomiphene and finally with recombinant FSH for an additional three cycles, whereas in the second arm, 85 patients were treated with recombinant FSH for 12 cycles. No difference in terms of miscarriages, ongoing pregnancies, and live-births was detected, whereas the number of multiple pregnancies was significantly higher during recombinant FSH treatment. There was no difference in cost between the two strategies *(83)*. Furthermore, considering the higher rate of multiple pregnancies caused by gonadotropin administration, electrocautery was considered the best choice in terms of the cost-effectiveness ratio *(83)*.

Metformin, an insulin-sensitizing drug used in type 2 diabetes, is an effective treatment to restore ovulatory menstrual cycles and to improve fertility in oligo-amenorrhoic women with PCOS after CC failure administered alone or added to CC. In addition, metformin, similarly to LOD but in contrast to gonadotropins, exerts beneficial effects at hormonal and metabolic levels, and does not require intensive hormonal and ultra-sonographic monitoring.

For these reasons, these two options have been carefully compared in a randomized controlled trial *(84)*. Specifically, 120 patients with PCOS underwent diagnostic laparoscopy followed by metformin or placebo for 6 months. At the end of the study, LOD and metformin yielded similar rates of ovulation, but metformin was more effective on other reproductive outcomes. In particular, the abortion rate was significantly lower in the metformin group and the pregnancy and live-birth rates were significantly higher. Analyzing the costs of two procedures, metformin administration was at least 20-fold less expensive then LOD *(84)*.

Based on these considerations, we believe that, at present, in an infertile anovulatory woman with PCOS, LOD should be performed only after failure of other treatments (lifestyle modifications, CC, metformin), or during laparoscopy performed for suspected or diagnosed organic factors of subfertility, such as endometriosis, uterine leiomyomas, and so on *(47)*.

CONCLUSIONS

LOD retains a place in the current treatment of PCOS in well-selected cases. It is a relatively simple procedure that provides an alternative treatment option for the infertile CC-resistant women with PCOS. However, LOD is a surgical procedure, and as such, it carries the usual risks of laparoscopic surgery. In a low percentage of cases, it can be complicated by pelvic adhesions and premature ovarian failure. Therefore, it is important to have good indications for the use of LOD, and to use a proper and meticulous technique in order to avoid complications.

Progress in understanding PCOS and effective new treatments seems to diminish the need for surgery and, eventually, this procedure will become a footnote of medical history (25).

FUTURE AVENUES OF INVESTIGATION

In the future, a well-designed randomized controlled clinical trial with a large sample size should identify the best surgical procedure and technique to induce ovulation in anovulatory women with PCOS. The primary end point should be the efficacy/safety ratio at short- and long-term. In other words, studies should not just evaluate reproductive outcomes (e.g., live-birth and pregnancy rates) but also adverse effects (e.g., surgical complications, ovarian sensibility to subsequent treatments, multiple pregnancy rate, miscarriage rate, and premature ovarian failure) in a view of managed care (cost–benefit analyses).

Recently, new diagnostic criteria for PCOS have been published (85), and even if with important limitations, they should be accepted by almost all researchers in order to homogenize the population studied. However, using these criteria, future studies should stratify the efficacy of the surgical induction of ovulation in anovulatory women with PCOS based on the different phenotypes, i.e., anovulation plus hyperandrogenism vs anovulation plus PCO, or in patients with PCOS who have different anthropometric characteristics, i.e., obese vs normal-weight women.

Finally, surgical procedures to induce ovulation should be assessed not only as "one-step" procedures in randomized comparisons within them and with medical treatments, but also as a part of more complex and specific therapeutical strategies.

KEY POINTS

- Surgical destruction of small amounts of ovarian tissue by creating a variable number of holes (drilling) in the ovarian capsule in anovulatory women with PCOS is associated with correction of the primary endocrine abnormalities, as well as a high rate of success in terms of menstrual cyclicity, ovulation, and pregnancy.
- Drilling is performed by electrocautery or laser, which yield similar results; however, laser is associated with fewer side effects than electrocautery.
- The surgical procedures are generally performed by a laparoscopic approach, are day-surgery procedures, and are considered as a second-line alternative after the failure of medical treatment with clomiphene citrate. They appear to be preferable in comparison to gonadotropins, but not to metformin.
- Further studies are needed to define the appropriate role that the surgical approach should have in the management of infertility associated with PCOS.

REFERENCES

1. National Institute of Clinical Exellence (NICE) of the British National Health Service. Available at: http://www.nice.org.uk/pdf/CG011niceguideline.pdf guideline 1.6.3.1. Last accessed on February 25, 2004.

2. Amer SA, Banu Z, Li TC, Cooke ID. Long-term follow-up of patients with polycystic ovary syndrome after laparoscopic ovarian drilling: endocrine and ultrasonographic outcomes. Hum Reprod 2002; 17:2851–2857.

3. Stein IF, Leventhal ML. Amenorrhea associated with bilateral polycystic ovaries. Am J Obstet Gynecol 1935;29:181–191.

4. Stein IF. Duration of fertility following ovarian wedge resection: Stein-Leventhal syndrome. West J Surg Obstet Gynecol 1964;72:237–242.

5. Greenblatt RB. Chemical induction of ovulation. Fertil Steril 1961;12:402–404.

6. Kistner RW. Induction of ovulation with clomiphene citrate. In: Berhman SH and Kistner RW, eds. *Progress in Infertility*. Boston, MA: Little, Brown and Co. 1968, p. 407.

7. Toaff R, Toaff ME, Peyser MR. Infertility following wedge resection of the ovaries. Am J Obstet Gynecol 1976;124:92–96.

8. Cohen J. Laparoscopic procedures for treatment of infertility related to polycystic ovarian syndrome Hum Reprod Update 1996;2:337–344.

9. Gjönnaess H. Polycystic ovarian syndrome treated by ovarian electrocautery through the laparoscope. Fertil Steril 1984;41:20–25.

10. Gjönnaess H. Ovarian electrocautery in the treatment of women with polycystic ovary syndrome (PCOS). Acta Obstet Gynaecol Scand 1994;73:407–412.

11. Campo S, Garcea N, Caruso A, Siccardi P. Effect of celioscopic ovarian wedge resection in patients with polycystic ovaries. Gynecol Obstet Invest 1983;15:213–222.

12. Portuondo J, Melchor J, Neyro J, Alegrea A. Periovarian adhesions following ovarian wedge resections or laparoscopic biopsy. Endoscopy 1984;16:143–145.

13. Mc Laughlin DS. Evaluation of adhesion reformation by early second-look laparoscopy following microlaser ovarian wedge resection. Fertil Steril 1984;42:531–537.

14. William R. Polycystic ovary syndrome and ovulation induction. Obstet Gynecol Clin North Am 2001;28:165–177.

15. Donesky B, Adashi E. Surgically induced ovulation in the PCO syndrome: ovarian wedge resection revisited in the age of laparoscopy. Fertil Steril 1995;63:439–463.

16. Adashi EY, Rock JA, Guzick D, Wentz AC, Jones GS, Jones HW Jr. Fertility following bilateral ovarian wedge resection: a critical analysis of 90 consecutive cases of the polycystic ovary syndrome. Fertil Steril 1981;36:30–35.

17. Buttram VC Jr. Vaquero C. Post-ovarian wedge resection adhesive disease. Fertil Steril 1975;26: 874–876.

18. Pirwany I, Tulandi T. Laparoscopic treatment of polycytic ovaries: is it time to relinquish the procedure? Fertil Steril 2003;80:241–251.

19. Gomel V, Yaralı H. Surgical treatment of polycystic ovary syndrome associated with infertility. Reprod Biomed Online 2004;9:35–42.

20. Tulandi T. Laparoscopic treatment of polycystic ovarian syndrome. In: Tulandi T, ed. *Atlas of Laparoscopic and Hysteroscopic Techniques for Gynecologists*. London: WB Saunders 1999, pp. 93–95.

21. Felemban A, Tan SL, Tulandi T. Laparoscopic treatment of polycystic ovaries with insulated needle cautery: a reappraisal. Fertil Steril 2000;73:266–269.

22. Gjönnaess H. Late endocrine effects of ovarian electrocautery in women with polycystic ovary syndrome. Fertil Steril 1998;69:697–701.

23. Huber J, Hosmann J, Spona J. Polycystic ovarian syndrome treated by laser through the laparoscope. Lancet 1988;2:215.

24. Daniell JF, Miller W. Polycystic ovaries treated by laparoscopic laser vaporization. Fertil Steril 1989;51:232–236.

25. Farquhar C, Lilford RJ, Marjoribanks J, Vandekerckhove P. Laparoscopic "drilling" by diathermy or laser for ovulation induction in anovulatory polycystic ovary syndrome. Cochrane Database Syst Rev 2005 Jul 20;(3):CD001122.

26. Dabirashrafi H. Complications of laparoscopic ovarian cauterization. Fertil Steril 1989;52:878.

27. Kovacs GT. Endoscopic surgical approach to the treatment of anovulation due to polycystic ovary syndrome—ovarian drilling. In: Sutton C and Diamond MP, eds. *Endoscopic Surgery for Gynaecologists*. London, UK: WB Saunders 1993, pp. 147–153.

28. Balen J, Jacobs HS. A prospective study comparing unilateral and bilateral laparoscopic ovarian diathermy in women with the polycystic ovary syndrome. Fertil Steril 1994;5:921–925.

29. Amer SA, Li TC, Cooke ID. Laparoscopic ovarian diathermy in women with polycystic ovarian syndrome: a retrospective study on the influence of the amount of energy used on the outcome. Hum Reprod 2002;17:1046–1051.

30. Malkawi HY, Qublan HS. Laparoscopic ovarian drilling in the treatment of polycystic ovary syndrome: how many punctures per ovary are needed to improve the reproductive outcome? J Obstet Gynaecol Res 2005;31:115–119.

31. Zullo F, Pellicano M, Zupi E, Guida M, Mastrantonio P, Nappi C. Minilaparoscopic ovarian drilling under local anesthesia in patients with polycystic ovary syndrome. Fertil Steril 2000;74:376–379.

32. Greenblatt E, Casper RF. Adhesion formation after laparoscopic ovarian cautery for polycystic ovarian syndrome: lack of correlation with pregnancy rate. Fertil Steril 1993;60:766–770.

33. Naether OG, Baukloh V, Fischer R, et al. Laparoscopic electrocoagulation of the ovarian surface in infertile patients with polycystic ovarian disease. Fertil Steril 1993;60:88–94.

34. Saravelos H, Li TC. Post-operative adhesions after laparoscopic electrosurgical treatment for polycystic ovarian syndrome with the application of Interceed to one ovary: a prospective randomized controlled study. Hum Reprod 1996;11:992–997.

35. Keckstein J. Laparoscopic treatment of PCOS. Baillière's Clin Obstet Gynecol 1989;3:563–581.

36. Rossmanith WG, Keckstein J, Spatzier K, Lauritzen C. The impact of ovarian laser surgery on the gonadotrophin secretion in women with polycystic ovarian disease. Clin Endocrinol (Oxf) 1991;34:223–230.

37. Aakvaag A, Gjonnaess H. Hormonal response to electrocautery of the ovary in patients with polycystic ovarian disease. Br J Obstet Gynaecol 1985;92:1258–1264.

38. Balen A, Tan SL, Jacobs H. Hypersecretion of luteinising hormone. A significant cause of infertility and miscarriage. Br J Obstet Gynaecol 1993;100:1082–1089.

39. Sumioki H, Utsunomyiya T, Matsuoka K, Korenaga N, Kadota T. The effect of laparoscopic multiple punch resection of the ovary on hypothalamo-pituitary axis in polycystic ovary syndrome. Fertil Steril 1988;50:567–572.

40. Alborzi S, Khodaee R, Parsanejad ME. Ovarian size and response to laparoscopic ovarian electrocauterization in polycystic ovarian disease. Int J Gynaecol Obstet 2001;74:269–274.

41. Lockwood GM, Muttukrishna S, Groome NP, Matthews DR, Ledger WL. Mid follicular phase pulses of inhibin B are absent in poycystic ovarian syndrome and are initiated by successful laparoscopic ovarian diathermy. A possible mechanism regulating emergence of the dominant follicle. J Clin Endocrinol Metab 1998;83:1730–1735.

42. Greenblatt E, Casper RF. Endocrine changes after laparoscopic ovarian cautery in polycystic ovarian syndrome. Am J Obstet Gynecol 1987;156:279–285.

43. Sakata M, Tasaka K, Kurachi H, Terakawa N, Miyake A, Tanizawa O. Changes of bio-active LH laser laparoscopic ovarian cautery in patients with PCOS. Fertil Steril 1990;53:610–613.

44. Pellicer A, Remohi J. Management of the PCOS by Laparoscopy. Karger Basel 1992.

45. Campo S, Felli A, Lamanna MA, Barini A, Garcea N. Endocrine changes and clinical outcome after laparoscopic ovarian resection in women with polycystic ovaries. Hum Reprod 1993;8:359–363.

46. Cohen BM. Laser laparoscopy for polycystic ovaries. Fertil Steril 1989;52:167–168.

47. Palomba S, Falbo A, Russo T. Zullo F. Ovulation induction in anovulatory patients with polycystic ovarian syndrome. Curr Drug Ther 2006;1:23–29.

48. Campo S. Ovulatory cycles, pregnancy outcome and complications after surgical treatment of polycystic ovary syndrome. Obstet Gynecol Surv 1998;53:297–308.

49. Li TC, Saravelos H, Chow MS, Chisabingo R, Cooke ID. Factors affecting the outcome of laparoscopic ovarian drilling for polycystic ovarian syndrome in women with anovulatory infertility. Br J Obstet Gynaecol 1998;105:338–344.

50. Amer SA, Banu Z, Li TC, Cooke ID. Long-term follow-up of patients with polycystic ovary syndrome after laparoscopic ovarian drilling: clinical outcome. Hum Reprod 2002;17:2035–2042.

51. Naether OGJ, Baukloh V, Fischer R, Kowalczyk T. Long-term follow-up in 206 infertility patients with polycystic ovarian syndrome after laparoscopic electrocautery of the ovarian surface. Hum Reprod 1994;9:2342–2349.

52. Dahlgren E, Johansson S, Lindstedt G, et al. Women with polycystic ovary syndrome wedge resected in 1956 to 1965: a long-term follow-up focussing on natural history and circulating hormones. Fertil Steril 1992;57:505–513.

53. Elting MW, Korsen TJM, Rekers-Mombarg LTM, Schoemaker J. Women with polycystic ovary syndrome gain regular menstrual cycles when ageing. Hum Reprod 2000;15:24–28.

54. Heylen S, Puttemans P, Brosens I. Polycystic ovarian disease treated by laparoscopic argon laser capsule drilling: comparison of vaporization versus perforation technique. Hum Reprod 1994;9:1038–1042.

55. Garcia JE, Jones GS, Wentz AC. The use of clomiphene citrate. Fertil Steril 1977;28:707–717.

56. Homburg R, Armar NA, Eshel A, Adams JM, Jacobs HS. Influence of serum luteinizing hormone concentrations of ovulation, conception and early pregnancy loss in polycystic ovary syndrome. BMJ 1988;297:1024–1026.

57. Sagle M, Bishop K, Ridley N, et al. Recurrent early miscarriage and polycystic ovaries. BMJ 1988;297:1027–1028.

58. Abdel Gadir A, Mowa R, Alnaser H, Alrashid A, Alonezi O, Shaw R. Ovarian electrocautery versus human menopausal gonadotrophins and pure follicle stimulating horone therapy in the treatment of patients with polycystic ovarian disease. Clin Endocrinol 1990;33:585–592.

59. Rimington MR, Walker SM, Shaw RW. The use of laparoscopic ovarian electrocautery in preventing cancellation of in-vitro fertilization treatment cycles due to risk of ovarian hyperstimulation syndrome in women with polycystic ovaries. Hum Reprod 1997;12:1443–1447.

60. Armar NA, McGarrigle HH, Honour J, Holownia P, Jacobs HS, Lachelin GC. Laparoscopic ovarian diathermy in the management of anovulatory infertility in women with polycystic ovaries: endocrine changes and clinical outcome. Fertil Steril 1990;53:45–49.

61. Kovacs G, Buckler H, Bangah M, et al. Treatment of anovulation due to polycystic ovarian syndrome by laparoscopic ovarian electrocautery. Br J Obstet Gynaecol 1991;98:30–35.

62. Dabirashrafi H, Mohamad K, Behjatnia Y, Moghadami-Tabrizi N. Adhesion formation after ovarian electrocauterization on patients with polycystic ovarian syndrome. Fertil Steril 1991;55:1200–1201.

63. Armar NA, Lachelin GC. Laparoscopic ovarian diathermy: an effective treatment for anti-oestrogen resistant anovulatory infertility in women with the polycystic ovary syndrome. Br J Obstet Gynaecol 1993;100:161–164.

64. Farhi J, Ashkenazi J, Feldberg D, Dicker D, Orvieto R, Ben Rafael Z. Effect of uterine leiomyomata on the results of in-vitro fertilization treatment. Hum Reprod 1995;10:2576–2578.

65. Colacurci N, Zullo F, De Franciscis F, Mollo A, De Placido G. In vitro fertilization following laparoscopic ovarian diathermy in patients with polycystic ovary syndrome. Acta Obstet Gynecol Scand 1997;76:555–558.

66. Tozer AJ, Al-Shawaf T, Zosmer A, et al. Does laparoscopic ovarian diathermy affect the outcome of IVF-embryo transfer in women with polycystic ovarian syndrome? A retrospective comparative study. Hum Reprod 2001;16:91–95.

67. Gjonnaess H, Norman N. Endocrine effects of ovarian electrocautery in patients with polycystic ovarian disease. Br J Obstet Gynaecol 1987;94:779–783.

68. Keckstein G, Rossmanith W, Spatzier K, Schneider V, Borchers K, Steiner R. The effect of laparoscopic treatment of polycystic ovarian disease by CO2-laser or Nd:YAG laser. Surg Endosc 1990;4:103–107.

69. Parsanezhad ME, Alborzi S, Zolghadri J, et al. Hyperprolactinemia after laparoscopic ovarian drilling: an unknown phenomenon. Reprod Biol Endocrinol 2005;3:31.

70. Szilagyi A, Hole R, Keckstein J, Rossmanith WG. Effects of ovarian surgery on the dopaminergic and opioidergic control of gonadotropin and prolactin secretion in women with polycystic ovarian disease. Gynecol Endocrinol 1993;7:159–166.

71. Tulandi T, Watkin K, Tan SL. Reproductive performance and three-dimensional ultrasound volume determination of polycystic ovaries following laparoscopic ovarian drilling. Int J Fertil Womens Med 1997;42:436–440.

72. van Wely M, Bayram N, van der Veen F, Bossuyt PM. Predictors for treatment failure after laparoscopic electrocautery of the ovaries in women with clomiphene citrate resistant polycystic ovary syndrome. Hum Reprod 2005;20:900–905.

73. Abdel Gadir A, Khatim MS, Alnaser HM, Mowafi RS, Shaw RW. Ovarian electrocautery; responders versus non-responders. Gynecol Endocrinol 1993;7:43–48.

74. Kriplani A, Manchanda R, Agarwal N, Nayar B. Laparoscopic ovarian drilling in clomiphene citrate-resistant women with polycystic ovary syndrome. J Am Assoc Gynecol Laparosc 2001;8:511–518.

75. Hayashi H, Ezaki K, Endo H, Urashima M. Preoperative luteinizing hormone levels predict the ovulatory response to laparoscopic ovarian drilling in patients with clomiphene citrate-resistant polycystic ovary syndrome. Gynecol Endocrinol 2005;21:307–311.

76. Amer SAK, Li TC, Ledger WL. Ovulation induction using laparoscopic ovarian drilling in women with polycystic ovarian syndrome: predictors of success. Hum Reprod 2004;19:1719–1724.

77. Duleba A, Banaszewska B, Spaczynski RZ, Pawelczyk L. Success of laparoscopic wedge resection is related to obesity, lipid profile and insulin levels. Fertil Steril 2003;79:1008–1014.

78. Stegmann BJ, Craig RH, Bay RC, Coonrod DV, Brady MJ, Garbaciak JA Jr. Characteristics predictive of response to ovarian diathermy in women with polycystic ovarian syndrome. Am J Obstet Gynecol 2003;79:1171–1173.

79. Palomba S, Falbo A, Orio F Jr. et al. Efficacy of laparoscopic ovarian diathermy in clomiphene citrate-resistant women with polycystic ovary syndrome: relationships with chronological and ovarian age. Gynecol Endocrinol 2006;22:329–335.

80. Donesky BW, Adashi EY. Surgical ovulation induction: the role of ovarian diathermy in polycystic ovary syndrome. Baillieres Clin Endocrinol Metab 1996;10:293–309.

81. Kovacs GT, Clarke S, Burger HG, Healy DL, Vollenhoven B. Surgical or medical treatment of polycystic ovary syndrome: a cost-benefit analysis. Gynecol Endocrinol 2002;16:53–55.

82. Bayram N, van Wely M, Kaaijk EM, Bossunyt PMM, van der Veen F. Using an electrocautery strategy or recombinant follicle stimulating hormone to induce ovulation in polycystic ovarian syndrome. BMJ 2004;328:1–5.

83. van Wely M, Bayram N, Bossunyt PMM, van der Veen F. An economic comparison of a laparoscopic electrocautery strategy and ovulation induction with recombinant FSH in women with clomiphene citrate-resistant polycystic ovary syndrome. Hum Reprod 2004;19:1741–1745.

84. Palomba S, Orio F Jr. Nardo LG, et al. Metformin administration versus laparoscopic ovarian diathermy in clomiphene citrate-resistant women with polycystic ovary syndrome: a prospective parallel randomized double-blind placebo-controlled trial. J Clin Endocrinol Metab 2004;89:4801–4809.

85. The Rotterdam ESHRE/ASRM-Sponsored PCOS consensus workshop group. Revised 2003 consensus on diagnostic criteria and long-term health risks related to polycystic ovary syndrome (PCOS). Hum Reprod 2004;19:41–47.

Index

Printed in the United States of America.